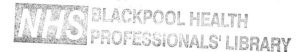

Rypins' Clinical Sciences Review

Rypins' Clinical Sciences Review

sixteenth edition

Edited by

Edward D. Frohlich, M.D.

Alton Ochsner Distinguished Scientist,
Vice President for Academic Affairs,
Alton Ochsner Medical Foundation;
Staff Member, Ochsner Clinic;
Professor of Medicine and of Physiology,
Louisiana State University School of Medicine;
Adjunct Professor of Pharmacology and
Clinical Professor of Medicine,
Tulane University School of Medicine,
New Orleans, Louisiana

With the Collaboration of a Review Panel

J. B. LIPPINCOTT COMPANY • Philadelphia

Acquisitions Editor: Richard Winters
Sponsoring Editor: Jody Schott
Production Editor: Virginia Barishek
Indexer: Maria Coughlin
Cover Designer: Leslie Foster Roesler
Production: Spectrum Publisher Services, Inc.
Compositor: Bi-Comp, Inc.
Printer/Binder: Courier Book Company/Kendallville

Sixteenth Edition

Library of Congress Cataloging-in-Publication Data

Rypins' clinical sciences review / edited by Edward D. Frohlich ;with
    the collaboration of a review panel. — 16th ed.
        p.   cm.
    Rev. ed. of : Rypins' medical boards review. 15th ed. Vol. 2,
Clinical sciences. c1989.
    Includes index.
    ISBN 0-397-51246-5
    1. Medicine—Examinations, questions, etc.   2. Medicine—Outlines,
syllabi, etc.   3. Clinical Medicine—examination questions.
I. Rypins, Harold, 1892–1939.   II. Frohlich, Edward D., 1931–
III. Rypins' medical boards review. Volume 2.   IV. Title: Clinical
sciences review.
    [DNLM: WB 18 R995]
R8.5.R964   1993
610'.76—dc20
DNLM/DLC
for Library of Congress   92-49956
                                                              CIP

*The editor, authors, and publisher have exerted every
effort to ensure that drug selection and dosage set forth
in this text are in accord with current recommendations
and practice at the time of publication. However, in view
of ongoing research, changes in government regulations,
and the constant flow of information relating to drug
therapy and drug reactions, the reader is urged to check
the package insert for each drug for any change in indications and dosage and for added warnings and precautions. This is particularly important when the recommended agent is a new or infrequently employed drug.*

Editorial Review Panel

Surgery

Ronald C. Elkins, M.D.
Chief, Section of Thoracic and Cardiovascular Surgery
University of Oklahoma Health Sciences Center
Professor, Department of Surgery
University of Oklahoma School of Medicine
Oklahoma City, Oklahoma

Internal Medicine

Edward D. Frohlich, M.D.
Alton Ochsner Distinguished Scientist,
Vice President for Academic Affairs,
Alton Ochsner Medical Foundation;
Staff Member, Ochsner Clinic;
Professor of Medicine and of Physiology,
Louisiana State University School of Medicine
Adjunct Professor of Pharmacology and
Clinical Professor of Medicine,
Tulane University School of Medicine
New Orleans, Louisiana

Obstetrics and Gynecology

Martin L. Pernoll, M.D., F.A.C.O.G., F.A.C.S.
Clinical Professor,
University of Kansas Medical School
Kansas City, Kansas
Hermann Hospital
Houston, Texas

Pediatrics

Margaret C. Heagarty, M.D.
Director of Pediatrics,
Harlem Hospital Center
Professor of Pediatrics,
College of Physicians and Surgeons
Columbia University
New York, New York

Public Health and Community Medicine

Richard H. Grimm, Jr., M.D., M.P.H., Ph.D.
Associate Professor,
Division of Cardiovascular Diseases, Department of Internal
Medicine, and Division of Epidemiology,
School of Public Health,
University of Minnesota School of Medicine
Minneapolis, Minnesota

Preface

After the editor of a multiauthored text finishes writing his own chapters, reviewing and editing the overall text, and attempting to coalesce the component chapters into an integrated volume that has its individual style and character, he settles back to put certain reflections about the book to pen and paper in the preface. With particular pleasure and great satisfaction I now complete this 16th edition of *Rypins' Clinical Sciences Review*. This is one of the few ongoing medical textbooks that will enjoy almost 65 years of renewed support by physicians preparing for licensure examination and a career of humane service. More personally, I am truly honored and flattered to have been the editor of this scholarly pursuit for more than 16 years by the time edition 17 will appear. What a remarkable experience I have been afforded every few years: to be provided the first opportunity to experience a broad personal ''updating'' of my knowledge on every aspect of fundamental and clinical experience by some of the most preeminent scholars, teachers, investigators, and clinicians in the world!

Clearly, our past performance has been nothing short of an outstanding success. This is attested by the long-standing confidence awarded by medical students and physicians desiring a comprehensive review prior to their sitting for licensure examinations. Over these years, if imitation is the sincerest form of flattery, many volumes have entered and left the bookstalls, but *Rypins'* continues to endure and to merit the confidence of its readers. As further evidence of the esteem in which this textbook is held, I continue to receive many letters and telephone calls from around the world, asking when the next edition is scheduled for publication and what will be new in the forthcoming edition.

This textbook was originally prepared for physicians planning to take state board medical licensure examinations. It consisted of short treatises or summaries in nine major areas of medicine, each followed by typical essay-type questions. This format remained rather constant throughout the first 12 editions. Multiple-choice questions and their answers were included in the 13th edition to help students prepare for the more recently introduced national board type of examination.

Most experts, teachers, students, and specialists in preparing examinations would agree that all examinations have their faults. Nevertheless, licensing examinations remain the only means available for objectively testing the knowledge and competence of individuals to practice the art and science of medicine. Coincidentally, these examinations and their scope and objectives have become more standardized, sophisticated, and expanded with the introduction of additional types of questions from the qualifying examination to national board examinations and the several examinations that test the overall knowledge of practicing physicians worldwide. Each state jealously (and justifiably so) guards its right to determine which physicians should be granted the privilege of practicing medicine within its borders. As a result, more than 50 jurisdictions have in the past prepared their own medical licensure examination. These examinations have varied so widely in kind, quality, and rate of failure of prospective practitioners that some states have refused to accept the licenses of others, placing serious obstacles in the way of interstate movement of physicians.

To resolve some of these difficulties, the Federation of State Medical Boards of the United States, after some years of study and research, developed a clinically oriented, reliable examination, the Federation Licensing Examination (FLEX), which is offered to any state board for use as its own licensing examination. It is prepared by a committee of the federation in collaboration with the National Board of Medical Examiners (NBME). Known by its acronym FLEX, this examination is given in all participating states of the United States twice a year on the same three days, in June and December.

By far the largest number of graduates from American medical schools take another series of examinations, not identical to the FLEX, that is offered in three parts by the NBME. The first is given after completion of the first two preclinical years in medical school; the second part, which focuses on clinical medicine, is taken after the second 2 years; and the third, taken after at least 6 months of the first postgraduate training year, is an objective test of general clinical competence. The U.S. Congress is constantly revising health manpower legislation that may affect medical licensure. The use by all states of these high-quality examinations, either under state board auspices or by a nationally constituted medical licensure examination, may help forestall legislation of a single federal licensing examination for graduates of American medical schools.

Nevertheless, federal licensing examinations seem to be unavoidable because of the need to determine the adequacy of the knowledge of graduate physicians who are educated and trained by foreign medical schools and who apply for license to practice medicine in the United States. Over the years, a number of types of examinations have been developed for foreign medical graduates. The first of these was the Educational Commission for Foreign Medical Graduates (ECFMG), a 1-day test, in English, which consisted of 300 well-chosen NBME multiple-choice questions. Five of every six questions came from the traditional clinical fields and one of every six from the basic medical sciences. Also included in the ECFMG examination was a 1-hour test designed to assess the graduate's understanding of the English language.

A second type of test, the Visa Qualifying Examination (VQE), was introduced under mandate by an Act of Congress in 1976. This law required all foreign medical graduates who are accepted for graduate training in the United States to pass the VQE before a visa to enter the United States would be issued. This examination was taken in three parts: the first in the basic sciences, the second in the clinical sciences, and the third in clinical and patient problems. Passing the VQE was declared equivalent to passing parts I and II of the standard NBME examination.

The VQE, however, was abandoned in favor of a revised format, the Foreign Medical Graduate Examination in the Medical Sciences (FMGEMS) and ECFMG English test. This examination takes place in two half-day sessions. The preclinical areas of medical inquiry are comprehensively and thoroughly reviewed on the first day. The second day includes an English language test and an examination of clinical knowledge.

Another area of medical licensure was the requirement for relicensure by state medical boards or by certain medical subspecialty organizations. In summary, therefore, a variety of examinations have been designed to determine medical knowledge and competence. These have undergone a tremendous evolution and growth in sophistication and in the demands they place on the fundamental knowledge of the professional physician.

In 1991, the Federation of State Medical Boards (FSMB) and the National Board of Medical Examiners (NBME) agreed to replace their respective examinations, the FLEX and NBME, with a new examination, the United States Medical Licensing Examination (USMLE). It appears that this new examination will satisfy the needs for state medical boards licensure, the national medical board licensure, and licensure examinations for foreign medical graduates. As indicated in the August 12, 1991, USMLE announcement, "it is expected that students who enrolled in U.S. medical schools in the fall of 1990 or later and foreign medical graduates applying for ECFMG examinations beginning in 1993 will have access only to USMLE for purposes of licensure." The announcement further outlines the phase-out of the last regular examinations for licensure, as indicated in Chapter 1.

It is apparent from these evolutionary developments in certification and board examinations that the examiners are desirous of making the process less complicated and confusing while devoting more attention to the construction of questions, thereby providing a more practical means for testing basic and clinical knowledge. This greater realism in testing relates to an increasingly interdisciplinary approach toward fundamental material and a more direct relevance accorded to practical clinical problems. This obviously adds to the difficulty experienced by those preparing for board or certification examinations. Students and physicians preparing for examinations must be aware of the interdisciplinary nature of fundamental clinical material, the common multifactorial characteristics of disease mechanisms, and the necessity to shift back and forth from one chapter to another in order to appreciate the less than clear-cut nature separating the pedagogic disciplines.

This brings us to the present 16th edition of *Rypins' Clinical Sciences Review,* which has dramatically changed with respect to the 15th edition. In this soft-cover edition we continue to use the same format begun in the 15th edition. The prerequisite to this textbook, *Rypins' Basic Sciences Review,* is also available in soft cover and discusses the basic preclinical sciences. This should provide the reader with a less "weighty" tome while reading, a greater ease in keeping up-to-date from one edition to the next, and a means for utilizing more directly the supplementary *Rypins' Questions and Answers for Basic Sciences Review* for the 16th edition. Additional innovations include key words, highlighted in bold italics, introduced to provide the reader with a valuable notation of terms critical to the topic under study and ready reference after using the index.

Certainly, a most valuable innovation is the participation of a new contributor to our review panel, Dr. Richard H. Grimm, a long-standing friend and colleague, who brings to the Public Health and Community Medicine chapter the broad perspective of a knowledgeable clinician, experienced epidemiologist and biostatistician, and a preeminent investigator from a major national team in this area. He joins our very strong mainstays and experienced "heavies" of the editorial review panel. Each of these contributors is widely recognized as an academic leader of the first order. All have been selected because of their ability to express and teach highly complex material in a simple and yet straightforward manner.

Each of these world-class teachers has drastically revised and updated his or her past material. The reader will find new material on molecular and cellular biology and immunology presented in a crystal-clear manner; this is integrated with the material of other chapters dealing with key pathophysiological and biochemical concepts and disease mechanisms, patient evaluation, management, and treatment. Note also the new tables, figures, and pedagogic text material.

Thus, we see a very dramatic and broadly revised 16th edition—a textbook markedly restructured in physical organization, content, and scientific material. We are all genuinely pleased with this new and exciting edition.

We are confident that this textbook will continue to be of value to all who are concerned with medical examinations—those who prepare the examination, those who must prepare and qualify for medical licensure, and those already licensed who are required to sit for relicensure examination. In addition, this textbook may be of value to the medical educator planning for courses in continuing medical education, to the medical student who is interested in reviewing material for specific course examinations, and to the practicing physician interested in gaining a quick resume of the present state of knowledge in a very specific area of medical pedagogy. This has been the text's aim for more than six decades: to present, in a clear and concise manner, the most comprehensive and up-to-date knowledge of the various fields of basic sciences and clinical medicine and to make the accompanying questions as pertinent and clinically oriented as possible. With respect to the questions that are appended to each chapter, it is suggested that the reader should not only review the rhetorical questions, but also consider carefully the multiple-choice questions. As indicated, these multiple-choice questions follow the style and format of the questions devised by the NBME, FLEX, and FMGEMS examinations. The questions in each chapter are followed by an answer key.

And what of the future of *Rypins'*? Well, this all depends on you, the readers. We always value your comments, suggestions, and needs. We sincerely hope that this textbook continues to merit your confidence and support. I am particularly grateful and flattered by the large number of personal comments and thoughts that you have had concerning the published material. All have been carefully considered, if not fully implemented. How kind many letters have been thanking us for our help in your intense and comprehensive preparation.

It is appropriate and gratifying to express to those who are so close to me personally and professionally my deep, personal appreciation for allowing me to put forth this new edition. I am truly grateful to my colleagues at the Ochsner Clinic and at the Alton Ochsner Medical Foundation for the opportunity, the time, and the ambience to pursue and complete this major academic challenge. Over the years, I have always valued the support and constant loyalty of an office staff that is a great source of personal satisfaction and appreciation. I am particularly grateful to my office ''mainstays'' and associates, Lillian Buffa, Caramia Fairchild, and Debby Smith. To each, I express my deep gratitude and appreciation for her secretarial support, manuscript preparation, telephone stress, and the general and indispensable help and advice. Clearly, my expression of appreciation is also in order to the publishing staff of J. B. Lippincott.

But, most of all, I again and always wish to express my deep love and inexpressible thanks to my wife, Sherry, and to my children, Margie, Bruce, and Lara. Only they know of their love and patience, their unselfish understanding of the time, effort, and commitment that is required to bring this idea and textbook to fruition. Without their support and encouragement it would have been impossible to organize, review, and get this material published within the planned schedule. It has been said that ''Medicine is a jealous mistress''; jealousy has been no part of my family's relationship with me, and endeavors such as this attest to their love and support. Indeed, it has been that loving understanding that has made this, and whatever else I do, worthwhile, possible, and personally rewarding and hence a labor of love.

Edward D. Frohlich, M.D.

Contents

Chapter 1   Medical Qualifying Examinations
Edward D. Frohlich

Types of Examinations   3
National Board of Medical Examiners   4
Federation Licensing Examination (FLEX)   7
Educational Council for Foreign Medical Graduates (ECFMG) Certification   9
Foreign Medical Graduate Examination in the Medical Sciences (FMGEMS)   9
Innovations in Formulating Test Questions   11
Five Points to Remember   11
Examples of Questions   12

Chapter 2   Surgery
Ronald C. Elkins

Response to Surgery   23
Wounds   24
Shock   29
Nutrition   30
Transplantation   31
General Conditions of the Extremities   32
Fractures and Dislocations of the Extremities   35
Soft-Tissue Sarcomas   42
Ear   43
Salivary Glands   43
Throat   43
Neck   44
Oral Cavity   44
Larynx   45
Nose   45
Thyroid   46
Parathyroids   46
Breast   47
Thorax   49
Lung   52
Gastrointestinal Tract and Abdomen   53
Genitourinary System   70
Questions in Surgery   75
Answers to Multiple-Choice Questions   82

Chapter 3   Internal Medicine
Edward D. Frohlich

Diseases of the Circulation   83
Diseases of the Hematopoietic System   101
Diseases of the Lungs   110
Diseases of the Kidneys   118
Diseases of the Esophagus, Stomach, and Intestines   121
Diseases of the Spleen, Pancreas, Gallbladder, and Liver   130
Metabolic and Endocrine Diseases   135
Infectious Diseases   141
Sexually Transmitted Diseases   148
Rheumatic Diseases, Connective Tissue Diseases, Vasculitides, and Related Disorders   155
Diseases of the Nervous System   161
Questions in Internal Medicine   170
Answers to Multiple-Choice and Matching Questions   178

Chapter 4   Obstetrics and Gynecology
Martin L. Pernoll

Obstetrics
Anatomy and Physiology of Female Sex Organs   184
Very Early Gestation   190
Physiologic Changes of Pregnancy   193
Prenatal Care   194
Physiology and Conduct of Labor   201
Normal Labor and Delivery   202
Analgesia and Anesthesia for Labor and Delivery   208
Complications of Pregnancy   209
Pathology of Labor and Puerperium   224
The Newborn   234

Gynecology
Disorders of the Lower Generative Tract   241
Benign Tumors of the Vulva   248
Invasive Malignancies of the Vulva   250
Cancer of the Vagina   251

Disorders of the Cervix   252
Disorders of the Uterine Corpus   255
Pelvic Infections   260
Endometriosis, Adenomyosis, and
    Dysmenorrhea   263
Gestational Pathology   267
Disorders of the Fallopian Tube   271
Disorders of the Ovary   271
Remote Effects of the Injuries of Childbirth and
    Gynecologic Therapy   275
Gynecologic Endocrinopathies   281
Infertility   286
Abnormal Sexual Development   290
Family Planning   293
Climacterium, Menopause, and Postmenopausal
    Syndrome   296
Questions in Obstetrics and Gynecology   297
Answers to Multiple-Choice Questions   310

Chapter 5   Pediatrics
Margaret C. Heagarty

Growth and Development   311
Nutrition   313
The Care of the Newborn   316
Pregnancy and Its Effects on the Fetus   316
Labor and Delivery and Their Effects on the
    Infant   317
The Normal Newborn   317
Diseases of the Newborn   321
Diseases of Children   323

Preventive Pediatrics   335
Questions in Pediatrics   336
Answers to Multiple-Choice Questions   338

Chapter 6   Public Health and Community Medicine
Richard H. Grimm, Jr.

Health Statistics   340
Epidemiology   346
Administration of Health Services   352
High-Priority Areas of Problem and
    Treatment   354
Economic Aspects of Health Care   367
Questions in Public Health and Community
    Medicine   370
Answers to Multiple-Choice Questions   374

Chapter 7   Psychiatry
Gordon H. Deckert and Ronald S. Krug

History   376
Evaluation   377
Nosology   381
Prevention   401
Treatment   402
Questions in Psychiatry   408
Answers to Multiple-Choice Questions   416

Index   417

sixteenth edition

Rypins' Clinical Sciences Review

Rypins' Clinical Sciences Review, 16th Edition, edited by Edward D. Frohlich. J. B. Lippincott Company, Philadelphia © 1993.

Medical Qualifying Examinations

Edward D. Frohlich, M.D.
Alton Ochsner Distinguished Scientist,
Vice President for Academic Affairs,
Alton Ochsner Medical Foundation;
Staff Member, Ochsner Clinic; Professor of
Medicine and of Physiology, Louisiana State
University School of Medicine; Adjunct Professor of
Pharmacology and Clinical Professor of Medicine,
Tulane University School of Medicine,
New Orleans, Louisiana

The testing of professional competence before certifying for public responsibilities is an age-old practice. In China, for example, candidates for public service were required to submit to special examinations at least 3,000 years ago, and the tests were said to be not unlike those employed today. In the United States the practice developed slowly, first as a kind of contribution by the profession itself to public welfare; later as a responsibility of the state. In New York State the problem arose in the early 19th century as far as the practice of medicine is concerned. At that time, the Legislature found that attempts to control the practice of "physic and surgery" in unorganized fashion had been most unsatisfactory, since charlatans and quacks abounded, and passed "an act to incorporate Medical Societies for the purpose of regulating the practice of Physic and Surgery in this state." This law provided for the establishment of a medical society in each county and gave to the practicing physicians themselves, thus legally organized, the power to grant licenses to qualified applicants and to regulate the practice of medicine in their counties.

Methods of testing varied. In general, tests were clinical and practical, limited to questions or discussions concerning the diagnosis and the treatment of diseases, for the candidates were chiefly those who had received their training as apprentices to practicing physicians. Not until nearly midcentury did the number of physicians who had had their education and training in medical schools predominate. Soon thereafter the states themselves assumed responsibilities for licensure and, consequently, for establishing formal testing procedures. With this development, Boards of Examiners, or similar bodies, were appointed to examine officially all applicants for fitness to practice the medical profession. Today, all 50 states, as well as the District of Columbia and the Commonwealth of Puerto Rico, have official medical licensing agencies.

The usual means of measuring knowledge is the formal written examination, and it has an important place in all educational programs. "Examination," the late President Eliot of Harvard once stated, "is the most difficult of the educational arts and its influence on both students and teachers may be very great.'' Indeed, intelligently and thoughtfully prepared examinations can be made a most valuable educational exercise in any course of study. They not only force students to review and stimulate them to keep up with their work, but if the examinations are well designed and the results are interpreted carefully, they also may serve to test the quality of teaching.

How effective are formal written examinations in testing professional competence? Perhaps not as effective as they are in an educational program. Nevertheless, they are the only practical means of assessing the competence of large numbers of applicants for professional licensure. Although this practice is not ideal and does not test for such essential attributes as ethical and moral standards, carefully designed tests do play a definite role in separating the qualified practitioner from the unqualified and, in doing so, protect the public from the charlatan and the incompetent.

Examinations for licensure, however, have not always kept pace with the remarkable advances in medical knowledge and the resultant changes in methods of training for the practice of medicine. For this reason, many of the examination methods employed in former years have become inadequate. Thus, the purpose of the licensing examination is not so much to test the candidate's general knowledge in such individual subjects as anatomy, pathology, medicine, and surgery as to determine his or her ability to apply this knowledge to the diagnosis and treatment of disease and to determine the candidate's general fitness to practice the art and the science of medicine. In the past, unfortunately, most licensing examinations failed miserably in this last category.

The existence of separate licensing boards in all the states, the District of Columbia and the Commonwealth of Puerto Rico, each setting its own type of qualifying examination for licensure, has led to great variation in the kind and quality of the examinations. This has worked against unity of procedures and standards and has made difficult the movement of physicians from one licensing jurisdiction to another. However, as will be described in more detail later, through the efforts of the Federation of State Medical Boards of the United States, a high quality examination—the Federation Licensing Examination (FLEX)—prepared by a special Federation committee for administration twice a year, has been offered to any state medical board that wishes to use the examination as its own licensing test. A measure of its success is shown by the fact that it has been used by nearly all states since 1973. The prerequisites for licensure still vary from one state to another; any physician interested in licensure in any specific state should write directly to the State Board of Medical Licensure of that state for specific requirements and information.

Another confusing element in the licensing procedure has been added by the establishment in a number of states of separate boards of examiners in the basic sciences. These tests are designed to be given to candidates for admission to all branches of the healing professions, not only medicine but such other areas as chiropractic and neuropathy. In these jurisdictions certification by the basic science boards is required before admission to the specific professional examination is granted.

In most instances the members of these boards are teachers of such subjects as general chemistry, physics, biology, and anatomy. The tests therefore are not specifically prepared for physicians who have had intensive training in the basic medical sciences that form an integral part of medical education. The purpose of this examination is to determine whether the candidate has had adequate training in the fundamental sciences considered essential for admission to the licensing examination of the particular healing art the applicant wishes to practice. At best these tests are elementary when compared with the comprehensive training in the basic medical sciences given in schools of medicine. The consequent repetition, in part at least, of an examination in basic sciences by the medical licensing boards in these states has complicated still further the licensing of physicians. Fortunately, the number of these basic science boards is diminishing, and the time appears not far off when they will be done away with.

Thus, with all their defects and deficiencies, examinations are essential to the licensing procedure. They form not only an essential part of any well-planned program of education but are also, when well constructed, the only generally satisfactory method thus far devised for determining the professional competence and fitness to practice for a large number of candidates. They constitute a dependable measure of coordinated thinking as well as a test of knowledge not to be gained in any other way. Examinations are therefore here to stay, and the objective of all boards of medical licensure must be to administer examinations that are as fair, comprehensive, and valid tests of fundamental knowledge and clinical competence as it is possible to make.

TYPES OF EXAMINATIONS

Essay Examination

Until rather recently many state boards of medical examiners employed the so-called essay examination, but it is no longer generally used in licensing tests. In this test a limited number of questions is asked, and the candidate answers each one in a short composition or dissertation. The essay examination emphasizes description, definition, explanation, and discussion. Symptoms, signs, abnormalities in function, pathologic changes, etiology, and the diagnosis and treatment of disease conditions are described, and discussed by the candidate, sometimes at considerable length.

The advantages of the essay test are that it gives candidates an opportunity to consider thoughtfully each of a limited number of problems posed, to reveal their ability to organize their answers, to demonstrate their skill at description, and to present evidence of general scholarship, writing ability, penmanship, spelling, composition, and neatness of execution. All of these qualities are desirable accomplishments, but not all of them are the particular attributes that define a physician's overall competence to practice medicine.

Among the disadvantages are the relatively long time it takes to grade essay answers, the difficulty the examiner has of being uniformly fair in grading answers to the same question on different papers and the frequent quandary the examiner finds himself or herself in when, because of poor penmanship or a lack of knowledge of English on the part of the candidate, he or she cannot interpret an answer. The grading of essay examinations is therefore slow, subject to considerable subjective variation in evaluation of answers, and occupies an excessive amount of an examiner's time.

Finally, in view of the continued rapid expansion of medical knowledge in every field, it is now recognized that a limited number of essay questions does not permit as adequate testing of the candidate's general knowledge as is desired. Occasionally, therefore, oral or practical tests have been used to supplement the written test. With the additional information that such tests provide, the examining boards feel more secure in certifying a candidate for licensure. The great difficulty with this type of individual test, however, is that it cannot be given within a reasonable time, nor can adequate numbers of examiners be provided when great numbers of candidates must be examined. At present, if given at all, these individual tests are limited to those states where the number of candidates is small.

Multiple-Choice Examination

In recent years more and more State Boards of Examiners have been turning to the objective, or multiple-choice, examination. In this type of test each question is so prepared that the candidate is faced with a problem, the correct answer to which is included in the question and must be selected and indicated on the answer sheet by making a mark in the appropriate place. The characteristic feature of these tests is that candidates answer the questions by blackening, with a special pencil on the answer sheet, the space they believe to indicate the correct answer. Although this is considered a written examination, no actual writing of sentences is required. This kind of test has two important advantages: A great many more questions covering a much wider range of subjects can be asked in a given time than is possible in the essay examination; and the answers can be graded more objectively and with greater speed and accuracy than in any other type of examination. Thus, the number of questions that can be asked in an allotted period can be increased from 8 or 10, or at most 12, in an essay test, to 100, 150, or even more, in the objective test, thereby effectively broadening the scope of the examination.

At first the objective, or multiple-choice, examination met with considerable disapproval on the candidate's part because the technique was so new and different, and on the examiner's part because the construction of valid, unambiguous, and reliable questions proved to be so difficult (far more difficult, in fact, than the preparation of essay questions). But with the passage of time the objective examination has come into its own as a valid, comprehensive, and dependable test of a candidate's knowledge and, when applied effectively, of his or her competence and ability. Moreover, this type of examination seems to be the most searching, valid, and comprehensive type of test to administer to large groups of candidates.

Many different forms of objective, multiple-choice questions have been devised to test not only medical knowledge but those subtler qualities of discrimination, judgment, and reasoning. Certain types of questions may test an individual's recognition of the similarity or dissimilarity of diseases, drugs, and physiologic or pathologic processes. Other questions test judgment as to cause and effect or the lack of causal relationships. Case histories or patient problems are used to simulate the experience of a physician confronted with a diagnostic problem; a series of questions then tests the individual's understanding of related aspects of the case, such as associated laboratory findings, treatment, complications, and prognosis. In this type of examination each question has only one correct response among a number of possible choices—most often one correct response out of five choices, although the ratio may be somewhat less or considerably more.

Ambiguity of questions is exceedingly rare because of the intensive review process by the examination committees before they are used. The preparation of objective or multiple-choice examinations is extremely difficult, for the work of the examiners, instead of consisting of the time-consuming and usually tiresome reading and grading of essay-type answers, shifts to the preparation of the many questions included in the tests. Because generally the objective is to construct questions with only one correct answer, the preparation of an examination is best done by a group, usually an examination construction committee. The members of each group or committee should be skilled in one basic or clinical science discipline. Usually each member prepares questions in advance of a committee meeting, at which each question will be subjected to a critical review. Doubtful items are revised, modified, or discarded and new items may be developed. All items not approved unanimously are discarded. An examination prepared in this way, which is the method used by the National Board of Medical Examiners, contains only material that has been thoroughly worked over and agreed upon as appropriate, free from ambiguity, and representative not only of important aspects of the subject but also of high standards of education.

SCORING OF MULTIPLE-CHOICE EXAMINATIONS

When objective multiple-choice examinations are used, the examinations are usually scored by electronic machines. To the casual observer, this machine scoring may look like a highly mysterious business. The answer sheets are loaded into the machine, a button is pressed, and the machine reads the sheets, matches the answers against an answer key, and punches the examinee's score into the automated machine data card. A manual check is also made to avoid the possibility of any technical error. Furthermore, these machines are not robots making their own decisions; they perform only in the way

that they are programmed to perform. The responsible examiners determine whether an individual should pass or fail.

A grade of 75 has been established as the passing score for the examinations of the National Board. But it does not follow that it is necessary to respond correctly to 75% of the items in order to obtain this grade. Indeed, the scoring procedure is such that usually a score of about 50% to 60% of the questions answered correctly results in a passing grade of 75. In arriving at the passing score, the distribution curve of all those taking an examination is given consideration.

Examinations of the multiple-choice type have certain advantages over the time-honored essay tests. Although essay tests may probe more deeply into a limited number of subjects, multiple-choice examinations sample a much greater breadth of medical knowledge. Because the answer sheets can be scored by machine, the grading can be accomplished rapidly, accurately, and impartially. With this type of examination it becomes possible to determine the level of difficulty of each test and to maintain comparability of examination scores from test to test and from year to year for any single subject. Moreover, of even greater long-range significance is the facility with which the total test and the individual questions can be subjected to thorough and rapid statistical analysis, thus providing a sound basis for comparative studies and the continuing improvement in the quality of the test itself.

NATIONAL BOARD OF MEDICAL EXAMINERS

In the years following the issuance of the Flexner Report on the medical schools of the nation [Flexner A: Medical Education in the United States and Canada, bulletin no. 4. New York, Carnegie Foundation for the Advancement of Teaching, 1910], it became evident that not only medical school programs, but also the licensing examinations of the various states, needed upgrading. One physician who took seriously the licensing examination matter was Dr. W. L. Rodman of Philadelphia, who, in 1915, founded the National Board of Medical Examiners (NBME). This board, a voluntary and unofficial examining agency, was organized "to prepare and to administer qualifying examinations of such high quality that legal agencies governing the practice of medicine within each state" could, at their discretion, "grant a license without further examination to those candidates" who had passed the

National Board examinations and had become Diplomates of the Board. The membership of the National Board of Medical Examiners has grown in strength and importance over the years and now includes representatives from the faculties of leading American medical schools and from the Association of American Medical Colleges, the American Medical Association, the Federation of State Medical Boards of the United States, the American Hospital Association, and various federal medical services.

The National Board, however, is in no sense a licensing agency, and the last interest this board could have would be the responsibility of licensing physicians on a national basis. It is the function of each individual state to determine who shall practice within its borders and to set the standards of medical practice in accordance with its own rules and regulations. As its name implies, the National Board is an examining board, and currently all but a few states are willing to issue licenses to practice medicine within their borders to holders of the National Board Diploma; a few states do so with minor additional requirements. In a majority of states the National Board Diploma is accepted for full licensure. In New York State, for example, in 1973 approximately 37% of all physicians licensed were licensed on the basis of their National Board qualifications. It goes without saying that the candidate preparing for licensure in a specific state should communicate directly with that state's Board of Medical Examiners to learn the requirements of that state.

Eligibility to take the National Board examinations is currently limited to candidates who are regularly enrolled as students in, or are graduates of, any approved medical school in the United States or Canada. Graduates of foreign medical schools are not admitted, although, before they may serve as interns or residents in any United States hospital, they must take and pass a special qualifying examination. The special testing procedures that are required of all foreign medical graduates will be discussed later.

The examination of the National Board of Medical Examiners has from the outset been given in three parts: Part I in the basic medical sciences, Part II in the clinical sciences, and Part III as a practical examination involving clinical and patient problems. Over the years, however, the examinations have not been static but have been changed in form and content to keep abreast of medical progress and changes in medical education. The examinations are prepared by special committees, one for each major basic science and clinical science field. These committees are selected with great care, and their members (usually six per committee) come from medical school faculties and the staffs of teaching hospitals all over the United States and Canada. Thus, the preparation of the examinations has been in the hands of leaders in the medical profession throughout the country, and the examinations themselves have reflected the progress and change occurring in the various fields of medicine and in science generally.

From carefully prepared essay tests in the various basic and clinical sciences the Board some years ago turned to the more efficient and valid objective, or multiple-choice tests in the different subjects. The Board also decided to change from the Part III practical examinations given at the bedside in hospital centers throughout the country to a new, unique objective test of clinical competence that is taken by all candidates. This has resulted in more universally uniform and valid testing of a physician's fitness to practice, effectively eliminating the lack of uniformity that characterized the bedside examinations carried out in many different centers. Not only has the National Board kept constantly abreast of progress in medicine and medical education, but it has actually been a leader in bringing about progressive change, especially in the quality of examination procedures.

Today the Part I and Part II examinations are set up and scored as total comprehensive objective tests in the basic sciences and clinical sciences, respectively. The format of each part is changed since it is no longer subject-oriented, that is, separated into sections specifically labelled Anatomy, Pathology, Medicine, Surgery, and so forth. Subject labels are therefore missing, and in each part questions from the different fields are intermixed or scrambled so that the subject origin of any individual question is not immediately apparent, although it is known in the National Board office. Therefore, if necessary, individual subject grades can be extracted.

Part I is a 2-day written test including questions in anatomy, biochemistry, microbiology, pathology, pharmacology, physiology, and a recently added discipline, behavioral sciences. Each subject contributes to the examination a large number of questions designed to test not only knowledge of the subject itself but also "the subtler qualities of discrimination, judgment, and reasoning." Questions in such fields as molecular biology, cell biology, and genetics are included, as are questions to test the "candidate's recognition of the similarity or dissimilarity of diseases, drugs, and physiologic, behavioral, or pathologic processes.'' Problems are presented in narrative, tabular, or graphic form, followed by questions designed to assess the candidate's knowledge and comprehension of the situation described.

Part II is also a 2-day written test that includes questions in internal medicine, obstetrics and gynecology, pediatrics, preventive medicine and public health, psychiatry, and surgery. The questions, like those in Part I, cover a broad spectrum of knowledge in each of the clinical fields. In addition to individual questions, clinical problems are presented in the form of case histories, charts, roentgenograms, photographs of gross and microscopic pathologic specimens, laboratory data, and the like, and the candidate must answer questions concerning the interpretation of the data presented and their relation to the clinical problems. The questions are ''designed to explore the extent of the candidate's knowledge of clinical situations and to test his [or her] ability to bring information from many different clinical and basic science areas to bear upon these situations.''

The examinations of both Part I and Part II are scored as a whole, certification being given on the basis of performance on the entire part, without reference to disciplinary breakdown. The grade for the part is derived from the total number of questions answered correctly, rather than from an average of the grades in the component basic science or clinical science subjects. A candidate who fails will be required to repeat the entire part. Nevertheless, as noted above, in spite of the interdisciplinary character of the examinations, all of the traditional disciplines are represented in the test, and separate grades for each subject can be extracted and reported separately to students, to state examining boards, or to those medical schools that request them for their own educational and academic purposes.

This type of interdisciplinary examination and the method of scoring the entire test as a unit have definite advantages, especially in view of the changing character of the curricula in modern medical schools. The old type of rigid, almost standardized, curriculum, with its emphasis on specific subjects and specified numbers of hours in each, has been replaced by a more liberal, open-ended kind of curriculum, permitting emphasis in one or more fields and corresponding deemphasis in others. The result has been rather wide variations in the totality of education in different medical schools. Thus, the scoring of these tests as a whole permits accommo-

dation to this variability in the curricula of different schools. Within the total score, weakness in one subject that has received relatively little emphasis in a given school may be balanced by strength in other subjects.

The rationale for this type of comprehensive examination as replacement for the traditional department-oriented examination in the basic sciences and the clinical sciences is given in the National Board Examiner:

> The student, as he [or she] confronts these examinations, must abandon the idea of ''thinking like a physiologist'' in answering a question labeled ''physiology'' or ''thinking like a surgeon'' in answering a question labeled ''surgery.'' The one question may have been written by a biochemist or a pharmacologist; the other question may have been written by an internist or a pediatrician. The pattern of these examinations will direct the student to thinking more broadly of the basic sciences in Part I and to thinking of patients and their problems in Part II.

Until a few years ago, the Part I examination could not be taken until the work of the second year in medical school had been completed, and the Part II test was given only to students who had completed the major part of the fourth year. Now students, if they feel they are ready, may be admitted to any regularly scheduled Part I or Part II examination during any year of their medical course without prerequisite completion of specified courses or chronologic periods of study. Thus, emphasis is placed on the acquisition of knowledge and competence rather than the completion of predetermined periods.

Candidates are eligible for Part III after they have passed Parts I and II, have received the M.D. degree from an approved medical school in the United States or Canada, and, subsequent to the receipt of the M.D. degree, have served at least 6 months in an approved hospital internship or residency. Under certain circumstances, consideration may be given to other types of graduate training provided they meet with the approval of the National Board. After passing the Part III examination, candidates will receive their Diplomas as of the date of the satisfactory completion of an internship or residency. If candidates have completed the approved hospital training prior to completion of Part III, they will receive certification as of the date of the successful completion of Part III.

The Part III examination, as noted above, is an objective test of general clinical competence. It occupies 1 full day and is divided into two sections, the first of which is a multiple-choice examination that relates to the interpretation of clinical data presented primarily in pictorial form, such as pictures of patients, gross and microscopic lesions, electrocardiograms, charts, and graphs. The second section, entitled Patient Management Problems, utilizes a programmed-testing technique (answer by erasure to uncover information or results of actions) designed to measure the candidate's clinical judgment in the management of patients. This technique simulates clinical situations in which the physician is faced with the problems of management presented in a sequential programmed pattern. A set of some four to six problems is related to each of a series of patients. In the scoring of this section, candidates are given credit for correct choices; they are penalized for errors of commission (selection of procedures that are unnecessary or are contraindicated) and for errors of omission (failure to select indicated procedures).

All parts of the National Board examinations are given in a great many centers, usually in medical schools, in nearly every large city in the United States, as well as in a few cities in Canada, in Puerto Rico, and in the Canal Zone. In some cities, such as New York, Chicago, and Baltimore, the examination may be given in more than one center.

The examinations of the National Board have become recognized as the most comprehensive test of knowledge of the medical sciences and their clinical application produced in this country. Approaching them in comprehensiveness and quality are the examinations, developed in close association with the National Board by a committee of the Federation of State Medical Boards of the United States, given twice a year under the auspices of the Federation in any state wishing to use them. These are known as the Federation Licensing Examinations or by the acronym FLEX. More will be said about these examinations later.

For years the National Board examinations have served as an index of the medical education of the period and have strongly influenced higher educational standards in each of the medical sciences. The Diploma of the National Board is accepted by 47 state licensing authorities, the District of Columbia, and the Commonwealth of Puerto Rico in lieu of the examination usually required for licensure and is recognized in the American Medical Directory by the letters DNB following the name of the physician holding National Board certification.

The National Board of Medical Examiners has been a leader in developing new and more reliable techniques of testing, not only for knowledge in all medical fields but also for clinical competence and

fitness to practice. In recent years, too, a number of medical schools, several specialty-certifying boards, professional medical societies organized to encourage their members to keep abreast of progress in medicine, and other professional qualifying agencies have called upon the National Board's professional staff for advice or for the actual preparation of tests to be employed in evaluating medical knowledge, effectiveness of teaching, and professional competence in certain medical fields. In all cases, advantage has been taken of the validity and effectiveness of the objective, multiple-choice type of examination, a technique the National Board has played an important role in bringing to its present state of perfection and discriminatory effectiveness.

FEDERATION LICENSING EXAMINATION (FLEX)

There have been several important developments in the field of medical qualifying examinations in recent years. The first significant achievement in the development of qualifying examinations was the introduction, in 1968, of the first Federation Licensing Examination (FLEX), prepared under the direction of the Examination Institute Committee of the Federation of State Medical Boards of the United States, Inc. Beginning in 1957, the Federation's Examination Institute Committee had held annual conferences designed to study examination procedures in the various states with the end in view of improving their quality and keeping them abreast of the continuing progress in medical education. As a result, there is general agreement to justify the continuation of this committee on a permanent basis.

At the present time this committee is charged: to provide state medical boards with high-quality, uniform, and valid examinations for purposes of evaluating clinical competence and qualification for licensure; to place licensure in a definite relation to modern medical education by updating state board examination procedures and providing flexibility; to establish uniform levels of examinations among the states; to create a rational basis for interstate endorsement; and to provide a basis for the management of the foreign medical graduate problem.

Following publication of their first complete report, in 1961, the Examination Institute Committee continued to hold special conferences and symposia at each annual Federation meeting, and to press forward in its efforts to develop an examination of high quality that would be acceptable to the various state medical boards. At first, it was believed that the Federation itself could set up an examination center, staffed by a medical director and a specialist in examination construction and preparation, that would be in competition with other examination centers, particularly the National Board of Medical Examiners, which had been functioning for more than 50 years. Since the cost was found to be prohibitive, the Examination Institute Committee consulted with the staff of the National Board of Medical Examiners, and the Federation Licensing Examination came into being. Thus, in 1967, the Federation of State Medical Boards gave the new examination its unanimous approval at its annual meeting; and in June 1968, candidates for licensure in six states took the first FLEX examinations. Since then, all but two states have accepted the FLEX examination as their own official licensing examination.

The FLEX is a uniform, valid, and reliable licensing examination, planned and prepared by FLEX Test Committees composed of Federation members and designed for use by any state medical licensing board. It is a 3-day examination given simultaneously by participating medical boards in the name of their own states twice a year, in June and December.

The arrangement with the National Board calls for making pools of already tested and validated objective questions in the six major basic medical science disciplines and the six major clinical fields available to the Test Committees composed of Federation members who represent the state medical boards that have decided to use the FLEX examination. From this collection of questions two subcommittees—one for the basic sciences and one for the clinical sciences—prepare the licensing examinations in these two fields. A third subcommittee selects the questions or problems to be given in the test of clinical competence.

This latter test is relatively new in licensing examinations in spite of the fact that such competence is the most essential requirement of a physician. A few state boards had attempted to solve the problem by requiring oral or practical tests in addition to the standard written tests, but for those boards that had a large number of applicants for licensure, individual tests of this kind were out of the question. The National Board of Medical Examiners had developed an ideal and unique practical test that had been used for some years with great success. This, the Federation's FLEX Committee (now called the FLEX Board) felt, met every need, and it was decided to add this practical test to those in the basic and clinical sciences. However, because of the many changes in the curricula of medical schools in this country, it was held that individual tests in anatomy, physiology, surgery, and so forth, were becoming outmoded. A comprehensive interdisciplinary examination that covered all basic medical science fields in one test and the clinical sciences in another was established. Questions in all of the important areas would be included in these tests; they would be "scrambled" without regard to discipline, but with all fields adequately represented. It was decided that about 90 questions each in anatomy, biochemistry, microbiology, pathology, pharmacology, and physiology would be mixed together in the basic sciences test, and about the same number of questions each in internal medicine, obstetrics and gynecology, pediatrics, preventive medicine and public health, psychiatry, and surgery would be mixed together in the clinical sciences test.

In each examination, the origin of the individual questions is known in the central office. Therefore, in spite of the scrambled character of the questions in the actual examination, it is possible to extract specific grades in each individual subject if these are needed. The FLEX Board felt, however, that each basic science and clinical science examination should be considered as a unit, with a single grade to be given for each entire test.

The examination in the basic sciences, given on the first day, is divided into three sections, A, B, and C, each lasting about 2½ hours, in which time some 180 questions must be answered, making a total of approximately 540 questions for the day. The clinical sciences examination, given on the second day, is presented in the same way.

On the third day the examination designed to test clinical competence is given. This test is divided into two sections that resemble in all details the two sections of Part III of the National Board examination. In the first section clinical material is presented in the form of pictures of patients or specimens, roentgenograms, electrocardiograms, and graphic or tabulated material about which searching questions are asked. In the second section a distinctive technique described as programmed testing is employed, the object being to assess the candidate's judgment in the sequential management of patients in a manner similar to that experienced in relation to his or her own patients in the course of studying their disease processes or injuries, evaluating findings, and planning treatment. A single overall grade is given to this entire part.

Because there will be many physicians who graduated from several to many years before appearing for this examination, the FLEX Board decided to provide, in addition to a single grade for each of the three parts (and of course, separate grades in each of the basic and clinical science subjects for those boards that might want them) a single overall grade for the entire examination, a grade that would give greater weight to the clinical, rather than the basic science, portion of the test. This is the so-called FLEX weight average. This average is developed by emphasizing the importance of the clinical parts of the examination, inasmuch as a weight of 1 is given to the basic sciences grade, a weight of 2 to the clinical sciences grade, and a weight of 3 to the clinical competence grade. How this weighted average is to be used will depend on the decision of each state medical board giving the FLEX examination. The FLEX Board recommends that a weighted average of 75 be the accepted passing grade.

Thus, there are now two important medical examinations for graduates of American and Canadian medical schools, those given by the National Board of Medical Examiners and those given under the auspices of the Federation of State Medical Boards of the United States. These two examinations do not conflict since their purposes are not exactly the same. The National Board examinations are designed to test the knowledge of students as they are learning medicine in medical schools today; these tests are focused on the student of today and the physician of tomorrow. The FLEX examination is designed to assess fundamental knowledge and, more especially, the clinical competence of the physician of today. A dual examination system has thus emerged, each examination important in its own right, each with a different objective and each aimed at its own clearly defined target.

EDUCATIONAL COUNCIL FOR FOREIGN MEDICAL GRADUATES (ECFMG) CERTIFICATION

The second significant achievement in the development of qualifying examinations was brought about as a result of the problems created by the ever increasing numbers of foreign-educated physicians, particularly from non-English-speaking countries, who were coming to the United States for further education and training, many of whom decided to remain in this country to practice. After a study by a committee representing the American Hospital Association, the American Medical Association, the Association of American Medical Colleges and the Federation of State Medical Boards of the United States, with the unofficial cooperation of the U.S. Department of State, the Educational Council for Foreign Medical Graduates (ECFMG) was created. The purpose of the Council is to develop and administer an evaluation procedure or qualifying

examination that will effectively ascertain the fitness of foreign medical graduates to serve as interns and residents in hospitals in the United States or to come to the United States to otherwise practice medicine. Also included for those who come from countries where English is not the spoken language is a 1-hour examination designed to assess comprehension of English vocabulary and language structure (the ECFMG English test).

It was only natural that the Council should turn to the National Board of Medical Examiners for advice and help. The result was that the examinations, given twice each year, were, and continue to be, prepared and scored by the National Board. Indeed, so close became the association between these two organizations because of this relationship, that the home office of the Council, formerly in Evanston, Illinois, was moved to Philadelphia, Pennsylvania, where it is now located. This is the same city in which the home office of the National Board is located.

The Council on Medical Education of the American Medical Association has adopted rules providing that no approved hospital in the United States can now employ as interns or residents any foreign-educated physicians who do not hold the ECFMG Certificate unless they already have a valid state license. In spite of some criticism (most of it unwarranted) of the Council as well as its sponsoring agencies in the first few years, the Council, after giving more than 315,000 examinations in 48 centers in the United States and Canada and in over 105 foreign countries, has fully justified its existence. Indeed, at the present time practically every state that will accept foreign-educated physicians for licensure requires that all these applicants be certified before being admitted to the licensing examination in that state.

FOREIGN MEDICAL GRADUATE EXAMINATION IN THE MEDICAL SCIENCES (FMGEMS)

Until 1976, all foreign medical graduates desiring to undergo postgraduate medical training in the United States were required to take the ECFMG examination. This comprehensive clinical examination permitted certification by the ECFMG for acceptance into an accredited graduate medical education training program in the United States. In 1976, the United States Congress enacted amendments to the Immigration and Naturalization Act (INA) that required all foreign medical graduates who desire entrance into the United States for postgraduate training (or to practice medicine) to pass a new Visa Qualifying Examination (VQE). If this examination, a 2-day comprehensive test of preclinical (basic) and clinical knowledge, was passed, a certificate was issued by the ECFMG. This document was required to obtain the necessary visa to enter the United States. Thus, a passing grade on the VQE was deemed equivalent to passing Parts I and II of the National Board Examinations, provided the candidate also demonstrated competence in oral and written English. In 1977 (and in subsequent years), there was an extremely high rate of failure of the basic sciences (day 1) of the VQE in comparison to the ECFMG examination (that had much fewer questions in the basic sciences area).

The VQE examination is no longer given; it has been supplanted by the Foreign Medical Graduate Examination in the Medical Sciences (FMGEMS). In addition, all candidates from foreign medical schools must also pass the ECFMG English test. Passage of both examinations is therefore required for ECFMG certification.

A word of definition of a "foreign medical graduate" (FMG) is necessary before discussing the FMGEMS test. An FMG is any physician whose medical degree of qualification was conferred by any medical school located outside the United States, Canada, and Puerto Rico. That medical school, however, must be listed in the *World Directory of Medical Schools,* published by the World Health Organization. Citizens of the United States who have completed their medical education in schools outside the United States, Canada, and Puerto Rico are defined as "foreign medical graduates" (FMGs). Alternatively, foreign nationals who have graduated from United States, Canadian, or Puerto Rican medical schools are not FMGs.

Thus, the ECFMG certification provides assurance to all directors of training programs of the Accreditation Council for Graduate Medical Education (ACGME) that the FMG applicant has fulfilled the minimum standards for medical knowledge and mastery of the English language necessary to enter their programs. This ECFMG certification is also prerequisite for licensure to practice medicine in most states of the United States. (Some states may require that the candidate also pass the FLEX examination.)

English Language Examinations

Two English language examinations are approved by the ECFMG. The *ECFMG English test* is administered twice yearly (in January and July) in the morning of the second day (prior to the clinical sci-

ence test) of the FMGEMS. The ECFMG states that examinees who take the clinical science component of the FMGEMS examination must also take the ECFMG English test that same day even if they have passed the English test at previous examinations. The only other English test that is acceptable to the ECFMG is an international or special administration of the *Test of English as a Foreign Language (TOEFL)*. The ECFMG emphasizes that this testing is with the provision that applicants have previously taken an ECFMG English test. There are a number of important requirements concerning these English tests as well as details concerning the medical science examination and the registration procedures. The applicant for all examinations of this nature, therefore, should not assume that the information concerning any of the examinations described in this textbook is the final word. It is strongly recommended that the applicant communicate directly with the testing agencies.

Medical Science Examination

As indicated previously, the examination is formulated by the ECFMG and the NBME and is given twice yearly, in January and in July, as 2 half-day sessions on 2 successive days. The questions on the first day relate to preclinical (basic) sciences and on the second day to the clinical sciences. The overall examination consists of approximately 950 test items constructed in a multiple-choice format. The preclinical science questions, about 500 items in number, are derived from the areas of anatomy, biochemistry, behavioral sciences, microbiology, pathology, pharmacology, and physiology. The second-day examination in the clinical sciences is preceded by the English test, which is followed by 450 question items drawn in approximately equal numbers from the disciplines of internal medicine, obstetrics and gynecology, pediatrics, preventive medicine and public health, psychiatry, and surgery. As indicated above, this new 2-day examination replaces the VQE and ECFMG examinations.

United States Medical Licensing Examination (USMLE)

In August 1991, the Federation of State Medical Boards (FSMB) and the National Board of Medical Examiners (NBME) agreed to replace their respective examinations, the FLEX and NBME, with a new examination, the United States Medical Licensing Examination (USMLE). This examination will provide a common means for evaluating all applicants for medical licensure. It appears that this new development in medical licensure will at last satisfy the needs for state medical boards licensure, the national medical board licensure, and licensure examinations for foreign medical graduates. This is because the 1991 agreement provides for a composite committee that equally represents both organizations (the FSMB and NBME) as well as a jointly appointed public member and a representative of the Educational Council for Foreign Medical Graduates (ECFMG).

As indicated in the USMLE announcement, "it is expected that students who enrolled in U.S. medical schools in the fall of 1990 or later and foreign medical graduates applying for ECFMG examinations beginning in 1993 will have access only to USMLE for purposes of licensure." The announcement further outlines the phase-out of the last regular examinations for licensure as follows:

NBME, Part I	September 1991
NBME, Part II	April 1992
NBME, Part III	May 1994
FLEX, Components 1 and 2	December 1993
Flex, Component 1 (repeaters only)	December 1994

The new USMLE will be administered in three steps. Step 1 will focus on fundamental basic biomedical science concepts with particular emphasis on "principles and mechanisms underlying disease and modes of therapy." Step 2 will be related to the clinical sciences with examination on material necessary to practice medicine in a supervised setting. Step 3 will be designed to focus upon "aspects of biomedical and clinical science essential for the unsupervised practice of medicine."

For further detailed information concerning this newest development in the evolution of the examination process for medical licensure (for graduates of both U.S. and foreign medical schools), the interested person should contact the USMLE Secretariat at 3930 Chestnut Street, Philadelphia, PA 19104, U.S.A. The telephone number there is (215) 590–9600.

INNOVATIONS IN FORMULATING TEST QUESTIONS

It is apparent from recent certification and board examinations that the examiners are devoting more attention in their construction of questions to more practical means of testing basic and clinical knowledge. This greater realism in testing relates to an increasingly interdisciplinary approach toward fundamental material and to the direct relevance accorded practical clinical problems. These newer approaches in testing will be incorporated into this text in the future. However, *Rypins' Questions and Answers for Basic Sciences Review*, 2nd edition, now includes questions that relate to these approaches.

Of course, the new approaches to testing add to the difficulty experienced by the student or physician preparing for board or certification examinations. The contributors to this book are acutely aware not only of the interrelationships of fundamental information with the basic science disciplines and their clinical implications but of the necessity to present their material clearly and concisely despite this complexity. For this reason, the questions provided at the end of each chapter are devised to test one's knowledge of specific material in that chapter. This permits the reader to identify areas for more intensive study. However, those preparing for examinations must be aware of the interdisciplinary nature of fundamental clinical material, the common multifactorial characteristics of disease mechanisms, and the necessity to shift back and forth from one chapter to another in order to appreciate the less than clear-cut nature separating the pedagogic disciplines.

FIVE POINTS TO REMEMBER

In order for the candidate to maximize chances for passing these examinations, a few commonsense strategies or guidelines should be kept in mind.

First, it is imperative to prepare thoroughly for the examination. Know well the types of questions to be presented and the pedagogic areas of particular weakness, and devote more preparatory study time to these weak areas. Do not use too much time restudying areas in which there is a feeling of great confidence and do not leave unexplored those areas in which there is less confidence. Finally, be well rested before the test, and if possible, avoid traveling to the city of testing just that morning or late the evening before.

Second, know well the format of the examination and the instructions before becoming immersed in the challenge at hand. This information can be obtained from many published texts and brochures or directly from the testing service (e.g., USMLE Secretariat and ECFMG's English Test from 3624 Market Street, Philadelphia, Pennsylvania 19104–2685 U.S.A.; cable: EDCOUNCIL; telephone: (215) 396–5900). In addition, the many available texts and self-assessment types of examinations are valuable for practice.

Third, know well the overall time allotted for the examination and its components and the scope of the test to be faced. These may be learned by a rapid review of the examination itself. Then, proceed with the test at a careful, deliberate, and steady pace without spending inordinate time on any single question. For example, certain questions such as the "one best answer" (questions 1 to 3 of "Examples of Questions" below) probably should be allotted 1 to 1½ minutes each. The "matching" type of questions (numbers 4 to 18) should be allotted similar time. The multiple "true-false" type should be given about 1½ minutes. Thus, each question of the five-component questions should be allotted approximately 20 seconds. With respect to the "recall" type of question, there is great need for logical judgment, for the candidate to infer an answer from the presentation of the data, and to discard illogical answers from the multiplicity of the choices. Further, the candidate should be aware that those questions containing the word *always* or *never* are unlikely to be wise choices; questions with words such as *may* and *could* are wiser selections.

Fourth, it follows that if a question is particularly disturbing, the candidate should note appropriately the question (put a mark on the question sheet) and return to this point later. Don't compromise yourself by so concentrating on a likely "loser" that several "winners" are eliminated because of inadequate time. One way to save this time on a particular "stickler" is to play your initial choice; your chances of a correct answer are always best with your first impression. If there is no initial choice, reread the question.

Fifth, allow adequate time to review answers, to return to the questions that were unanswered and "flagged" for later attention, and check every *n*th (e.g., 20th) question to make certain that the answers are appropriate and that you did not inadvertently skip a question in the booklet or answer on the sheet (this can happen easily under these stressful circumstances). There is nothing magical about these five points. They are simple and just make common sense. If candidates have prepared themselves well and follow the preceding commonsense points, the chances are they will not have to return for a second go-round.

EXAMPLES OF QUESTIONS

The following questions are presented as a guide to the physician preparing for examinations in the basic and clinical sciences. They offer the variety of types of multiple-choice questions that have been devised to provide objectivity in testing a large area of subject material that demands depth in knowledge and comprehension.

Objective Multiple-Choice Type

COMPLETION TYPE

The so-called completion-type item is the most common. Items of this type usually are placed together at the beginning of the test, as follows, with these directions:

Directions. *Each of the following questions or incomplete statements is followed by five suggested answers or completions. Select the one that is best in each case and blacken the corresponding space on the answer sheet.*

The following item illustrates this type, although obviously this question is rather easy.

Question 1:

To which one of the following systems of the body does the heart belong?

(a) The digestive system
(b) The central nervous system
(c) The circulatory system
(d) The endocrine system
(e) The musculoskeletal system

The correct answer, of course, is (c). To make this question somewhat more difficult and avoid naming the correct system among the choice, the circulatory system can be omitted and an alternative choice, "None of the above," substituted for it. Then the question will appear as:

Question 2:

To which of the following systems of the body does the heart belong?

(a) The digestive system
(b) The central nervous system
(c) The endocrine system
(d) The musculoskeletal system
(e) None of the above

The fifth choice, (e), now becomes the correct response. In this manner candidates are made to think of the various systems of the body and must know the right answer without its being suggested to them as one of the possibilities. In these examinations, the choice "None of the above" will appear and sometimes will be a correct and sometimes an incorrect response.

Another variant of the completion type of item is in the negative form, where all but one of the choices are applicable, and the candidate is asked to mark the one that does not apply. The following is an example:

Question 3:

All of the following are associated with prerenal azotemia EXCEPT:

(a) Shock
(b) Dehydration
(c) Pernicious vomiting
(d) Gastrointestinal hemorrhage
(e) Multiple myeloma

The correct answer is (e).

ASSOCIATION AND RELATEDNESS ITEMS

Items of a somewhat different nature may be used effectively, as, for example, in determining the candidate's knowledge of the action and the use of closely related drugs or the distinguishing features of similar diseases. There follow specific directions for items of this type with a group of items taken from a pharmacology test and another group from a medicine test. As illustrated in this group of items, the candidate must have well-organized information about a number of related drugs and is required to demonstrate considerable understanding of the differential use of these drugs.

Directions. *Each group of questions below consists of five lettered headings followed by a list of numbered words or phrases. For each numbered word or phrase, select the one heading that is related most closely to it.*

Questions 4–9:

(a) Quinidine
(b) Theophylline
(c) Amyl nitrite
(d) Glyceryl trinitrate
(e) Papaverine

4. Relaxes smooth muscle of the arterial system; causes fall in arterial pressure; commonly administered in tablets sublingually *Answer:* (d)
5. An opium alkaloid; direct vasodilator action;

used in instances of coronary occlusion and peripheral vascular disease *Answer:* (e)
6. Commonly effective in relieving symptoms of bronchial asthma *Answer:* (b)
7. The best for quick treatment of cyanide poisoning *Answer:* (c)
8. Increases the contractile force of the heart and is diuretic *Answer:* (b)
9. May be used in auricular fibrillation *Answer:* (a)

Questions 10–17:

(a) Coarctation of the aorta
(b) Patent ductus arteriosus
(c) Tetralogy of Fallot
(d) Aortic vascular ring
(e) Tricuspid atresia

10. Benefitted by systemic pulmonary artery anastomosis *Answer:* (c)
11. Most common type of congenital cyanotic heart disease *Answer:* (c)
12. Corrected surgically by resection and end-to-end anastomosis *Answer:* (a)
13. Possible cause of dysphagia in infants and children *Answer:* (d)
14. Wide pulse pressure *Answer:* (b)
15. Associated frequently with atrial septal defects *Answer:* (e)
16. A continuous murmur *Answer:* (b)
17. Hypertension in the arms and hypotension in the legs *Answer:* (a)

A further elaboration of association and relatedness items is considerably more searching and calls for a discriminatory understanding of a number of similar but distinguishable factors. For example, the following question reveals considerable information about the candidate's knowledge of the causes of hypoglycemia and the related functional disturbances: Four of the five situations in the numbered list below are common to one of the three functional disturbances designated by letters. The candidate is instructed to select one situation that is the exception and the functional disturbance common to the remaining four.

Question 18:

(a) Clinically significant hypoglycemia
(b) Clinically significant hyperglycemia
(c) Clinically significant glycosuria

(1) Overdose of insulin
(2) Functional tumor of islet cells

(3) Renal glycosuria
(4) Hypopituitarism
(5) von Gierke's disease

If the candidate selects (a) and (3), the correct answer, he or she demonstrates knowledge that (1), (2), (4), and (5) may produce clinically significant hypoglycemia; that (3) does not; and that no combination of four of the five conditions is associated with hyperglycemia or glycosuria. In other words, the possession of both positive and negative information is probed. Specific directions for handling this form of discriminatory question read as follows:

Directions. *There are two responses to be made to each of the following questions. There are three lettered categories; four of the five numbered items are related in some way to one of these categories. (1) On the answer sheet blacken the space under the letter of the category in which these four items belong. (2) Then blacken the space under the number of the item that does not belong in the same category with the other four.*

Items of this type may be used to determine knowledge of disease symptomatology, laboratory findings, or therapeutic procedures, as shown by the following:

Questions 19–21:

19. (a) Multiple neurofibromatosis (von Recklinghausen's disease)
    (b) Hemangioblastomas of the central nervous system
    (c) Multiple sclerosis

    (1) Neurofibromas of the skin
    (2) Meningeal fibromas
    (3) Congenital angiomas of the eye
    (4) Lipomas of subcutaneous tissue
    (5) Cystic disease of the pancreas

Answer: 1. (a)
         2. (5)

20. (a) Contraindications to saddle-block anesthesia
    (b) Contraindications to continuous caudal analgesia
    (c) Contraindications to local anesthesia

    (1) Deformity of the sacrum
    (2) Cutaneous infections
    (3) Perforated dura
    (4) Decreased perineal resistance
    (5) Prodromal labor

Answer: 1. (b)
         2. (4)

21. (a) Eosinophilia of diagnostic significance
    (b) Plasmacytosis of diagnostic significance
    (c) Lymphocytosis of diagnostic significance

    (1) Trichinosis
    (2) Multiple myeloma
    (3) Löffler's syndrome
    (4) Hodgkin's disease
    (5) Schistosomiasis

Answer: 1. (a)
         2. (2)

Another variant of the association and relatedness type of question is demonstrated by the following example from a test in public health and preventive medicine:

Directions. *Each set of lettered headings below is followed by a list of words or phrases. For each word or phrase blacken the space on the answer sheet under:*

A if the word or the phrase is associated with (a) *only*
B if the word or the phrase is associated with (b) *only*
C if the word or the phrase is associated with *both* (a) and (b)
D if the word or the phrase is associated with *neither* (a) *nor* (b)

Questions 22–26:

    (a) Maternal hygiene program
    (b) School health program
    (c) Both
    (d) Neither

22. Periodic physical examination *Answer:* C—(a & b)
23. Audiometer test *Answer:* B
24. Nutritional guidance *Answer:* C—(a & b)
25. Serologic test for syphilis *Answer:* A
26. Immunization against rubella *Answer:* B

QUANTITATIVE VALUES AND COMPARISONS

In general, questions in this category will call for an understanding of quantitative values rather than rote memory of the quantities themselves. The test committees have agreed that these examinations should contain a minimum of questions calling for the memorizing of absolute quantitative amounts. Actual figures will be found only where the details of the information are considered to be of such importance that they should be a part of the working knowledge that a practicing physician should have in mind without recourse to a reference book. Knowledge of the comparative significance of quantitative values may be called for by items such as the following:

Directions. *The following paired statements describe two entities that are to be compared in a quantitative sense. On the answer sheet blacken the space under:*

A if (a) is *greater than* (b)
B if (b) is *greater than* (a)
C if the two are *equal or very nearly equal*

Questions 27–31:

27. (a) The usual therapeutic dose of epinephrine
    (b) The usual therapeutic dose of ephedrine
    Answer: B
28. (a) The inflammability of nitrous oxide-ether mixtures *Answer:* A
    (b) The inflammability of chloroform-air mixtures
29. (a) The susceptibility of premature infants to rickets *Answer:* A
    (b) The susceptibility of full-term infants to rickets
30. (a) Life expectancy with glioblastoma of the occipital lobe
    (b) Life expectancy with glioblastoma of the frontal lobe *Answer:* C
31. (a) The amount of glycogen in the cells of Henle's loop in a diabetic *Answer:* A
    (b) The amount of glycogen in the cells of Henle's loop in a nondiabetic

Directions. *Each of the following pairs of phrases describes conditions or quantities that may or may not be related. On the answer sheet blacken the space under:*

A if increase in the first is accompanied by increase in the second or if decrease in the first is accompanied by decrease in the second
B if increase in the first is accompanied by decrease in the second or if decrease in the first is accompanied by increase in the second
C if changes in the second are independent of changes in the first

Questions 32–34:

32. (1) Urine volume
    (2) Urine specific gravity *Answer:* B

33. (1) Plasma protein concentration
    (2) Colloid osmotic pressure of plasma
    Answer: A
34. (1) Cerebrospinal fluid pressure
    (2) Intraocular pressure *Answer:* C

CAUSE AND EFFECT

A type of item that is especially applicable to some of the more elusive aspects of medicine and calls for an understanding of cause and effect is illustrated in the following type of questions:

Directions. *Each of the following sentences consists of two main parts: a statement and a reason for that statement. On the answer sheet blacken the space under:*

A if the statement and the proposed reason are *both true* and are *related* as cause and effect
B if the statement and the proposed reason are *both true* but are *not related* as cause and effect
C if the statement is *true* but the proposed reason is *false*
D if the statement is false but the proposed reason is *an accepted fact or principle*
E if the statement and the proposed reason are *both false*

Directions Summarized:

A = True True and related
B = True True and NOT related
C = True False
D = False True
E = False False

In situations that may be presented by this type of item, the right answer may sometimes be arrived at through good reasoning from an appreciation of the basic principles involved. The sample items are as follows:

Questions 35–39:

35. Herpes simplex usually is regarded as an autogenous infection BECAUSE patients given fever therapy frequently develop herpes. *Answer:* A
36. Cow's milk is preferable to breast milk in infant feeding BECAUSE cow's milk has a higher content of calcium. *Answer:* D
37. The corpus luteum of menstruation becomes the corpus luteum of pregnancy BECAUSE progesterone inhibits the activity of the anterior portion of the pituitary gland. *Answer:* B

38. The sinoauricular node serves as the pace-maker BECAUSE after its removal the heart fails to beat. *Answer:* C

39. A higher titer of antibody against the H antigen of the typhoid bacillus is a good index of immunity to typhoid BECAUSE any antibody to an organism can protect against disease caused by that organism. *Answer:* E

Question 40:

A modification of the true-false type of question that calls for careful thought and discrimination is the "multiple true-false" variety. In this question a list of numbered items follows a statement for which several possible answers are given and the candidate is required to select the appropriate response from a list of answers designated by letters:

40. Live virus is used in immunization against:
   1. Influenza
   2. Poliomyelitis
   3. Cholera
   4. Smallpox

Answers:
   A. Only 1, 2, and 3 are correct
   B. Only 1 and 3 are correct
   C. Only 2 and 4 are correct
   D. Only 4 is correct
   E. All are correct

STRUCTURE AND FUNCTIONS

Diagrams, charts, electrocardiograms, roentgenograms, or photomicrographs may be used to elicit knowledge of structure, function, the course of a clinical situation, or a statistical tabulation. Questions then may be asked in relation to designated elements of the same.

CASE HISTORIES

The most characteristic situation that confronts the practicing physician can be simulated by a clinical case history derived from a patient experience, which is followed by a series of questions concerning diagnosis, signs and symptoms, laboratory determinations, treatment, and prognosis. In answering these questions, much depends on arriving at the proper diagnosis, for, if an incorrect diagnosis is made, related symptoms, laboratory data, and treatment also will be wrong. These case history questions are set up purposely to place such emphasis on the correct diagnosis within a context comparable with the experience of actual practice.

Directions. *This section of the test consists of several case histories, each followed by a series of questions. Study each history, select the best answer to each question following it, and blacken the space under the corresponding letter on the answer sheet.*

The patient is a 21-year-old white man with a complaint of malaise, cough, and fever. The present illness had its onset 10 days prior to admission with malaise and a nonproductive cough, followed in 24 hours by a temperature varying from 100° F to 101° F that persisted up to the time of admission. On about the fourth day of illness the cough became more severe, producing scant amounts of white viscid sputum. Three days prior to admission, paroxysms of coughing began, followed sometimes by vomiting. Chilly sensations were noted but no frank shaking chills. Anterior parasternal pain on coughing has been present since the fifth day of illness.

On physical examination the temperature is 101° F; the pulse rate 110 beats per minute; the respiratory rate 32 per minute; and the blood pressure 108 mmHg systolic, 60 mmHg diastolic. The patient is well developed and well nourished, appears to be acutely but not chronically ill, and is dyspneic but not cyanotic.

Positive physical findings are limited to the chest and are as follows:

Vocal and tactile fremitus and resonance are within normal limits. In the left axilla a few fine rales are heard, and the bronchial quality of the sounds is increased, although the intensity is normal.

Blood findings are reported as follows:

White blood count, 3,400 (polymorphonuclears 30%, lymphocytes 62%, monocytes 5%, eosinophils 3%).

Roentgenogram of the chest reveals an increase in the density of the perihilar markings with ill-defined areas of patchy, soft, increased radiodensity at both bases and in the left upper lung field.

Questions 41–45:

41. Which one of the following is the most likely diagnosis?
   (a) Tuberculosis
   (b) Pneumococcal pneumonia
   (c) Primary atypical pneumonia *Answer:* (c)

(d) Coccidioidomycosis
(e) Bronchopneumonia
42. Which one of the following is the most likely additional physical finding?
   (a) Splenomegaly
   (b) Signs of meningeal irritation
   (c) Pleural friction rub
   (d) Frequent changes in distribution of chest findings *Answer:* (d)
   (e) Signs of frank lobar consolidation
43. Which one of the following laboratory findings is consistent with the diagnosis?
   (a) Elevation and further increase of cold agglutinins *Answer:* (a)
   (b) Positive blood culture
   (c) Marked leukocytosis with the beginning of recovery
   (d) Positive sputum examination
   (e) Positive skin test
44. Which one of the following is the therapy that should be given?
   (a) Bed rest and streptomycin
   (b) Bed rest and penicillin
   (c) Streptomycin and paraaminosalicylic acid
   (d) Bed rest and Aureomycin *Answer:* (d)
   (e) Psychotherapy and physical rehabilitation
45. Which one of the following is the probable outcome of this disease in this patient if untreated?
   (a) The fever will subside spontaneously by crisis
   (b) Recovery will be gradual, with relapse not unexpected. *Answer:* (b)
   (c) Empyema will develop
   (d) Residual fibrosis will appear with healing
   (e) Lung cavitation will not be unexpected

Objective examinations permit a large number of questions to be asked, for 150 to 180 in each subject can be answered in a 2½-hour period. Because the answer sheets are scorable by machine, the grading can be accomplished rapidly, accurately, and impartially. It is completely unbiased and percentile, since the human element is not a factor. Of long-range significance is the facility with which the total test and individual questions can be subjected to thorough and rapid statistical analyses, thus providing a sound basis for comparative studies of medical school teaching and for continuing improvement in the quality of the test itself. Furthermore, multiple-choice written examinations have certain advantages of real benefit to the candidate, to the medical school, and, ultimately, to state boards of medical examiners.

Review Questions

Following are examples of review questions. In those relating to the basic sciences in particular, an attempt has been made, in most of them at least, not merely to call for information based on recollection of past study but rather to relate the questions to practical clinical or patient problems. These questions are rhetorical in nature and would require an essay-type answer. The reviewer is presented these questions primarily as an overall suggestion of important areas for study and review.

QUESTIONS IN THE BASIC SCIENCES

Describe or diagram the conduction pathways of the heart. Indicate the sites of pathology or disturbances in the presence of:

   (a) Paroxysmal tachycardia
   (b) Adams-Stokes syndrome
   (c) Heart block after myocardial infarction

Diagram the anatomy encountered in doing a tracheotomy.

What neurologic structures are found at the cerebellopontine angle, both within and outside of the brain, where pathology might be reflected in clinical symptoms?

A patient has sustained fractures of the lower left ribs posteriorly. What subjacent structures might be injured? What studies should be performed to determine the extent of the injury?

Diagram a cross section of the spinal cord at the level of L2, indicating major tracts. Indicate the blood supply to the cord at this level.

Name five congenital defects that may be detected at birth and give their embryologic derivation.

Diagram the abdominal aorta with its major branches. Indicate site of occlusion for Leriche syndrome.

Describe the embryologic development of the pituitary gland. Diagram its relationship to surrounding structures.

Diagram the relationship of the pancreas to the duodenum with its duct system. Describe its embryology.

Diagram the tracheobronchial tree, showing the major lung segments. Where will a foreign body aspirated into the tracheobronchial tree most frequently lodge?

Discuss the role of progesterone in pregnancy.

What is intermittent claudication? What is its cause?

What is meant by the specific dynamic action (SDA) of food? What is the significance of SDA in prescribing a diet for an obese patient?

Describe briefly the functions of the hypothalamus.

Define *each* of the following:

(a) Conditioned reflex
(b) Jaundice
(c) Orthopnea
(d) Emphysema
(e) Tidal air
(f) Heartburn

Name and discuss the factors responsible for the tonic activity of the respiratory center.

Explain why pulmonary edema develops first in dependent parts of the lungs.

Discuss the role of bile in fat digestion.

What is the origin of bilirubin found in the serum?

In a patient with jaundice and a mild anemia, what five *biochemical* determinations would, in your opinion, be most effective in the differential diagnosis? Explain your choices.

Define a vitamin.

Under what circumstances can hypervitaminosis develop? List the clinical and biochemical manifestations of any hypervitaminosis.

The following proteins may be found in human serum. Define four of the six listed below, list the methods by which they may be detected and explain their clinical significance:

(a) Cryoglobulin
(b) Myeloma protein
(c) Siderophilin (transferrin)
(d) Macroglobulin
(e) Cold agglutinin
(f) Haptoglobin

Define a *buffer system*. Give an example of a buffer system important in clinical medicine and explain the operation of the system in:

(a) Metabolic acidosis
(b) Respiratory alkalosis

What are the clinical manifestations of hypokalemia? What electrocardiographic changes are frequently associated with hypokalemia? List three clinical states in which hypokalemia is a common finding.

Define four of the following:

(a) Methemoglobin
(b) Thyroglobulin
(c) Respiratory quotient
(d) Pasteur effect
(e) Nitrogen balance
(f) Intrinsic factor

In advising a community hospital that is about to establish a clinical diagnostic radioisotope laboratory, what radioactive chemical compounds would you recommend? List the compounds (*not* just elements) and give at least *one* use for *each*.

Name three microorganisms sensitive to penicillin and three resistant to penicillin as it is administered in clinical practice.

Define the terms *anamnestic response* and *booster effect*. How are these principles applied to artificial immunization?

List three infections in which disease is caused primarily by the toxin of the infecting microorganism.

Name a vaccine in which the immunizing principle is a modified toxin.

Describe two laboratory tests for the diagnosis of syphilis. How may these tests be modified by antiluetic therapy?

Name two microorganisms that may induce cavitating disease of the lung. Describe briefly the morphology and the staining characteristics of each.

What streptococcus is associated with "streptococcal" sore throat? What distinguishes this microorganism on blood agar culture? What are three possible sequelae of untreated streptococcal pharyngitis?

Name three bacteria that are frequently associated with meningitis. For each of the three types of meningitis, list an antimicrobial drug that is effective in its treatment.

What is the etiologic significance of a pneumococcus in the throat culture of an adult patient with pharyngitis? In the sputum of a patient with pneumonia? In the nasopharynx of a child with otitis media?

List three cultural or biochemical characteristics of pneumococcus.

What is Sabin's vaccine? Are its antigenic constituents living or dead? Name one constituent of the vaccine in addition to those that are intended for immunization. Does the vaccine prevent infection?

Classify the etiologic agent of "Asiatic influenza."

Which antimicrobial agents are effective in the treatment of uncomplicated influenza?

What is the most frequent cause of death in influenza?

Name two microorganisms frequently implicated in the fatal termination of influenza.

Describe three characteristics by which viruses differ from bacteria.

Identify three diseases caused by rickettsia.

What are selective media? Give the name of one such medium and its purpose. Of what value is penicillinase in diagnostic bacteriology?

Name two diseases that may be prevented or modified by the parenteral injection of antibody.

Name two diseases in which antibody must be used for optimal treatment.

What is the significance of:

(a) An elevated serum ASO (antistreptolysin O) titer
(b) An elevated serum heterophile antibody titer
(c) An elevated cold agglutinin titer in the serum

Compare infectious hepatitis and serum hepatitis with respect to:

(a) Etiologic agent
(b) Epidemiology
(c) Incubation period

Indicate for *each* of the following organisms whether it is sensitive or resistant *in vitro* to penicillin and tetracycline:

Streptococcus pyogenes
Neisseria gonorrhoeae
Neisseria meningitidis
Klebsiella pneumoniae
Hemophilus influenzae
Brucella abortus

Name three vaccines that contain living and three that contain dead infectious agents, listing also the microorganisms they contain. How would you test for the efficacy of immunization with any one of these agents (without exposing your patient to disease)?

List three gram-positive and three gram-negative bacteria. For *each* organism listed, give a brief description of its morphology.

Cite two laboratory characteristics of the staphylococci that are most commonly pathogenic for humans. What is the drug of choice for treating most staphylococcal infections acquired outside the hospital?

Name three diseases in humans caused by spirochetes. What are the names of the etiologic agents of these diseases?

Briefly discuss the most common gross pathology of an adenocarcinoma of the right hemicolon and contrast it with that most often seen in the descending colon. Correlate these gross findings with the usual initial symptom complex of each.

Which of the following is the most frequent site of carcinoma of the colon?

(a) The cecum
(b) The splenic flexure
(c) The sigmoid
(d) The rectum

Which of the following figures most nearly represents the percentage of carcinoma of the colon and the rectum that are detectable by digital rectal examination?

(a) 10%
(b) 2%
(c) 20%
(d) 50%

A 55-year-old woman is admitted to the hospital with complaints of tiredness, weakness, progressive enlargement of the abdomen and continuous mild generalized abdominal discomfort for "some time." No further reliable history is obtainable. Physical examination reveals a middle-aged woman with obvious recent wasting. The blood pressure is 130/80 mmHg; pulse 80 beats per minute and regular; temperature 97° F. The *only* other significant physical finding is an enlarged, tense abdomen exhibiting shifting dullness and fluid wave. (A routine urinalysis has revealed no significant abnormality, nor has an electrocardiogram.)

In the absence of other significant physical findings, what two conditions would you consider most probable in your provisional diagnosis?

What one simple and practical procedure, utilizing the clinical laboratory, would best aid in the differential diagnosis between the two?

Indicate the characteristic clinical laboratory findings elicited by this procedure for *each* of the two conditions that you have mentioned.

Very briefly discuss cancer of the lip under the following headings:

(a) Sex incidence
(b) Location
(c) Gross pathology
(d) Microscopic pathology
(e) Spread
(f) Prognosis

In cases of pernicious anemia, name:

(a) The fundamental defect involved in the pathogenesis
(b) Three laboratory findings indispensable to a diagnosis of pernicious anemia
(c) Three accessory laboratory findings that confirm the diagnosis

The following phrases are descriptive of characteristics of certain neoplasms. In *each* case, name a neoplasm to which the phrase might correctly pertain:

   (a) A tumor that has a high mortality but rarely, if ever, metastasizes
   (b) A serotonin-secreting tumor that may produce spells of flushing of the skin
   (c) An invasive tumor of the skin that rarely, if ever, metastasizes
   (d) A neoplasm that may be mistaken for eczema
   (e) A malignant neoplasm originating from the placenta
   (f) A neoplasm associated with intermittent episodes of hypertension

A man, age 55 years, has had a recent myocardial infarction. Anticoagulant therapy is ordered.

What drug should be used for rapid anticoagulant effect, and what laboratory procedure should be used to check the result?

What drug should be used for long-term anticoagulant effect, and what laboratory test should be used for its control? Give the normal values for this test and the range of values optimal for the patient receiving anticoagulant therapy.

Discuss briefly the pathology of bronchogenic carcinoma, indicating usual sites of primary origin, histologic types, and method of spread.

List five common sites of metastasis of bronchogenic carcinoma, arranging them in order of frequency.

Following overindulgence in food and alcohol, a man, age 30, develops sudden severe epigastric pain with moderate rigidity and tenderness of the upper abdomen. There are nausea, vomiting, cyanosis, abdominal distention, rapid pulse, and shock.

Indicate two conditions that should be considered and laboratory findings that would aid in the differential diagnosis.

Describe clinical features that should suggest that a skin lesion is a malignant melanoma.

Describe briefly the histopathology of malignant melanoma.

Indicate method of spread and prognosis.

Name three diseases that can be transmitted by blood or blood products from donor to recipient.

What precautions should be taken to prevent such transmission?

QUESTIONS IN THE CLINICAL SCIENCES

A patient is admitted to a hospital unconscious immediately following an automobile accident. The neurologic examination is normal. Consciousness is not regained. Two hours later respirations are irregular, the left pupil is a little dilated, and the right arm is tonic. In another hour the right side of the face begins to twitch. The right arm is spastic, and the left pupil is fully dilated. Respirations are very irregular and slow. (Consider unmentioned phenomena to be normal.)

Write the letters *a* and *b* on your answer paper. After *each* letter write the *number* preceding the word or the expression that best completes the statement.

   (a) At this time the diagnosis is:
      1. Depressed skull fracture
      2. Intracranial hematoma
      3. Subdural hematoma
      4. Epidural hematoma
   (b) The immediate procedure should be:
      1. Lumbar puncture
      2. Neurologic consultation
      3. Electroencephalogram
      4. Angiogram
      5. Temporal trephine

Outline the procedure to be followed in the evaluation of a severe injury of the pelvis.

What basic information must you have to order and manage intelligently a patient's fluid intake for the few days following a major abdominal surgical procedure during which oral fluids cannot be taken in adequate amounts?

Following a cholecystectomy for gallstones but with no previous history of jaundice, a patient drains bile from the incision. This drainage gradually becomes less and finally ceases after 2 weeks. Concomitantly, the patient becomes jaundiced and develops periodic attacks of chills and fever. The stools become somewhat lighter in color but are not clay colored.

What conditions would you consider in the differential diagnosis?

What laboratory tests or diagnostic procedures, if any, would definitely confirm your diagnosis?

Should this patient be operated upon?

If operation is indicated, when should it be performed?

List the procedures you might employ if necessary to arrive at the diagnosis of a lesion of the lung that has been noted on an anteroposterior chest x-ray film.

What means would you use to manage the problem presented by the elderly, frail, weak individual who has great difficulty in getting rid of copious mucoid tracheobronchial secretions in the immediate postoperative period?

A 65-year-old man with chronic bronchitis and emphysema has a combined abdominal-perineal resection of the rectum and the sigmoid colon for carcinoma. During the immediate postoperative period he is being treated with an indwelling urethral catheter and an indwelling nasogastric tube. By the fourth postoperative day the patient's temperature has gradually risen since operation to 103° F by rectum.

What significance, if any, is the amount of fever?

What should be done in an attempt to explain it?

Peptic ulcers of the duodenum are treated surgically by a variety of procedures. Indicate the rational basis for the treatment of his lesion by:

(a) Vagotomy with pyloroplasty
(b) Subtotal gastric resection
(c) Gastroenterostomy

Outline your management of a patient presenting himself with a history of painless hematuria lasting for 1 day, 1 week ago.

Given a patient with severe hypertension, list some of the changes in the fundus of the eye that you would likely encounter in doing an ophthalmoscopic examination.

A 55-year-old woman with atrial fibrillation due to rheumatic heart disease experiences a sudden severe pain in the left leg. When she is seen at the hospital 4 hours later the pain is still present. The leg is cooler than the right from the knee down, and the skin is blanched. The toes can be moved, but sensation in the lower leg is decreased. Pulsation can be felt over the left common femoral artery at the level of Poupart's ligament on the left, but none below this level.

What is the clinical diagnosis?

At what specific point is the lesion most likely located?

What recommendations for management do you make?

A 32-year-old white man is found to have hypertension of 190 mmHg systolic and 100 mmHg diastolic on routine examination. What are the possible causes of this, and what clinical and laboratory findings would help in identifying these causes?

A 28-year-old Puerto Rican woman, the mother of children 6 and 8 years of age, complains of weakness, slight fever, anorexia, and hemoptysis. How should this situation be managed from the diagnostic and therapeutic standpoints? What is the most likely diagnosis, and what are the implications with respect to this patient's family?

Discuss the management of *each* of the following clinical situations:

(a) Congestive failure in a child with acute rheumatic pancarditis
(b) Paroxysmal ventricular tachycardia
(c) Premature ventricular beats in a patient with acute myocardial infarction

A 3-year-old child has a generalized convulsive seizure and is rushed to you in the emergency room of a hospital. Tabulate the common causes and give the clinical and laboratory findings of *each* cause mentioned.

Indicate briefly the clinical significance of *each* of the following:

(a) Bence Jones protein in the urine
(b) A positive heterophil agglutination test
(c) A high blood alkaline phosphatase
(d) A high blood acid phosphatase
(e) A positive porphobilinogen in the urine

A moderately obese middle-aged woman presents herself complaining of recurrent belching and a sense of a lump and burning in the substernal area. These symptoms occur especially when she stoops over or after a heavy meal, and when she goes to bed at night. Discuss differential diagnosis and treatment.

Outline the clinical and laboratory differential diagnosis of hematuria in an elderly male.

A middle-aged female patient with rheumatoid arthritis has been under long-term treatment with steroids. She now requires operation for acute appendicitis. What are the implications of the prior steroid therapy in such a situation, and how would you manage the medical aspects of the case?

Tabulate briefly the major indications and contraindications for use of each of the following:

(a) Oral hypoglycemic agents
(b) Nitrogen mustard
(c) Parenteral iron preparations
(d) Intravenous aminophylline
(e) Intravenous ACTH

A young adult man has anorexia, vomiting, and mild nausea for a few days and then notes dark urine and light stool. Discuss clinical and laboratory differential diagnosis and therapy.

Name one subjective complaint and one objective indication for estrogenic hormone in the management of a woman after her menopause.

A 9-year-old girl experiences prolonged vaginal bleeding. Examination reveals breast and vulvar development and a 6 cm by 9 cm tumor in the pelvis. What would you suspect?

What two complaints warrant a suspicion of gonococcal infection in the female? Indicate two procedures, either of which would confirm the diagnosis.

A 60-year-old nulliparous woman, 9 years postmenopausal, reports serous to bloody vaginal discharge on several occasions in the past month.

Indicate two probabilities.

How would you establish the diagnosis?

What two possibly predisposing factors would you consider when suspecting vaginitis is due to *Monilia?*

What would confirm that diagnosis?

What treatment would you prescribe?

A patient, gravida I, with uterus approximately term size, states that she cannot be more than 30 weeks pregnant. What three possibilities would you consider?

The child survived delivery by section when profuse antepartum bleeding was due to placenta previa. Name three possible causes if menstruation fails to occur by the sixth month postpartum.

What two observations noted during labor warrant a suspicion that defibrination of maternal blood may occur?

How can you determine if this is occurring?

If undetected, what could be the result?

Name three laboratory procedures that might be indicated repeatedly during the prenatal care of a normal patient.

Name three disadvantages inherent in "deep" general anesthesia for delivery at term.

List the activities of the U.S. Public Health Service.

What health hazards may be encountered in a boys' summer camp?

What voluntary agencies are active in the field of cardiovascular disease, and what are some of their activities?

What immunizations should be recommended for travelers to the Middle East and Africa?

What is meant by *each* of the following terms:

(a) Crude death rate
(b) Standardized death rate
(c) Infant mortality rate
(d) Birth rate

What services are offered by local health departments to the practicing physician?

Discuss health hazards in industry, and outline methods of preventing them.

Discuss health facilities provided by unions.

Rypins' Clinical Sciences Review, 16th Edition, edited by Edward D. Frohlich. J. B. Lippincott Company, Philadelphia © 1993.

2

Surgery

Ronald C. Elkins, M.D.
Chief, Section of Thoracic
and Cardiovascular Surgery
University of Oklahoma Health Sciences Center

Professor, Department of Surgery
University of Oklahoma School of Medicine
Oklahoma City, Oklahoma

In this chapter will be discussed, first, those subjects common to all branches of surgery and, second, the surgical lesions encountered in various organs and anatomic sites.

RESPONSE TO SURGERY

Homeostasis is maintained in the normal person by a system of autoregulatory control mechanisms. The stress of accidental injury, sepsis, or major surgery initiates a complex sequence of events designed to restore health. This response mobilizes every system of the body. The stress of surgery triggers the same pattern of response as major trauma but to a lesser extent.

The neuroendocrine system functions as the afferent pathway for the stimuli associated with injury and also initiates the neural and hormonal responses designed to facilitate the repair of the injury and diminish the injury response. Preexisting disease, medications, and starvation alter both the afferent pathway and the neural and hormonal responses.

The primary stimuli are tissue injury and pain, hemorrhage and hypovolemia, hypoxia and acido-sis, and emotional factors. Secondary stimuli and modifiers include temperature, glucose, blood volume replacement, immobilization and bed rest, and preexisting disease and medications.

Significant injury or major surgery is associated with the release of the following pituitary hormones: adrenocorticotropic hormone, antidiuretic hormone, growth hormone, prolactin, and gonadotropin. Sympathetically mediated hormone release includes the following: catecholamines, glucagon, insulin, and activation of the renin-angiotensin system.

The time course of metabolic response to injury has been categorized into four phases. The transition between these is imprecise and the duration of each phase varies. The first phase has been identified as the "ebb" phase and is characterized by the need to conserve circulating blood volume and recover from shock. With prompt resuscitation and avoidance of shock, the ebb phase can be curtailed or even avoided. On the other hand, failure of hemostasis leads to continuing shock and death. After resuscitation the ebb phase is followed by the "flow" phase; usually this transition occurs 24 to 36 hours after injury. The flow phase is characterized by a period of general catabolism. This period can last from 1 day to 10 to 14 days, depending on the severity of injury. The flow phase is followed by a period of anabolism, which has been called the "anabolic" phase. This phase is characterized by a sense of well-being and improvement. Protein synthesis and weight gain are slow, and patients with significant injury may take weeks to restore the deficits associated with the catabolism that follows a major injury. Following the anabolic phase, when wound healing has been completed and protein stores have been restored, the patient frequently progresses to a "fat" phase. With inactivity and the increased caloric intake associated with the anabolic phase, considerable weight gain and a significant increase in adipose tissue can occur.

WOUNDS

Wound healing follows a similar time course as described for the metabolic effects following injury. Within hours after a patient has been wounded, a process of phagocytosis and neovascularization begins; this is followed by repair and epithelialization. Collagen deposition begins within a few days and continues. Collagen realignment occurs over a period of weeks to months and is followed by devascularization and collagenolysis and eventually a permanent scar. Wound strength is dependent on collagen synthesis and knowledge of this process affects surgical management. In a clean surgical wound, no collagen is present during the first 3 to 4 days, and wound strength is dependent on either sutures or other closure devices. Between 3 and 10 days, wound strength increases rapidly, then more slowly for 6 weeks. Complete healing and final composition of the wound is not complete for at least 1 year.

Hydroxyproline and *hydroxylysine* are amino acids identified in the collagen molecule, but in no other biologic protein that has been studied except for minute amounts in complement. The enzyme peptidyl proline hydroxylase is responsible for the hydroxylation of proline. Ascorbate has been identified as a necessary cosubstrate in this system. The rate of hydroxyproline formation from ^{14}C-labelled proline in healing wounds has been used as an index of the rate of collagen synthesis.

The collagen molecule is stabilized by polymerization, and there is good evidence that cross linkage between the three helices in the molecule is important in fibrogenesis.

In addition to collagen, the healing wound contains considerable quantities of *proteoglycans* (mucopolysaccharides). These substances are largely polysaccharides composed of chains of repeating disaccharide units that are in turn composed of glucuronic acid or iduronic acid and a hexosamine. The units are called glycosaminoglycans, they rarely exist free in the body, but instead couple with proteins to form proteoglycans. The hexosamine fraction gives a metachromatic staining reaction to healing wounds. This reaction reaches a peak on the fifth or sixth day after wounding and thereafter gradually subsides. The role of proteoglycans in the process of wound healing is not well understood, but it appears that they play an important role in collagen fiber formation by binding polymer chains of collagen by electrostatic interactions. Fiber orientation and size may be influenced by the characteristics of specific proteoglycans.

The relation between deficiencies in various nutrients and wound healing has been studied extensively. Blood flow adequate to provide a sufficient quantity of oxygen and removal of metabolic end products is certainly necessary. Hypoproteinemia is probably a significant factor only where local edema occurs and interferes with blood flow.

Collagen synthesis and wound healing are suppressed by corticosteroids, but collagen synthesis and tensile strength can be returned to normal by the administration of vitamin A.

The type of suture material used influences wound healing, inasmuch as all sutures are foreign bodies. Absorbable sutures elicit a greater inflammatory response than nonabsorbable sutures. Both cellular and humoral factors are responsible for the absorption. No suture material produced for clinical use is devoid of tissue reaction, although inert metals and plastics stimulate a minimal reaction. The eventual fate of nonabsorbable sutures is encapsulation. In the presence of infection, nonabsorbable sutures act as foreign bodies and perpetuate the infection until they are extruded or removed. However, monofilament sutures are less conducive to infection than are multifilament sutures of the same material.

Efforts to regulate the process of fibroplasia or accelerate the process of healing have not been rewarding to date. Cleanly incised wounds that are properly sutured will heal unless infection supervenes. Bleeding points must be ligated carefully, because the development of a hematoma predisposes to infection. Careful obliteration of dead space is necessary to minimize the collection of serum in the wound.

Traumatic wounds that are associated with a large amount of contamination and destruction of soft tissue should be debrided. If the wounds are seen early and cleaned properly, primary closure may be feasible. The use of antibiotic therapy in conjunction with debridement has markedly reduced the massive infection rates previously seen in contaminated wounds and has permitted early secondary closure and plastic procedures heretofore impossible.

In wounds that are unsutured, or in wounds with loss of substance, there is initial retraction of the wound margins owing to the elasticity of the normal skin. As the process of healing progresses, contraction of the wound occurs and narrows the size of the defect. Primitive mononuclear cells in the healing tissues may differentiate into fibroblasts or myofibroblasts. Both can form collagen fibers, but the myofibroblast also has contractile properties. These properties are thought to play a part in the process of wound contraction.

Infection

Infection of surgical wounds is the result of bacterial contamination either from the patient's internal environment (including the skin) or from breaks in surgical technique (*e.g.*, from the surgical team). Two primary factors are significant in the pathogenesis of infections: (1) the dose of bacterial contamination and (2) the resistance of the patient. In order to better understand and reduce the frequency of this serious complication, wounds are classified according to the degree of contamination into clean, clean-contaminated, heavily contaminated (or dirty), and infected. In clean wounds, the only source of contamination from within the patient is the skin. In clean-contaminated wounds, the contamination is from the skin plus an additional source, such as: opening the appropriately prepared colon, the small intestine or the preoperatively cleansed stomach, the not obviously infected biliary tree, and so forth. The final two categories are self-explanatory. In any event, infection of the surgical wound is a complex problem in which the number and virulence of the microbes involved are related to host factors such as the presence of dead and devitalized tissue and hematoma or seroma formation. At operation, the surgeon can unfavorably influence the balance in favor of infection by rough handling of tissues, causing foci of necrosis by including large amounts of fat in clamped and ligated blood vessels; using too large ligature and suture material; poor aseptic technique; imperfect hemostasis; and imperfect approximation of the wound.

In current practice, antimicrobial prophylaxis is indicated in clean-contaminated wounds only when foreign bodies are deliberately inserted or for anticipated prolonged procedures. This consists of the preoperative intravenous administration of a suitable broad-spectrum agent. Additionally, the antimicrobial must be given during operation in dosage sufficient to maintain a blood level considered sufficient for that agent. Postoperative administration is generally not indicated except in instances of established infection.

The early stage of the inflammatory response in soft tissue is known as **cellulitis**. This may subside spontaneously or may progress to formation of an abscess. Extension of the infection along the course of the lymphatics is manifested by the development of red streaks with local tenderness. The regional lymph nodes become tender and enlarged. These conditions are known as **lymphangitis** and **lymphadenitis**. The *Streptococcus pyogenes* is the organism most frequently causative of cellulitis, lymphangitis, and lymphadenitis. It does this by virtue of its production of hyaluronidase and streptokinase. Contrarily, the *Staphylococcus* is more likely to produce localized abscesses.

Erysipelas is a special type of cellulitis also usually caused by the *Streptococcus pyogenes* and characterized by a red, raised advancing margin.

Treatment of cellulitis consists of local application of heat, adequate immobilization, and elevation. In addition, antimicrobial agents, such as penicillin and the broad-spectrum antibiotics, often are of value in arresting the spread of the infection and in shortening the course of the disease. In the modern treatment of infection the antimicrobials hold a very prominent place. The surgeon chooses the antimicrobial on the basis of the organisms he believes will most likely be present in a given situation, which choice is based on clinical judgment aided by Gram stains of smears. Cultures should always be obtained and antimicrobial therapy adjusted according to the proven sensitivity of the predominant organisms.

TETANUS

Tetanus is an infection caused by a strict anaerobe, *Clostridium tetani*. It is found in puncture wounds and in wounds in which there is dead tissue or poor blood supply. The organisms are found in the excreta of animals, especially cows and horses; hence, wounds contaminated by street dirt and fertilized soil are more susceptible to infection by the tetanus organism.

The organism produces an exotoxin that is absorbed by the peripheral nerves and carried to the spinal cord. The sensory nerves react to the slightest stimuli, and the hypersensitive motor nerves carry impulses that produce spasms of the muscles they supply. The extensor muscles in spasm produce a convulsive contraction, with the head pulled back, called opisthotonos. Death occurs from asphyxia, due to diaphragmatic spasm or exhaustion.

Meticulous wound care is the greatest prerequisite for tetanus prophylaxis. This includes irrigation, thorough debridement of dead and devitalized tissues, and the removal of foreign bodies.

Table 2-1 is a guide to the use of active and passive tetanus immunization prophylaxis following the recommendations of the United States Public Health Service Committee on Immunization Practices. In all patients who have not previously had a complete course of immunizations (three or more injections of tetanus toxoid), tetanus toxoid is given. In patients with clean minor wounds, the interval since the last dose should not exceed 10 years. In all other wounds this period must not exceed 5 years. An accurate history is essential, and if there is any doubt, the patient needs an immunizing course. Basic immunization with adsorbed toxoid requires three injections; the second injection is given 4 to 6 weeks after the first, and the third is given 6 to 12 months later.

Antibiotic treatment and surgical debridement do not give adequate protection against tetanus. Thus, the immunization status of all patients with contaminated wounds must be ascertained and appropriate treatment should be initiated.

GAS GANGRENE

Gas gangrene infection results following injuries in which there are destruction and death of soft tissue.

TABLE 2-1. Guide to Tetanus Prophylaxis in Wound Management

HISTORY OF TETANUS IMMUNIZATION (DOSES)	CLEAN MINOR WOUNDS		ALL OTHER WOUNDS	
	Tetanus Toxoid	Tetanus Immune Globulin	Tetanus Toxoid	Tetanus Immune Globulin
Uncertain	Yes	No	Yes	Yes
0–1	Yes	No	Yes	Yes
2	Yes	No	Yes	No*
3 or more	No†	No	No‡	No

 * Unless wound is more than 24 hours old.
 † Unless more than 10 years have elapsed since the last dose.
 ‡ Unless more than 5 years have elapsed since the last dose.

These tissues serve as a culture medium for the growth of the anaerobic gas-forming organisms. Gas gangrene spreads rapidly along fascial planes, destroying large segments of soft tissue, especially muscle. It is a serious infection requiring prompt and radical treatment. This consists of wide excision of the involved part, with amputation if necessary. It also includes the use of massive doses of antitoxin and penicillin. Good results have been reported with the use of oxygen under pressure. The patient is placed in a sealed tank, and oxygen is supplied under 3 atm of pressure.

NECROTIZING FASCITIS

Necrotizing fascitis is a serious infection characterized by extensive necrosis of the superficial fascia with widespread undermining of surrounding tissue and severe toxicity. Although it may be seen following surgical wounds, in most instances the infection follows comparatively mild injury outside the hospital. A variety of microorganisms, including anaerobes, have been cultured. The diagnosis depends on the presence of widespread necrosis of the superficial fascia rather than on the causative organism. Treatment consists of adequate drainage, thorough debridement, and antimicrobials effective against both streptococci and penicillinase-producing staphylococci.

CARBUNCLE

The carbuncle is a soft-tissue infection, usually staphylococcal in origin, in which there is diffuse destruction of the subcutaneous tissues with the development of multiple sinuses presenting on the skin surface. Antistaphylococcal antibiotics, administered parenterally in adequate doses, may abort the infection and allow it to subside spontaneously. However, with the formation of extensive slough and pus, operative excision of the area or incision and drainage is necessary. In these cases the resulting defects may be so massive as to require subsequent skin grafting.

Bite Wounds

RABIES

In all patients who have sustained animal bites or have been in contact with bat feces, rabies prophylaxis must be considered. The decision for or against rabies prophylaxis is based on the severity of the wound and the availability of the animal for observation and autopsy purposes to substantiate the diagnosis of rabies. Prophylaxis consists of a course of duck embryo vaccine and the administration of rabies antiserum. Hyperimmune rabies immune globulin (HRIG) obtained from human volunteers is available, and is the treatment of choice in patients bitten by a rabid animal. The recommended dose of HRIG is 20 IU/kg.

INSECT BITES

Bees, wasps, and hornets inject a venom that may cause sensitization, and in sensitized people, anaphylaxis that may be fatal. The black widow spider venom is a neurotoxin that causes severe muscle spasm; death may occur. The brown spider bite produces ischemic necrosis and a slough that may necessitate skin grafting.

SNAKE BITES

The poisonous snakes in the United States are, with the exception of the coral snake, pit vipers. The venom is both neurotoxic and hemolytic. The bite is painful, and fang marks are the first external evidence. Swelling, pain, and ecchymosis rapidly follow. The use of a tourniquet to impede venous and lymphatic return but not arterial flow as an emergency measure is important. Definitive treatment is early excision of the bite wound; this can remove most of the venom and eliminates the need for antiserum. The defect is repaired by either a local flap or a graft.

Frostbite

Frostbite results from prolonged exposure to cold. Depending on the degree of cold and the length of exposure, the damage may range from the most minimal superficial changes all the way to frank gangrene. Fingers, toes, hands, feet, and ears are the common sites of involvement. Rapid warming of the frostbitten tissue using warm water (40° C to 44° C) for a period sufficient to return the tissue temperature to normal is important. In minor degrees of frostbite, complete recovery will occur; however, in extensive injury, gangrene may set in and require local amputation after demarcation has been established. Paresthesias may follow this injury. Sympathectomy early after severe frostbite has not been shown to reduce the amount of tissue loss; yet, when paresthesias are present, sympathetic block may give relief. Sympathectomy is indicated for treatment of late sequelae of frostbite including chilblain and causalgia.

Amputations

Among the indications for amputation are extensive infection, gangrene, and malignant tumor. It is indicated also in cases of extensive trauma with so much destruction of bone or soft tissues that preservation or conservation of the part is impracticable. On rare occasions, amputation is carried out as an elective procedure in order to improve the function of a part for cosmetic reasons, or to facilitate nursing care. Primary amputation is carried out early after injury when there is irreparable tissue damage or loss of viability. In selecting the site of amputation, in general, one attempts to preserve as much of the extremity as possible. Considerations that alter this are the suitability of the level for fitting a functional prosthesis, resistance of the tissues at the stump to long-term trauma and cosmetic ones. In the upper extremity length is particularly important. At least 7.5 cm of radius and ulna are necessary for a functioning prosthesis if the elbow joint is to be preserved, and a similar length of humerus is needed at the shoulder. Amputation through the flare of the humeral condyles should be avoided. Above all, however, if there is the possibility of salvage of anything resembling a functioning hand everything possible should be done to preserve it. In amputation of digits or portions of digits articular cartilage should be removed. Amputation through the carpus or tarsus is generally unsatisfactory.

In the lower extremity transmetatarsal amputation leaves a very satisfactory functioning foot. Weight-bearing stumps such as that left by the Syme's amputation at the ankle or the Gritti-Stokes at the knee are satisfactory. Amputations through the leg are best done at the junction of the upper and middle third. Amputation through the femur may be carried out at any site. Supracondylar amputation, which is largely tendinous, is particularly satisfactory, and a minimum of 5 cm below the greater trochanter is necessary for satisfactory fitting of a lower limb. If a patient has had an amputation through the femur on one side every effort should be made to preserve the knee joint should amputation become necessary on the other side.

In diabetics conservative amputation is frequently possible. Either amputation of a toe or transmetatarsal amputation yields good functional results. When wet gangrene with systemic manifestations of sepsis is present, either in diabetics or patients with arteriosclerosis, refrigeration along with use of a tourniquet and antimicrobial therapy will permit control of sepsis. Thereafter, guillotine amputation with skin traction and secondary closure is the treatment of choice.

Burns

Burns are classified according to their severity. *First-degree burns* involve only the superficial layers of the skin and are marked by erythema. *Second-degree burns* are somewhat deeper, and blisters or bullae develop. In *third-degree burns* there is destruction of all layers of the skin, and a granulating surface results. Burns are also classified according to the extent of surface area involvement. A convenient method of estimating this is by the *rule of nines*. In the adult, the entire head accounts for 9% of the body surface area; the anterior and posterior surfaces of the torso are each 18%; the upper extremity is 9%; the lower extremity, 18%; and the entire genitalia, 1%. In infants and children, this formula is modified in keeping with the proportionately larger surface area of the head.

Mortality rate depends upon the age of the patient and the surface area involved, particularly in deep second- and third-degree burns. Large amounts of serum are lost to the body in the burn wound by exudation from the surface. Early mortality in burns is the result of burn shock. This is controlled by the replacement of lost extracellular fluid and electrolytes. At present we use a continuous infusion of lactated Ringer's solution and 5% dextrose in water, adjusting the rate according to urinary output, hematocrit, pulse rate, blood pressure, and state of consciousness. A minimal output of urine of 30 ml to 50 ml per hour must be maintained. Hypertonic sodium solutions may be useful in extensive, deep burns in the aged and very young patient, permitting reduction in the total volume of fluid administered and thereby reducing the risk of pulmonary edema. The concentration of sodium chloride or lactate is twice that of its concentration in body fluids.

Local treatment of the burn wound consists of gentle cleansing with mild soap solutions followed by isotonic sodium chloride and debridement. Adequate analgesia and, in some instances, general anesthesia are required. Following this, one of the following agents is applied and continued: 0.5% silver nitrate solution, Sulfamylon ointment, or silver sulfadiazene ointment. These agents have reduced the mortality rate from burn sepsis, particularly in patients with 30% to 50% body surface burns. Mafenide acetate is the best agent available for local treatment of the contaminated burn wound, particularly those with questionable subeschar bacterial growth.

Early excision and grafting of burn wounds has been shown to reduce the mortality and morbidity of extensive burns. Temporary substitutes for autografts of skin include allografts of preserved cadaver skin. In addition to this a number of promising skin substitutes are in the process of clinical investigation.

First- and second-degree burns should be healed in a period of 10 to 14 days. Burns of the face may involve the upper respiratory tract; tracheostomy and assisted respiration may be necessary in these cases.

The Control of Bleeding

Nothing is more important in surgery than the ability of the surgeon to control hemorrhage, either in wounds or at operation. In addition to the skill of the surgeon, the control of bleeding depends upon the complex process of coagulation of blood, local vascular factors, and a balance between coagulation and fibrinolysis.

Defects in the clotting mechanism most often encountered by the surgeon are thrombocytopenia, vitamin K deficiency, hemophilia (Factor VIII deficiency), and those of iatrogenic cause such as the administration of heparin or the coumarin drugs.

The local vascular factors that influence the control of bleeding include such things as the ability of a cut blood vessel to contract, the state of the vascular bed with regard to the existing degree of vasodilatation or vasoconstriction, and the hydrostatic pressure within the vascular bed. Capillary oozing under normal circumstances is controlled by the agglutination of platelets. Defects in platelet function can result in excessive bleeding from capillaries. An artery that is completely transected will contract, its lumen will be narrowed, and clot will form at the end, with control of bleeding. If the same artery is partially transected, it cannot contract; hemorrhage will continue to the point of near-exsanguination. Surrounding scar tissue or sclerosis of the vascular wall will also limit contraction of the blood vessel and increase the amount of hemorrhage. This is frequently the case in arterial bleeding from chronic duodenal ulcer. Anesthetic agents such as cyclopropane may cause vasodilatation and increased blood loss. Bleeding is also more profuse in patients with arterial or portal hypertension.

Disseminated intravascular coagulation is a syndrome that may complicate shock, massive hemorrhage, general sepsis, septic abortion, prolonged use of the pump oxygenator, and large cavernous hemangiomas. As the name implies, there is diffuse intravascular coagulation that results in a depletion of the factors essential for clot formation. Fibrinogenopenia, thrombocytopenia, prothrombinemia, and a deficiency in Factors V and VIII are all noted. Split fibrin products are likely to be found in the blood, and activation of the fibrinolytic system is likely to be present. Bleeding is the clinical manifestation. The process usually follows release of thromboplastic material into the circulation. Treatment is directed toward relief of the underlying disease state and the maintenance of capillary blood flow. Fresh whole blood, cryoprecipitate, and intravenous fluids are indicated to maintain plasma volume, and if myocardial function is impaired an inotropic agent such as dopamine may be indicated. Heparin has been used to prevent intravascular coagulation, but it must be given cautiously while monitoring the levels of platelets and fibrinogen. Epsilon aminocaproic acid may be utilized if the patient has exaggerated fibrinolysis.

SHOCK

Shock is characterized as inadequate blood flow to vital organs or the inability of the body cell mass to metabolize nutrients normally. In either case, decreased tissue oxygenation and the retention of metabolites will follow. Depending on the effectiveness of compensatory mechanisms and treatment, failure in function of major organ systems will lead to death. A reduction in circulating blood volume may be absolute in terms of hemorrhage or may be relative owing to an increased capacity of the vascular bed. At times a combination of factors will intensify the physiologic abnormality. Clinically, shock is most frequently seen in patients with massive hemorrhage, burns, acute myocardial infarction with heart failure, or bacterial sepsis.

The concepts of cause and pathogenesis of shock are changing; however, a number of basic mechanisms cause the shock state.

1. Reduction of blood volume (hypovolemic shock)
2. Failure of the myocardium (cardiogenic shock)
3. Redistribution hypovolemia due to alteration of the vascular bed (septic shock, anaphylactic shock, and neurogenic shock)
4. Failure of the cell to utilize oxygen delivered to it despite normal or near normal blood flow (septic shock)

The appropriate management of shock involves an accurate diagnosis and appropriate understanding of the pathophysiology associated with the patient's clinical condition.

Hypovolemic Shock

Patients with acute blood loss (usually greater than 15% of their circulating blood volume), patients with chronic blood loss or plasma loss such as a burn patient, or patients with loss of extracellular and intracellular fluid and electrolytes will present with signs and symptoms of the clinical syndrome of shock, depending on the rate of volume of fluid loss and the rapidity of loss. The neurohumoral compensatory mechanisms activated by the volume loss are responsible for the signs of shock, and if therapy is not instituted and continued volume loss is not prevented, end-organ failure can occur, leading to patient death. Prompt resuscitation with appropriate fluids will usually reverse the process. On occasion end-organ failure such as cardiac or renal dysfunction can require specific therapy.

Cardiogenic Shock

Hypotension associated with myocardial failure or "pump failure" is the result of acute myocardial ischemia, arrhythmia, or chronic progressive myocardial failure. Obviously, diagnosis and appropriate management are critical for survival. Intensive care and appropriate invasive monitoring with judicious fluid administration, appropriate anti-arrhythmic agents, inotropic therapy, or mechanical support of the circulation will reverse the shock state and permit patient survival. The use of a Swann-Ganz catheter with appropriate monitoring of pulmonary artery pressure, pulmonary capillary wedge pressure and cardiac output, as well as calculation of systemic and pulmonary vascular resistance, will enhance one's ability to select the appropriate therapy for the patient.

Neurogenic Shock

Spinal cord injury is associated with acute loss of sympathetic control of the peripheral vascular system. This loss of ability to control peripheral vascular resistance is associated with hypotension and can lead to end-organ failure if not recognized and treated. The pathophysiologic mechanism is related to an acute increase in the vascular space and can be treated by increasing the circulating vascular volume or the use of an alpha-adrenergic agent such as neosynephrine to increase the peripheral vascular resistance.

Septic Shock

Shock associated with sepsis is the most difficult to diagnose and treat. Although much has been learned about the pathophysiology of this disease state, there are many unanswered questions. Septic shock is associated with infection and is most frequently seen in the chronically ill, aged, or debilitated patients, or patients with a compromised immune system. Patients who develop septic shock outside the hospital are usually found to have infection involving the genitourinary system. In hospitalized patients, frequently the source of infection is an indwelling intravascular catheter. The hemodynamic response in septic shock is a spectrum with low cardiac output at one end and high cardiac output with reduced peripheral vascular resistance at the other. Throughout the clinical course, there appears to be a reduced uptake and utilization of oxygen at the cellular level irrespective of the adequacy of oxygen delivery. Successful management always involves identification of the source of the sepsis and aggressive therapy. This may involve drainage of a contained abscess, removal of infected intravascular catheters, or major surgical procedures as indicated. Treatment of the hemodynamic instability will involve fluid resuscitation and inotropic support as indicated by appropriate hemodynamic monitoring. Appropriate antimicrobial therapy is always indicated and should be instituted as soon as appropriate cultures have been obtained and the therapy should be altered or changed based on the culture data.

In septic shock the most important aspect of therapy is the control of infection; however, attention to the maintenance of adequate tissue perfusion is also essential.

NUTRITION

Inasmuch as many surgical patients are unable to eat or drink for varying periods, they must be protected against serious alterations in body composition by parenteral therapy. Over short periods, changes in water and electrolyte balance are of little importance. However, all too frequently a short-term problem turns into one requiring protracted parenteral support. Under these circumstances caloric intake, along with sufficient fat, protein, and

vitamins, becomes significant. The routine use of flow sheets, upon which intake and output are charted on a cumulative as well as a daily basis, will be helpful in management. The source, composition, and volume of all known losses and increments should be individually noted.

Daily basal requirements of an average-sized adult man in the temperate zone are: water, less than 2,000 ml; sodium chloride, 2 g to 3 g; calories, 1,600. Insensible water loss through skin and lungs increases with fever and increased environmental temperature. With vomiting, diarrhea, fistulas, and so forth, losses of water, sodium chloride, potassium, and bicarbonate increase. The latter losses are measurable and should be replaced in equal volume of water and concentration of salts. Most abnormalities in electrolyte concentration are iatrogenic, resulting either from improper ingestion of fluid by the patient, or most often, incorrect replacement by the surgeon.

In the prolonged vomiting of pyloric obstruction, hypochloremic–hypokalemic alkalosis usually develops. Treatment with sodium and potassium chloride will restore the potassium and chloride deficits as well as the acid–base imbalance. Sodium will be excreted by the kidneys.

The symptoms and signs of specific electrolyte deficits are at times characteristic:

Hyponatremia is manifested by restlessness and mental confusion with delusions or hallucinations.

Hypokalemia results in decreased tone and contractility of smooth, striated, and cardiac muscle. Adynamic ileus may be present. The electrocardiogram shows a depressed S-T segment, a prolonged QT interval, and small T waves fused with V waves.

Hypochloremia, most frequently secondary to vomiting, paradoxically causes nausea and vomiting.

Hypocalcemia increases muscle tone and irritability leading to tetany. Early symptoms include perioral numbness and tingling of the digits.

Intravenous Hyperalimentation

In patients who are unable to use their alimentary tract for the maintenance of their nutritional state, intravenous hyperalimentation has been shown to be a suitable substitute. The technique is also applicable to patients in whom for one reason or another it is desirable to rest the alimentary tract. The feeding mixture consists of a hypertonic solution of glucose and amino acids, vitamins, and minerals infused into the superior vena cava through a catheter placed usually percutaneously into the subclavian vein or internal jugular vein. Each 1,000 ml contains approximately 1,000 kcal. Twice a week solutions of fat (Intralipid) are given in order to prevent essential fatty acid deficiency. The infusate, 2,500 ml to 3,000 ml in volume, is delivered slowly over a 24-hour period. Nitrogen equilibrium, positive nitrogen balance, weight gain, and growth are possible when this route is used as the sole source of food. The complications include sepsis caused by both bacteria and fungi, of which *Candida albicans* is most frequent. Prophylaxis is most important, consisting of care in the insertion of the catheter and strict asepsis in the dressing of the skin at the point of puncture as well as in the preparation and changing of solutions. Complications resulting from catheter placement include pneumothorax, hemothorax, hydrothorax, injury of the subclavian artery, air embolism, and catheter breaks. Arrhythmias may occur if the catheter enters the heart and perforation of the myocardium has been reported. Metabolic complications include hypophosphatemia, hyperosmolarity, nonketotic hyperglycemia, convulsions, and coma. In diabetics, ketoacidosis may develop. When the intravenous hyperalimentation is stopped, rebound hypoglycemia may occur. Deficiencies of trace elements have also been reported. Prevention, of course, consists of the addition of these elements to the solution.

Peripheral veins can also be used for intravenous feeding by using less concentrated solutions of amino acids and glucose with added fat. Eventually, however, thrombosis occurs.

Another approach to the management of patients with small intestinal fistulas, Crohn's disease, or the short bowel syndrome is the use of elemental diets for feeding. A number of commercially prepared mixtures of medium-chain triglycerides, protein hydrolysates, glucose, minerals, and vitamins, in variable proportions, are available. Some of the preparations contain no fat. Most of the preparations are unpalatable and may require a small polyvinyl feeding tube if they are to be given for prolonged periods.

TRANSPLANTATION

Burgeoning interest in tissue and organ transplantation has given rise to the development of a series of new specialties in biology, including transplantation immunology, transplantation genetics, transplantation pathology, and transplantation surgery. A new vocabulary has evolved, and the field becomes increasingly complex. Certain tissues such as aorta, bone, cartilage, and fascia are transplanted as dead tissues. They are replaced by the process of creeping substitution and are called **homostructural** grafts. The transplantation of complex organs, however, involves the maintenance of viability by connecting the blood vessels of the transplant to those of the host. This is a **homovital** graft. With the exception of grafts between identical twins, such grafts will undergo necrosis through a recognizable sequence of steps, and this process is called rejection.

A second graft from the same donor is rejected faster—a second-set response. This can be likened to the anamnestic response familiar in classical immunology.

The phenomenon of rejection is caused by antigenic differences between host and graft. The strength and number of antigens in a given case will alter the speed of rejection. Cellular aspects of rejection are prominent in terms of the infiltration of lymphocytes. Humoral factors, not at first apparent, are now proving also to play a significant role in the process of rejection.

Allografts of skin have been used for many years in the management of burns in infants; usually they were obtained from the mother and were permitted to take as lifesaving measures to control evaporative water loss and infection. Today, xenografts as well as allografts are used as biologic dressings.

Immunosuppressive agents are used to ablate or retard rejection. They include (1) azathioprine—an antimetabolite originally used in cancer chemotherapy, (2) corticosteroids, (3) cyclosporin, (4) antilymphocyte globulin or antithymocyte globulin, and (5) monoclonal antibodies.

Transplantation of all organs and tissue has been investigated and dramatic breakthroughs during the past 5 years have allowed the transplantation of heart, liver, lung, and pancreas to become clinical realities. Because these organs are single vital organs and require brain death for their recovery, the availability of donors has limited the clinical use of these lifesaving procedures.

Renal transplantation continues to be the most common organ transplant, allowing many patients with chronic renal failure a new life-style. As the understanding of transplant immunology increases, our ability to control rejection and avoid the complications of infection, accelerated atherosclerosis, and other causes of transplant failure, the outlook for the transplant recipient will improve.

GENERAL CONDITIONS OF THE EXTREMITIES

Lower Extremities

LEG

Ulcers. The most common ulcer of the lower extremities results from venous stasis secondary to deep thrombophlebitis with reversal of flow between the deep and superficial venous systems. The valves in the communicating veins are incompetent. The skin of the lower medial leg develops a brawny induration that is brownish in color, the result of accumulation of hemosiderin pigment. Usually varicosities of the greater saphenous system are also present. Extreme or neglected cases may show circumferential ulcers. The diagnosis is made on the basis of the history and physical findings. It is confirmed by venography, which shows recanalized channels with destroyed valves and flow from deep to superficial veins. Treatment consists of stripping of the superficial varicosities, along with ligation of all incompetent communicating veins. Ulcers are treated by the application of split-thickness skin grafts after excision of devitalized skin and the scarred base of the ulcer.

Ulcers on the legs and feet may also occur as a result of syphilis or arteriosclerosis obliterans. Luetic ulcers are mainly of historical interest. Ulcers resulting from decreased arterial flow will be considered subsequently.

Varicose Veins. Abnormally dilated veins, seen most frequently in the lower extremities, are spoken of as varicose veins. Varicosities appear more frequently in women than in men, occurring most often following pregnancy and in those engaged in occupations demanding that the patient be on her feet for long periods. In some patients there is a familial tendency toward varicosities; in others the varicose veins are the result of deep thrombophlebitis. The valves in the involved veins become incompetent. The Trendelenburg test is used to demonstrate such incompetency of the valves. This is carried out by applying a tourniquet to the upper thigh, with the patient lying supine with the leg elevated and the veins empty. Upon the patient's standing and removal of the tourniquet, the entire vein fills immediately from above. With the tourniquet in place and the patient erect, rapid filling from below indicates incompetence of valves in the com-

municating veins. Application of the tourniquet at different levels will help to localize these channels.

The treatment of varicose veins involves either high ligation—with multiple excision of segments in which incompetent communicating veins are present—or stripping of the entire varicose vein. Injection therapy with sclerosing solution is frequently used to enhance the cosmesis following stripping. The sclerotherapy is used to obliterate small residual varicose veins after stripping and ligation of incompetent perforating veins. In patients with a history of thrombophlebitis or with stasis changes in the skin, a period of compression with elastic bandages or well-fitting elastic stockings is a useful test to indicate whether the stripping of varicose veins will be tolerated or will give satisfactory symptomatic results. Perthes' test also may be used to determine the competency of the deep veins. It is carried out by placing a rubber tube tourniquet snugly around the lower thigh. Then the patient is asked to walk or exercise the leg. If the deep veins are competent, contraction of the calf muscles will suck the blood in the superficial varices through the communicating veins into the deep veins, and the varicose veins will become less prominent. On removal of the tourniquet the veins will refill from above.

Venous Thrombosis (Phlebitis). In this condition the veins are involved by intravascular clotting. Phlebitis has been divided into two types.

Thrombophlebitis. By this is meant an acute inflammatory reaction in the wall of the vein associated with production of a thrombus within the vein. This type of phlebitis is seen in the puerperal period, postoperatively, after trauma, and in debilitating disease such as myocardial infarction or cancer. In its most common form it is known as milk leg. There is marked swelling of the leg because of obstruction of the deep venous circulation and the edematous white leg is called *phlegmasia alba dolens.* The entire lower extremity is swollen, pale, and cold. This is the result of reflex arterial spasm and can be improved by lumbar sympathetic block. More extensive involvement of the venous system leads to a dusky purple discoloration of the skin associated with painful swelling. This condition, called *phlegmasia cerulea dolens,* is a much more serious manifestation with gangrene as a potential sequela. Treatment may include direct removal of venous thrombi by thrombectomy and anticoagulant therapy, usually introduced by the use of heparin intravenously, either by continuous drip or intermittent injection, preferably the former. The clotting time is monitored with the objective of maintaining it at approximately twice normal. The activated partial thromboplastin time has generally supplanted the clotting time as a measure of heparin dosage.

Heparin is usually continued for 7 to 14 days followed by one of the coumarin drugs. Since at least 48 hours is necessary before a significant effect on the clotting mechanism is observed, whichever drug is selected is begun several days before heparin is to be discontinued. Stopping heparin abruptly may be followed by a rebound increase in clotting potential. For this reason the dose is gradually reduced over a 48- to 72-hour interval. The coumarin drugs are continued for a variable time, usually 3 months. The prothrombin time is used to adjust dosage and optimally is kept at twice normal.

Phlebothrombosis. This is another type of intravascular clotting, seen most often following abdominal operations. It probably results from a slowing of the blood flow in the veins. It occurs without symptoms in the veins of the calf and the thigh. Often the first indication is pulmonary embolism. Careful examination may show calf tenderness, slight increase in calf diameter, and calf pain on dorsiflexion of the foot (Homans' sign). Frequently all signs are absent. In this type of intravascular clotting there is a minimal reaction in the walls of the veins, and the clot is soft and loosely attached to the intima. It is complicated by pulmonary embolism, which is frequently the first manifestation of the process. The diagnosis of phlebothrombosis should be confirmed by venography.

In patients with suspected pulmonary embolism, further confirmation of the diagnosis should be obtained by isotopic injection and pulmonary scanning. The most certain means of diagnosis, however, is pulmonary angiography. Recurrent pulmonary embolism in a patient receiving adequate anticoagulant therapy is an indication for interruption of the inferior vena cava either by ligature or insertion of an intracaval filter to trap further emboli. In the postpartum female both ovarian veins must also be ligated. Septic thrombophlebitis with embolization is an indication for complete interruption of the vena cava. Anticoagulant therapy is also given to prevent further intravascular clotting. It may be necessary for these patients to wear supporting stockings or bandages to prevent swelling when they are back on their feet.

A number of prophylactic measures have been shown to be effective in the prevention of clot formation in the veins following operation. They are elevation of the legs during and after operation, low-dose heparin therapy given subcutaneously and prophylactic use of the coumarin drugs. Devices for intermittent compression, using a series of inflatable balloons during operation and in the early postoperative period, are also effective. Early ambulation, relied upon by some, is not as effective for prophylaxis of thrombophlebitis as it is in improving respiratory mechanics. The exercise is also of nutritional help in attaining positive nitrogen balance.

Peripheral Arterial Disease

Arteriosclerosis Obliterans. This is a degenerative disease occurring in older people, and in diabetics at a younger age. Its clinical manifestations are those of impaired arterial flow. In the muscles, intermittent claudication—pain on activity relieved by rest—constitutes the clinical picture. Impending gangrene, manifested by rest pain, rubor on dependency, and extreme pallor on elevation, is another means of presentation. Atrophy of the distal fat pads on the plantar surface of the toes, loss of growth of hair, thin shiny skin, and actual necrosis of the distal toes may all be seen. The onset may be gradual or abrupt. Arteriography is the most important method of study. Noninvasive methods are also useful. These include evaluation of the flow signal and determination of ankle blood pressure by means of doppler flowmetry and pulse volume recordings. Frequently segmental occlusion is seen. This may be correctable by direct surgical means. Bypass grafting, preferably using autologous veins, or short thromboendarterectomy yields good results. Anastomoses to increasingly small vessels are surprisingly effective in salvage of limbs. Lumbar sympathectomy is used in patients with signs of sympathetic overactivity—particularly excessive sweating—or in an effort to prevent gangrene of the skin. Arterial flow in muscle is not improved by sympathectomy.

Thromboangitis Obliterans (Buerger's Disease). There is considerable question as to whether this exists as a clinical and pathologic entity. As originally described, it is a syndrome in which there is hypersensitivity to tobacco with venous and arterial spasm, followed by thrombosis. Its onset is in the third decade of life, and migratory venous thrombosis may be the first clinical manifestation. Involvement of middle-sized vessels and associated nerves by an inflammatory process is supposedly characteristic. Involvement of vessels in the upper extremities and viscera are end stages. Complete avoidance of tobacco is the most important therapeutic measure. These patients should be studied by arteriography if gangrene threatens.

Raynaud's Syndrome. This syndrome defines a condition characterized by episodic attacks of constriction of the arteries and arterioles of the extremities, especially the fingers, followed by cyanosis and rubor upon warming. The syndrome usually occurs in women and rarely begins after the age of 40. Symptoms are almost always bilateral. Careful evaluation has shown that an associated connective tissue disease has been proven or strongly suspected in 80% of the patients. Preganglionic sympathectomy has been utilized when loss of tissue was threatened; however, long-term results were unsatisfactory. The best results have been obtained from drugs that decrease neuromuscular synaptic transmission (*e.g.*, reserpine, guanethidine, or phenoxybenzamine).

Peripheral Embolization. The breaking off of a thrombus on the myocardial wall or a valve may lead to its passing through the arterial circulation until it lodges in a vessel. Sudden obliteration of arterial flow to a part results in pain, pallor, anesthesia and, depending upon the extent of collateral circulation, gangrene. The level depends upon the point of occlusion of the arterial circulation, as well as upon the condition of the arterial bed with regard to primary degenerative changes. Immediate embolectomy is the treatment of choice, followed by anticoagulant therapy. Removal under local anesthesia is usually possible and Fogarty catheters (long plastic catheters with inflatable balloons of varying dimension) passed proximally and distally are valuable adjuncts in the complete removal of clots. Major arterial occlusion may occur without gangrene, but the end results are best when normal flow is restored. The temptation to treat such patients with sympathetic block and anticoagulation should be avoided.

Arteriovenous Fistula. This is a communication—usually traumatic in origin—between artery and vein, shunting arterial blood into the venous system, in which there is a lower pressure. It is evidenced clinically by swelling of the extremity, associated with the increased collateral circulation and a continuous bruit heard over the fistula. The cardiovascular effects are often severe. Increased blood volume, diminished pulse pressure, cardiac hypertrophy, and increased local venous pressure occur. Digital pressure over the fistula causes an increase in peripheral resistance, resulting in a temporary rise of blood pressure with a decrease in pulse rate. This is called the Nicoladoni-Branham's sign. Modern treatment consists of the restoration of arterial flow by excision and grafting. Quadruple ligation after suitable collaterals have developed is of historic interest only.

Arterial Aneurysm. The most frequent type of aneurysm in civilians is the result of arteriosclerotic weakening of the wall. The vessels most frequently involved are the abdominal aorta below the renal arteries, the common iliacs, the femorals, and the popliteals. Aneurysms of the thoracic aorta are most frequently traumatic from deceleration tears in high-speed automobile accidents. Syphilitic aneurysms are still seen but are less common than prior to penicillin therapy for syphilis. Spontaneous rupture and occlusion are serious complications, and in most instances repair by resection and grafting is indicated. Traumatic aortic aneurysm is treated by excision and direct suture and when necessary by insertion of a prosthesis.

Upper Extremities

HAND

Paronychia. This is an infection between the nail and the eponychium usually caused by *Staphylococcus aureus*. It usually arises from a hangnail or from too vigorous manicuring. Elevation of the eponychium by incising it at the nail edge will drain a small abscess in the early stages. Infection can progress around the base of the nail between the eponychium and the nail, later extending underneath the nail to form a subungual abscess. The eponychium should be incised and turned back, and the base of the nail should be excised in order to provide adequate drainage.

Distal Closed Space Infection, or Felon. An infection of the pulp of the palmar surface of the distal phalanx of the finger is very common. It usually arises from injury. Because of the anatomic characteristic of this space, a small infection may rapidly shut off the blood supply and lead to necrosis of the pulp and extension of the infection to the bone. To drain the abscess adequately, all of the septa between the dermis and the periosteum of the distal phalanx must be cut. Bilateral incisions may be necessary, but through-and-through drains should be avoided. Bone involvement is treated conservatively and bone removed only if it is free in the abscess cavity.

Tenosynovitis of the Flexor Tendon Sheaths. Flexor tendon sheaths of the index, the middle, and the ring fingers end at the distal palmar crease, but those of the fifth finger and the thumb extend upward to the bursae at the wrist. Infection of these sheaths is usually a result of penetrating injury. It is characterized by pain, swelling, and immobility. The finger is held in slight flexion, and attempts to extend it are terribly painful. Early incision and drainage on the lateral sides of the finger are indicated if necrosis of the tendon is to be avoided. Infections of the fifth finger and the thumb spread to involve the radial and ulnar bursae. In postoperative care, splinting from the forearm to the fingertips, hot wet dressings and a synthetic penicillin not destroyed by penicillinase such as methicillin, oxacillin, or dicloxacillin are indicated. Through-and-through irrigation using antimicrobial solutions is also used by some. The solution is introduced through a catheter placed in the proximal portion of the tendon sheath and removed through a catheter in the distal portion.

Infections of the Palmar Spaces. The palmar spaces are hypothetical areas in the palm lying between the metacarpal bones and the overlying tendons and palmar fascia. They are infected by direct implantation or extension of infection from tenosynovitis or from infections along the lumbrical muscles arising under calluses at the distal part of the hand. The thenar space lies to the thumb side of the middle metacarpal, and the middle palmar space lies to the ulnar side. Infection of these spaces is characterized by swelling of the palm and marked swelling of the loose tissue of the dorsum of the hand. Drainage of the middle palmar space is obtained through the web between the middle and the fourth fingers. Drainage of the thenar space is through the web between the thumb and the index finger.

Mouth Wounds of the Hand. Frequently these wounds are sustained by a blow of the fist in which the teeth lacerate the skin, usually over the fingers or the knuckles. Anaerobic organisms are implanted in the contused lacerated wound. These give rise to an extensive necrotizing suppurative infection unless checked by early adequate treatment. This consists of thorough cleansing and debridement. The wound is left open, and the extremity is elevated and splinted. Prophylactic antibiotics using broad-spectrum agents effective against both aerobic and anaerobic microorganisms are also given.

Treatment of Infections of the Fingers and Hand. In all the infections of the finger, the tendon sheaths and the palmar spaces, intensive antibiotic therapy may abort the infection if given early. Incision and drainage may be necessary only if the infection does not subside before suppuration takes place. Incision and drainage for infection of the major spaces should be done under general anesthesia using a tourniquet to ensure a bloodless field.

SHOULDER

Acute Subdeltoid Bursitis. This is a fairly common and very painful condition of the shoulder. It often follows moderate trauma, such as prolonged use of the arm in unaccustomed activities, but may occur without any history of such injury. A deposit of amorphous calcium soaps is found within the bursa when it is exposed at operation. Injuries to adjacent tendons—particularly the supraspinatus and long head of the biceps, followed by chronic tendonitis—are frequent associated lesions.

On roentgenographic examination, one may find evidence of calcium deposition in the region of the bursa. The acute pain may be relieved by infiltration of the area with a local anesthetic agent such as procaine. Injection of a corticosteroid is helpful in certain patients. Local heat and adequate sedation are also of value. Complete immobilization of the shoulder is undesirable, because fixation may result. This is especially likely to occur following repeated acute attacks in which the patient refuses to move the shoulder because of pain. In such cases it is necessary to carry out manipulation under anesthesia in order to break up the adhesions and permit return of function to the shoulder. At times excision of the calcified mass is necessary, but such areas may disappear spontaneously under treatment. X-ray therapy has been used in certain cases with satisfactory results. Anti-inflammatory agents may also be helpful.

In addition to the bursae about the shoulder, other sites may be involved, such as those over the olecranon process and the ischial tuberosity and beneath the Achilles tendon. Effusion into the prepatellar bursa is known as ***housemaid's knee***.

FRACTURES AND DISLOCATIONS OF THE EXTREMITIES

By definition a fracture is a disruption in the continuity of bone. Fractures can be described as ***simple***—a single fracture line, or as ***comminuted***—multiple fracture lines and bone fragments. Either of these injuries may be nondisplaced (in anatomic position) or displaced. The fracture may be described as ***open*** if an external penetrating injury communicates with the fracture or the fracture fragments pierce the skin in the course of injury. Thus, fractures are classified into simple or compound, displaced or nondisplaced, open or closed. These distinctions are very important as they influence treatment and prognosis.

Upper Extremities

CLAVICLE

Fracture of this bone usually occurs at the junction of the middle and the outer thirds. The proximal fragment is drawn upward by the sternocleidomastoid muscle. The outer fragment is carried downward, inward, and forward by the weight of the shoulder. The fracture is reduced by lifting the shoulder upward, outward, and backward. It usually can be held in a satisfactory position by the use of a posterior figure-of-eight dressing of plaster or a posterior clavicular T splint. Delayed union or nonunion is almost unknown in this region. Immobilization for 4 weeks usually suffices.

Greenstick fractures are partial fractures without significant displacement and may be managed by the use of a Velpeau dressing, an axillary pad, or a sling and swathe dressing.

HUMERUS

Fractures of the Greater Tuberosity. This is a frequent complication accompanying dislocation of the shoulder. Under any circumstances the displacement usually is not great, and satisfactory position may be obtained by the use of an axillary pad, a sling and swathe dressing, or by use of an abduction splint.

Fracture of the Anatomic Neck. Fracture of the anatomic neck or of the lesser tuberosity of the humerus is uncommon. Prolonged immobilization of fractures of the upper end of the humerus is undesirable. Active and passive motion should be started after 10 days.

Fracture of the Surgical Neck. The upper fragment is abducted, and the lower fragment is drawn upward and inward into the axilla. At times, the fragments may be impacted with very little displacement. In contrast with dislocation of the shoulder, the contour of the shoulder is maintained because the humeral head is still in place. With adequate anesthesia, reduction usually can be accomplished by abduction of the arm, bringing the lower fragment outward to meet and engage the upper fragment. Following reduction the arm may be brought to the side. In some instances an axillary pad and a sling and swathe dressing may suffice for fixation. An alternative method of treatment of stable fracture of the surgical neck of the humerus is the so-called hanging cast. This consists of a plaster cast from the upper portion of the arm to the metacarpal heads. The elbow is at 90 degrees of flexion, and the forearm is in midposition with regard to pronation and supination. A supporting sling goes around the neck and is passed through a ring incorporated at the wrist. The long tendon of the biceps must be intact if this method of management is to be successful. The patient is instructed to keep the arm hanging freely as much of the time as possible. While he or she is in bed, about 2.25 kg of traction are maintained through a second ring formed at the elbow. This method permits abduction and circumduction exercises relatively early, thereby preventing disabling shoulder stiffness.

Separation of the Upper Humeral Epiphysis. This injury results in a deformity similar to that of a fracture of the surgical neck of the humerus. Accurate reduction is necessary in order to minimize interference with growth of the bone. Following reduction of the separation, a dressing similar to that used for fracture of the surgical neck of the humerus is satisfactory.

Dislocation of the Shoulder. This injury usually follows acute abduction of the arm, with resultant tearing of the head of the humerus through the weak inferior portion of the capsule of the joint. The displaced head then comes to lie in the subglenoid position but rarely remains there. Instead, it is carried forward to lie in the subcoracoid position, which is the most common location for the head following dislocation in this region. More rarely the humerus may be displaced even further medially, and the head then occupies the subclavicular position. Posterior dislocation of the humerus is extremely rare and upward displacement almost unknown. Under adequate anesthesia this dislocation is reduced readily by either the Cooper or the Kocher method. In the Cooper method the foot is placed in the axilla, while gentle traction is maintained on the outstretched hand and forearm. Moderate adduction and internal and external rotation in association with traction usually result in prompt replacement of the dislocation. In the Kocher maneuver, the elbow is flexed to a right angle, and the humerus is rotated outward as far as possible. With external rotation maintained, the elbow is carried medially, and then the hand is brought to the point of the opposite shoulder. A Velpeau or axillary pad, a sling and a swathe dressing provide adequate immobilization following reduction. After a week or 10 days a simple sling should suffice; however, abduction of the arm should be avoided for a period of 6 to 8 weeks.

Following initial dislocation of the shoulder, subsequent dislocations are much more likely to occur, and eventually dislocation may take place as the result of extremely minor trauma. Under such circumstances, an operative procedure to prevent such recurrence is desirable.

Fracture of the Shaft of the Humerus. This fracture may be complicated by radial nerve injury, inasmuch as the nerve follows a winding course about the shaft of the humerus. This injury is manifested by the presence of wristdrop. Following reduction of the fracture, a hanging plaster cast may be applied. Union usually is obtained in 6 to 8 weeks, though delayed union or nonunion of the shaft of the humerus occasionally results. An abduction cast or an intramedullary pin also may be used in the management of fractures of the shaft of the humerus.

Fractures of the Lower End of the Humerus. The most common fracture in the lower end of the humerus is supracondylar. This occurs usually in children and results in posterior displacement of the distal fragment. Satisfactory reduction usually can be accomplished by flexing the elbow acutely and at the same time bringing the distal fragment forward into line with the upper. For older children, a lateral hyperflexion plaster dressing holding the arm in this position may be applied, provided that the radial pulse is not obliterated as the result of swelling. *Volkmann's ischemic contracture* is a dreaded complication of supracondylar fractures treated by acute flexion. If the radial pulse is weak or disappears the arm should be extended beyond 45 degrees, and as the swelling subsides it may be returned to acute flexion of 45 degrees or greater. It may be preferable to resort to traction. In young children, flexion of the elbow may be maintained by the use of Jones's position, in which the wrist is suspended by a short sling about the neck. In general, this dressing will be satisfactory for most fractures in the region of the lower end of the humerus, though occasionally displacement is such that open reduction will be necessary. Fractures in this region occasionally are associated with ossifying hematoma. This is the development of a calcified mass in the soft tissues as a result of calcium deposit in the hematoma. Bone formation may take place. As a rule, these ossifying hematomas tend to disappear gradually over a time.

Dislocations of the Elbow. Though anterior and lateral dislocations of the elbow may occur, the common deformity in this injury is that of posterior displacement. This is manifested by prominence of the olecranon posteriorly, loss of the lower humeral posterior concavity, and fullness in the antecubital fossa. Reduction is accomplished under anesthesia by hyperextension and traction. Immobilization by means of a right-angle splint for 1 week, followed by use of a sling for another week or 10 days, should suffice.

FOREARM

Fractures Through the Olecranon Fossa. These often are associated with sufficient displacement that results from pull of the triceps tendon, to necessitate open reduction. Otherwise, immobilization in moderate extension for a period of several weeks is required.

Fracture of the Head of the Radius. This fracture is often associated with comminution and tearing of the orbicular ligament, so that the fragments lie either free in the joint or outside the orbicular ligament. Fractures of this type are treated best by excision of the head of the radius, though linear or compression fractures may be managed by simple immobilization for a few days, followed by guarded function. Other fractures of the radial head requiring operation are marginal fractures with displacement toward the elbow joint, fracture involving more than one third of the articular surface of the radial head, and fractures of the neck with angulation.

Fractures of the Shafts of the Radius and Ulna. Fracture of only one bone of the forearm usually may be reduced without undue difficulty, inasmuch as the other serves as a splint. However, fracture of both bones of the forearm with displacement sometimes presents a problem in reduction. Occasionally, open reduction must be accomplished. Intraosseous pins frequently are employed to maintain reduction. Unless satisfactory reduction is obtained, the interosseous space may be narrowed, thus interfering with supination and pronation. Synostosis between the radius and ulna may also occur, similarly limiting function. The interosseous space can be preserved by applying padded board splints and incorporating them in the cast. Following reduction it is necessary to immobilize the hand, the wrist, and the elbow in order to avoid loss of position.

Colles' Fracture. This is a fracture of the radius at the suprastyloid level that often is associated with a fracture of the styloid process of the ulna. This is an extremely common site of bone injury. It results from a fall on the outstretched hand. In the typical displacement there is a silver-fork deformity, the distal fragment of the radius being displaced upward and backward. The articular surface of the radius is displaced upward, and the interstyloid line lies at right angles to the forearm. Reduction usually is accomplished readily, and immobilization is maintained for 4 weeks with plaster splints or a cast. In splinting these cases, the wrist frequently is held in a position of moderate flexion and ulnar deviation. Reduction is deemed adequate when length is normal and the distal articular surface of the radius has regained palmar deflection.

HAND AND WRIST

Fractures of the Carpals. These injuries are not common. The only one of particular interest is that of the scaphoid. Frequently it is missed, inasmuch as there is no significant displacement, and roentgenographic examination often is not undertaken at the time of the initial injury. Instead, a diagnosis of sprain of the wrist is made, and the patient is treated for such an injury. Careful roentgenographic examination, including oblique views at the time of the accident, should reveal the nature of the injury. This is a common site for nonunion. Therefore, prolonged immobilization in a plaster cast for 12 weeks or more should be carried out, including immobilization of the proximal phalanx of the thumb and utilization of a small amount of radial deviation in order to impact the fragments.

Fractures of the Metacarpals. These fractures usually result from a blow with a closed fist. Healing takes place readily, and satisfactory position can be obtained by pressure over the flexed proximal phalanx. Diagnosis in this injury usually can be made by the local tenderness at the fracture site and the presence of a dropped knuckle when the patient tries to make a fist.

Fractures of the Phalanges. Often these injuries are associated with insignificant displacement and are treated readily by simple immobilization with a padded tongue depressor or a plaster splint. However, the displacement occasionally is such that a satisfactory position is obtained only by elastic or spring traction utilizing a banjo splint.

Dislocation at the metacarpophalangeal or the interphalangeal joints is quite evident on physical examination. Usually, reduction is accomplished readily, and immobilization by means of a tongue depressor splint for a period of a week to 10 days should suffice.

VERTEBRAL COLUMN

The usual injury to the vertebral column results from forcible flexion of the spine, such as may result from a fall from a height, jolting of the patient while riding in a car, and so on. The region most commonly involved is the lumbar or lower thoracic spine. As a rule, there is no cord damage, and the patient's only complaint is of pain. On examination there are tenderness and localized muscle spasm. However, the diagnosis must be made by roentgenographic studies, and lateral views of the spine especially demonstrate the compression deformity of the vertebral body. The treatment consists of rest in bed for 2 to 3 weeks followed by ambulation, with the patient wearing a back brace for support until the fracture is stable. Hyperextension, previously used, requires a long period of disability and does not give better results than the simpler method of management. Occasionally the articular facets also are damaged, and fracture–dislocation results. This is a much more serious injury and frequently is associated with damage to the cord, which is likely to be permanent. Cord damage is evidenced by findings on neurologic examination and the presence of bloody spinal fluid, associated at times with evidence of block. Prompt reduction of the fracture–dislocation is necessary in order to minimize the damage to the nervous system. Operative treatment may be necessary to accomplish this reduction. In the lower spine, extension may be obtained by the application of traction to the lower extremities. In the cervical region, extension may be obtained by the use of traction through the skull. In either circumstance it must be prolonged, and, even after the patient is allowed out of bed, partial immobilization is necessary for several months, by means of either a neck or a back brace, as the case may be.

In patients who have sustained head injuries from automobile accidents or falls from a height, fracture of the cervical spine should be suspected until excluded by satisfactory roentgenograms. The head and neck should be immediately immobilized with sandbags until roentgenograms have been reviewed.

Fracture of the Coccyx. This is a rare injury, and only gross deformity requires correction. Often healing—whether by bony or by fibrous union—will be satisfactory, but occasionally pain persists. In these circumstances, excision of the coccyx is justified, inasmuch as this bone serves no useful purpose.

Herniated Nucleus Pulposus. This injury may follow a fall or attempts at lifting heavy objects. There is pain in the back with radiation down the leg, usually along the course of the sciatic nerve. The reflexes are altered, and sensory impairment can be elicited. The pain is produced by pressure of the herniated cartilaginous disk on the spinal nerves. Roentgenographic examination, including myelography or magnetic resonance imaging, will demonstrate the herniated disk.

Treatment has consisted of conservative management by bed rest and mild sedation or of operative removal of the herniated disk.

PELVIS

Fractures of the pelvis result from a fall from a height, a direct blow, or a crushing injury. Common sites for fracture of the pelvis include the symphysis and the rami of the pubis and the ischium. These may be bilateral, and, in addition, there may be fractures of the sacrum and the ilium. Pressure over the greater trochanters or the crests of the ilia is likely to give rise to pain at the fracture site. The diagnosis must be made by roentgenographic examination. The amount of displacement usually is not great, and satisfactory union results. Frequently there are soft-tissue injuries of serious degree. The most common of these is a tear of the bladder or the urethra. This is manifested by inability to void or by the passage of bloody urine. A tear of the bladder may be demonstrated by instillation of sterile salt solution through a catheter and subsequent inability to recover all this fluid, or by instillation of a radiopaque solution such as sodium iodide and x-ray demonstration of the extravasation. A tear of the bladder must be repaired promptly by operative means. A tear of the urethra should be managed with a suprapubic cystostomy. The patient is re-evaluated at 6 weeks following injury, and if urinary continuity is demonstrated with the presence of stricture, a urethrotomy can be performed. If complete disruption remains and there is no urinary continuity, surgical correction of the defect can be performed at 3 months. Tears of the vagina and the rectum are less common. Fractures of the pelvis should be managed by bed rest for 6 to 8 weeks. Approximation of the fragments can be assisted by the use of a tight binder or sling. In fractures extending through the acetabulum it may be necessary to use both a binder and traction on one or both lower extremities.

Lower Extremities

FEMUR

Fracture of the Neck of the Femur. This fracture usually occurs in elderly persons. It is a common site for nonunion, and even after apparently satisfactory union has occurred, avascular aseptic necrosis of the head of the femur may develop. The diagnosis is suspected on the basis of the history and physical examination and confirmed by roentgenograms. The history usually is a fall in an elderly person who subsequently is unable to rise. The lower extremity is externally rotated, abducted, and the heel cannot be lifted from the bed. Shortening may be obvious on inspection, or it may be slight and only demonstrated by measurement. In impacted fractures the patient may be able to walk, the posture may be normal, and the heel may be lifted from the bed. The degree of displacement is important with respect to the frequency of avascular necrosis and consequently, to treatment.

In the usual case the greater trochanter will lie above *Nelaton's line* (a line drawn from the anterior–superior spine of the ilium to the ischial tuberosity). There is also shortening of the horizontal line of *Bryant's triangle*. (This triangle is formed by one line projecting downward from the anterior–superior spine of the ilium perpendicular to the table. The second side is formed by a line passing from the anterior–superior iliac spine to the greater trochanter. The third side is a line joining the first two at the level of the table.) Since this fracture occurs in the elderly, death frequently results from intercurrent infection, such as bronchopneumonia. For this reason, older methods of treatment, such as the application of an abduction plaster cast or the use of balanced traction, have been displaced by internal fixation after adequate reduction. In some older patients immediate resection of the femoral head and neck with insertion of a prosthesis may be indicated.

Intertrochanteric Fracture of the Femur. This fracture occurs frequently in the elderly from a direct fall on the hip. The blood supply is excellent and delayed or nonunion is almost unknown. The fracture is unstable with considerable shortening and external rotation. The fracture should be reduced under anesthesia with fixation by means of a nail and plate such as the Jewett blade plate.

Dislocations of the Hip. These are uncommon. The displacement of the head of the femur may be either anterior or posterior to the acetabulum. The latter is the more common deformity. In this injury the patient lies with the knee and the hip flexed and the leg rotated internally, so that the affected extremity overlies the normal side. There is apparent shortening, and the foot on the involved side rests on the opposite instep. Occasionally there is sciatic nerve injury.

In anterior dislocations the extremity is abducted and rotated externally. The head of the femur is palpable in the groin. As a rule, the deformity in either condition is reduced readily under adequate anesthesia. The knee and the hip are flexed. With traction in this position, and with internal and external rotation, abduction, and adduction, the head of the femur usually returns readily to the acetabulum (methods of Bigelow and Allis). In posterior dislocations of the hip, the deformity at times may be reduced without anesthesia by placing the patient prone on a table with the thighs extending over the edge at right angles. The knee on the affected side is flexed. The weight is applied to the calf. As the muscles gradually tire, spontaneous reduction may occur.

Following reduction of a dislocation of the hip, the patient should be kept in bed for a period of 2 to 3 weeks. The ankles may be strapped loosely together during this time, or simple Buck's extension may be applied to the involved extremity. Weight bearing may be begun after this time if extreme range of motion is not undertaken. Prolonged follow-up is indicated because of the possible occurrence of avascular necrosis of the head of the femur and of arthritis.

Congenital Dislocation of the Hip. This deformity occurs much more frequently in the female than in the male. It may not be recognized until the age of about 1 year, because the first symptom is a limp when the child starts to walk. It may be a bilateral deformity. There is shortening of the extremity as shown by the displacement of the greater trochanter above Nelaton's line. On roentgenographic examination the head of the femur may be deficient, and the acetabulum may be malformed. Treatment should be begun as early as possible. Initially, reduction may be obtained under anesthesia. Then the child is dressed in a wide abduction plaster cast for a period of many months. If closed reduction is unsatisfactory, operative therapy is indicated. If conservative treatment is unsatisfactory, some form of reconstruction ultimately must be undertaken.

Fracture of the Shaft of the Femur. This fracture may occur anywhere in the shaft and may be transverse, spiral, or comminuted. The principal deformity is one of shortening and angulation. In most cases, satisfactory reduction can be obtained and the definitive treatment carried out by the use of balanced traction (Russell). Either skin or skeletal traction may be used. In the latter, a Thomas or a Hodgen splint with a Pierson attachment may be used. Alternate forms of treatment consist of closed reduction and immobilization by means of a plaster spica, or open reduction and internal fixation by means of a bone plate or by intramedullary nail.

In supracondylar fractures of the femur the distal fragment is displaced posteriorly and may damage the vessels and the nerves in this region to such an extent that vascular occlusion and gangrene set in. In order to accomplish reduction of the fracture in this area, the hip and knee must be well flexed. Though the actual progress of healing must be followed by repeated roentgenologic examinations, one should anticipate a period of immobilization of 8 to 12 weeks.

PATELLA

Fracture of the patella may be either transverse or comminuted. In either event, the bony injury is associated with a tear of the quadriceps tendon. For this reason, open reduction with repair of the laceration and approximation of the fragments is necessary, unless the roentgen films show no significant displacement of the fragments and the power of extension of the extremity is maintained. In badly comminuted fractures, excision of the patella fragments and tendon suture give good results. Following operation, the knee should be immobilized for about 6 weeks in plaster in almost complete extension, though weight bearing may be begun after 4 weeks.

KNEE

Injuries to the knee joint are of particular interest to surgeons responsible for the care of athletic teams. Football players are especially liable to incur serious injuries to the knee joint. Injuries to the collateral ligaments of the knee, particularly the medial collateral ligament, are the most frequently seen major injury. They may occur alone or in combination with injuries of the semilunar cartilages or the cruciate ligaments. Early repair of major injuries of the knee is an important new concept, which has reduced the disability incident to these injuries. Early exercise of the muscles around the knee joint also contributes to the lessened disability.

Injuries of the menisci can be evaluated by arthrography, in which air and an absorbable contrast media are injected into the joint. Arthroscopy is also useful for evaluating tears of the menisci as well as of the cruciate ligaments. A great many operations on the knee joint formerly requiring open operation are now done through the arthroscope. For example, torn menisci and foreign bodies can be removed, synovectomy is feasible, and so forth. The disability produced by arthroscopic procedures is much less than with open operation.

TIBIA

A common site for fracture of the tibia is at the junction of the lower and the middle thirds. Frequently, there is an associated fracture of the fibula, though this may occur at a different level. Because of the subcutaneous position of the tibia in this region, compounding is seen frequently. Under fluoroscopic guidance and with adequate anesthesia, satisfactory reduction usually can be obtained and the position maintained by means of plaster splints or a plaster cast extending from the toes to the upper thigh. Occasionally it may be necessary to resort to open reduction and internal fixation by means of a bone plate or an intramedullary pin.

This is a common site for delayed union, but ultimate union is to be anticipated. If adequate healing has not taken place after 8 to 12 weeks, a walking caliper splint should be used.

Fractures of the upper portion of the tibia may extend into the joint (plateau fracture) with downward displacement of a portion of the weight-bearing surface. This may be associated with a fracture of the head or the neck of the fibula. If there is no displacement in a plateau fracture of the tibia, the injury may be treated by immobilization in plaster. If there is displacement of the joint surface, open reduction and internal fixation may be necessary in order to obtain a satisfactory weight-bearing surface. Fractures of the upper portion of the fibula occasionally are associated with footdrop as a result of damage to the peroneal nerve as it curves about the neck of the fibula.

ANKLE

Pott's Fracture. This is a common fracture in the region of the ankle, with the foot in eversion and abduction. As a result the internal malleolus is torn off, and the fibula is fractured, usually at a level somewhat above the external malleolus. Lateral displacement of the foot results. This is known as *bimalleolar fracture*. Occasionally the posterior lip of the tibia is also torn away, resulting in a *trimalleolar fracture* with posterior displacement of the foot. Swelling is marked in this injury, and the deformity is evident. Roentgenologic examination is essential, and prompt reduction of displaced fractures is desirable. Satisfactory closed reduction can frequently be accomplished with fixation in a plaster cast for 6 to 8 weeks. If the fracture is unstable, open reduction and internal fixation are necessary. In either case, fractures involving joint surfaces require anatomic reduction.

A *sprain* is a more common injury in the region of the ankle. However, this normally results from inversion of the foot. There is no bony deformity, and the tenderness lies in the region of the ligaments that are injured, usually below, and anterior to, the external malleolus.

If fractures of the lower portion of the lower extremity are well reduced and adequately immobilized by plaster, a walking iron may be incorporated in the cast to permit weight bearing during the period of healing. This minimizes the disability and promotes healing.

OS CALCIS

Fracture of the os calcis results from a fall from a height, the individual landing on his or her feet and suffering a crushing injury of the os calcis. Comminution is frequent, and there is flattening of the bone with decrease in Böhler's angle. ***Böhlers angle*** is the angle formed by the axis of the subtalar joint and the superior surface of the tuberosity. Accurate reduction of these fractures is extremely difficult and often impossible. With minimal displacement, simple immobilization for several weeks should suffice. However, if there is marked flattening of the os calcis, skeletal traction through the posterior and inferior fragment may be necessary in order to improve the position.

Joint Replacement

Prosthetic joints have been developed to replace interphalangeal joints, metacarpophalangeal joints, the hip joint, knee joint, and scapulohumeral joint. The usual indications are avascular necrosis and rheumatoid arthritis. Considerable rehabilitation has been accomplished with these measures in patients otherwise incapacitated by their joint disease.

DELAYED UNION OR NONUNION OF FRACTURES

Delayed union of a fracture is prolongation of healing beyond the time that normally would be required for union to occur at that particular site. Nonunion is indefinite delay in healing. Certain fracture sites are particularly likely to develop delay in union. Among these are fractures at the junction of the lower and the middle thirds of the tibia, the neck of the femur, and the carpal scaphoid. Factors that contribute to delay in union include inadequate reduction, for example, undue separation of the fragments or interposition of soft tissue; improper immobilization, which permits excessive movement; and poor blood supply. The position of the fracture relative to the point or points of entry of the nutrient artery and the extent of periosteal injury are both important in the development of delayed union or nonunion of fractures. Rarely, constitutional disease may contribute to delay in union.

Delayed union should be prevented insofar as possible by adequate reduction and fixation of the fragments at the time of the original injury. However, once it has developed, delayed union may be managed by the following: (1) prolonged immobilization, such as in a carpal scaphoid fracture; (2) application of splints that permit active use of the parts to improve the blood supply—for example, a walking caliper splint; (3) physiotherapy; (4) drilling of the fracture site; and (5) the use of bone grafts to bridge the fracture site.

SOFT-TISSUE SARCOMAS

Soft-tissue sarcomas present challenging problems in diagnosis and treatment. Most of them arise in areas in which early diagnosis and treatment should be simple. Despite this, they are frequently large and have been present for months before the patient seeks medical advice. In some instances, that advice is poor, in that simple reassurances are offered on the fallacious assumption that a given lump is a lipoma or some other innocent lesion. Obviously at some point in their clinical evolution all soft-tissue sarcomas should be curable by wide local excision. Nevertheless, the curability rate in many histologic types is low, and amputational surgery is necessary for local control of the growth. The end results of treatment depend on (1) the "biologic potential" of the tumor in terms of its speed of growth and capacity to invade blood vessels and thereby to metastasize to distant sites; (2) resistance of the host; (3) the anatomic site of occurrence; and (4) the type and adequacy of treatment. The only clue to the biologic potential of a given soft-tissue sarcoma is its histologic grade and the size of the tumor. It is therefore most important to assess this by preliminary biopsy before the method of treatment is decided upon, if the tumor is greater than 3 cm in diameter.

These tumors arise from the mesenchymal supporting tissues. Exact classification may be difficult, but an expert tumor pathologist can usually provide the surgeon with a reasonable assessment of the biologic aggressiveness of a given sarcoma: (1) *Fibrosarcoma*—extreme variability in the degree of malignancy, metastasizes infrequently to lymph nodes and is radioresistant. (2) *Malignant fibrous histiocytoma*—many of the previously unclassified soft-tissue sarcomas and anaplastic fibrosarcomas fall into this group. The growth pattern is variable, as is the degree of malignancy. Metastasis to lymph nodes is infrequent. (3) *Liposarcoma*—also variable in behavior, is frequently moderately radiosensitive. (4) *Synovial sarcoma*—arises in the region of joints, but direct connection to synovial membrane is infrequent. In children its behavior is more benign than in adults. This type metastasizes to regional lymph nodes with greater frequency than other sarcomas. (5) *Rhabdomyosarcoma*—embryonal form in children may respond to combined surgical removal and chemotherapy. In adults it is highly malignant. (6) *Malignant schwannoma*—tumor of nerve sheath origin, seen alone or in patients with von Recklinghausen's disease. Local persistence following removal is frequent; metastasis to the lungs is usually late. (7) *Kaposi's sarcoma*—of vascular origin, it is frequently multicentric. Individual lesions can be controlled with radiotherapy or surgical excision. The recognition and apparent increase in frequency of the acquired immunodeficiency syndrome (AIDS), of which Kaposi's sarcoma is a feature, has extended our experience with this lesion. However, whether it occurs independent of alterations of the immune system is undetermined at this time.

Because the growth of soft-tissue sarcomas is expansile, an adventitious capsule tends to form at its periphery; however, this is never complete. The temptation to shell them out must be resisted if the objective of operation is wide removal. Since the tendrils of tumor extending beyond the adventitious capsule usually cannot be seen by the surgeon, adequate removal consists of removal of surrounding normal tissues. In the instance of tumors encroaching upon major blood vessels or nerves, amputation may be necessary for local control of the tumor unless it is believed that radiation therapy, or radiation therapy combined with chemotherapy, or chemotherapy alone will suffice for the local control of a given inadequately removed sarcoma. Experience with embryonal rhabdomyosarcoma of childhood, which has demonstrated a greatly increased cure rate by the combined use of surgery, radiation therapy, and chemotherapy, has served as a model for efforts to cure other high-grade soft-tissue sarcomas as well. High-dose radiation therapy alone is also in use.

EAR

Ménière's Syndrome

Ménière's syndrome is characterized by attacks of vertigo, nausea, and vomiting, along with progressive loss of hearing and tinnitus in one ear. Occasionally the opposite ear becomes involved. The underlying pathology consists of hydrops of the vestibular and cochlear labyrinth. It should be differentiated from other causes of vertigo, particularly those cases that arise from decreased blood flow in the basilar artery.

Facial Nerve Paralysis

Facial nerve paralysis results from (1) direct extension of acute or chronic otitis media; (2) invasion by malignant tumors of the parotid glands; (3) operative trauma; (4) fractures of the temporal bone; (5) lesions of the central nervous system; and, most frequently, (6) undetermined causes as an isolated lesion (Bell's palsy).

Central lesions causing paralysis of the facial nerve differ from peripheral lesions in that the fibers of the chorda tympani nerve are involved in the latter. For this reason, in peripheral lesions there is loss of sense of taste, the eyelids cannot be closed completely, and the brow cannot be wrinkled.

SALIVARY GLANDS

The major salivary glands include the parotid, submaxillary, and sublingual glands. Minor salivary glands are distributed throughout the submucosa of the buccal mucous membrane and tongue.

Suppurative infection involves primarily the parotid; it is caused by staphylococci and occurs in dehydrated, debilitated patients. Treatment consists primarily of the synthetic penicillin drugs to which nearly all staphylococci are sensitive. If suppuration occurs, incision and drainage are necessary.

In Sjögren's syndrome, enlargement of the parotid gland results from lymphocytic infiltration. This must be differentiated from the congenital anomaly (frequently misclassified as a neoplasm) papillary cystadenoma lymphomatosum. Primary lymphosarcoma occurs but is unusual.

Primary tumors are seen in both major and minor salivary glands. The most common site for neoplasia is the parotid gland. The ''rule of 80s'' concerning the parotid gland states that 80% of parotid neoplasms are benign, of which 80% are pleomorphic adenomas (benign mixed tumors), and 80% are located in the superficial (lateral) lobe. The ratio of benign to malignant lesions is somewhat lower in the submaxillary and sublingual glands, approaching 50 : 50.

In 5% of cases, mixed tumors are malignant. The mucoepidermoid tumors are malignant but may be very low grade and therefore quite curable by surgical removal. The cylindromatous variant of adenocarcinoma is a distinctive tumor with a long clinical course. It characteristically invades nerve sheaths, and for this reason local recurrence after surgical removal is the rule. Poorly differentiated adenocarcinoma, epidermoid carcinoma, and undifferentiated carcinoma all occur; they are generally of high malignancy and infrequently cured.

THROAT

Vincent's Angina (Trench Mouth)

Vincent's angina, more commonly known as *trench mouth,* is caused by two organisms—a spirochete and a fusiform bacillus. It is characterized by one or more painful ulcers, usually found on the tonsils, the gums, the faucial pillars, the buccal membrane of the cheeks, and the pharyngeal wall. These ulcers are undermined, have sharp irregular edges and bleed easily. If they are present on the gums, pyorrhea results. The diagnosis depends on the foregoing clinical picture and on the finding of the two organisms on a smear obtained from the ulcer. Treatment consists of perborate gargles, penicillin, or 5% neoarsphenamine in glycerin applied directly to the ulcer. Penicillin lozenges are of value.

Peritonsillar Abscess (Quinsy)

An infection of the peritonsillar tissues with abscess formation, peritonsillar abscess is more common in adults than in children. Symptoms are (1) pain, usually radiating to the ear of the affected side; (2) fever; (3) malaise; and (4) great difficulty in swallowing. Examination reveals swelling or bulging of the tonsil and the soft palate and cervical adenitis. Treatment consists of incision and drainage of the abscess when it is pointing. Hot saline throat irrigations are helpful before and after incision. The incision should be made at the junction of an imaginary line along the free border of the anterior pillar at its most bulging point and at another line along the free edge of the soft palate.

Ludwig's Angina

Ludwig's angina is an acute inflammatory process involving the cellular tissues of the floor of the mouth and the submaxillary region of one or both sides of the neck. Symptoms include pain in the floor of the mouth, difficulty in swallowing and talking, and excessive salivation. The tongue is elevated, and there is brawny induration beneath the jaw. Dyspnea and edema of the glottis may necessitate tracheostomy. Treatment consists of bed rest, intravenous fluids, chemotherapy—preferably penicillin in large doses—and incision and drainage when indicated.

Retropharyngeal Abscess

An accumulation of pus between the posterior wall of the pharynx and the vertebral column, retropharyngeal abscess is most common in young children. The staphylococcus is the microorganism usually found in cultures of the abscess. Signs of general sepsis are present, with local symptoms of dysphagia, dyspnea, aphonia, cough, and regurgitation. The head is in an extended position, and the mouth is open. Palpation reveals a soft, fluctuant swelling of the posterior pharynx that occasionally is palpable at the sides of the neck. Unless prompt diagnosis is made and treatment instituted, the prognosis is grave.

NECK

Branchiogenic Cysts

Branchiogenic cysts arise from embryonic remnants of the branchial clefts. Although they may appear in childhood, they are more frequently seen after puberty and may first be evident in the fifth and sixth decades of life. They arise anterior to the sternocleidomastoid muscle, although the highest ones arise anterior to the tragus of the ear. Treatment of these cysts consists of complete excision. If they become secondarily infected, or are incompletely drained or removed, a fistula may develop.

Thyroglossal Cysts

Congenital cysts that arise in the midline of the neck as a cystic remnant of the thyroglossal duct, these cysts may be seen in the region extending from the suprasternal area to the suprahyoid area. Remnants of thyroid tissue are frequently present. The cysts are lined by stratified squamous, pseudostratified columnar, or ciliated columnar epithelium. Lymphoid tissue is also usually prominent. The thyroglossal duct originates in the foramen cecum at the base of the tongue and frequently passes through the hyoid bone. Treatment involves excision of the cyst and its associated tract, which may include removal of the midportion of the hyoid bone and the foramen cecum.

Lymph Node Enlargements in the Neck

In former years tuberculosis lymphadenitis was the most frequent cause of enlarged cervical lymph nodes. Since the compulsory pasteurization of milk and the destruction of tuberculous herds, this is no longer so. In childhood, lymphadenitis related to regional infection in tonsils, gums, or middle ear is most frequent. In girls in the late teens to 20s, metastatic carcinoma from the thyroid is the most likely explanation for persistent cervical lymph node enlargement. In middle-aged and older males metastatic carcinoma from the upper digestive or respiratory tract is common.

Malignant lymphoma including *Hodgkin's disease* is an additional cause of lymph node enlargement. The staging of Hodgkin's disease is important in deciding upon the correct course of therapy. Lymphography and abdominal exploration are the methods whereby staging is accomplished. Splenectomy, liver biopsy, and lymph node biopsy of the most suspicious periaortic nodes on lymphography are the basis for histologic grading. In women the ovaries and tubes should be mobilized and transposed behind the uterus. Radiation therapy in adequate dosage is now known to be curative in early stages, whereas combination chemotherapy is of considerable value in systemic disease.

ORAL CAVITY

Carcinoma of the Tongue

Found predominantly in the male, carcinoma of the tongue usually is of the squamous-cell type and occurs along the edges. These lesions present as ulcerating infiltrating areas, often with palpable metastatic involvement of the regional cervical lymph nodes at the time that patient is first seen. Predisposing factors in the development of carcinoma of the tongue include chronic irritation from poor dental care, poorly fitted dental plates, chronic inflammation, pipe smoking, leukoplakia, and syphilis.

Surgical excision is recommended for small lesions that occupy the anterior third of the tongue. If cervical lymph nodes are suspiciously enlarged, combined jaw-neck resection should be done. For larger cancers and lesions that involve the posterior third of the tongue, radiation therapy is usually indicated.

Carcinoma of Buccal Mucosa

Squamous-cell carcinoma arising from the buccal mucosa is treated by wide local removal. If lymph nodes are clinically involved, combined resection of the primary lesion and radical neck dissection is indicated. A variant known as verrucous carcinoma, seen in tobacco chewers, seldom metastasizes, but it may extend entirely through the cheek to the skin surface.

Carcinoma of Floor of the Mouth

Carcinoma in this area frequently requires resection of both mandibular rami if surgical treatment is elected. Primary reconstruction should be performed to avoid the crippling deformity that may otherwise result. Lymph nodes metastases are frequent in this anatomic site of origin, and when clinical evidence of lymph node involvement is present, primary surgical treatment is indicated.

Gingival Carcinoma

Either primary surgical resection or radiation therapy with a supervoltage source is indicated for gingival carcinoma, again depending to a great extent on the status of the regional lymph nodes.

Cancer of the Lips

On the lower lip any sore that does not promptly heal should be considered squamous-cell cancer until proven otherwise by biopsy. On the upper lip the usual malignant lesion is basal-cell carcinoma. Metastases from squamous-cell carcinoma of the lower lip to regional lymph nodes occur in approximately 10% of cases. For this reason elective node dissection is not indicated. The curability of squamous-cell carcinoma is high, even when lymph node metastases exist. For lesions that require sacrifice of most of the lower lip along with extensive recon-

struction, primary radiation therapy should be elected instead of surgery.

LARYNX

Overuse of the voice may cause fibrotic nodules on the vocal cords with resultant hoarseness. Epidemiologically the use of tobacco and alcohol is associated with the development of squamous-cell carcinoma of the larynx. These tumors are classified according to the exact site and extent of involvement along with the status of the regional nodes. Cancer limited to the vocal cord with continued mobility of the cord is curable in over 90% of cases by radiation therapy. More extensive lesions are treated by partial or total laryngectomy. Whether or not neck dissection is done depends on the exact anatomic area of involvement as well as the clinical status of the lymph nodes.

NOSE

Sinusitis

The paranasal sinuses may be involved in acute or chronic infectious or allergic process or by neoplasia. Acute or chronic infectious processes are the most common forms, and the symptoms vary according to the sinus or group of sinuses involved. Headache or periodic pain and nasal discharge are the usual complaints. Suppurative sinusitis may arise (1) as a complication of the common cold; (2) from contaminated water that enters a sinus of a swimmer; (3) from obstruction to the sinus ostia by intranasal foreign bodies, polyps, neoplasms, or a deviated septum; (4) from an infected tooth; and (5) from rapid changes in barometric pressure, as in an aerosinusitis. One or all of the sinuses may be involved.

The diagnosis is made by (1) inspection and palpation, which may reveal swelling and tenderness over the involved sinus; (2) intranasal examination, which may reveal pus in the middle meatus if the anterior sinuses (frontal, maxillary, and anterior ethmoid) are involved or in the sphenoethmoid recess if the posterior sinuses (posterior ethmoids, and sphenoids) are involved; (3) transillumination; (4) roentgenologic examination; and (5) diagnostic puncture of a maxillary sinus.

Acute sinusitis, whether of viral or bacterial origin, is treated primarily by antibiotics and usually responds well. Chronic maxillary sinusitis may require drainage by maxillary sinusotomy in the canine fossa (Caldwell-Luc). Acute ethmoid sinusitis may cause orbital cellulitis.

The most frequent malignant tumor of the maxillary sinuses is squamous-cell carcinoma; salivary gland tumors also occur. Radical maxillectomy combined with radiation therapy is the treatment for squamous-cell carcinoma. The operation includes exenteration of the orbit.

THYROID

Goiters may be nodular or diffuse and toxic or nontoxic. The most common is the diffuse nontoxic gland caused by iodine deficiency that occurs in endemic goiter belts. With the public acceptance of iodized table salt, the incidence of iodine deficiency in these areas has been decreased greatly. Such glands are removed only when pressure symptoms appear or for cosmetic reasons.

Nodular goiters usually are removed because of the significant incidence of carcinoma in such glands. Carcinoma occurs in 10% to 20% of solitary nodules.

Nontoxic goiters produce pressure symptoms because of their size, causing dyspnea, hoarseness, dysphagia, and disfigurement. Toxic goiters are characterized by overproduction of thyroxine, and the symptoms are nervousness, sweating, tremor, loss of weight, exophthalmos, and an increase of body metabolism.

The functional status of the thyroid gland is evaluated by determination of the plasma level of thyroxine (T_4), triiodothyronine (T_3), uptake of red-blood cells, or the ^{131}I uptake.

Patients with diffuse toxic goiter (Graves' disease) are treated by subtotal thyroidectomy, prolonged use of antithyroid drugs or with ^{131}I. The decision is based on the age of the patient and the preference of the physician. Generally in patients under 35 years of age ^{131}I should be avoided. Patients to be operated on should be restored to a euthyroid state by the use of antithyroid drugs such as propylthiouracil in adequate dosage. Iodine, as potassium iodide or Lugol's solution, is given for 10 to 14 days before operation. The procedure used today is subtotal thyroidectomy. Some patients are treated with propylthiouracil for 1 to 2 years in the hope that a permanent remission will result. The recurrence rate is 30% to 40%. Therapeutic use of radioactive iodine is reserved for patients over 35 years of age. Fear of the development of thyroid cancer is the reason for avoiding radioactive iodine

therapy in the young, however, there are no published reports of the development of thyroid cancer in the patients treated for hyperthyroidism with ^{131}I.

Carcinoma of the thyroid (papillary, follicular, or Hürthle cell carcinoma) is treated by total thyroidectomy and removal of any clinically involved nodes. Radioactive iodine has proved to be of benefit after total thyroidectomy.

Thyroiditis

Thyroiditis is a rather obscure group of nonspecific inflammations of the thyroid encountered occasionally by the surgeon. Hashimoto's disease, or struma lymphomatosa, signifies a firm gland infiltrated with lymphocytes. The process is usually seen in middle-aged women; it is bilateral and associated with reduced thyroid function. The titer of autoantibodies to thyroglobulin is usually high in Hashimoto's disease. Riedel's struma is an unusual process that consists of a woody hard fibrosis involving the surrounding muscles as well as the thyroid. Subacute granulomatous thyroiditis is frequently made manifest by acute pain in the lower neck, dysphagia, and so forth. Frequently it can be dramatically improved by corticosteroid therapy. Thyroidectomy sometimes is necessary to relieve pressure symptoms or to exclude malignancy.

PARATHYROIDS

Parathormone has a dual function; first, it mobilizes calcium from bone; second, it increases renal tubular excretion of phosphate. Excessive parathormone secretion is seen in hyperplasia of the parathyroid glands and in functioning tumors. Benign adenoma greatly exceeds carcinoma in frequency. Clinically, two pictures are produced by parathormone excess. Most frequent is renal calculus formation or nephrocalcinosis. The second is osteitis fibrosa cystica (von Recklinghausen's disease of the bone). Frequently seen today are examples of parathormone excess without clinical manifestations, diagnosed by the increased serum calcium concentrations found on routine screening study. Duodenal ulcer and pancreatitis are also seen with parathormone excess. Primary hyperparathyroidism is usually caused by an adenoma, but hyperplasia may also be causative. Differentiation between the two may be difficult. Secondary hyperparathyroidism is caused by renal failure. Hyperplasia of the parathyroids with hyperparathyroidism occurs as a feature of both type I and type II multiple endocrine neoplasia.

Hypoparathyroidism is seen either as a congenital process or, more commonly, as a complication of operations on the thyroid gland. It is manifested early by paresthesias of the lips and digits. There may be signs of increased neuromuscular excitability (positive Chvostek's or Trousseau's sign) and frank tetany. Tetany is due to hypocalcemia, resulting from hypophosphaturia and hyperphosphatemia. Treatment consists of vitamin D and a high-calcium diet. Dihydrotachysterol (A.T. 10), which possesses the properties of both vitamin D and parathormone, is reserved for prolonged cases. Parathormone may be used for brief periods.

BREAST

Examination

Breast examination should be conducted in a well-lighted room with the assistance of a chaperone. Inspection in the sitting position may demonstrate subtle changes that may be significant, such as irregularities in contour, changes in the configuration or axis of the nipple or dimpling of the skin. These may be further accentuated by having the patient raise her arms over her head, bend forward with the hands supported, or by contraction of the pectoral muscles. Palpation should be conducted with the side to be examined elevated by a pillow, feeling the breast tissue against the chest wall. The patient should be instructed in self-examination, which should be done once a month preferably at the end of the menstrual period.

Mammography and xeroradiography are screening techniques of value in demonstrating some early cancers of the breast. Based on the increased frequency of breast cancer in woman survivors of the atomic bombing of Hiroshima, and the increased frequency of breast cancer in women with pulmonary tuberculosis who had repeated fluoroscopic examinations of the chest, as well as in theoretical models, mammography and xeroradiography have been used in more restricted manner than formerly. Routine screening is now advised only in women age 40 or older. Younger women should have mammography only when they have one or more factors increasing their risk of breast cancer. These "risk factors" include, in decreasing order of importance, cancer of one breast; a family history of breast cancer in siblings or on the maternal side of the family, the presence of fibrocystic disease or nodular breasts, nulliparity, first pregnancy after age 30, and early menarche.

Fibroadenoma of the Breast

A benign tumor, usually occurring in a girl in her late teens or 20s, fibroadenoma of the breast manifests itself by the appearance of a solitary lump, usually associated with little or no discomfort. The tumor appears to be well encapsulated, freely movable, and not attached to the skin and the subcutaneous tissue. Treatment consists of simple excision of the tumor. Complete removal is not followed by recurrence.

Fibrocystic Disease (Chronic Cystic Mastitis)

Fibrocystic disease, or chronic cystic mastitis, encompasses a group of lesions that may start during the second decade of life, increasing in frequency until the time of the menopause. It is extremely frequent, and few women in our society escape it completely. Clinically, it presents as discomfort in one or both breasts, usually most severe before the menstrual period (mastodynia). Dominant masses may or may not form. On palpation, in the absence of a mass, irregular areas of shotty induration are found. Pathologically, microcysts without epithelial hyperplasia but with increased prominence of periductal connective tissue are the earliest lesion. Macrocysts are frequent (blue-domed cysts of Bloodgood), as is sclerosing adenosis, in which increasing fibrosis in lobules gives rise to a bizarre appearance sometimes mistaken for cancer. Lobular hyperplasia also occurs as do intraductal papillomas. At times there may be doubt about the presence or absence of a dominant mass. Needle aspiration in some instances will be followed by disappearance of the questionable mass. If not, biopsy is justified. Obvious macrocysts should be aspirated. Clear fluid seldom shows cells on cytologic study, but bloody fluid should always be examined.

The relationship between fibrocystic disease and cancer has long been debated. Patients with a biopsy showing fibrocystic disease have an increased frequency of subsequent breast cancer as compared with similar women without such a history.

Duct Papilloma

In general duct papilloma are quite small and often cannot be felt on examination of the breast. These lesions usually manifest themselves by the appearance of intermittent bleeding from the nipple. Their relation to cancer is not clear-cut, but when they can be localized by compression of the duct their removal is indicated. Although Paget's disease of the nipple, which is intraductal carcinoma with invasion, may present without a palpable mass, seldom indeed will a patient with *only* a bloody discharge from the nipple have cancer.

Carcinoma of the Breast

Carcinoma of the breast is now the most frequent lethal cancer in women. Although occurring usually in middle and older age groups, it is not unknown in the 20s. It is almost always unilateral. Except on rare occasions the presenting symptom is a painless lump that has developed insidiously. In contrast with fibroadenoma, these tumors are not readily movable and show early evidence of infiltration and fixation to the surrounding structures. This is manifested by dimpling of the skin, retraction or deviation of the nipple, and elevation of the breast. As the disease progresses, the overlying skin becomes involved to such an extent that there is frank infiltration with development of edema and an orange-peel type of skin. Extension inward leads to fixation of the breast to the pectoral muscles and eventually to the chest wall. Along with the local extension, there is a lymphatic spread of the disease. The axillary nodes are involved early. They become enlarged, hard, and eventually, matted together. The lymphatic drainage of the breast also may lead to enlargement of the supraclavicular nodes and those in the thorax along the course of the internal mammary vessels. Eventually, widespread metastasis takes place with involvement of bone, liver, lungs, and the brain. Unfortunately, local pain is a very late symptom in the disease. In untreated cases ulceration often takes place with secondary infection, purulent and foul drainage, and repeated episodes of hemorrhage.

Treatment of the patient with breast cancer should be individualized. Therapy may include surgery, radiation therapy, or chemotherapy, in combination or as single modalities. In general, surgical removal of the breast and an axillary lymph adenectomy is indicated in Stage I or Stage II breast cancer. The pectoral major muscle is not removed unless fixation to this muscle is present. If these nodes show no evidence of metastatic spread at the time of operation, about 80% to 90% of the patients will survive 5 years. On the other hand, if these nodes are involved at the time of operation only about 35% to 45% will survive that long.

Partial mastectomy is practiced by some for management of Stage I cancer, and partial mastectomy combined with radiation therapy is advocated by others for Stage I and Stage II.

When the initial biopsy is done, tissue should be assayed for the presence of estrogen receptor protein. When significant levels are present, alteration of hormonal balance is likely to be beneficial in treatment of patients with disseminated disease. Progesterone receptor analysis will further refine the indications for hormone therapy or ablation.

X-ray therapy has been used both preoperatively and postoperatively, but controlled studies have not shown prolonged survival in the treated group. Generally, radiation therapy is reserved for the treatment of recurrent or metastatic disease. The role of surgical or roentgen castration in premenopausal women who have this disease is debatable, but is contraindicated when the cancer is estrogen receptor negative.

In patients who are inoperable by virtue of locally extensive disease (including inflammatory carcinoma; the presence of proved supraclavicular lymph node metastases; large, bulky ulcerated and fixed lesions; extensive edema; satellite skin nodules, etc.), treatment will be by radiation therapy, alteration of hormonal balance and chemotherapy, alone or in combination. Surgical treatment will be limited to debulking, if at all.

Disseminated or recurrent breast cancer requires palliative treatment, which may be very effective in some patients. Prognostic factors, in addition to estrogen and progesterone receptor status, include the length of the "free interval" (the length of time between treatment and evidence of recurrence or metastatic disease) and the site and extent of metastases.

Chemotherapy may provide effective palliation in over 50% of women with disseminated breast cancer. New agents are under continual investigation, and improved results can be anticipated.

In this disease cure can be expected only with early recognition and prompt treatment. Therefore, all women should undergo frequent careful physical examinations. However, during the intervals they should examine their own breasts each month and report immediately for attention if any lump develops. As previously indicated, in women with significant "risk factors" for breast cancer and in women over 40 years of age, mammography should be done yearly. It is also indicated in the follow-up of women who have been treated for breast cancer.

Paget's disease of the breast should be considered a special form of carcinoma in which there is an eczematoid lesion of the nipple and the areola with an associated carcinoma beneath. The management of this condition is the same as that of any carcinoma of the breast.

Sarcoma of the Breast

Sarcoma is an uncommon type of malignant neoplasm in the breast. It occurs usually in middle-aged women and appears as a mass in the breast, normally undergoing rather diffuse enlargement. *Cystosarcoma phyllodes* (giant fibroadenoma) is the most common sarcomatous lesion. It consists of both epithelial elements and a stroma that may contain smooth muscle as cartilage. In approximately 20% of cases the stroma will contain malignant areas. Axillary metastases are infrequent. The lesions are usually large but not fixed to skin or chest wall. Other sarcomas, including all cell types, also occur. Axillary metastasis is seldom found, and the prognosis, as in other sites, depends on the grade of the tumor. Simple mastectomy is the usual treatment.

THORAX

Trauma

ALTERATIONS IN BASIC PHYSIOLOGIC MECHANISMS

An understanding of the alterations in basic physiologic mechanisms is vital to the treatment of patients with chest trauma.

Inspiration is the result of expansion of the intrathoracic space by movement of the chest wall out and up and of the diaphragm down. Because the intrapulmonary airways are an open system and are at atmospheric pressure, air moves passively into the lungs. With expiration, the chest wall relaxes and the lungs collapse, expelling the air from within the alveoli and bronchi. The lungs remain expanded during expiration as the intrapleural pressure remains less than atmospheric while intrabronchial and alveoli pressure is atmospheric. Coughing is an essential function that clears secretions from the airways. Failure to clear such secretions leads to obstruction of bronchioles and atelectasis.

The most common injury secondary to thoracic trauma is a fractured rib. A nondisplaced fractured rib is important because it cannot be splinted and respiratory movement produces increased discomfort. Because of the pain, the patient will "splint" the chest on the injured side and maintain his or her minute ventilatory volume by increasing the rate of breathing. Because coughing requires maximal in-

halation with forced exhalation initially against a closed glottis, this produces significant pain. The injured patient voluntarily suppresses the cough reflex and without an effective cough, secretions accumulate and atelectasis develops. If the atelectatic segments are secondarily infected, pneumonia supervenes and in the elderly or the patient with respiratory compromise, this can become life-threatening. Management of rib fractures is based on adequate but judicious control of pain.

Frequently, penetrating wounds of the thorax cause **pneumothorax** or **hemothorax,** or a combination of both. The effect is similar. If one pleural space is filled with air or blood, respiratory exchange may be embarrassed seriously. This burden can be tolerated by the patient unless the air or the blood causes displacement of the mediastinum toward the normal side, thereby further hindering respiration and impairing venous return to the heart.

Treatment consists of insertion of a thoracostomy tube attached to either a water seal drainage bottle or to a suction apparatus. When air in the pleura is under tension (tension pneumothorax), immediate aspiration is lifesaving.

Defects in the chest wall give rise to an open pneumothorax. Aeration of the lung on the involved side is impossible in these circumstances. The heart and the mediastinal structures move from side to side with each respiratory movement (mediastinal flutter). Emergency measures require that the defect be closed immediately.

Crushing injuries of the thoracic cage in which there are multiple rib fractures ("flail chest") create paradoxic respiration, that is, collapse of the chest wall with inspiration and expansion with expiration. Flail chest producing respiratory embarrassment, as judged by inspection and the finding of a low oxygen tension and a high carbon dioxide tension in arterial blood, is splinted today by use of a cuffed endotracheal tube and use of a volume-cycled mechanical ventilator.

Of great importance in all chest injuries is maintenance of an open airway and the clearing of bronchial secretions.

With severe thoracic injuries pulmonary contusion is very likely to occur. If suspected, arterial blood gases should be monitored. A falling Pao_2 or a rising $Paco_2$ are indications for ventilatory support with a volume-cycled ventilator. The O_2 in inspired air (Fio_2) is raised in increments to a maximum of 60% depending on response of the Pao_2. If elevated inspiratory pressure and Fio_2 fail to correct abnormalities in blood gases, positive end expiratory pressure (PEEP) should be instituted also, in increments from 5 cm to 15 cm of H_2O, depending on response.

Because the use of PEEP can impede venous return and reduce cardiac output, its use at higher levels (>7 cm of H_2O) or in critically ill patients should be monitored with a Swan-Ganz catheter so that appropriate adjustments can be made to maintain the patient's hemodynamic state.

CARDIAC TAMPONADE

Penetrating wounds of the heart that are not immediately fatal may result in death by cardiac tamponade. A relatively small amount of bleeding into the pericardial sac may embarrass the diastolic filling of the heart, giving rise to a classic triad of symptoms—increased venous pressure, distant heart sounds, and increased diastolic blood pressure with narrowed pulse pressure.

Treatment consists of immediate pericardial aspiration, followed by operation if bleeding continues. The pericardium is exposed by a median sternotomy incision.

Cardiac Arrest

The cessation of the heartbeat can be caused by many factors, but essentially two mechanisms are involved: (1) simple arrest occurs with potassium intoxication, severe hypoxemia, or hypercapneia; and (2) ventricular fibrillation most frequently attends acute myocardial infarction, but may be seen with hypothermia and hypoxia. Treatment must be rapidly and skillfully executed in order to be effective. An adequate airway must be provided by removal of vomitus or other foreign material and by keeping the tongue forward. Next, artificial respiration is instituted, preferably by an anesthesia machine using oxygen, but if this is not available, by mouth-to-mouth technique. Cardiac output is maintained by closed-chest cardiac massage at a rate of 80 to 100 per minute. Intravenous infusion of Ringer's lactate solution should be started, if necessary, by cutdown. The mechanism of arrest is determined by obtaining an electrocardiogram. If the heart is beating weakly and ineffectively, epinephrine is added to the intravenous infusion. If an effective heartbeat does not return, calcium chloride should be injected into the heart. If the heart is in standstill, epinephrine should be injected into the right ventricular cavity. If ventricular fibrillation is present, the defibrillator must be used. Metabolic acidosis develops rapidly and should be combated

by adding sodium bicarbonate to the intravenous infusion. If blood loss was responsible for the cardiac arrest, blood is rapidly transfused.

Open cardiac massage is seldom used today except when cardiac arrests develops during thoracotomy. If heart action does not return with closed-chest massage in patients who are in the operating room, open massage may be effective.

Heart and the Great Vessels

Great strides have been made in the surgical correction of congenital and acquired lesions of the heart and the great vessels. The development and refinement of pump oxygenators that permit total cardiopulmonary bypass without an unacceptable physiologic insult permit more leisurely and extensive intracardiac manipulations. This was essential to the expansion of this field and constitutes one of the fascinating chapters in the history of modern surgery. Common lesions that are amenable to surgical techniques will be listed and described briefly.

Patent Ductus Arteriosus

The persistence of the embryologic shunt from aorta to pulmonary artery is associated with symptoms caused by left heart strain and pulmonary hypertension. There is a classic machinery murmur heard to the left of the sternum. The treatment of choice is ligation and division of the ductus.

Coarctation of the Aorta

Coarctation of the aorta is a narrowing of the arch of the aorta just past the origin of the left subclavian artery. It may range from severe stricturing incompatible with life to minor degrees of narrowing. The clinical picture may range from symptoms of heart failure to the incidental finding of hypertension in the upper extremities. In most cases there is hypotension in the trunk and the legs. Death results from heart failure or cerebrovascular accidents.

Surgical treatment entails resection of the narrowed segment and end-to-end anastomosis, grafting, or a subclavian flap angioplasty in the neonate.

Tetralogy of Fallot

The tetralogy of Fallot is a complex anomaly including pulmonary valve stenosis, overriding of the aorta, interventricular septal defect, and hypertrophy of the right ventricle. Its presence is obvious in infancy or early childhood because of the cyanosis (blue baby).

Treatment of this complex lesion evolves around the size of the pulmonary arteries and the age or size of the patient. In the symptomatic infant (severe cyanosis or hypercyanotic spells) with small pulmonary arteries a palliative systemic to pulmonary artery shunt is performed. This can be performed by use of a plastic tube graft or direct anastamosis of the subclavian artery to the pulmonary artery. In the child with normal or near normal size pulmonary arteries, total correction, consisting of closure of the ventricular septal defect and relief of the pulmonary stenosis, is accomplished using cardiopulmonary bypass.

Atrial Septal Defects

Atrial septal defects must be differentiated from a patent foramen ovale that is a normal defect in up to 25% of adult hearts. Because of its slitlike opening, the patent foramen ovale permits shunting only from right to left. Left-to-right shunting of blood is characteristic of atrial septal defects, but is also seen with anomalous pulmonary veins and atrioventricular canal malformations. The atrial septal defects are divided into ostium secundum and ostium primum types. The former is the more frequent and more readily repaired. Mitral and tricuspid insufficiency accompany ostium primum defects and atrioventricular canals. The diagnosis of ostium secundum defect is seldom made early in life because the symptoms and physical signs are not sufficiently distinct. With the passage of time a soft systolic murmur is heard in the second or third left intercostal space along with fixed splitting of the second pulmonic sound. Pulmonary blood flow is increased and eventually pulmonary hypertension develops. Repair is indicated when the shunt is large and the volume of flow in the pulmonary circuit is one and one half to two times greater than the systemic circuit.

Ventricular Septal Defects

Ventricular septal defects are frequent congenital anomalies of the heart comprising 20% to 30% of all cases of congenital heart disease. Because of the great difference in resistance between the pulmonary and systemic vascular beds, the left-to-right shunt is likely to be very large, depending on the size of the defect. The volume of blood flow in the pulmonary and systemic circuits is determined by cardiac catheterization. As in atrial septal defects,

when pulmonary blood flow is one and one half to two times systemic flow, operation is indicated. Severe pulmonary hypertension, seldom seen in children, is a contraindication.

Transposition of the Great Arteries

Transposition of the great arteries is one of the more common serious anomalies. In the lethal form there is no communication between the pulmonary and systemic circuits. Palliative procedures are directed toward increasing the communication in order to allow intracardiac mixing so that oxygen tension is increased in the systemic circuit. Nonoperative opening of the foramen ovale by balloon fracture is one method; the Blalock-Hanlon operation is another.

Definitive correction of this lesion can be accomplished by the arterial switch procedure (Jatene) or by an intra-atrial procedure (Senning or Mustard). In many centers definitive correction is being accomplished in the first week of life, prior to a fall in pulmonary vascular resistance and while the left ventricle can support the systemic circulation.

Congenital or Acquired Valvular Lesions

Congenital or acquired valvular lesions are the result of either rheumatic valvulitis or arteriosclerosis. In some instances direct repair (such as mitral commissurotomy) of damaged valves is possible; in others the damage to valves is so extensive that repair is not feasible. In the latter situation, resection and replacement by homografts, xenografts, or prosthetic valves gives good functional results, provided that the myocardium remains in good condition. Multiple replacements are frequently necessary; however, the use of homografts or pulmonary autografts for replacement of the aortic valve may last for the life of the patient.

Other Congenital Lesions

Many of the less common congenital lesions are now corrected with relatively low mortality. These include total anomalous pulmonary venous connection, endocardial cushion defects, tricuspid atresia and other forms of hypoplastic right heart syndromes corrected by use of the Fontan procedure, truncus arteriosus, and some forms of single ventricle. Patients with hypoplastic left heart syndrome can be palliated by the Norwood procedure, although in some centers neonatal cardiac transplantation is being utilized in management of this rapidly fatal cardiac abnormality.

Myocardial Revascularization

The main indication for myocardial revascularization is intractable angina pectoris not responsive to medical therapy. Coronary and cardiac angiography permit an exact assessment of the state of the coronary arteries and the myocardium. Satisfactory examination is essential for the selection of patients for myocardial revascularization procedures. Most frequently used today are direct anastomoses between the internal mammary artery to a coronary artery and bypass vein grafts to the aorta and diseased coronaries, as indicated. Some surgeons perform multiple bypasses using both internal mammary arteries. Although this procedure remains controversial, there is agreement that patients with left main coronary disease, three-vessel disease with abnormal wall motion, and certain subsets of two-vessel disease are best treated surgically.

Pulmonary Embolism

Pulmonary embolism often occurs during a postoperative or postpartum period. It results from a breaking off of a segment of thrombus in the venous circulation, the separated portion then being swept into the heart and carried into one of the pulmonary arteries, where it lodges. The symptoms of pulmonary embolism consist of a sudden onset of chest pain, cough, bloody sputum, dyspnea, and extreme anxiety. If the embolism is large, cardiovascular collapse occurs, and death occurs promptly. In cases of small emboli, spontaneous recovery usually takes place, although repeated pulmonary embolism is common, and eventually death may result. Although the symptoms and signs may be typical, great difficulty in differential diagnosis between pulmonary embolization and acute myocardial infarction exists. Inasmuch as the therapy for the one condition differs from that for the other, a need exists for rapid and accurate methods of establishing the correct diagnosis. Selective pulmonary angiography is the most accurate method of making the diagnosis of pulmonary embolism. In patients who are in shock, pressure studies using the Swan-Ganz catheter should be carried out rapidly. In proved instances, embolectomy is indicated. In patients who are not in shock, ventilation–perfusion scan of the lungs is the initial investigative procedure of choice. If there is no evidence of thrombophlebitis, venograms of the lower extremities are indicated.

Treatment consists of continuous intravenous infusion of heparin. The objective is to maintain the activated partial thromboplastin time at twice control levels. In patients who have recurrent pulmonary emboli while receiving adequate heparin therapy, one of the filters (Mobin-Udin or Greenfield) should be inserted into the inferior vena cava by way of the right jugular vein. Open operation is reserved at present for ligation of the inferior vena cava for septic embolization.

LUNG

Pulmonary complications significantly increase the morbidity and mortality of many major surgical procedures. Frequently these complications can be avoided by careful preoperative assessment of the patient's pulmonary function and careful attention to those disorders that tend to increase the risk of respiratory failure. Emphysema, asthma, chronic bronchitis, a significant smoking history, or a history of dyspnea with exertion are all associated with an increased risk of postoperative pulmonary failure.

Adult Respiratory Distress Syndrome

Adult respiratory distress syndrome (ARDS) is frequently associated with septic shock, multiple organ trauma, long bone fractures, overzealous fluid administration, or other causes of pulmonary edema. The morphologic changes within the lung irrespective of the etiology of ARDS are the same. The pulmonary response to injury includes endothelial and alveolar membrane injury, interstitial edema, accumulation of proteinaceous exudate within the alveolar air space, loss of alveolar type II cells, decreased surfactant, and progressive atelectasis. Without vigorous therapy, this entity has a very high mortality. However, judicious use of ventilatory support, proper oxygen therapy, and the use of PEEP have significantly reduced the mortality of ARDS.

Tumors of the Lung

BRONCHIAL ADENOMA

There are two histologic types of bronchial adenoma. The cylindromatous variety, which resembles the similar tumors of salivary gland origin, and the carcinoid type. The latter may secrete serotonin and cause the carcinoid syndrome. Both lesions are really low-grade carcinomas and may metastasize. When metastasis occurs it is most frequently to regional lymph nodes and liver.

BRONCHOGENIC CARCINOMA

Bronchogenic carcinoma is one of the most frequent cancers in men and is increasing in women. The correlation between smoking and lung cancer appears to be irrefutable evidence of a causative relationship. The most frequent symptoms are cough, hemoptysis, weight loss, and weakness. All of these are late manifestations, and by the time they appear the tumor is usually incurable. The diagnosis is at times made on incidental chest roentgenogram. In addition to chest roentgenography, sputum cytology, and bronchoscopy with biopsy are usually done for diagnosis. The fiberoptic, flexible bronchoscope extends the range of visibility of the examination. When combined with brush biopsy the diagnostic accuracy is considerably enhanced. Treatment consists of pulmonary resection, the extent depending on the location and size of the primary lesion.

At times bronchogenic tumors have an endocrine function, producing a parathormone-like substance, an antidiuretic hormone, and even an inappropriate adrenocorticotropic hormone (ACTH) secretion that causes the clinical manifestations of Cushing's syndrome.

Tuberculosis

The antituberculous drugs have made possible a direct attack on the disease process. Surgical emphasis has shifted from thoracoplasty to resection in instances in which the lung involvement is confined and the disease is not controlled by chemotherapy alone.

Empyema

Empyema may be a complication of pneumonia, particularly in children. It is common during epidemic influenza and may occur from contiguous infection (tuberculosis, gangrene, abscess of the lung) or from chest wounds.

The most common organism is the pneumococcus. The streptococcus causes a virulent form. Staphylococcus, *Haemophilus influenzae,* Friedlander's bacillus and the colon bacillus are rarely the primary invaders. If there is communication with an abscessed, gangrenous, or bronchiectatic lung, the pus is foul. Empyema is rarely bilateral. It may be encapsulated. Physical examination, roentgenograms, and aspiration give the diagnosis.

The treatment of empyema requires a bacteriologic diagnosis of the causitive organism, selection of an appropriate systemic antibiotic, and adequate drainage of the pleural space. Occasionally, an early postpneumonia empyema can be successfully treated with one or more thoracentesis. In those patients with thick pus or in whom the empyema has become loculated, their pleura space must be drained with chest tubes or open drainage. Occasionally, thoracotomy and decortication will be necessary to restore pulmonary function due to encasement of the lung by the inflammatory process.

Lobar or Lung Atelectasis

Occasionally, a main or lobar bronchus will become plugged with thick mucus, which the patient cannot clear with coughing. With obstruction of the bronchus, the residual air within the distal alveoli will be absorbed and the obstructed lung will collapse and opacification will be seen on the chest x ray. Bronchoscopy with aspiration of the mucous plug is curative. The clinical signs of atelectasis are an increased respiratory rate, absence of breath sounds, fever, and tachycardia.

GASTROINTESTINAL TRACT AND ABDOMEN

Abdomen

ABDOMINAL INJURY

Two types of abdominal injury are seen; the first, the result of blunt forces; the second, penetrating injuries from stab wounds or gunshot wounds.

Blunt Injury. The usual cause today is automobile accidents. Properly worn seat belts minimize such injuries, but if the force is sufficient, may actually cause them. Industrial accidents, falls, sports injuries, and so forth, are less common causes. Frequently blunt injuries of the abdomen are seen in association with multiple-organ injury, especially of the brain, as well as injuries of the thorax and osseous fractures. Lacerations of the spleen and liver are frequently associated with fractures of overlying ribs. Both result in hemorrhage; shock is frequent. The pancreas, despite its protected location, may also be injured. Contusion or laceration may cause extravasation of pancreatic juice with resulting pancreatitis and pseudocyst formation. Elevation of serum amylase is a usual accompaniment of such injuries. Tears in the mesentery and blowout injuries of the small intestine occur. The most frequent site of intestinal injury is at the duodenojejunal juncture. Renal injuries are seen with all types of abdominal trauma, but for some reason are particularly common in football players. A distended bladder may be ruptured by a seat belt or kick, so also may a gravid uterus. Fractures of the pelvis may cause secondary lacerations of the bladder or urethra. Displaced fractures of the pelvis are prone to tear large pelvic veins with resultant potentially exsanguinating hemorrhage.

When intra-abdominal injury is suspected, but the indications for abdominal exploration are not clear, aspiration is useful. A small midline incision below the umbilicus with insertion of a small peritoneal dialysis catheter is often preferred. Aspiration of blood that does not clot is a significant finding. If no aspirate is returned, isotonic saline is injected, aspirated, and examined microscopically for leukocytes, red cells, amylase, and bile.

Stab Wounds. The decision whether or not to perform surgical exploration of a stab wound is made primarily on the basis of signs of peritonitis or of bleeding. An abdominal tap with irrigation is a useful diagnostic supplement as well as exploration of the wound to determine whether the peritoneum has been entered. However, there is no universal agreement about the latter possible diagnostic procedure.

Gunshot Wounds. All gunshot wounds of the abdomen should be operated on. The extent of injury is related to the velocity of the missile; high-velocity missiles produce great tissue damage, while injury from low-velocity missiles is much less. Fortunately in civilian life the latter are most frequently seen. Holes in the small intestine are usually debrided and closed. Small puncture wound of the colon with minimal contamination may also be closed. More extensive injuries, however, as well as a greater degree of contamination or questionable viability of tissues are all indications for exteriorization.

HERNIA

A hernia is a protrusion of a viscus through the wall of the cavity that ordinarily confines it. Several terms are used to describe various types of hernias. A *reducible* hernia is one in which the contents may be returned entirely to the cavity that ordinarily contains them. This is not possible in an *irreducible* or *incarcerated* hernia, usually because of the development of adhesions between the contents and the hernial sac or between the visceral surfaces of the contents themselves. Incarcerated hernias can be either acute or chronic. A painful acutely incarcerated hernia should be suspected of being *strangulated* until proven otherwise by early operation. A strangulated hernia is one in which the blood supply of the viscus is interfered with so that gangrene ultimately results. A *congenital* hernia is one present at birth and is almost always inguinal or umbilical in type. An *acquired* hernia develops somewhat later in life.

Hernias are described also according to their location. The most common type of hernia is one in the *inguinal* region. It is more common in the male. There are two types, *direct* and *indirect*. An indirect hernia is one in which the sac opens at the internal inguinal ring and passes down the course of the inguinal canal anterior to the structures of the spermatic cord. The neck of the sac lies lateral to the inferior (deep) epigastric artery and vein. If sufficiently large, it then emerges through the external inguinal ring and may actually continue down along the cord into the scrotum. In the female the sac passes along the course of the round ligament of the uterus into the labium majus. The sac is the unobliterated processus vaginalis and follows the course of descent of the testicle and the round ligament.

A direct inguinal hernia is a protrusion directly through the posterior wall of the inguinal canal medial to the deep epigastric vessels. It may also present through the external inguinal ring and usually manifests itself as a rounded swelling of limited size, in contrast with the elongated tubular course of the indirect type. This type represents a bulging of all the structures of the abdominal wall, and, although it may present at the external ring, it does not descend into the scrotum. The direct inguinal hernia usually is seen in older men and is the result of a weakening of the fascial structures. Direct inguinal hernias do not occur in women because of the excellent support of the posterior wall of the inguinal canal.

A *femoral hernia* passes through the femoral canal. Therefore, the sac lies below Poupart's ligament, slightly lateral to the pubic tubercle and medial to the femoral vein, upon the pectineus muscle. The sac may present at the fossa ovalis and be directed upward over Poupart's ligament. In such cases it may be confused with an inguinal hernia. Also, it may be difficult at times to distinguish it from enlarged inguinal lymph nodes in that region.

An *umbilical* hernia is a defect in the region of the umbilicus. A small defect in this area is not uncommon, but usually it fills with scar tissue as the child develops, especially if the hernia is kept reduced by means of adhesive strapping or a truss. Umbilical hernias also are common in older women. In children especially, umbilical hernia often is associated with separation of the rectus muscles, known as diastasis of the recti. An *incisional* hernia occurs at the site of a previous operative wound and frequently is the result of postoperative infection. This is a type of ventral hernia.

There are various types of internal hernias in which the viscera protrude through openings within the abdominal cavity and, therefore, are not manifested externally. A protrusion through the obturator foramen, an *obturator* hernia, is an example of this type.

An *epigastric* hernia is a small nodular mass in the midline of the upper abdomen that results from protrusion of the preperitoneal fat along the course of a vessel penetrating the linea alba. These hernias contain no peritoneal sac.

A *diaphragmatic* hernia is a protrusion of abdominal contents upward through the diaphragm into the thorax. Almost always, these are left-sided, since the right side of the diaphragm is protected by the liver. They may be congenital or acquired. Trauma is the most frequent cause of the latter.

As a rule the diagnosis of hernia is made readily by the demonstration of a mass in one of the locations described. This mass often transmits an impulse on coughing or on straining. If reducible, the defect in the abdominal wall is demonstrable. Diaphragmatic hernia can be demonstrated by the finding of peristalsis in the thorax on auscultation, the roentgenographic demonstration of intestinal gas patterns or the presence of barium following the administration of a barium meal.

Incarceration and strangulation of hernias constitute surgical emergencies. A strangulated hernia, implying an interference with the blood supply of the contents of the sac, in addition presents a picture of constant severe pain and a tense, tender hernial sac. An attempt may be made to reduce such a hernia by placing the patient in a reclining position with the hips elevated and the knees and hips flexed. With the patient relaxed it may be possible to reduce the hernia by gentle manipulation. This procedure is known as taxis. In attempts to reduce an incarcerated or strangulated hernia, at times the mass is returned to the abdominal cavity en bloc or en masse; therefore, the trouble is not relieved, because the constricting ring of the neck of the hernial sac still imprisons the viscera.

In infants, indirect inguinal hernias are usually not associated with significant abnormalities in the musculoaponeurotic supporting structures. Removal of the patent processus vaginalis is sufficient to cure the hernia and simple closure of the wound in layers is all that is necessary. If the conjoined tendon is sutured to Poupart's ligament anterior to the spermatic cord, a *Ferguson herniorrhaphy* will have been done. When the internal inguinal ring is significantly stretched, a defect in the transversalis fascia of varying size will be present and reconstruction of the posterior wall of the inguinal canal will be necessary. The spermatic cord may be mobilized and the conjoined tendon sutured to Poupart's ligament posterior to the cord, constituting a *Bassini* repair. In large indirect inguinal hernias and in direct inguinal hernias the posterior wall of the inguinal canal is deficient. The *Halsted* herniorrhaphy corrects this by suturing both the conjoined tendon and external oblique aponeurosis posterior to the spermatic cord leaving the cord in a subcutaneous position. The preferred operation by many for large indirect inguinal hernias and direct inguinal hernias is the *McVay* repair. In this operation the transversus aponeurosis is sutured posterior to the cord to Cooper's ligament medially, and the transversalis fascia laterally. A relaxing incision in the rectus sheath is necessary to relieve tension on the suture line. The anterior preperitoneal approach of Henry is favored by some.

Esophagus and Diaphragm

CARCINOMA OF THE ESOPHAGUS

The manifestations of carcinoma of the esophagus are difficulty in swallowing and weight loss. Roentgenograms obtained during the ingestion of barium and direct esophagoscopic examination will usually establish the diagnosis. In some instances, patients with preexisting esophagitis develop cancer and the diagnosis is more difficult. It arises anywhere in the esophagus, but involvement of the lower third is most frequent. Early lymph node metastasis, not uncommonly at some distance from the primary tumor, limits curability. In the middle third, invasion of the carina of the trachea may accentuate pulmonary symptoms. Bronchoscopy is essential for the evaluation of lesions in this area. Esophageal carcinoma is usually a squamous-cell carcinoma, however, adenocarcinoma is frequently seen in the lower third. Squamous-cell carcinoma is treated with adjuvant chemotherapy, radiotherapy, and surgical resection. Adenocarcinoma is treated by surgical resection. Those patients with demonstrated distal metastasis are treated with dilatation and placement of an intraesophageal stent or occasionally by an intestinal bypass.

DIVERTICULUM OF THE ESOPHAGUS

Traction diverticula are usually not symptomatic. The most important pulsion diverticula are those arising at the pharyngoesophageal juncture. Regurgitation of undigested food, gurgling in the neck, and dysphagia are the usual symptoms. When visualized radiographically, they present in the left lower neck. Excision with closure of the mucosal and muscular defect is the recommended treatment. Cricopharyngeal myotomy should also be done.

Diaphragmatic Hernia

Hernias about the esophageal hiatus are of two types—the "sliding" and the paraesophageal. The former is an acquired widening of the right diaphragmatic crus associated with weakening of the esophageal attachments to the diaphragm, permitting the esophagocardiac junction to slide up and down with changes in posture and intra-abdominal pressure. Pressure studies show the presence of a functional lower esophageal sphincter that may become incompetent in the presence of a sliding type of hiatus hernia. In some instances it is incompetent in the absence of a hiatus hernia. When incompetence develops, reflux of gastric juice leads to esophagitis. Muscle spasm, ulceration, and scarring with stricture formation eventually result. Once a fixed stricture develops treatment is much more difficult; therefore, patients who do not respond promptly to medical therapy should be advised that operative treatment is indicated. The operations in greatest favor today are the Nissen fundoplication, Belsey Mark IV repair, or Hill repair. Each of these repairs produce satisfactory results, providing the technical details are carefully observed. When duodenal ulceration and gastric hypersecretion are present along with reflux esophagitis, control of hypersecretion is an essential part of the operative treatment.

The paraesophageal hiatal hernia produces symptoms due to entrapment of a portion or all of the stomach within the hernia sac. Operative repair is indicated to avoid these complications of bleeding, incarceration, and strangulation.

Subdiaphragmatic Abscess

An abscess in this location is secondary to infection elsewhere in the peritoneal cavity, such as acute appendicitis. Fever and leukocytosis persist. There may be discomfort in the region of the abscess, and tenderness usually can be elicited by pressure or jarring over the abscess. Pain may be referred to the shoulder. Fluoroscopic examination reveals limitation of movement and elevation of the diaphragm and a sterile pleural effusion.

The treatment for this disease is adequate drainage. This may be done in some instances by means of a catheter passed by a radiologist under ultrasound control. Should this not result in cure, open surgical drainage will then be necessary.

Stomach and Duodenum

GASTRIC ULCER

The etiology of benign gastric ulcer is not completely understood. Pyloric obstruction is a factor contributing to increased antral stimulation of gastrin, which in turn plays a part in the pathogenesis of benign gastric ulcer. Prepyloric ulcers have the same secretory pattern as duodenal ulcers. The resting level of acid production in most benign gastric ulcers is low, but in prepyloric as in duodenal ulcer the fasting level is increased. Acute gastric ulcers occur as complications of sepsis, burns, extensive fractures, and so forth. A relation to acid secretion is doubtful. Nevertheless, in vulnerable patients, constant neutralization with antacids has proved to be effective prophylaxis. Cimetidine, raniditine, or other H_2 receptor inhibitors may be less so.

The surgical treatment of gastric ulcer usually consists of partial gastrectomy with gastroduodenostomy or gastrojejunostomy. When pyloric obstruction is present, pyloroplasty or gastrojejunostomy may suffice. If the ulcer is not removed, four-quadrant biopsy is mandatory to exclude cancer. Prepyloric ulcers should be treated similarly to duodenal ulcer, as should other gastric ulcers in which fasting hyperacidity exists or in which a scar of active or healed duodenal ulcer is present. Acute gastric ulcer is usually manifested by massive hemorrhage. Treatment is directed toward control of hemorrhage and removal or healing of the ulcerative process. Many benign gastric ulcers will heal with conservative therapy, which is empirical inasmuch as the etiology is usually not clear-cut. The recurrence rate is high; this, along with the difficulty in differentiating benign gastric ulcer from ulcerating cancer, is a strong indication for surgical management.

GASTRIC CARCINOMA

Carcinoma of the stomach has decreased in frequency in the United States for reasons that are unclear. It occurs twice as often in men as it does in women. It usually appears at the age of 45 or beyond and is characterized by rather indefinite digestive symptoms—indigestion, malaise, lack of appetite, and so forth. As the disease progresses, it produces more marked symptoms—obstruction when the tumor becomes large enough to obstruct the pyloric end of the stomach, bleeding, anemia, and the presence of a mass in the epigastrium. Many patients with gastric carcinoma have pain that may be almost exactly like that of peptic ulceration. Carcinomatous ulcers may not be distinguishable from benign ulcers. The combined use of roentgenograms, gastric analysis, gastric cytology, and gastroscopy with biopsy increase diagnostic accuracy. In a good laboratory the frequency of false-positive reports on gastric cytology is practically zero. Neither the location of the ulcer nor roentgenographic criteria are as useful in diagnosis as formerly believed.

Surgery is the only known method of cure for carcinoma of the stomach. The prognosis usually is poor because the patients are referred for operation when complete removal of the tumor is no longer possible. The extent of the stomach to be removed depends upon the operative findings, but as a rule a very radical gastrectomy is performed, including also the areas of lymphatic extension; that is, the gastrohepatic and greater omentum and the lymphatic areas of drainage around the pylorus and around the left gastric vessels. Some authors believe that a total gastrectomy should be performed in all cases in which carcinoma is present or suspected. The principle behind this theory is the radical excision of the tumor, but there is no convincing evidence that such radical operation produces better results, and the morbidity associated with total gastrectomy is much greater than with subtotal resection of the stomach.

DUODENAL ULCER

Duodenal ulcer is generally associated with acid and pepsin hypersecretion, particularly in the interdigestive phase. With recurring exacerbations of the ulcer and healing, changes that produce organic complications may take place. Indications for surgical therapy are these symptoms: (1) bleeding; (2) obstruction of the pylorus; (3) intractability, that is, unsatisfactory response to medical treatment; and (4) perforation.

In the treatment of perforation of a duodenal ulcer, early operation with closure of the perforation or plugging of the perforation with an omental graft is indicated. It has been found that the results depend upon the lapse of time between perforation and the performance of surgery. Thus, those who are operated upon soon after perforation have an excellent prognosis, whereas those who have had a continuing leak over a period of 12 hours or more have generalized peritonitis and a less favorable prognosis. Patients with a prolonged history of ulcer disease prior to perforation may be treated by a definitive operation to control the ulcer diathesis, providing severe peritonitis is not present. In patients with few or no preceding symptoms, closure of the ulcer with an omental flap is the operation of choice. Conservative treatment of perforated ulcers is associated with a higher mortality risk than is operative treatment.

Because duodenal ulcers are believed to be the result of the action of the acid and pepsin of gastric juice upon the mucosa of the duodenum, operations have been proposed that would reduce the secretion of this juice in order to cure the ulcer. Some operations are designed to remove the factors that stimulate the production of gastric juice. One of these entails division of the vagus nerve (vagotomy), thereby blocking the impulses that produce the nervous phase of the stimulation of gastric juice. Another consists of removal of the gastric antrum, which is the area of the stomach in which the acid-stimulating hormone gastrin is produced. Other operations may remove not only the antrum but also a fairly generous portion of the body of the stomach. In such a case, not only is the hormonal stimulating area (antrum) removed but also a large part of the stomach—that part in which the cells that produce gastric acid juice are located. These various factors that are concerned with the production of acid gastric juice may be combined in a single operation. Thus, the vagus nerve may be divided and partial gastrectomy performed.

In those operations in which the vagus nerve is divided, some form of drainage of the stomach must be provided, because the vagus nerve not only influences the secretion of gastric juice in the stomach but also serves as the motor nerve to the stomach.

Heineke-Mikulicz pyloroplasty, Finney pyloroplasty, and Jaboulay pyloroplasty are all used as drainage procedures, as is gastrojejunostomy. If gastrojejunostomy is undertaken it should be placed close to the pylorus in order to provide good drainage of the antrum.

Highly selective (or parietal cell) vagotomy is under investigation at present. Since it spares the innervation of the pylorus (nerves of Latarjet) a drainage procedure is unnecessary. It is hoped that this operation will result in minimal disturbance of gastric physiology while controlling the ulcer diathesis. At present, the early excellent results of this procedure appear to be sustained. If this proves to be correct on further follow-up, highly selective vagotomy will supplant other operations that are all associated with physiologic deficits that are undesirable.

The operation that has been most effective, in that the rate of recurrence of ulcers is lowest after it, is truncal vagotomy with antrectomy. Subtotal gastrectomy is no longer justifiable.

Operations that ablate the pyloric mechanism may lead to the *dumping syndrome*. This syndrome is characterized by a feeling of faintness, sweating, palpitations, and nausea coming on during or shortly after the ingestion of food. The cause appears to be related to the rapid passage of hyperosmolar liquids into the duodenum or jejunum. Fluid passes from the vascular compartment into the intestinal lumen. The symptoms result from distention of the intestine and reduction in plasma volume. Hypoglycemia is seen in certain patients but not until some time later. Treatment is directed at reducing the hyperosmolarity of the material leaving the stomach; fat is increased, carbohydrate decreased, and liquids are given between meals. This syndrome was seen in severe form more frequently when radical subtotal gastrectomy was the operation of choice. It leads to crippling nutritional depletion, so every effort should be made to avoid it by the selection of operations that are less likely to produce it.

STRESS ULCER

Stress ulcer refers to acute gastroduodenal ulceration that occurs after shock, sepsis, complicated operations, burns, serious fractures, and head injuries. The etiology is uncertain, but gastric hypersecretion is not present. Ischemia appears to play a part, but back diffusion of hydrochloric acid has also been incriminated. In spite of the apparent decrease in hydrochloric acid secretion, prophylaxis with antacids and, to a lesser extent, the H_2 receptor inhibitors cimetidine and ranitidine has been effective in reducing the frequency of this complication.

Gallbladder and Bile Ducts

CHOLELITHIASIS

Calculus cholecystitis is a chronic disease, frequently subject to acute exacerbations, known as *biliary colic*. This disease usually occurs during middle life and is more common in females than males. It often follows pregnancy. Stasis and infection probably predispose to gallstone formation, but probably of greater importance are abnormalities in the composition of bile. Most important is maintenance of a normal ratio between bile salts and phospholipid (lecithin) and cholesterol. An increase in cholesterol or a reduction in the bile salt pool is a potential cause of a derangement in this association. The bile salt pool can be reduced by resection or bypass operations on the ileum. The type of bile salt is important since lithocholate is insoluble and deoxycholate is soluble. In experimental studies in which chenodeoxycholate has been fed to patients with asymptomatic stones there has been evidence of decrease in size and disappearance of stones after prolonged feeding.

CHOLECYSTITIS

Acute Cholecystitis. If a stone obstructs the cystic duct, an attack of acute biliary colic results. In general, these attacks occur at night and are more likely to follow a dietary indiscretion, such as overeating. The pain is severe and is present in the epigastrium or the right upper quadrant. However, in addition, it frequently radiates to the back, the scapular region, or the right shoulder. Nausea and vomiting are common. During the attack, in most cases, tenderness occurs in the region of the gallbladder, and there is some muscle guarding. As a rule these attacks subside in a few hours with the aid of analgesics and atropine or similar drugs. Residual soreness in the region of the gallbladder often persists for 1 or 2 days after the attack has subsided.

Although these acute attacks may subside, not infrequently the stone becomes so impacted in the cystic duct that it cannot be released spontaneously. In addition to the factor of obstruction, bacterial infection sets in, with marked fever and leukocytosis. Frank pus forms in the gallbladder, and eventually gangrene of the gallbladder wall occurs. However, this process is much slower than such a development in acute appendicitis. Unless operative intervention is resorted to, perforation of the gallbladder may take place, with the development of peritonitis, either spreading or localized. Occasionally the perforation takes place into an adjacent viscus, such as the stomach, the duodenum, or the colon, with a resulting internal biliary fistula.

The following conditions must be considered in differential diagnosis: (1) acute appendicitis, (2) perforated peptic ulcer, (3) acute pancreatitis, (4) renal colic or pyelitis, (5) pneumonia, (6) coronary artery occlusion, and (7) salpingitis.

Chronic Cholecystitis. During the intervals between the acute exacerbations there may be no symptoms at all, or a sense of fullness and distention in the upper abdomen may be present, with a tendency toward belching. There may actually be some epigastric distress. These symptoms usually occur after large meals or ones containing fatty foods.

During the acute episode, the finding of gallstones and a dilated gallbladder on ultrasound evaluation is confirmatory evidence of acute cholecystitis; however, all of the previously mentioned diagnoses can occur in a patient with asymptomatic gallstones. Oral cholecystography continues to be an effective diagnostic test for the presence of gallstones. This test should be performed during a quiescent period, usually 6 weeks after an acute attack.

The ideal treatment consists of cholecystectomy as an elective procedure between attacks of acute biliary colic. Should an attack of colic fail to subside promptly with administration of narcotics and atropine, continuous gastric suction drainage and intravenous fluids, operation is indicated. Occasionally, because of obliteration of normal anatomic planes, the best procedure will be cholecystostomy, though usually it is possible to remove the gallbladder even during an acute attack.

COMMON DUCT OBSTRUCTION

If a stone reaches the common duct and is unable to pass the ampulla of Vater, obstructive jaundice results. There may be upper abdominal distress, nausea, and vomiting, or the patient may present little in the way of symptoms aside from icterus. However, there frequently is associated infection, with chills and fever. The stools become clay colored as the result of the absence of bile pigments, and the urine is very dark. The direct van den Bergh reaction is immediate. The degree of jaundice may be measured either by the indirect van den Bergh determination or by the icterus index. Bilirubin and bile salts appear in the urine.

In prolonged jaundice the prothrombin level falls, and hemorrhagic tendencies develop. This results from failure of absorption of vitamin K from the intestinal tract, because this vitamin requires the presence of bile salts for absorption. In preparing these patients for operation, it is necessary to make repeated determinations of the prothrombin level and to supply vitamin K parenterally or to administer it by mouth in conjunction with bile salts, so as to provide for its absorption. In addition, the hepatic damage associated with jaundice should be combated by providing these patients with a high-calorie, high-protein, high-carbohydrate, and high-vitamin diet that is low in fat content. Treatment consists of choledochostomy and removal of the stones. Ordinarily the gallbladder also is removed at this time. Prior to removal of the drainage tube, patency of the ductal system should be demonstrated by means of a cholangiogram.

Frequently a common duct stone has a ball-valve-like action, producing bouts of fever, chills, and jaundice (Charcot's intermittent hepatic fever). A progressive relentless jaundice should suggest the possibility of carcinoma, primary in the ductal system or in the head of the pancreas.

When cholecystectomy is performed, the status of the common bile duct with regard to the presence of stones or tumor must be clarified. The duct is exposed and carefully palpated. Operative cholangiography should be considered an essential part of the operation. The pancreas is also gently palpated. If the common bile duct is dilated, the pancreas is abnormal, there is a history of jaundice, and particularly if stones are seen or felt, the common bile duct must be opened and explored. Inspection of the interior of the bile duct with either the flexible or the rigid choledochoscope is an essential feature of such exploration. When the common bile duct contains sludge or if stones in hepatic ducts cannot be removed, sphincteroplasty should be considered. Occasionally a common duct drainage procedure will be necessary, either a choledochojejunostomy or choledochoduodenostomy.

Tumors within the common duct will require resection (pancreatoduodenectomy) or bypass operation. Biopsy should be taken, if feasible, particularly if resection will *not* be done.

Pancreas

ACUTE PANCREATITIS

Though the etiology of this condition is not understood clearly, it often has been surmised that it results from reflux of bile into the pancreatic ducts, with resultant activation of the pancreatic enzymes and subsequent autodigestion of this organ. Others believe that the significant factors in the etiology of acute pancreatitis are obstruction of the pancreatic duct and the presence of an actively secreting gland. The obstruction may occur at the ampulla because of edema or a common duct calculus when there is a "common channel" shared by the common and the pancreatic ducts.

This disease manifests itself by the sudden onset of severe upper abdominal pain, commonly associated with nausea and vomiting. The pain may be referred to the back. On examination one finds tenderness and muscle guarding over the region of the pancreas; if the disease progresses, these findings become more diffuse, and generalized distention sets in. There is a moderate febrile response, frequently with tachycardia that is out of proportion to the temperature elevation. Polymorphonuclear leukocytosis is present. However, the distinctive laboratory finding in this disease is the prompt elevation of the serum amylase and lipase levels. These values usually show a definite increase within a few hours of the onset of the disease, and though the former may return to normal after 24 hours, the latter usually is elevated for several days.

There are two distinct types of acute pancreatitis that are of great importance, because the prognosis is so different in the two. The first is known as the *acute edematous or interstitial type.* This is marked by an intense edema of the retroperitoneal tissues in the region of the pancreas. There is an outpouring of free peritoneal fluid, which is bile tinged and at times somewhat hemorrhagic in character. There are yellowish white areas of fat necrosis, most marked in the region of the pancreas. This condition is usually a mild self-limited disease and carries with it a low mortality. However, in contrast, acute *hemorrhagic or necrotizing pancreatitis* is marked by areas of frank hemorrhage and necrosis that frequently destroy almost the entire pancreas. This type is extremely serious and carries with it a high mortality.

In the milder cases, if one can rule out a catastrophe such as perforated peptic ulcer, conservative treatment is justified. This includes the use of a nasogastric tube with continuous suction drainage, intravenous fluids, and supportive measures, such as transfusions. On the other hand, in the more severe cases, or in those in which the diagnosis cannot be made with certainty, surgical exploration is justified. The purpose of operation is first to confirm or refute the diagnosis, secondarily, if bile-tinged hemorrhagic peritoneal fluid is present, cholecystostomy should be done and the lesser peritoneal sac should be drained.

The operative measures used in patients with *chronic pancreatitis* are directed toward correction of the specific etiologic factors involved. Since there is a high incidence of related gallbladder or common duct stones, or both, cholecystectomy and removal of stones from the common duct may give relief. Transduodenal sphincterotomy is done if the sphincter of Oddi is spastic or fibrotic. If the pancreatic duct is obstructed close to the sphincter and is otherwise normal, caudal pancreaticojejunostomy should be considered. When multiple points of obstruction of the duct of Wirsung produce the "chain-of-lakes" appearance, lateral pancreaticojejunostomy may give relief. It may be easier, as well as more effective, to carry out 95% pancreatectomy.

CYSTS

Three types of pancreatic cysts are seen: (1) congenital, (2) pseudocysts, and (3) neoplastic. Of these the pseudocyst is most common. Congenital cysts are of little clinical importance except when they are multiple and part of the systemic disease, cystic fibrosis. Pseudocysts follow leakage from a disrupted major pancreatic duct in which the secretory products become walled off. This is caused by blunt or penetrating injuries or acute necrotizing pancreatitis. Cysts without a persistent communication with the pancreatic ductal system can be cured by simple drainage. These are infrequent, however, and a more reliable method of management is drainage to the stomach or jejunum by cystogastrostomy or Roux-en-Y cystojejunostomy.

CARCINOMA OF THE PANCREAS

Usually the head is involved in pancreatic carcinoma. Unfortunately, there are few symptoms early in this disease. However, as it progresses to involve the region of the common duct, obstructive jaundice sets in, is usually relentless, and gradually increases in intensity. The stools become acholic, and the urine is dark. Frequently, the icterus is associated with extreme itching that is almost intolerable and may be the most distressing feature of the disease. Other symptoms include vague indigestion, nausea, vomiting, weight loss, and, eventually, cachexia.

Epigastric discomfort often is present, but severe pain is not ordinarily a feature early in this disease. The differential diagnoses include carcinoma of the ampulla of Vater, ductal carcinoma, calculous common duct obstruction, and hepatitis. The usual roentgenograms are seldom diagnostic, although widening of the duodenal loop, straightening of the descending duodenum, and the "reversed-three" signs are suggestive. Newer procedures include endoscopic retrograde pancreatogram, hypotonic duodenography, and selective angiography. A distended gallbladder in the presence of obstructive jaundice suggests carcinoma of the head of the pancreas, whereas a contracted gallbladder suggests calculous common duct obstruction (Courvoisier's law).

Carcinoma arising in the body or tail of the pancreas is usually asymptomatic until invasion of somatic nerve fibers leads to pain. The pain is nonspecific in character and the usual roentgenograms and laboratory studies are negative, leading to prolonged delays in diagnosis. Selective angiography will frequently show encasement of vessels with irregularity of contour and size. Ultrasonography and computerized tomography may outline a mass. With newer techniques the diagnosis may be suspected earlier, leading to exploratory operation, but it is unlikely that many such tumors will be found to be surgically resectable.

ISLET CELL ADENOMA

These tumors are derived from β-cells that are responsible for insulin secretion. They become manifest by virtue of hyperinsulinism provoked by fasting. Together they explain ***Whipple's triad***. This includes (1) central nervous system symptoms of weakness, nervousness, alterations in mood or personality, and at times convulsions and coma; (2) blood sugar of 50 mg (or less)/100 ml; and (3) prompt relief of symptoms following oral glucose or its administration by vein. The tumors are too small to be felt on physical examination and can easily be missed by palpation at the time of operation. The injection of contrast material into pancreatic arteries may show a tumor blush, but in many instances angiographic study is negative so it cannot be relied upon. The lesions may be multiple, and hyperplastic β-cells may be present throughout the pancreas (nesidioblastosis). The diagnosis is confirmed by determination of plasma insulin levels by radioimmu-

noassay in the fasting state. The tolbutamide tolerance test is also of value.

Treatment consists of removal of the adenoma or adenomas. Most lie in the body and tail of the pancreas. Mobilization of the gland facilitates palpation. If no discrete tumor is found, the surgeon may resort to near-total pancreatectomy. The results in this situation are variable, but not as good as when an adenoma is found. Insulinomas may be malignant.

ULCEROGENIC TUMORS (NON-BETA-CELL TUMORS, ZOLLINGER-ELLISON SYNDROME)

Some tumors of the pancreatic islets are associated with the secretion of a gastrinlike substance that induces maximal and continued secretion of hydrochloric acid by the stomach. This results in ulcers of the stomach and duodenum that are atypical in location and refractory to the usual medical and surgical methods of treatment. Diarrhea is a frequent associated symptom. The most important laboratory procedure for substantiation of the diagnosis is the finding of elevated levels of gastrin in the serum as determined by the radioimmunoassay technique. At times calcium infusion or secretin stimulation will be necessary to bring out the presence of increased gastrin secretion. Gastric analysis shows increased volume and acidity without further increase when histamine is given. The tumors may be benign or malignant, but the most important feature of surgical treatment is total gastrectomy. Solitary and resectable tumors should be removed, but this is rarely a substitute for total gastrectomy. Surprisingly regression of metastases has followed total gastrectomy and the subsequent nutritional state remains very good. In some children growth and development have been perfectly normal after total gastrectomy for the Zollinger-Ellison syndrome, even though metastases to liver were present.

Another syndrome caused by secretion of a humoral agent by a pancreatic tumor consists of watery diarrhea, hypokalemia, and gastric hypochlorhydria or achlorhydria (WDHA syndrome or pancreatic cholera). The active agent appears to be vasoactive intestinal peptide. Removal of the pancreatic tumor is curative.

Spleen

INDICATIONS FOR SPLENECTOMY

Rupture of the Spleen. This injury results either from a fall from a height, the individual landing on his or her feet or buttocks, or from direct trauma to the region of the spleen, as in an automobile accident. The patient complains of severe left upper quadrant pain, frequently with reference to the left shoulder. There are tenderness and muscle guarding in the left upper quadrant, and shifting dullness may be demonstrable. Leukocytosis is promptly evoked. If the bleeding is severe, a shocklike picture results. Abdominal paracentesis should demonstrate blood in the peritoneal cavity. Scanning the spleen using 99m technetium sulfur colloid is a useful diagnostic procedure; it is of particular help in instances of subcapsular bleeding as is computed tomography (CT) scan with the use of concurrently administered contrast agents. Angiography is also of value.

Treatment consists of surgical exploration as promptly as possible. Splenectomy, formerly routine surgical treatment is now avoided, whenever possible, particularly in children. This change is the result of the increased incidence of rapidly fatal infection by encapsulated bacteria, especially pneumococcus following splenectomy. If a splenectomy is necessary in childhood, pneumococcal vaccine should be used as prophylaxis against infection. Prophylactic antibiotics are advised for children and others at high risk. Large amounts of blood should be available for transfusion during operation in order to maintain the patient in satisfactory condition.

The most common indication for splenectomy today is trauma.

Congenital Hemolytic Icterus. This disease is due to a congenital tendency to form abnormally shaped red blood cells (spherocytes) that are more fragile than normal. The spleen filters out and destroys these abnormal cells, producing a hemolytic type of jaundice. Occasionally, the hemolyzed pigments are excreted in the bile in sufficient quantity to form pigment stones in the common bile duct; splenectomy is curative.

Idiopathic Thrombocytopenic Purpura. This is a bleeding tendency characterized by a low platelet count and prolonged bleeding time. Bleeding may occur into the skin, the kidneys, the gastrointestinal tract, or the brain. In children, idiopathic thrombocytopenic purpura usually is an acute self-limited process that responds promptly to corticosteroids. In adults it follows a chronic course, with frequent remissions and exacerbations. In the absence of a response to corticosteroids splenectomy is indicated. It is also indicated when, after a satisfactory response, it is impossible to withdraw corticosteroids without an exacerbation. This is true re-

gardless of age, although the need arises more frequently in adults than in children.

Hypersplenism. Enlarged spleens occasionally are hyperactive, causing a decrease in one or all of the cellular blood elements. When there is associated active bone marrow, splenectomy may be of benefit.

Other Indications. Tumors or cysts of the spleen are uncommon but may cause pressure symptoms and should be removed.

Liver

PORTAL HYPERTENSION

Increased pressure in the portal bed may result from an intrahepatic (cirrhosis) or an extrahepatic (thrombosis of the portal or splenic vein) block. Naturally occurring collateral venous channels between the portal circulation and the inferior vena cava proximal to the liver form as nature's effort to bypass the block. Peptic erosion, or rupture of such collateral veins in the esophagus, gives rise to serious gastrointestinal hemorrhage, with death following rapidly if the hemorrhage is not controlled. Emergency treatment consists of control of hemorrhage by esophageal balloon tamponade. During this time studies of hepatic function are carried out. The tendency today is to carry out portacaval shunt or a distal splenorenal shunt early in the course of bleeding from varices resulting from hepatic outflow block of cirrhosis. Extrahepatic portal bed block frequently occurs in childhood; if conservative measures fail, endoscopic sclerotherapy is a useful temporizing measure. Splenorenal shunt is not possible until growth has progressed to the point at which a splenic vein has developed of sufficient size to effectively decompress the portal bed when anastomosed to the renal vein. If splenectomy has already been done, a shunt should be created between the vena cava and superior mesenteric veins either by end-to-side anastomosis between the inferior vena cava and the superior mesenteric vein or by use of a so-called H graft using a Dacron prosthesis between the same vessels.

An alternate shunting procedure is the Warren operation of central splenorenal shunt in which the spleen is left in place, and the central end of the divided splenic vein is anastomosed to the renal vein. The operation is technically difficult, but Warren reports satisfactory reduction in portal pressure without the usual deleterious effect of portal-systemic shunting.

Another complication of increased portal pressure is splenomegaly and hypersplenism. When there is appreciable depression of the cellular elements of the blood despite active bone marrow, splenectomy and splenorenal shunt are indicated.

Intestines

INTESTINAL OBSTRUCTION

Intestinal obstruction may be either mechanical (dynamic) or paralytic (adynamic). Mechanical obstruction results from any factor, extrinsic or intrinsic, that encroaches on the lumen of the bowel. These factors include tumors, adhesions, hernias, volvulus, and intussusception; the obstruction may be either partial or complete. The patient suffers intermittent crampy abdominal pain. Peristalsis is visible and audible, and the crampy pain may be correlated with bouts of borborygmus. On auscultation, peristalsis is heard in rushes, and the note frequently is high pitched, metallic, and tinkling. Distention is evident. Vomiting is frequent, and the vomitus actually may be intestinal in character. As a result of repeated vomiting, dehydration, electrolyte deficits, and alterations in acid–base balance may be present. A survey film of the abdomen reveals distention. If the film is taken with the patient in the erect or lateral recumbent position, it reveals air and fluid levels in the gut (stepladder pattern). Constant severe pain in contrast to simple intermittent crampy pains should suggest strangulation of the bowel.

When the diagnosis of mechanical obstruction of the small intestine is made, the patient should be prepared for operation. A tube is inserted into the stomach, and continuous suction is begun. An intravenous infusion of isotonic sodium chloride or Ringer's lactate solution and 5% glucose is begun. The urine output is monitored and should reach a minimum of 25 ml/hour with a falling specific gravity before operation is performed. Ketosis, if present, should be corrected. At operation the obstructive mechanism is determined and relieved. If necrotic bowel is found, it must be removed. Primary anastomosis is desirable, but operative decompression of distended small intestine is essential if a primary anastomosis is done. If the bowel is decompressed without intestinal resection, it is best done without opening the intestine, thereby greatly decreasing the risk of infection. Closed decompression is accomplished by the passage of the Leonard tube (a special long rubber tube containing a coiled spring to facilitate its passage). If this is not available, a long rubber tube with a condom containing mercury at the end is passed by way of a jejunostomy.

During the course of colonic obstruction by a carcinoma, the intraluminal pressure rises gradually. Under these conditions the ileocecal valve usually remains competent. As the intraluminal pressure rises, the tension on the wall of the segment with the largest diameter is greatest. Capillary and venous blood flow are reduced until necrosis occurs with catastrophic results unless prevented by surgical decompression. Transverse colostomy is recommended if the obstructing lesion is distal to the right colon. Because of dissatisfaction with cecostomy or right-sided colostomy most right-colon obstruction lesions are treated with primary resection.

Adynamic (paralytic) ileus results from reflex loss of tone and peristalsis of the muscle of the intestinal tract. It occurs, to greater or lesser degrees, following intraperitoneal operations depending on the degree of trauma from handling, heat, drying, and so forth. It may also result from compression fractures of the spine, retroperitoneal hematoma formation, renal calculi, pneumonia, or certain drugs that inhibit parasympathetic function. Hypokalemia also may produce adynamic ileus. In contrast to mechanical obstruction, no peristaltic sounds are heard on auscultation. Painless distention is present, but vomiting soon develops and reoccurs until recovery.

APPENDICITIS

Acute inflammation of the vermiform appendix is caused most frequently by obstruction of the lumen, usually by a fecalith and occasionally by kinking. A short closed-loop obstruction leads to rising intraluminal pressure, erosion of the lining, inflammation, and, unless the obstruction is spontaneously relieved, perforation. Epidemic appendicitis has been reported in institutionalized children, presumably by inflammatory swelling of the lymphoid tissue in the mucosa, caused by a microorganism, possibly a streptococcus.

Perforation of the appendix will lead to peritonitis either with localized abscess formation or with generalized peritonitis. Bacterial culture will demonstrate a mixed infection with both gram-positive and gram-negative bacteria.

The first symptom of this disease is poorly localized abdominal discomfort. Frequently the patient feels that a good bowel movement will relieve the distress, but neither passage of flatus nor stool gives relief. Anorexia, nausea, and vomiting soon follow. The pain increases in intensity and becomes localized when the inflammatory process involves the parietal peritoneum. The temperature is seldom over 100° F until peritonitis develops. The leukocyte count rises, and there is a shift to the left of the differential leukocyte count. On physical examination, the most important finding is localized tenderness. Muscle spasm may be prominent when the anterior abdominal wall is involved, but both tenderness and increased muscle tone may be difficult to demonstrate when the appendix lies retrocecally. When the appendix lies in the pelvis or with pelvic peritonitis, tenderness on rectal examination will also be found.

Perforation of the appendix most frequently is followed by localized abscess formation in the right iliac fossa or pelvis. Less frequently, an abscess can occur in the right subphrenic space. Neglected abscesses may result in secondary perforation with involvement of the general peritoneal cavity. Complicated appendicitis is associated with an increased mortality and is most frequently seen in the elderly or in children under 5 years of age.

Other complications of acute appendicitis are intestinal obstruction and septic pyelophlebitis. The latter may lead to liver abscess formation, usually multiple. The mortality rate is high in the latter event.

The differential diagnosis should include acute mesenteric adenitis, bleeding graafian follicle, acute gastroenteritis, acute diverticulitis involving the sigmoid or Meckel's diverticulum, renal colic, pyelitis, biliary colic, perforated peptic ulcer, salpingitis, and pneumonia.

Though many cases of acute appendicitis no doubt subside spontaneously, the mortality in delayed treatment is extremely high, and that of prompt operation is minimal. Operation should be undertaken within the first few hours of the onset of the disease. If perforation has already taken place, and an abscess is present, nothing more than simple drainage may be feasible at the time of operation. Following such a procedure, a regimen for postoperative peritonitis should be followed, including continuous gastric suction drainage and intravenous fluids. Antibiotic therapy has greatly reduced the mortality in such cases.

Recurrent or chronic appendicitis is a term that should be reserved for cases of intermittent appendiceal colic, resulting in most cases from a fecalith that intermittently obstructs the appendiceal lumen. Not infrequently, one such attack fails to subside spontaneously and goes on to the typical changes described above with secondary bacterial invasion. When the diagnosis of recurrent appendicitis can be made with reasonable certainty, interval appendectomy is warranted.

POLYPOSIS OF THE INTESTINAL TRACT

Familial Polyposis. This disease is characterized by innumerable polyps of the colon and rectum and is inherited as a Mendelian dominant. The polyps usually appear at puberty and cause bleeding from the rectum, diarrhea, tenesmus, or, less commonly, intestinal obstruction. The most serious complication is malignant change in the polyps. Most untreated patients die before the age of 50 from carcinoma of the colon. Treatment consists of colectomy and ileoproctostomy, or total colectomy and ileostomy.

Gardner's Syndrome. This is a variant of familial polyposis, also inherited as a Mendelian dominant, that is associated with osteomas of the skull, multiple sebaceous cysts of the scalp, and desmoid tumors. It involves both large and small intestines, and lesions of the second portion of the duodenum close to the ampulla of Vater have been reported with some frequency. The age at which it is expressed is earlier than polyposis coli, but it also has an inexorable tendency toward malignant change.

Peutz-Jegher's Syndrome. This is a familial disease in which there is an association between hamartomatous polyps of the gastrointestinal tract and pigmented spots on the lips, buccal mucosa, and hands. These polyps do not undergo malignant change. The small intestine contains more polyps than other portions of the gastrointestinal tract, but the entire tract may be involved. Symptoms arise from intussusception, which may spontaneously reduce or progress to intestinal obstruction.

Nonfamilial Polyps of the Colon. Nonfamilial adenomatous polyps of the colon may be single or multiple, pedunculated, or sessile. Whether benign polyps undergo malignant change remains conjectural, but both benign and malignant polyps occur. There is a correlation between size and malignancy; for example, pedunculated polyps less than 1 cm in diameter have nearly a zero frequency, whereas the likelihood of a polyp 4 cm or more in diameter being malignant is nearly 30%.

The villous adenoma (papillary adenoma) is a polyp of glandular origin with a great tendency to undergo malignant change. Larger lesions may be associated with significant losses of water, sodium, and potassium.

Juvenile polyps, as the name implies, are lesions seen predominantly in the first decade of life. They are hamartomas and are not associated with cancer. The presenting symptoms are bleeding and, less frequently, abdominal pain.

MALIGNANT TUMORS OF THE SMALL INTESTINE

Cancer of the small intestine is rare. It is manifested by bleeding or obstruction, or both. Adenocarcinoma tends to encircle and obstruct the bowel. Smooth muscle tumors are bulky and polypoid with central ulceration, which gives rise to bleeding. Carcinoid tumors in the small intestine metastasize with greater frequency than carcinoids elsewhere in the alimentary tract; they also give rise to obstruction.

Carcinoid Syndrome. A symptom complex consisting of episodic flushing of the skin, abdominal cramps, diarrhea, and asthma, carcinoid syndrome is caused by a serotonin-secreting argentaffin tumor that has metastasized to the liver. The primary growth is located most commonly in the gastrointestinal tract, particularly in the distal ileum. The benign, nonfunctioning carcinoid tumor occurs preponderantly in the appendix. The diagnosis of a functioning carcinoid tumor is made by the detection of abnormal amounts of the breakdown product of serotonin (5-hydroxyindoleacetic acid) in the urine. Surgical excision of the primary lesion is indicated. Carcinoid tumors of the tracheobronchial tree can also cause the carcinoid syndrome.

CARCINOMA OF THE COLON AND RECTUM

The large intestine is a frequent site of carcinoma. The type of lesion and the symptoms differ greatly on the two sides of the colon. In the left side of the colon a constricting ringlike lesion is found. Associated with it are symptoms of mechanical obstruction, including alternating constipation and diarrhea, crampy abdominal pain, and distention of the bowel. Blood may be noticed in the stools, and sometimes there is alteration in their caliber as the result of the constriction. On the other hand, in the right side of the colon the lesions are bulky and cauliflowerlike in nature and are less likely to encircle the bowel. In addition, the liquid character of the fecal material on this side also diminishes the likelihood of obstructive symptoms. In this region blood loss is marked, and a profound anemia develops. This and the associated weakness may be the earliest symptoms of the disease in this area.

There may be some discomfort in the region, and a mass may be palpable.

Carcinoma of the rectum presents symptoms that resemble more closely those of carcinoma of the left side of the colon. The change in caliber of the stools, alternating diarrhea and constipation, loss of blood and mucus, and tenesmus all should suggest this lesion. Carcinoma of the rectum and the sigmoid comprises the largest percentage of neoplasms in the large bowel. However, in recent years the frequency of carcinomas of the right side of the colon has been steadily increasing. Digital examination of the rectum and sigmoidoscopic examination remain important in diagnosis. The rigid instrument should probably be used only for examination of the rectum itself and appropriate biopsy of lesions therein. The flexible sigmoidoscope is practical for regular office use. The bowel is prepared with two commercially prepared disposable enema kits with good cleansing and the procedure can be expeditiously performed. Barium and air-contrast x-ray studies continue to play an important role in the diagnosis of colonic disease, but their diagnostic accuracy is greatly enhanced by the flexible colonoscope. In the hands of those suitably trained in its use it is a safe and accurate examination. The entire colon can be inspected, biopsies can be performed, and pedunculated polyps up to 5 cm in diameter may be removed. Its use has also been important in the evaluation of inflammatory bowel disease.

Carcinoma of the colon and rectum are treated primarily by surgical removal. The prognosis to a great extent is dependent upon the stage of the disease at the time of treatment. Dukes' classification, as modified by Astwood and Coller, is the one in general use. It is as follows: stage A, invasion to the muscularis; stage B, invasion to the serosa; stage B_2, invasion of pericolonic fat, no lymph node metastases; stage C, invasion to the serosa, lymph node metastases present; and stage C_2, invasion of pericolonic fat, lymph node metastases present.

While cancer of the colon is moderately radioresponsive it is not, with few exceptions, radiocurable. Preoperative radiation therapy has been studied in cancer of the rectum. The results vary between different series, but significant reduction in size is usually possible, thereby facilitating operation for large cancers.

Below the pectinate line the epithelium becomes squamous in character. Therefore, carcinoma occurring in the anal canal or the anus is a squamous-cell lesion, in contrast to adenocarcinoma of the bowel. Carcinoma in this area manifests itself as a persistent ulcer. Diagnosis is established readily by biopsy. Both wide surgical excision and radiation therapy have been used in the treatment of this lesion, but surgical removal is preferable. Metastases involve the inguinal lymph nodes as well as inferior mesenteric and hypogastric lymph nodes.

DIVERTICULAR DISEASE OF THE COLON

In older persons diverticula of the large intestine are very common. They occur most often in the region of the sigmoid and the descending colon but may appear anywhere in the colon. Though frequently asymptomatic, they may undergo acute inflammatory changes, giving rise to pain, fever, leukocytosis, tenderness, and a mass. The inflammatory change in the bowel wall may be sufficient to encroach on its lumen and result in partial obstruction. In some ways the clinical picture resembles that presented by malignant disease in this area. A barium enema demonstrates the irregular constricted lesion. The roentgenologist may or may not be able to establish the nature of the constricting lesion, and, indeed, carcinoma and diverticulitis may coexist.

Mild cases of acute diverticulitis may respond to conservative treatment consisting of rest of the intestinal tract, parenteral fluids, and antispasmodic drugs such as atropine and phenobarbitol. Antimicrobial agents are also of value in limiting the infection. If the process subsides completely, nothing more need be done. However, recurrent bouts of diverticulitis should lead to resection of the involved area. Frequently, diverticulitis progresses to the point of perforation with the development of a localized abscess. If the abscess forms in the mesentery, resection and anastomosis are feasible and preferable to drainage. Abscesses other than these will require adequate drainage and proximal colostomy. Resection will subsequently be necessary. Perforation into adjacent viscera, including bladder, small intestine and vagina, leads to fistula formation. This is also an indication for surgical resection.

Hemorrhage from diverticulosis occasionally occurs. This appears most often in the hypertensive older patient. Bleeding from the rectum in profuse amounts is the outstanding symptom.

Selective angiography of the superior and inferior mesenteric arteries is most useful in delineating the site of bleeding. Although diverticula are more frequent in the sigmoid, massive bleeding is frequent from lesions on the right side. For this reason total colectomy and ileorectostomy may be necessary.

In those patients with chronic gastrointestinal blood loss and in whom lesions can be demonstrated by angiography, segmental colon resections can be performed. However, bleeding is likely to recur from failure to recognize preexisting lesions or the development of new lesions. Utilizing the flexible colonoscopy and either electrocoagulation or photocoagulation these lesions can be obliterated nonoperatively, and improved results are being obtained.

ULCERATIVE COLITIS

Ulcerative colitis is a chronic disease subject to acute exacerbations. The etiology is unknown, though the disease appears to be more common in nervous, high-strung individuals. Relapses may be related to periods of emotional upset or nervous tension.

The disease is marked by diarrhea containing blood, pus, and mucus. There are marked weight loss and anemia. During exacerbations the patient may be critically ill with high temperature, leukocytosis, and tachycardia. Death from peritonitis may result during such a period.

The process begins in the rectum and spreads proximally to successively involve the colonic mucosa. Skip areas do not occur. Involvement, mainly of the mucosa, consists of crypt abscesses, ulcerations, pseudopolyp formation, and healing.

On direct inspection of the rectal mucosa, a velvety appearance is seen. There are multiple tiny ulcers that bleed readily from trauma. A barium enema may demonstrate a fuzzy appearance of the mucous membrane, and in late stages the bowel is contracted and rigid.

Differential diagnosis includes consideration of specific diseases, such as amebic and bacillary dysentery. Crohn's disease of the colon is the most frequently seen inflammatory lesion of the large intestine to be confused with idiopathic ulcerative colitis. The cobblestone appearance of the mucosa, presence of granulomas and transmural involvement are distinguishing features of Crohn's disease. It may be segmental, and skip areas may also be present as well as involvement of the small intestine.

Every effort should be made to control the disease by medical management, including adequate rest and bland diet from which all foods irritating to the patient's bowel have been excluded. Corticosteroid therapy has been shown to increase the frequency of remissions and to shorten the periods of activity of disease. Mild cases may be controlled in this way. However, many will continue to have so much trouble that surgery becomes necessary. The procedure of choice combines ileostomy and colectomy. Rarely the disease process quiets down sufficiently after ileostomy to permit restoration of bowel continuity. Complications of ulcerative colitis include profuse hemorrhage, perforation, obstruction, arthralgia, uveitis, necrotizing pyoderma, and cancer. Toxic megacolon is a complication that frequently necessitates emergency colectomy. Cancer of the colon occurs with greater frequency and at an earlier age in patients with ulcerative colitis. The longer a patient suffers from ulcerative colitis, the greater is the risk of cancer.

REGIONAL ENTERITIS (CROHN'S DISEASE)

Regional enteritis, or Crohn's disease, is an inflammatory disease of the intestinal tract, which usually, but not always, involves the terminal ileum. Skip areas occur, with involvement of jejunum, colon, duodenum, stomach, and even the esophagus. As noted above many cases involving the colon have been erroneously called idiopathic ulcerative colitis. The process is characterized by involvement of all layers of the wall of the intestine, granuloma formation with predominantly a giant-cell response, and skip areas. The regional lymph nodes are strikingly involved. The etiology is unknown, but the condition may be the result of lymphatic obstruction. Symptoms consist of diarrhea, weight loss, fever, and crampy abdominal pain. Blood, pus, and mucus may be found in the stool. The acute form may be mistaken for appendicitis.

Treatment is conservative unless one of the complications appears—perforation, fistula formation, obstruction, or intractability. If operation becomes necessary, resection of the diseased intestine is done, if possible. Other options include bypass procedures such as ileostomy or ileocolostomy in exclusion. Recurrences are common.

ISCHIORECTAL ABSCESS

The causative agent in ischiorectal abscess usually is the colon bacillus. It reaches the ischiorectal fossa as the result of extension of an infection in an anal crypt outward into the perirectal space. The disease is manifested by pain, tenderness, induration, and redness on one side or the other of the anus. Eventually, fluctuation is demonstrable. The temperature is elevated, and there is leukocytosis. Treatment consists of adequate incision and drainage. Frequently the patient is left with a fistula-in-ano following this procedure, which requires cor-

rection by secondary operation. Supralevator abscess is most frequently caused by diverticular disease of the colon.

FISTULA-IN-ANO

Fistula-in-ano results from extension of infection in an anal crypt outward into the subcutaneous tissues. Having reached this area the infection eventually appears beneath the skin in the perianal region and usually drains spontaneously. Then the patient is left with either a fistula that persistently drains a small amount of pus, and perhaps fecal material, or is subject to recurrent bouts of superficial healing of the external opening, with subsequent formation of an abscess that opens spontaneously at the site of the previous opening. Treatment of the condition consists of complete excision of the tract, with division of the external sphincter or a portion of it, if necessary, to obtain complete removal. The wound is packed open and allowed to heal secondarily by granulation tissue.

HEMORRHOIDS

Hemorrhoids are protruding masses of tissue in the region of the anal canal, usually associated with dilation of the venous plexus beneath. Contributing factors in the development of hemorrhoids include back pressure such as results from pregnancy, constipation, and straining at stool. The term *external hemorrhoids* is reserved for those hemorrhoids that rise below the pectinate line and the term *internal hemorrhoids* for those rising above this level. Frequently the two types are combined and are known as mixed hemorrhoids. Hemorrhoids may be asymptomatic or give rise to various complaints. Internal hemorrhoids may excite a mucoid discharge. They may prolapse at the time of stool and have to be replaced. They are eroded readily and give rise to rectal bleeding, which is bright red in color. Hemorrhoids may be associated with itching. External hemorrhoids occasionally undergo thrombosis with the development of a painful, tender, bluish swelling at the anal margin. Finally, internal hemorrhoids may prolapse and become strangulated, ulcerated, and gangrenous.

The treatment for hemorrhoids in general is surgical excision, which usually calls for sharp dissection and suture, though occasionally the clamp and cautery method is used. Thrombosis of an external hemorrhoid is relieved readily by incision of the thrombosed hemorrhoid with the clot being shelled out under local anesthesia. Surgical excision is the preferred treatment. Though bleeding in hemorrhoids usually is small in amount, its continuance over a long time may give rise to definite secondary anemia. Sigmoidoscopic examination should always be carried out before hemorrhoidectomy is done.

FISSURE-IN-ANO

Fissure-in-ano is a longitudinal ulceration at the opening of the anal canal. Almost always these ulcerations are located in the midline. Fissure-in-ano is associated with pain and bleeding at the time of defecation, and the pain persists for some time thereafter. There is usually spasm of the sphincter muscle that is responsible for the pain. The usual treatment is excision with packing of the wound. Division of the external sphincter is usually necessary.

RECTAL PROLAPSE

Rectal prolapse is a herniation of the rectum through the anus. It usually occurs in older individuals. The primary etiologic factors are as follows: (1) weakening of the muscular and ligamentous support of the pelvic floor, (2) dilation of the anal sphincters, and (3) redundancy of the rectum and the sigmoid. Very often, surgical correction is followed by recurrence. The difficulty of successfully correcting this lesion by operative means is attested to by the number of different operations that have been devised. Any operation to control rectal prolapse should include resection of the prolapsing and redundant bowel, reduction in the size of the anus, plastic reconstruction and reinforcement of the perineal floor, transabdominal suspension and fixation of the prolapsed bowel to the pelvis, obliteration of the cul-de-sac, or repair of the perineal sliding hernia.

Adrenal Glands

The indications for surgery of the adrenals are (1) tumors or hyperplasia of the adrenal medulla or cortex and (2) palliation in metastatic carcinoma of the breast.

TUMORS OF THE ADRENAL MEDULLA

Neuroblastomas arise from nerve cells. They have no endocrine function and are more common in infants and children than in adults. Treatment is surgical excision.

Pheochromocytoma is an endocrine tumor that arises from chromaffin cells and produces norepinephrine and epinephrine. The chief symptom is persistent or paroxysmal hypertension. If untreated, the patient dies from a complication of hypertension or from congestive heart failure. Ten percent of these tumors arise in an extra-adrenal location, primarily along the paravertebral sympathetic chain. A small percentage are malignant. When bilateral pheochromocytomas are present, they are likely to be familial. The thyroid gland may harbor a medullary carcinoma with amyloid stroma in this situation (Sipple's syndrome).

The diagnosis today is based on the quantitative assay of catecholamines and their metabolic products in the urine. Treatment consists of surgical removal. Preparation with dibenzyline and adequate hydration is helpful.

TUMORS OF THE ADRENAL CORTEX

A number of interesting syndromes result from hyperplasia and tumors of the adrenal cortex. Newborn females may present with the adrenogenital syndrome. This is the result of adrenal–cortical hyperplasia with overproduction of androgens. The hyperplasia in turn results from a defect in cortisol production. Clinically pseudohermaphroditism is the main presenting clinical feature. Precocious puberty in the first few years of life is the presentation in males. The administration of cortisol will correct the defect.

Cushing's syndrome results from hyperplasia of the adrenal cortex; both cortisol and androgen secretion are increased. In males, moon facies, a buffalo hump, truncal obesity with wasting of the extremities, thinning of skin, and so forth, are the presenting signs. The same signs are present in the female, plus hirsutism, deepening of the voice, and amenorrhea. The cause is basophilic adenoma of the anterior lobe of the pituitary. Treatment is by removal of the adenoma, which is frequently microscopic in size.

Cushing's disease results from a functioning adenoma or, more frequently, carcinoma of the adrenal cortex. The distinction between adrenal hyperplasia and tumor is important because the treatment of the latter is removal of the adrenal tumor.

HYPERALDOSTERONISM

A primary increase in secretion of aldosterone is seen in some functioning cortical adenomas or with cortical hyperplasia. The manifestations are hypertension, muscular weakness, metabolic alkalosis, hypokalemia, suppressed plasma renin activity, and increased potassium and aldosterone excretion. These findings must be documented in the absence of diuretic therapy, chronic vomiting (or laxative abuse), or renal arterial disease.

PALLIATION FOR ADVANCED CANCER

Total adrenalectomy will provide temporary benefit to many patients with hormone-dependent meta-static carcinoma. This therapy is reserved until castration, radiation, and hormone therapy are no longer helpful. Its greatest use has been in cancer of the breast.

Pediatric Surgery Involving the Digestive Tract

ESOPHAGEAL ATRESIA

The most common form of esophageal atresia consists of discontinuity between proximal and distal esophagus; the proximal esophagus ends blindly, and a fistula is present between the distal esophagus and the trachea. The infant appears to salivate excessively. A tube cannot be passed into the stomach if intubation is attempted. Barium swallow is contraindicated, for it will be regurgitated into the tracheobronchial tree. The preferred treatment is early repair through an extrapleural approach.

INTESTINAL ATRESIA

The absence of swallowed vernix cells in the meconium (Farber's test) indicates intestinal atresia. Such atresias occur most frequently in the ileum and the duodenum. Abdominal roentgenograms confirm the diagnosis. There is a characteristic "double bubble" on the roentgenogram in duodenal atresia. The type of operation depends upon the site of the atresia: in the duodenum, either duodenojejunostomy or gastroenterostomy with accompanying pyloroplasty; elsewhere, end-to-end anastomosis using interrupted fine nonabsorbable sutures is the procedure of choice. The extremely dilated proximal segment is resected and the distal segment distended by injecting saline solution.

IMPERFORATE ANUS

Imperforate anus usually is diagnosed at birth when the absence of an anal opening is apparent. If this defect is not recognized for 36 to 48 hours, the infant presents a picture of colon obstruction.

The common anorectal abnormalities may be grouped as follows: (1) anal stenosis due to incomplete rupture of the anal membrane; (2) imperforate anal membrane; (3) imperforate anus with the rectum ending in a blind pouch some distance from the anal dimple—with associated rectovesical, rectourethral, or rectoperineal fistulas in males, and rectovaginal or rectoperineal fistulas in females in a large percentage of cases; and (4) normal anus and lower rectum, with the rectal pouch ending blindly. The treatment varies with the type of abnormality. The third type is much more common than the others. Treatment depends partly upon the distance separating the rectum from the anus. This can be determined by means of a roentgenogram with the infant inverted and a marker on the anal dimple. If the pouch is low or an anal membrane is present primary anal repair is feasible. When the pouch is high a transverse colostomy is performed with elective repair after the baby is 1 year of age. With larger structures more satisfactory positioning of the rectum in relation to the puborectalis sling is possible.

MECONIUM ILEUS

Meconium ileus, caused by impacted meconium as a part of a picture of cystic fibrosis and pancreatic insufficiency, is a form of intestinal obstruction in the newborn with a high mortality rate. Vomiting frequently begins on the first day and is associated with abdominal distention, caused partly by palpable masses of meconium within the dilated loops. Roentgenograms characteristically reveal distended loops of intestine that vary in size. There is a mottled appearance due to inspissated meconium. Volvulus of the involved segment is also frequent. Diagnosis is confirmed by a contrast enema, which confirms a distal unused microcolon with obstruction of the cecum and terminal ileum by inspissated meconium. Use of meglumine diatrizoate (Gastrografin) may not only prove diagnostic but therapeutic, as it may assist in mobilizing the meconium and allow evacuation. This procedure may need to be repeated on several occasions to allow complete evacuation. Anatomic defects that are demonstrated will require surgical correction.

PYLORIC STENOSIS

Hypertrophic pyloric stenosis represents a form of pyloric obstruction resulting from hypertrophy of the pyloric muscle. It occurs most commonly in first-born male infants, 2 to 4 weeks of age. The etiology is uncertain. Diagnosis is confirmed by palpation of an olive-sized, firm tumor in the right upper quadrant and by roentgenograms of the stomach. Vomiting may be propulsive and is usually free of bile. Operation consists of dividing the thickened pyloric muscle (Ramstedt operation).

MALROTATION

Incomplete rotation of the midgut, due to peritoneal bands across the duodenum, causes duodenal obstruction in infants. The mesentery of the small intestine is elongated and its fixation to the posterior parietes is shortened, because of this, midgut volvulus is frequent. Operation consists of freeing the bands lateral to the duodenum and untwisting the midgut in a counterclockwise direction.

INTUSSUSCEPTION

Intussusception is the telescoping of a portion of intestine into another segment. It is the most common cause of obstruction in childhood. The etiology is unknown in most cases. The most common type is ileocolic. The clinical picture consists of a triad of signs: (1) abdominal cramps, (2) a mass in the right lower quadrant, and (3) blood in the stool.

Reduction of the intussusception may be achieved by operation or by barium enema. If reduction is not accomplished, the blood supply to the gut is compromised, and gangrene develops.

CONGENITAL MEGACOLON

Hirschsprung's disease consists of colon obstruction appearing in infancy or childhood and due to abnormal distal colonic function. Peristaltic waves are ineffective in the involved segment because of the absence of ganglion cells in Auerbach's myenteric plexus. The rectum and the rectosigmoid are involved most commonly.

The diagnosis will be suspect if barium studies of the colon and rectum show constriction of the distal aganglionic segment and dilatation of the proximal colon. The diagnosis is established by deep biopsy of the rectal wall that shows absence of ganglion cells in the myenteric plexus.

Considerable abdominal distention may occur, particularly in older children. In these cases, large fecal masses within the colon may be felt through the abdominal wall.

Treatment consists of resection of the aganglionic segment. It may be necessary to perform a prelimi-nary colostomy in infants when obturation or obstruction is present. It is important that the colostomy be done at a point where the colon is normally ganglionated.

GENITOURINARY SYSTEM

Hematuria

Hematuria may be:

1. Urethral from (a) calculus, (b) instrumentation or trauma, (c) acute urethritis, or (d) new growths. Gross blood may be visible at the meatus; though the voided specimen contains blood, the catheterized specimen does not.
2. Prostatic from: (a) calculus, (b) trauma, (c) instrumentation, (d) hypertrophy, or (e) tumor. The urine usually contains blood clots at the end of micturition.
3. Vesical from: (a) papilloma, (b) carcinoma or other tumors, (c) stones or foreign bodies, (d) ulceration, or (e) inflammation. The urine contains clots, mostly at the end of micturition.
4. Ureteral from: (a) calculus, (b) neoplasm, (c) inflammation, or (d) trauma. The bleeding often is slight, and the clots formed in the ureter may appear in the urine as wormlike casts.
5. Renal from: (a) calculus, (b) tuberculosis or other bacterial infections, (c) papilloma, (d) other neoplasms, (e) trauma, (f) chemical poisoning, (g) blood disease, or (h) essential hematuria.

In hematuria from systemic disease, such as nephritis secondary to fever, albumin and casts also are found in the urine. Moderate microscopic hematuria following renal colic is almost pathognomonic of a calculus.

The Kidneys

CALCULUS

A large staghorn calculus anchored in the substance of the kidney does not give rise to obstruction and therefore rarely produces colic. There is rather a dragging ache in the loin. However, pyuria, gross or microscopic hematuria and crystalluria are present. A smaller stone in the pelvis or the ureter is likely to give rise to obstruction. This is characterized by acute agonizing pain in the back and loin, often referred along the course of the ureter to the bladder and the external genitalia. Nausea, vomiting, chills, and fever may be present. Unless the ureter is obstructed completely, red blood cells and leukocytes usually can be seen in the urine. Urgency and dysuria often are present. If the calculus is of long duration, chronic or recurrent infection is frequent, and the chief complaints may be those of pyelitis or pyelonephritis.

The history, physical examination, urinalysis, and survey film of the abdomen usually establish the diagnosis. On cystoscopic examinations and catheterization of the ureters, the obstruction may be demonstrated, and scratch marks appear on a wax-tipped ureteral bougie. Differential diagnosis includes acute appendicitis, acute biliary colic, and penetrating or perforating peptic ulcers. The milder pain in acute appendicitis and the characteristic initial and subsequent locations of the pain, plus the absence of roentgenographic and urinary tract findings, help to establish the diagnosis of the disease. In biliary tract disease the history of preceding attacks, fatty-food indigestion, and radiation of the pain to the right scapula and shoulder, associated with local tenderness over the gallbladder area, aid in distinguishing this disease from renal calculus. Usually in peptic ulcer there is a typical history of gastric pain exacerbated by hunger and eased by the ingestion of food prior to the onset of penetration or perforation.

Small stones may pass through the ureter, with morphine being given for pain and drugs of the atropine group being given in an attempt to relax the ureter. Frequently, also, hot baths give the patient great comfort during the passage of the calculus. If the stone becomes impacted in the ureter, it may be dislodged at times by ureteral manipulation through the cystoscope. Larger calculi require surgical removal by incising the renal pelvis or the ureter. Extremely large stones at times require surgical removal through the renal cortex. If the calculus has been associated with distention of long standing, the kidney is damaged beyond repair. Removal by percutaneous passage of a nephroscope containing an ultrasonic probe for lithotripsy is now feasible in some cases. Following lithotripsy the fragments are removed by forceps and irrigation. It requires the collaborative efforts of the interventional radiologist and the urologist. Recently, ureteral and smaller renal stones have been treated with external lithotripsy. Using water as a conducting medium, and focusing shock waves on the stone, stone fracture can be accomplished in many patients and if the fragments pass, surgical removal is avoided.

HYDRONEPHROSIS

Hydronephrosis is distention of the renal pelvis and calices secondary to obstruction somewhere in the course of the urinary tract, giving rise to back pressure. If the distention is of sufficiently long standing, there is secondary atrophy of the renal parenchyma. The obstruction may be due to (1) angulation or kinking of the ureter, (2) structure, (3) aberrant vessels, (4) calculus, (5) neoplasm, (6) trauma, (7) pressure from external growths, (8) prostatic enlargement, or (9) retroperitoneal fibrosis. It is seen more frequently in women than in men. In the mild form there is discomfort in the region of the kidney. In ureteral catheterization a large amount of urine is obtained on entering the renal pelvis. Hydronephrosis may be demonstrated both by intravenous urography and retrograde pyelography. Hydronephrosis often is associated with secondary bacterial infection, and the primary symptoms then are those of pyelonephritis.

Treatment depends entirely on the cause of the obstruction. Removal of the causative factor usually will result in relief of the hydronephrosis. If the obstruction has been of long standing, and the renal parenchyma is largely destroyed, nephrectomy at times will be necessary. Retroperitoneal fibrosis usually results in bilateral ureteral obstruction. To relieve the obstruction both ureters must be mobilized and transposed to an intraperitoneal position.

INFECTIONS OF THE KIDNEY

Perinephric Abscess. This condition may result from a primary infection, probably blood-borne, or from secondary infection of the urinary tract or extension from an adjacent focus of infection in the kidney. The infection usually lies behind the kidney, though it may involve an extensive area in the retroperitoneal region above and below the kidney. The colon bacillus is a frequent offending organism. If allowed to go untreated, the abscess may dissect well downward toward the pelvis in the retroperitoneal space or upward into the thorax and rupture into the pleural cavity.

The symptoms consist of deep-seated pain in the flank, often radiating downward and increased by pressure, together with local tenderness over the kidney and muscular rigidity. As the result of muscular spasm, the spine may be quite rigid. High temperature and leukocytosis are present, and there may be visible fullness on the involved side overlying the kidney. Redness and edema are seen occasionally. The abscess is likely to be so deep that fluctuation cannot be demonstrated. Unless there is associated pyelonephritis, the urine is likely to be normal. Perinephric abscess often is recognized only late in the course of the disease. Any patient who has a persistent fever and leukocytosis should be examined carefully for evidence of this condition. The obliteration of the psoas shadow on a supine film of the abdomen is a strongly suggestive finding.

As soon as the diagnosis can be established, adequate drainage should be carried out through a posterior approach.

TUBERCULOSIS

Tubercle bacilli may reach the kidney from the bloodstream, the lymphatics, or the lower urinary tract. Renal tuberculosis may be one manifestation of the miliary form of the disease. This occurs commonly in children. Primary involvement of the renal parencyhma is unilateral as a rule and is more common in young women than in men. If the parenchyma alone is involved, there are no specific findings in the urinary sediment. However, as soon as the lesion drains into the renal pelvis, the urine contains blood, pus, and tubercle bacilli. Renal tuberculosis may result also from extension of the disease upward from the lower urinary tract. This type is more common in men and is often bilateral.

There is bladder irritability with urgency, frequency, and polyuria. Hematuria may be profuse without apparent cause. Pyuria is present, and the urine usually contains no bacteria other than tubercle bacilli. There is discomfort in the lumbar region and local tenderness. General symptoms of tuberculosis, such as an evening rise in temperature, loss of weight, night sweats, and weakness, may be present. On cystoscopic examination there are redness, swelling, and retraction of the ureteral orifice. Occasionally, tuberculous ulcers of the bladder may be seen. Diminished renal function eventually results. X-ray examination may show calcified deposits in the parenchyma. Both the intravenous urogram and the retrograde pyelogram show distortion of the pelvis, the calices, and the ureter. Complications include extension of the infection to involve the perinephric area or downward extension to involve the ureter and the bladder. This often results in secondary involvement of the opposite kidney. Mixed infections may ensue eventually. Stricture formation may lead to pyelonephritis.

Irritability of the bladder without adequate explanation and sterile pyuria suggest the possibility of renal tuberculosis. Evidence of the disease may be found elsewhere, as in the bladder, the epididymis, and the seminal vesicles. Demonstration of the tubercle bacilli in the urine smear, culture, or guinea pig inoculation establishes the diagnosis.

Treatment with antituberculous drugs for a minimum of 2 years is indicated. Surgery is reserved for complications such as abscess formation, a destroyed kidney, and so forth.

TUMORS OF THE KIDNEY

Hypernephroma (clear-cell carcinoma) is the most common renal tumor. Usually it occurs in the male in midlife. Embryoma (Wilms' tumor), in contrast with hypernephroma, occurs in children, frequently manifesting itself during the first year of life. Other malignant tumors include papillary carcinoma and epithelioma of the renal pelvis, carcinoma, and sarcoma. Occasionally the kidney also is the site of metastatic carcinoma.

Benign tumors of the kidney include cortical adenoma, papilloma, papillary cystadenoma, angioma, and simple or solitary cysts of the kidney. Polycystic disease of the kidney is benign in the true sense of the term. However, the prognosis is poor, because eventually there is so much destruction of renal parenchyma that renal insufficiency develops.

The cardinal symptoms of renal tumor are hematuria, a mass, and pain. Nonspecific symptoms such as cachexia, anemia, and weight loss usually are late manifestations of the disease. Hematuria may be intermittent and therefore demands early and complete investigation. An intravenous urogram and retrograde pyelogram demonstrate deformity of the renal pelvis and the calices. Angiography is extremely helpful, particularly in smaller tumors that do not encroach on the renal collecting system.

If there is no roentgenographic evidence of widespread metastases, exploration should be carried out and nephrectomy performed, if this is feasible. Though some of the malignant lesions, such as embryoma, are radiosensitive, the best results in the treatment of malignant tumors of the kidney have followed early nephrectomy. Benign lesions often can be corrected by local removal or partial nephrectomy. Though repeated aspiration of the cysts in polycystic disease of the kidney has been tried, up to the present time no satisfactory treatment has been discovered.

Wilms' tumor (embryoma of the kidney) is the most common abdominal tumor in childhood. These tumors are highly malignant and may reach a large size. Metastases are first noted in the lungs.

The mass is painless. There is usually associated low-grade fever.

Treatment consists of excision in association with radiation and chemotherapy. Addition of the latter two modalities has greatly improved survival rates.

RUPTURE OF THE KIDNEY

Kidney rupture results from direct trauma. There are local pain and tenderness with splinting of the overlying muscles. The adjacent ribs may be fractured. Blood is found in the urine. On ureteral catheterization, origin of the bleeding from the damaged kidney can be confirmed. In most cases conservative treatment will suffice. If there is evidence of extensive and continued hemorrhage, nephrectomy may be necessary to control the bleeding. Intravenous urography is useful in evaluating the extent of injury and in deciding if an operation is necessary. In patients with multiple organ injury, tears in the kidney may be present. At operation a retroperitoneal hematoma will be present. There is a tendency for bleeding from minor tears, as well as some major ones, to be tamponaded by the peritoneum and fascia with clot formation and cessation of bleeding. Formerly, nonexpanding hematomas were not explored, but it is now believed that the hematoma should be explored, with control of bleeding and reconstruction of damaged major vessels. Even disruption of the renal artery and vein may be tamponaded. If the disrupted renal artery and vein are not repaired pyelography will show absence of function and renal scanning with ^{131}I hippurate will show lack of perfusion. A delayed complication of a perinephric hematoma may be hypertension. This elevated pressure can be normalized by nephrectomy or removal of the encapsulating hematoma.

Prostate

BENIGN HYPERTROPHY

Benign hypertrophy of the prostate is extremely common in men over 50. In many cases of hypertrophy obstructive symptoms of some degree develop, and some ultimately develop carcinoma. The etiology is unknown. The hypertrophy is composed of both glandular and fibrous tissue elements. The prostatic urethra becomes elongated and distorted. As a result of obstruction at the internal meatus, the bladder wall undergoes hypertrophy, trabeculation, and dilatation. There is increasing residual urine. Secondary infection ultimately results, involving primarily the bladder. However, as the obstruction gradually involves the upper urinary tract, hydroureter and hydronephrosis set in. Secondary infection also occurs here and, finally, renal insufficiency. The symptoms include diminution in force and size of the urinary stream, delay in starting, frequency, nocturia, bouts of acute retention requiring catheterization, and incontinence due to overflow. When chronic cystitis and pyelonephritis develop, the picture of infection is evident. Rectal examination reveals an enlarged firm prostate. Catheterization may be difficult because of elongation and distortion of the prostatic urethra. However, hypertrophy of the prostate gland is best demonstrated by cystoscopic examination. In chronic retention with back pressure of long standing, one should guard against sudden decompression of the bladder by catheterization. Unless decompression is gradual, edema and congestion of the bladder and kidney result, with gross hematuria, suppression of urine and uremia that may be fatal.

Treatment. Obstruction to the outlet of the bladder may be relieved surgically by four procedures: (1) suprapubic prostatectomy, (2) perineal prostatectomy, (3) retropubic prostatectomy, and (4) transuretheral resection. Transuretheral resection especially has attained widespread popularity. It consists of removal of the obstructing prostate through a cystoscope by electrosurgery. In advanced disease with uremia, a preliminary period of preparation is frequently desirable, including catheter drainage or suprapubic cystotomy, chemotherapy, and increased fluid intake.

CARCINOMA

The symptoms of carcinoma of the prostate may be minimal or absent at first, or may resemble those of simple hypertrophy if the malignant mass leads to obstruction of the outlet of the bladder. However, on rectal examination, the prostate is firm, hard, nodular, and asymmetrical. If the disease is advanced, there may be evidence of fixation to the surrounding structures. If seen early, prostatectomy may be carried out. The acid phosphatase should be measured, elevation is usual with extension and metastasis. Metastasis occurs to the regional lymph nodes, the spine, and the pelvic bones. Pain from bony metastasis may be the first symptom of the disease. Radiation therapy has no permanent value. In inoperable cases or in patients with pain from bone metastasis, excellent palliative results may be obtained by bilateral orchiectomy and the use of estrogenic agents. If prostatic obstruction is sufficiently severe suprapubic cystostomy or transurethral resection may be required.

Scrotum and Genitalia

Common enlargements include hydrocele, hernia, acute orchitis, epididymitis, tuberculosis, syphilis, malignant neoplasms, and varicocele.

HYDROCELE

Hydrocele is a cystic enlargement of the tunica vaginalis. It may occur at any age. Frequently it is entirely asymptomatic except for the presence of the mass. It may be quite tense or cystic in nature. Transillumination usually confirms the diagnosis. The cystic swelling may obliterate the outlines of the testicle and the epididymis. Aspiration yields a clear fluid. Occasionally, hydrocele may involve a portion of the spermatic cord instead of surrounding the testis.

Repeated aspirations are of palliative value only. The procedure of choice is surgery, consisting of opening the sac and everting it about the testicle.

SCROTAL HERNIA

Usually scrotal hernia can be demonstrated proceeding downward from the inguinal canal into the scrotum above the testis. Often it is reducible, transmits an impulse when the patient coughs, increases when he stands and may be tympanitic and demonstrate peristalsis on auscultation if it contains bowel. It does not transmit light on transillumination.

VARICOCELE

An undue enlargement or varicosity of the pampiniform plexus, varicocele is more common on the left side than on the right. Occasionally it is associated with a dragging, aching sensation in the testis on that side. The discomfort may be diminished by the use of adequate support. On examination, the varicosity is evident along the structures of the cord above the testicle. This is most marked in the erect posture. Frequently, it has been described as feeling like a bag of worms. Treatment consists of excision of the varicose portion of the plexus.

STRICTURE OF THE URETHRA

Stricture of the urethra is usually the end result of a gonorrheal infection. On the other hand, it may fol-low trauma to the urethra, as in fracture of the pelvis. Repeated dilatation of the stricture by a sound usually will maintain an adequate passage, but it may be necessary to resort to transurethral division of the stricture.

ACUTE ORCHITIS

Acute orchitis may follow mumps or other infectious disease or, occasionally, trauma. The onset is usually rather sudden. The pain is extremely severe and may radiate to the groin and the back. The disease may be sufficiently severe to produce systemic symptoms. The testis is swollen, hard, and tender. An associated history of trauma or parotitis may establish the nature of the orchitis.

ACUTE EPIDIDYMITIS

Acute epididymitis is a common complication of gonorrheal urethritis. There is a sudden onset of pain and tenderness, frequently with associated systemic symptoms. The epididymis is swollen and tender; the testis also may be involved. A history of gonorrhea and the finding of gonococci in the urethral discharge establish the diagnosis in the usual type.

Tuberculosis occurs in young adults. There is likely to be evidence of tuberculosis elsewhere, especially in the prostate and the seminal vesicles. The epididymis is hard and nodular with coalescent swelling. Sinuses may develop, and tubercle bacilli may be isolated from the pus in these sinuses.

Acute epididymitis may also complicate prostatectomy or instrumentation of the urethra (including catheterization).

TORSION OF THE TESTIS

Torsion of the testis refers to a twisting of the testis and terminal spermatic cord interfering with blood flow and leading to gangrene if detorsion is not performed within 4 hours of the sudden onset of pain that heralds the onset of torsion. Presumably there is an elongated mesorchium attaching the testis to the epididymis. There is a tendency toward bilaterality; therefore, bilateral orchiopexy should be performed at the time of detorsion.

SYPHILIS

A gumma manifests itself as a unilateral, hard, freely movable painless mass in the testis. The history of the primary and the secondary lesions, a positive serologic test, and the prompt response to antiluetic therapy establish the diagnosis.

CARCINOMA OF THE TESTIS

Carcinoma of the testis is a disease of young adult life. The treatment and prognosis vary with the histologic type; therefore, accurate classification is important. The clinical manifestation is, in all forms, the presence of an enlarging tumor that is usually not tender. When such a lesion is found, operation should be performed through an inguinal incision with high ligation of the cord structures and removal when the presence of a tumor is confirmed on gross inspection. Seminoma is then treated by irradiation therapy to the preaortic area and the hilum of both kidneys. Embryonal carcinoma is treated by surgical removal of the lymph nodes. Teratomas are treated by removal of the testis alone. The trophoblastic tumors may be associated with gynecomastia and increased urinary excretion of chorionic gonadotropins. The tumors are highly malignant and infrequently cured.

CRYPTORCHIDISM

On examination the scrotum is found to be empty on the involved side. The testis may lie anywhere along the course of the inguinal canal or in the retroperitoneal tissues. It is likely to be small and underdeveloped if the individual is an adult. If the disease is bilateral, sterility is almost always present. Inguinal hernia is often associated. If the condition is not corrected early—before the onset of puberty—atrophy of the testis results, and a high incidence of malignant transformation takes place in these retained testes. For these reasons, the condition should be corrected early in life. Although replacing the testis in the scrotum does not alter the tendency toward cancer, it does permit palpation and earlier diagnosis. Some good results have been recorded following the use of pituitary gonadotropins; however, in general, it is necessary to resort to operation with movement of the testis down into the scrotum, anchoring it in this position while healing takes place.

PHIMOSIS

A condition in which the prepuce is elongated and the opening is so constricted that retraction cannot take place, phimosis results in retention of secretions with irritation and secondary infection. Occasionally the opening is so small that the urinary flow is obstructed, with subsequent dilatation of the urinary tract above it. Rarely, cystitis and vesical calculus result. In adults an epithelioma may be found. The treatment for phimosis is circumcision; however, if extensive acute infection is present, the more conservative procedure of making a dorsal slit in the prepuce until the infection is under control is indicated.

PARAPHIMOSIS

In paraphimosis the tight retracted prepuce is constricted behind the glans. There are swelling, edema, pain and, at times, ulceration and gangrene. Early reduction of the paraphimosis may be carried out by manipulation. However, it frequently is necessary to make a dorsal slit in the prepuce in order to accomplish this. Circumcisions should be carried out unless infection is so extensive that the procedure must be deferred.

QUESTIONS IN SURGERY

Review Questions

By what process does the healing of wounds take place?

Name two amino acids found only in collagen.

What functions have been attributed to mucopolysaccharides in wound healing?

Name five local factors that interfere with wound healing. Which one is the most important?

Why is catgut used as ligature and suture material in contaminated wounds?

Discuss the prophylactic and active treatment of tetanus.

What are the indications for rabies prophylaxis?

What is the difference in the clinical manifestations of bites by the black widow spider and the brown spider?

Describe the modern definitive treatment of poisonous snake bites.

Discuss the systemic and local factors of importance in the coagulation of blood.

Discuss the predisposing factors to disseminated intravascular coagulation.

Define and discuss surgical shock, cardiac shock, and septic shock.

What are the daily water and salt requirements of normal man?

Discuss the diagnosis and treatment of water intoxication.

What are the complications of intravenous hyperalimentation?

What alternatives to intravenous hyperalimentation exist for nutritional maintenance in patients with small intestinal fistulas?

What is the pathogenesis of stasis ulceration of the leg?

Discuss the diagnosis and treatment of acute thrombophlebitis and phlebothrombosis. What is phlegmasia cerulea dolens?

How can you determine whether peripheral arterial insufficiency is surgically correctable?

Discuss the management of an embolism to the common femoral artery.

What is Branham's sign?

Discuss the pathogenesis and prevention of Volkmann's ischemic contracture.

Give the indications for amputation of an extremity.

What are the areas of election for amputation of the forearm? the leg? the thigh?

Discuss the treatment of burns.

Describe paronychia and give its treatment.

What is a felon? How is it treated?

What are the anatomic boundaries of the mid-palmar space?

Discuss the rejection of allografts.

What agents have been used to prevent the rejection of an allograft (homograft)?

Discuss the management of a liposarcoma 10 cm in diameter arising in the lateral portion of the thigh.

Discuss delayed union and nonunion of fractures. What are the frequent sites of nonunion?

Describe the most common fracture of the clavicle and its treatment.

Describe fracture of the surgical neck of the humerus; give its complications and treatment. How is it differentiated from dislocation of the shoulder joint?

Describe the primary and secondary positions of dislocations of the shoulder joint. Give Kocher's method of reduction.

What are the common complications of fracture of the shaft of the humerus? Give the treatment of the fracture and the complications.

What symptoms suggest a herniation of an intervertebral disk? What is the treatment for a patient with a herniated disk?

Differentiate fracture of the lower extremity of the humerus from dislocation of the elbow and its treatment.

Describe the appearance of posterior dislocation of the elbow and its treatment.

What is a Colles' fracture?

Describe intracapsular fracture of the femur and its treatment.

How is congenital dislocation of the hip diagnosed?

Describe fracture of the shaft of the femur. Describe the treatment.

Give the treatment of fracture of the patella.

Give the diagnosis and the treatment of fracture of the tibia.

Describe Pott's fracture and its treatment.

How is dislocation of the semilunar cartilage diagnosed and treated?

Describe the common fractures of the true pelvis. What are the common complications, and how are they treated?

What are the indications for insertion of a prosthetic joint?

How would you treat surgical parotitis?

What is the most frequent tumor seen in the parotid gland?

How would you treat a peritonsillar abscess?

What is the most likely cause of a persistently enlarged lymph node in the deep cervical chain in a 25-year-old woman?

Discuss the staging of Hodgkin's disease.

Is elective lymph node dissection indicated in cancer of the lower lip?

Describe the preparation for surgery of the patient with thyrotoxicosis.

State the possible results of accidental but serious injury to the parathyroids occurring during thyroidectomy.

Describe the syndrome associated with hyperparathyroidism.

What are the physical signs of breast cancer?

Discuss the pathology, the diagnosis, the routes of metastasis, and the treatment of carcinoma of the breast. Describe the palliative measures available in advanced mammary carcinoma.

What is paradoxic respiration? Explain its significance.

What is the treatment of a patient with a flail chest resulting in respiratory embarrassment?

Discuss the signs, the symptoms, and the treatment of cardiac tamponade.

Describe the management of acute cardiac arrest.

What are the components of the tetralogy of Fallot?

What is the most accurate method of establishing the diagnosis of pulmonary embolism?

Where do bronchial adenomas most frequently metastasize?

What are the advantages of fiberoptic bronchoscopy?

Give the causes, diagnosis, and treatment of thoracic empyema.

What is the preferred treatment of carcinoma of the lower third of the esophagus? The middle third?

Describe the treatment of pharyngoesophageal pulsion diverticulum.

What are the two types of hiatal hernia? Describe their differences.

Discuss blunt and penetrating wounds of the abdomen.

What are the indications for surgery for duodenal ulcer?

Under what conditions should a definitive operation for control of ulcer disease be used in patients with a perforated duodenal ulcer?

Describe the physiologic basis for the common operations for duodenal ulcer.

How should a patient with the Zollinger-Ellison syndrome be treated?

Discuss the etiology, the symptomatology, the differential diagnosis, and the treatment of chronic cholecystitis. Give the clinical picture and the treatment of acute gallstone colic; of empyema of the gallbladder.

What substance has been used for the dissolution of gallstones *in vivo?*

Why is vitamin K given in the treatment of patients with icterus?

Give the etiology, the clinical picture, and the treatment of acute pancreatitis.

What is Whipple's triad? Of what is it a diagnostic finding?

What laboratory tests are used for the confirmation of the diagnosis of islet cell adenoma?

Give the differential diagnosis of carcinoma of the head of the pancreas.

Give the signs and symptoms of rupture of the spleen. What is the treatment? What are commonly accepted indications for splenectomy?

What is the rationale of the portacaval shunt operation? What are the indications and contraindications for its use?

What are the causes of subdiaphragmatic abscess?

Describe the management of a patient with mechanical obstruction of the ileum arising from an adhesive band.

How would you treat a patient with complete obstruction of the sigmoid colon resulting from cancer?

What is the cause of acute appendicitis? Give the symptoms and signs in the order of their usual appearance. Give the differential diagnosis and the surgical treatment.

What are the indications for operation in terminal ileitis? What is the operation of choice?

Contrast Peutz-Jegher's syndrome with familial polyposis of the colon.

What are the indications for colonoscopy?

Why is barium by mouth contraindicated in a patient with carcinoma of the colon?

Describe the treatment of carcinoma of the rectum.

Give the clinical picture and treatment of acute diverticulitis of the colon.

Give the causes, the diagnosis, and the treatment of ischiorectal abscess; fistula-in-ano; hemorrhoids.

Give the pathology, the symptomatology, the complications, the diagnosis, and the treatment of carcinoma of the rectum.

Differentiate indirect inguinal hernia and describe its anatomic features; direct inguinal hernia; femoral hernia.

What is a sliding hernia? Discuss its treatment.

Discuss management of a patient with pheochromocytoma.

What are the clinical manifestations of an aldosteronoma?

What is the Farber test?

Discuss the management of imperforate anus.

What is the pathogenesis of congenital megacolon?

Of what is hematuria a symptom?

Give the symptoms of ureteral calculus and the conditions to be considered in the differential diagnosis.

What are the symptoms that would suggest benign hypertrophy of the prostate?

What is a transurethal resection of the prostate, and for what is it performed?

What is cryptorchidism? Discuss its treatment.

Classify the causes of hematuria.

Give the clinical picture, the differential diagnosis, and the treatment of renal calculus.

Discuss the pathogenesis, the pathology, the diagnosis, and the treatment of hydronephrosis.

What is the treatment of Wilms' tumor (embryoma of the kidney)?

Give the causes, the diagnosis, and the treatment of perinephric abscess.

What are the common causes of intestinal obstruction in the newborn?

Describe the diagnostic features of duodenal atresia.

Contrast the clinical pictures of hypertrophic pyloric stenosis and duodenal atresia.

What is the triad of signs that make up the clinical picture of intussusception in children?

What is the basic defect in congenital megacolon?

Discuss common tumors of the kidney and give their diagnosis, routes of metastasis, and treatment.

Differentiate prostatic hypertrophy and carcinoma of the prostate. What are the early symptoms, the complications, and the treatment?

List the common causes of enlargement of the scrotum.

Give the diagnosis and the treatment of hydrocele.

Differentiate the common causes of enlargement of the epididymis and of the testis.

Give the diagnosis and treatment of undescended testis.

Describe phimosis and paraphimosis and their treatment.

Multiple-Choice Questions

Select the *best* answer for each question. Answers are at the end of this chapter.

1. Hyperkalemia is most likely to occur:
   (a) With prolonged vomiting
   (b) In renal failure
   (c) With functioning adrenal cortical tumors
   (d) In Boeck's sarcoidosis
   (e) In the Zollinger-Ellison syndrome
2. All of the following are well-recognized inciting factors in thrombophlebitis except:
   (a) Prolonged bed rest
   (b) Driving an automobile for long distances
   (c) Pelvic tumors
   (d) Brain tumors
   (e) Pelvic operations
3. Raynaud's disease:
   (a) Is most frequent in males
   (b) Is associated with hypertrophy of the volar carpal ligament
   (c) Causes prolonged conduction time in the median nerve
   (d) Is caused by spasm of small arteries
   (e) Is frequent in the tropics
4. The most frequent complication of delayed treatment of a felon is:
   (a) Spread to flexor tendon sheaths
   (b) Necrosis of the skin overlying the distal phalanx
   (c) Osteomyelitis of the distal phalanx
   (d) Septicemia
   (e) None of the above
5. In Colles' fracture of the wrist,
   (a) The usual mechanism is a fall on the outstretched hand.

   (b) A "silver-fork" deformity is characteristic.
   (c) Reduction implies restoration of length and palmar deflection of the distal articular surface of the radius.
   (d) Initial fixation in a long arm cast is essential.
   (e) All are correct.
6. Neoplasms occur most frequently in which of the following salivary glands?
   (a) Submaxillary
   (b) Parotid
   (c) Sublingual
   (d) Buccal
   (e) Lingual
7. A 13-year-old girl develops exophthalmos, nervousness, diarrhea, and weight loss following the death of her mother. Her blood pressure is 170/90. The most likely diagnosis is:
   (a) Multiple endocrine adenoma (MEA), type II
   (b) A pheochromocytoma
   (c) Graves' disease
   (d) Retroorbital pseudotumor
   (e) None of the above
8. If the diagnosis is MEA type II, which of the following confirmatory findings would be least likely?
   (a) Elevated serum thyrocalcitonin
   (b) Elevated urinary metanephrins
   (c) Elevated serum calcium
   (d) Low serum phosphorus
   (e) Elevated T_4
9. Of the following pathological findings in the breast, which is *least* likely to be precancerous?
   (a) Fibroadenoma
   (b) Intraductal papilloma
   (c) Sclerosing adenosis
   (d) Lobular hyperplasia
   (e) Cancer of one breast
10. A 6-year-old underdeveloped boy is seen because of signs of heart failure. He also has hypertension in the arms, but not in the legs and prominent notching of the lower rib margins. The most likely diagnosis is:
    (a) Patent ductus arteriosus
    (b) Tetralogy of Fallot
    (c) Pulmonary stenosis
    (d) Patent interventricular septal defect
    (e) Coarctation of the aorta
11. Open drainage of empyema is indicated only:

(a) In streptococcal infections

(b) When the pus is thick

(c) When the mediastinum is fixed

(d) In bilateral disease

(e) When thoracostomy tube drainage is ineffective

12. Cricopharyngeal myotomy is used in the surgical correction of pharyngoesophageal pulsion diverticulum in order to:

(a) Better expose the neck of the diverticulum

(b) Restore normal pressure relationships and thereby prevent recurrence

(c) Prevent narrowing of the esophagus at this point

(d) Eliminate the risk of infection

(e) All are correct

13. Positive findings in suspected subphrenic abscess include:

(a) Fixation of the diaphragm

(b) Sterile pleural effusion above the abscess

(c) Absent Litton's signs

(d) Elevation of the diaphragm

(e) All of the above

14. A previously healthy 17-year-old male has had an appendiceal abscess drained. The appendix was not removed. Future management should consist of:

(a) Long-term antibiotic therapy

(b) Roentgenograms of the small intestine and colon

(c) Regular physical examination

(d) Weekly complete blood counts

(e) Interval appendectomy at 3 months

15. A 45-year-old man is brought to the emergency room when he fainted after vomiting an undetermined amount of bright red blood. The history and physical examination were uninformative. Laboratory studies: WBC 9,600; RBC 3,200,000; hemoglobin 9 g/100 ml; hematocrit 32%. The *next* diagnostic procedure should be:

(a) Selective angiography

(b) Upper gastrointestinal roentgenograms

(c) Barium enema

(d) Endoscopic examination of esophagus, stomach, and duodenum

(e) None of the above

16. Which of the following is most supportive of the diagnosis of the Zollinger-Ellison syndrome?

(a) 12-hour gastric secretion of 800 ml

(b) Serum gastrin level of 1,000 nanograms percent

(c) Basal acid output of 12 ml/hour

(d) A history of recurrent ulcer following three presumably satisfactory ulcer operations

(e) Multiple ulcers of duodenum and jejunem

17. Whipples triad, useful in the diagnosis of insulinoma of the pancreas, consists of:

(a) Central nervous system symptoms, fasting blood sugar of 50 mg/100 ml, relief following ingestion of glucose

(b) Central nervous system symptoms, fasting blood sugar of 50 mg/100 ml, relief following intravenous glucagon

(c) Abdominal pain, fasting blood sugar of 50 mg/100 ml, relief following ingestion of glucose

(d) Abdominal pain, high serum insulin, relief following the ingestion of glucose

(e) Fasting nausea and vomiting, positive tolbutamide test, relief following intravenous glucagon

18. A 49-year-old woman has been treated with steroids for idiopathic thrombocytopenic purpura, with return of the platelet count to normal. Following discontinuance of steroids, thrombocytopenia recurs. Treatment at this time should consist of:

(a) Splenectomy

(b) Repeat steroid administration, if good response continues indefinitely

(c) Give azathioprine for 1 week then recommend splenectomy

(d) Repeat steroids, and if no response initially, increase the dosage

(e) None of the above

19. The most frequent adverse effect following otherwise successful portacaval shunting for bleeding esophageal varices in the cirrhotic patient is:

(a) Progressive hepatic failure

(b) Intolerance to fats

(c) Meat intoxication

(d) Recurrent bleeding

(e) Lactic acidosis

20. Treatment of intestinal obstruction caused by cancer of the rectosigmoid is best accomplished by:

(a) Decompressive colostomy

(b) Decompression by passage of a long intestinal tube, subsequent resection

(c) Immediate resection

(d) Ileostomy

(e) All of the above

21. A 13-year-old boy experiences sudden severe pain in the right testis. On palpation there is exquisite tenderness. The most likely diagnosis is:
    (a) Spontaneous hemorrhage
    (b) Torsion
    (c) Strangulated hernia
    (d) Epididymitis
    (e) Seminoma of the testis

For the following, answer:
    (a) If 1, 2, and 3 are correct
    (b) If 1 and 3 are correct
    (c) If 2 and 4 are correct
    (d) If only 4 is correct
    (e) If all are correct

22. Which of the following play an important role in wound healing?
    (1) Zinc
    (2) Vitamin C
    (3) Copper
    (4) Cobalt

23. A properly positioned Swan-Ganz catheter will permit determination of:
    (1) Left atrial pressure
    (2) Right atrial pressure
    (3) Pulmonary artery pressure
    (4) Right ventricular pressure

24. Complications of intravenous feeding include:
    (1) Nonketotic hyperglycemic coma
    (2) Hyperphosphatemia
    (3) Hyperosmolarity
    (4) Hypercalcemia

25. Characteristic of renal allograft rejection is:
    (1) Lymphocytopenia
    (2) Bradycardia
    (3) Polyuria
    (4) Rising serum creatinine

26. Patients with intermittent claudication:
    (1) Most frequently have a block in the superficial femoral artery
    (2) Will most likely require an amputation within 5 years of onset
    (3) Should be encouraged to exercise
    (4) Should have an immediate arteriogram

27. Causative in embolization of major arteries is:
    (1) Mural thrombus following myocardial infarction
    (2) Ventricular aneurysm
    (3) Cardiac myxoma
    (4) Patent ventricular septal defects

28. In a 50-year-old woman with a 35% body surface burn of the trunk:
    (1) Mortality is mainly secondary to burn shock
    (2) The severity of infection can be lessened by topical use of sulfamylon
    (3) Systemic antimicrobials are of greater efficacy than are topical agents
    (4) Either lactated Ringer's solution or isotonic sodium chloride solution will be effective in combatting burn shock

29. Nonunion is frequent in fractures of:
    (1) The carpal scaphoid
    (2) The lower third of the tibia
    (3) The neck of the femur
    (4) Intertrochanteric fractures

30. Joint replacement is useful in crippling arthritis involving which of the following joints?
    (1) Metacarpophalangeal
    (2) Hip
    (3) Scapulohumeral
    (4) Knee

31. Thyroglossal duct cysts are characterized by:
    (1) Location beneath the anterior margin of the sternocleidomastoid muscle
    (2) Absence of thyroid tissue in the wall
    (3) Disturbances in thyroid function
    (4) A tract extending through the hyoid bone to the foramen cecum

32. Pleomorphic adenoma (mixed tumor) of the parotid gland:
    (1) Is best treated by superficial lobectomy
    (2) Frequently requires removal of the facial nerve for adequate treatment
    (3) Has a tendency to locally recur following removal
    (4) Frequently metastasizes to cervical lymph nodes

33. Which of the following are indicative of inoperability in patients with breast cancer?
    (1) Inflammatory cancer
    (2) Satellite skin nodules
    (3) Parasternal nodules
    (4) Involved axillary lymph nodes

34. Signs of cardiac tamponade include:
    (1) Small pulse pressure
    (2) Hypertension
    (3) Distended neck veins
    (4) Bradycardia

35. Useful methods of study in suspected traumatic splenic rupture include:
    (1) Scanning with 99m technetium sulfur colloid
    (2) AP and lateral roentgenograms
    (3) Arteriography
    (4) Ultrasound scanning

36. A 21-year-old man is operated upon for acute appendicitis, the appendix, and cecum are normal but the terminal ileum is acutely inflamed. Which of the following statements is correct?
    (1) The appendix should be removed.
    (2) A right hemicolectomy is acceptable treatment.
    (3) The likelihood of developing chronic regional enteritis is small (less than 25%).
    (4) A course of Asulfadine should be given postoperatively.
37. Continuous neutralization of gastric acidity with antacids is indicated in which of the following clinical situations?
    (1) Perforative appendicitis with localized peritonitis treated by appendectomy
    (2) A patient with a 40% body surface burn
    (3) Following acute myocardial infarction
    (4) A patient comatose, but responsive to painful stimuli following severe head injury
38. A 68-year-old man is suspected to have a carcinoma of the body of the pancreas. Which of the following studies will be helpful in substantiating the diagnosis?
    (1) Serum amylase concentration
    (2) Selective angiography
    (3) 99m technetium sulfur colloid scans
    (4) Computerized tomography
39. Which of the following is precancerous?
    (1) The polyps of Peutz-Jeghers syndrome
    (2) Juvenile polyps of the colon
    (3) A solitary pedunculated adenomatous polyp 5 mm in diameter of the midsigmoid
    (4) Villous adenomas of the rectum
40. Useful studies in the diagnosis of renal cell carcinoma include:
    (1) Angiography
    (2) Intravenous pyelography
    (3) Nephrography
    (4) Urine cytology

Each set of lettered headings below is followed by a list of numbered words, phrases, or statements. For each numbered word, phrase, or statement the correct response will be:
    (A) If the item is associated with (a) only
    (B) If the item is associated with (b) only
    (C) If the item is associated with *both* (a) and (b)
    (D) If the item is associated with neither (a) nor (b)

    (a) Carcinoma of the lip
    (b) Carcinoma of the tongue
41. Is (are) radiosensitive
42. Causally related to exposure to sunlight
43. Elective lymph node dissection frequently employed in treatment
44. Highly curable even if cervical lymph nodes are involved
45. Metastases present in 60% or more of patients

    (a) Papillary cancer of the thyroid
    (b) Follicular cancer of the thyroid
46. Frequent multicentric foci in both lobes
47. Cervical lymph node metastases in over 50% of patients
48. Vein invasion and blood born metastases a significant factor
49. Radiosensitive
50. Highly lethal

    (a) Sliding hiatus hernia
    (b) Paresophageal hiatus hernia
51. Only indication for repair is esophagitis
52. Require truncal vagotomy for adequate repair
53. Necrosis of the gastric wall may occur

    (a) Familial polyposis of the colon
    (b) Gardner's syndrome
54. Polyps also occur in the small intestine with some frequency
55. Age of expression usually latter part of the second or the third decade of life
56. Osteomas of the cranial bones
57. Death from cancer inevitable if untreated
58. Usual treatment total colectomy and proctectomy

    (a) Angiodysplasia of the colon
    (b) Diverticular disease of the colon
59. Occult anemia
60. Precancerous
61. Treated by surgical resection when the diagnosis is made
62. Massive bleeding
63. Fistula formation

    (a) Meconium ileus
    (b) Duodenal atresia
64. Farber test positive
65. Double-bubble sign
66. Complicated by volvulus
67. Early operation desirable

(a) Benign prostatic hypertrophy
(b) Carcinoma of the prostate
68. Elevated acid phosphatase
69. May require transurethral resection
70. Most frequently starts in posterior lobe
71. Elevated alkaline phosphatase

ANSWERS TO MULTIPLE-CHOICE QUESTIONS

1. (b)	**5.** (e)	**9.** (a)	**13.** (e)	**17.** (a)	**31.** (d)	**45.** (B)	**59.** (A)
2. (d)	**6.** (b)	**10.** (e)	**14.** (e)	**18.** (d)	**32.** (b)	**46.** (A)	**60.** (D)
3. (d)	**7.** (c)	**11.** (c)	**15.** (d)	**19.** (c)	**33.** (a)	**47.** (A)	**61.** (D)
4. (c)	**8.** (e)	**12.** (b)	**16.** (b)	**20.** (a)	**34.** (b)	**48.** (B)	**62.** (C)
				21. (b)	**35.** (b)	**49.** (D)	**63.** (B)
				22. (a)	**36.** (b)	**50.** (D)	**64.** (B)
				23. (e)	**37.** (c)	**51.** (A)	**65.** (B)
				24. (b)	**38.** (c)	**52.** (D)	**66.** (A)
				25. (d)	**39.** (d)	**53.** (B)	**67.** (C)
				26. (b)	**40.** (A)	**54.** (B)	**68.** (B)
				27. (a)	**41.** (C)	**55.** (A)	**69.** (C)
				28. (c)	**42.** (A)	**56.** (B)	**70.** (B)
				29. (a)	**43.** (B)	**57.** (C)	**71.** (D)
				30. (e)	**44.** (A)	**58.** (C)	

Rypins' Clinical Sciences Review, 16th Edition, edited by Edward D. Frohlich. J. B. Lippincott Company, Philadelphia © 1993.

3

Internal Medicine

Edward D. Frohlich, M.D.*

Alton Ochsner Distinguished Scientist,
Vice President for Academic Affairs,
Alton Ochsner Medical Foundation;
Staff Member, Ochsner Clinic; Professor of
Medicine and of Physiology, Louisiana State
University School of Medicine; Adjunct Professor of
Pharmacology and Clinical Professor of Medicine,
Tulane University School of Medicine,
New Orleans, Louisiana

DISEASES OF THE CIRCULATION

The *heart* is a muscular pump that has the function of distributing blood through the systemic and pulmonary circulations. Its efficiency may be impaired by damage to the (1) valves; (2) myocardium, endocardium, or pericardium; (3) coronary arteries; (4) conduction system; and (5) peripheral vessels. Initial symptoms of patients with cardiac disease result primarily from myocardial ischemia, from disturbances in myocardial contractility, or from abnormal cardiac rate or rhythm.

Since publication of the last edition an endocrine role of the heart has been demonstrated. Thus the

* The author acknowledges the following physicians in the Department of Medicine of the Ochsner Clinic who have reviewed sections of this chapter: Drs. Archie W. Brown, C. Braddock Burns, Richard L. Hughes, Fred E. Husserl, George A. Pankey, Robert J. Quinet, James W. Smith, Hector O. Ventura, and Robert S. Zimmerman. Each of these very knowledgeable and experienced clinicians has reviewed the material for his subspecialty area (hematologic, pulmonary, neurologic, renal, infectious disease, rheumatologic, gastroenterologic, cardiovascular, and endocrine areas, respectively). I am truly grateful to them for their time-consuming and important contributions to this chapter.

atrium (and in certain circumstances the ventricle) produces a polypeptide hormone, the atrial natriuretic factor. Overfilling of the circulation and distention of the atrium releases the hormone and permits natriuresis and diuresis. The potential clinical significance of this factor is apparent for such clinical conditions as cardiac failure, hypertension, and paroxysmal atrial tachycardia, but the details await further study.

A correct and complete diagnosis is essential for the proper management of the patient. As outlined by the New York Heart Association, the diagnosis should consider:

1. Etiology: congenital, rheumatic, hypertensive, atherosclerotic, infective, or unknown
2. Structural abnormalities: chamber enlargement (*i.e.,* dilatation, hypertrophy), valvular involvement, myocardial infarction, pericardial involvement
3. Physiologic function: dysrhythmia, myocardial perfusion, or congestive heart failure
4. Functional reserve impairment: degree of activity to elicit symptoms

The most common variety of cardiac disease in the infant relates to a congenital defect in development; in the adolescent and young adult, valvular cardiac disease, often due to degenerative (myxomatous) mitral valve prolapse syndrome and less often rheumatic fever, and in the older adult, atherosclerosis and hypertension.

For the sake of simplicity, most pathologic or functional disturbances will be discussed only with the etiologic class in which they are most characteristic, even though they may occur also in other types of cardiac disease.

Congenital Cardiac Disease

Significant cardiovascular abnormalities occur in approximately 8 births in 1,000. With appropriate medical and surgical management most of these children may be cured or dramatically improved. The most frequent occurrences are atrial septal defect, patent ductus arteriosus, coarctation of the aorta, ventricular septal defect, and tetralogy of Fallot. Other entities such as single ventricle, valvular atresias, pulmonary stenosis, persistent truncus arteriosus, and common atrioventricular canal have less than 5% incidence in the patients diagnosed with congenital heart disease (Table 3-1).

The pathogenesis of congenital defects in the development of the heart is unknown, except that a significant number are apparently the consequence of maternal rubella during the first trimester of pregnancy. Rubella immunization is a major factor in the declining incidence of congenital heart disease. Evidence is accumulating that other illnesses of the mother, especially viral diseases, may have a similar result during the critical first 3 months of pregnancy. Other potential causes include ionizing irradiation, hypoxia, intake of several categories of drugs (including alcohol and tobacco), and deficiency or excess of several vitamins. Maternal lupus erythematosus during pregnancy has been linked to complete cardiac block in the infant.

At this time it is important to indicate the many measures available to prevent or minimize develop-

ment of congenital cardiac diseases. These measures include avoidance of teratogenic drugs; appropriate use of radiographic equipment; and detection of abnormal chromosomes in fetal cells obtained by amniocentesis or by chorionic villus biopsy (*e.g.,* Down's, Turner, or trisomy syndrome).

Many patients with congenital heart disease have two features in common: (1) history of early onset of cardiac symptoms such as birth as a "blue baby," a loud murmur with a thrill along the left sternal border, and the occurrence of cyanosis with intense dyspnea upon exertion early in childhood—polycythemia and clubbing of fingers are likely to occur in patients with long-standing cyanosis; (2) failure of normal growth and development; (3) rapid heart rate (160 to 180 beats per minute); (4) pulmonary wheezing; and (5) diminished urinary output.

A clinical classification of congenital heart disease based on the presence or the absence of cyanosis is commonly employed:

I. Without Cyanosis
  A. No shunt (normal pulmonary perfusion)
    With right ventricular predominance: valvular pulmonic stenosis, pulmonary artery stenosis, or primary pulmonary hypertension
    With left ventricular predominance: idiopathic hypertrophic aortic stenosis, valvular subaortic stenosis, or coarctation of the aorta
  B. Left-to-right shunt (increased pulmonary perfusion)
    With right ventricular predominance: atrial septal defect with or without mitral stenosis
    With left ventricular predominance: ventricular septal defect, patent ductus arteriosus
II. With Cyanosis
  A. Right-to-left shunt (normal or decreased pulmonary perfusion)
    With right ventricular predominance: tetralogy of Fallot
    With left ventricular predominance: tricuspid atresia or Ebstein's anomaly of the tricuspid valve
  B. Right-to-left and left-to-right shunts (increased pulmonary perfusion). Complete transposition of great vessels

Another lesion not included in the above classification is congenital cardiac block, which may occur in the absence of any other abnormality. Before the various congenital lesions are discussed, it is neces-

TABLE 3-1. Incidence of Defects in Patients Diagnosed with Congenital Heart Disease

CONGENITAL DEFECT	INCIDENCE (%)
Ventricular septal defect	30.0
Atrial septal defect	9.8
Patent ductus arteriosus	9.7
Pulmonic stenosis	6.9
Aortic coarctation	6.8
Aortic stenosis	6.1
Tetralogy of Fallot	5.8

sary to emphasize the importance of antibacterial prophylaxis in all affected patients in order to prevent bacterial endocarditis.

The most common congenital heart disease lesions are:

1. *Ventricular Septal Defect.* Interventricular septal defects usually are small in size. The harsh systolic murmur and thrill at the left margin of the sternum are in striking contrast to the usual absence of cyanosis or other evidence of impaired cardiac efficiency. In other instances there may be an overactive heart with biventricular enlargement, an accentuated pulmonic component of the second sound. ECG evidence of left ventricular hypertrophy, and increased pressure within the pulmonary circuit. The 2D-echocardiogram reveals evidence of left, right, and ventricular volume overload (*i.e.,* hyperdynamic left ventricle). Moreover, anatomical localization of all ventricular septal defects is facilitated by the use of 2D-echocardiography and Doppler color-flow technology. All gradations of severity may exist, and the septal defect may be complicated by other defects such as patent ductus, atrial septal defects, pulmonic stenosis, and coarctation of the aorta. Sometimes the treatment is surgical if a moderate or large amount of the left ventricular output is shunted to the right side, although in other patients spontaneous closure of the defect may occur.

2. *Patent Ductus Arteriosus.* The congenital lesion is most common in premature infants and is more frequently encountered in individuals born at high altitudes. Patients with this lesion should be considered for subendocarditis prophylaxis. The presence of a continuous loud machinerylike murmur in the pulmonic area is virtually diagnostic of this condition. Usually there is a thrill and moderately elevated systolic and depressed diastolic blood pressure. Because of the higher pressure in the systemic aorta, the direction of the blood shunt is from the aorta into the pulmonary artery. The increased volume of blood in the pulmonary circuit increases the work of the right ventricle, and the increased volume of blood returning from the lungs increases the load on the left ventricle so that both sides of the heart are involved. Cyanosis is absent in uncomplicated instances. Elimination of the shunt by surgical ligation of the patent ductus is a highly successful procedure, particularly when done in childhood and reduces the risk of infective endocarditis. In recent years pharmacologic therapy with indomethacin (a prostaglandin synthetase inhibitor) has met with some success in certain instances in infants with patent ductus arteriosus.

3. *Atrial Septal Defect.* This is also a common congenital cardiac defect and may be classified according to location in the atrial septum: the ostium secundum defect, located at the fossa ovale; and the ***ostium primum defect,*** located at the low atrial septum (the endocardial cushion defect). ***The sinus venosus defect*** is located in the upper septum and is frequently associated with partial anomalous pulmonary venous return. A *patent* ovale persists in a significant percentage of adults, but shunting of the blood does not occur with normal atrial pressures, and no symptoms result. Persistent ostium secundum, midseptal or cephalad in location, permits a left-to-right shunt because the left atrial pressure is higher than the right. A systolic murmur due to increased pulmonary flow results, with splitting of the second sound that does not vary with respiration. Increased pressure within the pulmonary arterial system may be evident from fluoroscopic examination and becomes apparent on the ECG later in the disease. The ECG usually shows right-axis deviation and incomplete right bundle branch block. Surgical repair is successful. The 2D-echocardiogram and color-flow Doppler can be used to localize the defects and calculate the shunt. Persistent ostium primum (frequently associated with Down's syndrome), one margin of the opening being made up of tissue between the atrioventricular (A-V) valves, is technically much more difficult to repair. Symptoms usually appear in childhood, with a systolic murmur and evidences of left as well as right ventricular hypertrophy. Mitral or tricuspid regurgitation may be present and favors the diagnosis of ostium primum defect. Pulmonic stenosis may be present and result in a right-to-left shunt.

4. *Coarctation of the Aorta.* In the usual type of coarctation, the narrowing of the aorta occurs at the point where the ligamentum arteriosum is attached near the origin of the left subclavian artery. This anomaly is associated with a bicuspid aortic valve in 25% of patients and occasionally with a patent ductus arteriosus. It is generally discovered during examination of an adolescent or a young adult with hypertension,

and is more common in male than female patients. When there is very weak or unobtainable pulse and blood pressure below the diaphragm, the diagnosis is practically established. The murmur (produced at the point of narrowing of the aorta) ordinarily is neglected until the basic diagnostic findings have been discovered. Sometimes coarctation is discovered by the radiologist who notices "scalloping" or "notching" of the lower borders of the ribs. This is produced by the enlarged intercostal arteries, which serve to "detour" circulation around the coarctation. A plastic operation on the aorta produces a dramatic cure. It should not be delayed since the aorta loses its elasticity steadily as the patient becomes older. In 5% to 10% of the operated patients there may be recurrent narrowing of the coarctation in infancy. This problem may be treated effectively with balloon angioplasty. The major complications of coarctation include severe hypertension, congestive heart failure, aortic rupture or dissecting aneurysm, infective endarteritis or endocarditis, and cerebral hemorrhage.

5. *Pulmonary Stenosis.* This congenital valvular lesion varies in severity and degree and may be associated with an atrial septal defect, resulting in a right-to-left shunt. It may lead to heart failure in infancy or cause difficulty only in later life. A systolic murmur in the pulmonic area, splitting of the second sound and right ventricular hypertrophy are found, and the stenosis is verified on cardiac catheterization. The treatment is surgical in the severe form; however, mild pulmonary stenosis requires no treatment other than antibiotic prophylaxis for bacterial endocarditis. More recently, balloon angioplasty by means of cardiac catheterization has been performed in milder degrees of severity or prior to surgery.

6. *Tetralogy of Fallot.* This is a combination of four defects: (a) pulmonic stenosis, (b) dextroposition of the aorta, (c) ventricular septal defect, and (d) hypertrophy of the right ventricle. Indeed, "tetralogy" is the most common cyanotic congenital anomaly in the adult. The clinical features include spells of hyperpnea, cyanosis, and syncope. However, the most characteristic diagnostic feature is continuous cyanosis, which nevertheless is compatible with life to adult years. There may be a harsh systolic murmur at the left sternal border, but the location and the intensity of the murmur are variable. The M-mode echocardiogram demonstrates aortic enlargement, aortic septal discontinuance, and aortic overriding. The 2D-echocardiogram shows right ventricular outflow narrowing and horizontal orientation. Usually the ECG shows right-axis deviation. Secondary polycythemia is usually present. The major complications of tetralogy are bacterial endocarditis and a high incidence of brain abscess. Complete surgical reconstruction is possible with mortality rates of less than 10% in children. The most important factor in assessing candidacy for primary repair is the size of the pulmonary artery. Marked hypoplasia is a contraindication for early corrective repair. When total surgical correction is possible, an operation to produce an anastomosis between the pulmonary artery and the systemic aorta or one of the great systemic arteries (the Blalock-Taussig procedure) will greatly improve the efficiency of the patient's cardiorespiratory system by increasing the blood flow through the pulmonary circuit and relieving hyperemia.

7. *Eisenmenger Complex.* This consists of a ventricular septal defect with a right-to-left or bidirectional shunt. The latter results from elevated pulmonary arterial pressure. This is differentiated from the tetralogy of Fallot, in which there is evidence of pulmonic stenosis. Cyanosis is not as severe.

In practically all instances of congenital heart disease, confirmation of the clinical diagnosis by such technical procedures as cardiac catheterization and angiocardiography will be desired before any operation is attempted.

8. *Ebstein Anomaly (of Tricuspid Valve).* This is manifested by a downward displacement of a malformed tricuspid valve into an underdeveloped right ventricle. On auscultation the first heart sound is widely split and multiple systolic clicks may be present because of vibrations of the saillike anterior leaflet of the valve. Tricuspid regurgitation may occur. The ECG will show peaked P waves with right bundle branch block and Wolff-Parkinson-White syndrome in 25% of cases. The echocardiogram shows a large anterior leaflet of the tricuspid valve with delayed closure, a small right ventricle, and a large atrialized right ventricle. The treatment is surgical repair.

Valvular Cardiac Disease

This group of cardiac lesions now represents a decreasing portion of all instances of acquired cardiac disease because of recognition and prophylaxis of rheumatic fever and the prevention of its recurrence. Although not all chronic valvular cardiac disease is due to rheumatic fever, a significant proportion is a characteristic sequela of rheumatic carditis. About half of all patients with valvular disease present a definite history of acute rheumatic fever. The common factor is regarded as a sensitivity reaction to the Group A β-hemolytic streptococcus, which produces its damage without actually being present in the heart. There is evidence to suggest that a hereditary factor may determine the susceptibility to rheumatic heart disease. During the acute phase there is pancarditis, with pericarditis, myocarditis (Aschoff bodies), and endocarditis. The first two ordinarily resolve, leaving chronic endocarditis with scarring of the valves.

The mitral valve is the valve most commonly affected (over two thirds of patients), and aortic stenosis is present in one fourth of patients with valvular disease.

In *mitral insufficiency (mitral regurgitation)* there is regurgitation of blood through the incompetent mitral valve when the left ventricle contracts. Consequently the typical murmur is halosystolic in timing. It is heard best at the apex and transmitted to the axilla and is "blowing" in character. The left ventricle usually is enlarged as demonstrated by palpation, percussion, and by x-ray examination. Unless acute in onset, or complicated by stenosis, the condition is often well compensated, and the prognosis is fairly good. However, symptomatic patients (functional class III or IV), despite vigorous trials with medical therapy, should be considered for surgery. Moreover, patients with lesser symptoms who have early evidence of myocardial dysfunction (*e.g.,* increased systolic left ventricular diameter) may also benefit from surgery.

The etiology of *mitral valve prolapse (Barlow's syndrome, click–murmur syndrome)* is poorly understood. It most often occurs in otherwise healthy young women (idiopathic mitral valve prolapse syndrome). However, it is also noted in men, with atrial septal defect, with Marfan's syndrome, and after myocardial infarction; sometimes it appears to be familial. Patients may be asymptomatic or have atypical chest pain or dysrhythmias. On physical examination there is a normal-sized heart, and a midsystolic click that may be followed by a late systolic murmur. The ECG may show specific ST-T changes, and the QT interval may be long. Chest roentgenogram is normal except for straightening of the thoracic spine in some patients. Echocardiography may be diagnostic, demonstrating a bowing of the posterior mitral valve leaflet occurring late in systole. In general, mitral valve prolapse has a benign course. However, the presence of redundant, thickened mitral valve leaflets by echocardiogram is associated with increased risk (10%) of sudden death, infective endocarditis, and cerebral ischemic events as compared with mitral valve prolapse of redundant leaflets treated effectively with β-adrenegic receptor blocking drugs. The risk of endocarditis, especially in patients with ballooning and diseased valve leaflets, is treated with antibacterial prophylaxis, particularly if a murmur is present.

Pure *mitral stenosis* occurs in 40% of patients with rheumatic heart disease. The stenosis interferes with filling of the left ventricle because of the narrowed valve. Therefore, the typical murmur is middiastolic, low pitched, diminuendo, and best heard at the apex. Often it is associated with a rough, crescendo, presystolic murmur, terminating in a sharp first sound and accompanied by a fine apical thrill. If atrial fibrillation (AF) intervenes, the presystolic murmur disappears. The pulmonic component of the second sound usually is accentuated and split, and the first sound at the apex is loud and sharp. There may also be an opening snap at the lower left sternal border. The x ray shows transverse enlargement with prominence of the left atrium and the pulmonary artery segment. The ECG shows right ventricular preponderance. The echocardiogram is diagnostic, revealing thickened mitral valvular leaflets and anterior movement of the posterior leaflet during diastole. AF, peripheral emboli, and cardiac decompensation are common as late manifestations. The narrowed mitral valve interferes with the inflow of blood from the left atrium into the left ventricle. In time the left atrial pressure increases, the chamber enlarges, and the pressure is transmitted back to the pulmonary circulation. Pulmonary congestion and exertional dyspnea may result. Orthopnea, paroxysmal nocturnal dyspnea, cough, and hemoptysis may follow. In a more advanced stage, increased pulmonary pressure occurs with arteriolar changes, increased resistance to blood flow, and relative pulmonary valvular insufficiency. Dilatation and failure of the right ventricle may cause tricuspid insufficiency. Evidence of right ventricular failure may appear with increased venous pressure, distended neck veins, engorged liver, and peripheral edema.

The ultimate prognosis is guarded. In patients with pure mitral stenosis, mitral comissurotomy has proved to be a highly satisfactory procedure if the valve leaflets are pliable. Replacement of the valve by a prosthesis has proved to be a satisfactory procedure but is associated with a greater operative mortality (5%). Surgical correction is not contraindicated by the presence of pulmonary hypertension.

Aortic stenosis is found more frequently in older patients, and calcification of the valve is a common occurrence. Isolated aortic stenosis is rarely due to rheumatic heart disease. Multiple valve disease including aortic stenosis suggests a rheumatic etiology. In patients under the age of 65 congenital bicuspid aortic valve is the most common cause of aortic stenosis. In patients over 65 years, the cusps may be sclerotic and calcified secondary to arteriosclerosis. The left ventricle hypertrophies without much dilatation in the early stages. Deficient cerebral blood flow, with fainting, syncope, and dizziness, is frequent. Anginal pain may occur. Cardiac failure or sudden death may follow with frequent incidence of ventricular dysrhythmias. A harsh or a musical systolic ejection murmur at the aortic area, transmitted to the vessels of the neck, is the classical sign. There is an accompanying thrill and a reduced aortic second sound. The narrow pulse pressure and pulsus tardus are characteristic. The treatment of severe aortic stenosis is valve replacement and is indicated when it becomes symptomatic, thereby indicating significant hemodynamic impairment. Aortic valvuloplasty is another means for repair of stenosis in those patients who are not considered for surgical repair.

The characteristic finding of **hypertrophic cardiomyopathy (HCM)** is inappropriate myocardial hypertrophy, often involving the interventricular septum of a nondilated ventricle. There is a dynamic pressure gradient in the subaortic area, which divides the left ventricle into a high-pressure apical region and a lower-pressure subaortic region. Hence the term **idiopathic hypertrophic subaortic stenosis (IHSS)** was originally suggested. However, not all patients have obstruction to ventricular outflow. For this reason, HCM is more appropriate. The etiology is now believed to be genetic. Anatomically, HCM is a cardiomyopathy characterized by an asymmetric and thickened ventricular septum. The septal cells are hypertrophied, abnormal in shape and arrangement. If outflow obstruction occurs it is apparently due to anterior motion of the mitral valve into the outflow tract. Although many patients are asymptomatic and referred because of murmur or ECG findings, patients may have dyspnea, angina, syncope, and palpitations. The most characteristic pathophysiological abnormality in HCM is not systolic, but diastolic, dysfunction. The myocardial disease is characterized by abnormal stiffness of the left ventricle during diastole, which impairs left ventricular filling. This results in increased left ventricular end-diastolic pressure, causing pulmonary congestion and dyspnea in the presence of normal systolic function. On physical examination there is a left ventricular impulse and a left ventricular ejection or regurgitant murmur at the lower left sternal border or apex. The murmur radiates poorly if at all to the carotids, as distinguished from prominent radiation in aortic stenosis. The murmur characteristically increases on Valsalva maneuver and in the upright position. ECG often shows left ventricular enlargement. The chest roentgenogram is commonly normal. Echocardiography is often virtually diagnostic, demonstrating an enlarged septum and systolic anterior motion of the mitral valve. The course is quite variable. Endocarditis prophylaxis is indicated. **Beta-adrenergic blocking drugs** or verapamil is often useful in decreasing outflow obstruction. Digitalis may enhance obstruction. Ventral septal myotomy or a myectomy may be indicated if symptoms are severe and propranolol is not uniformly effective.

Aortic regurgitation may occur as a result of rheumatic heart disease, but it also may be of syphilitic origin as well as associated with rheumatoid spondylitis, Marfan's syndrome, trauma, and bacterial endocarditis. The findings are (1) a soft, high-pitched diastolic murmur in the aortic area transmitted to the left border of the sternum; (2) left ventricular dilatation and hypertrophy; (3) lowered diastolic pressure with a wide pulse pressure; (4) to-and-fro arterial bruits (Duroziez's sign); (5) pistol-shot femoral artery sound; (6) water hammer pulse; and (7) capillary pulsation. There is usually a systolic murmur at the aortic area which, combined with the diastolic murmur, gives a to-and-fro murmur. The left ventricle hypertrophies and may compensate for this defect for many years, but when decompensation occurs it is likely to progress rapidly. Valve replacement is effective therapy.

Pulmonic stenosis has already been discussed in the section on congenital heart disease.

Tricuspid insufficiency occurs most frequently as a result of cardiac dilatation and failure—relative tricuspid insufficiency. Organic insufficiency is the result of rheumatic fever, endocarditis often associated with intravenous drug abuse, Ebstein anomaly, and carcinoid syndrome. Rheumatic tricuspid insufficiency is usually associated with disease of other valves as well. It produces a systolic murmur at the lower end of the sternum accentuated with respiratory inspiration, marked cardiac enlargement to the right, palpable systolic venous pulse in the neck veins, and a palpable expansile pulsation of the liver. Tricuspid stenosis is relatively infrequent and seldom recognized by clinical means but can be associated with carcinoid tumors.

Infective (Bacterial) Endocarditis

Traditionally, distinction has been made between "acute" and "subacute" endocarditis. Although recent years have revealed less sharpness in this separation, there is probably still some clinical value in its consideration.

Acute bacterial ("ulcerative") endocarditis is a rapidly progressive infection of the endocardium associated with destruction of the affected valves and with signs and symptoms of a fulminating infection. Its differentiation from subacute bacterial endocarditis is primarily on the basis of the virulence of the invading pyogenic organism. Hemolytic streptococci, *Haemophilus influenzae,* staphylococci (*aureus, epidermidis*), pneumococci, gonococci, *Pseudomonus aeruginosa*, or fungi, may be the infecting organisms. Prompt and vigorous treatment with antibiotics and valve replacement have made recovery possible in a large number of cases.

Subacute bacterial endocarditis is much more common than the acute type. Alpha-hemolytic streptococci and nonhemolytic streptococci are the most common infecting agents. The infection usually is superimposed upon diseased mitral and aortic valves. Symptoms include (1) fever, (2) chills, (3) malaise, (4) fatigue, and (5) development of complaints of embolic and progressive valvular involvement. Anemia is common. Emboli originating from the valvular vegetations may produce splanchnic, renal, or cerebral infarcts; other embolic phenomena include petechial hemorrhages in the skin and mucous membranes and splinter hemorrhages beneath the nails. Tender Osler's nodes of the fingertips also occur. The diagnosis is suggested by protracted fever in a patient with a valvular defect, particularly if petechial hemorrhages or gross embolic phenomena (including flank pain), marked anemia, microscopic hematuria, and a palpable spleen are present. Repeated blood cultures are positive in about 90% of cases. Vigorous treatment with penicillin will result in a bacteriologic cure in the majority of cases; in the case of infection with

penicillin-resistant organisms, combinations of bactericidal antibiotics such as penicillin plus gentamicin may be necessary. Surgical intervention is indicated in patients with infective endocarditis in the presence of refractory valve infection, persistent congestive heart failure, and recurrent major systemic embolization. Complications of endocarditis include cardiac failure, myocardial abscess, and myocarditis; neurological symptoms from embolization and mycotic aneurysms; and renal sequelae, including infarction, glomerulonephritis, and abscess formation.

Endocarditis (usually acute) in narcotic addicts using intravenous drugs is increasing. More recently it has been observed in patients with acquired immunodeficiency syndrome (AIDS). Staphylococcus is the predominant organism, and the right side of the heart is frequently involved with tricuspid insufficiency and pulmonic lesions; aortic valvular involvement is not uncommon, however.

Bacterial endocarditis may result from dental and other surgical procedures, gastrointestinal (GI) or genitourinary infections, and in patients with rheumatic or congenital cardiac disease. When such procedures are undertaken these patients should be protected by antibiotics in therapeutic doses. Culture-negative endocarditis may be related to noninfective endocarditis; prior antimicrobial therapy; Q fever; fungi; acid-fast bacteria; chlamydia; viral etiologies; and uremia.

Prosthetic valvular endocarditis may be associated with the development of fever with or following detection of a new cardiac murmur. Several complications are peculiar to prosthetic valvular endocarditis: gradual development of cardiac failure in a patient with a ball-type device (Starr-Edwards), increased incidence of emboli because of increased frequency of fungal infection, or abscess of an annulus.

Pericarditis, an inflammation of the pericardium, is clinically manifested by substernal, sharp, knife-like chest pain that may radiate to left supraclavicular, shoulder, and neck areas; fever; and pericardial effusion. It may be due to a variety of causes including viruses, bacteria, fungi, collagen vascular disease, uremia, trauma, or it may be of unknown etiology. It may be acute, subacute, recurrent, or chronic in nature. The most common virus causing pericarditis is Coxsackie B; however, Coxsackie A, echovirus, mumps, and Epstein-Barr (mononucleosis) have all been implicated. Bacterial pericarditis results from hematogenous dissemination of organisms from another focus of infection or from direct extension from the lung or esophagus. Streptococci, meningococci, mycobacteria, and gonococci all may produce pericarditis. Positive physical findings include a pericardial friction rub. Diagnosis may be difficult if signs and symptoms are absent—but if clinically suspected may be confirmed by chest x ray, echocardiogram, ECG (concave S-T segment elevation), pericardiocentesis and, if necessary, surgical exploration, which may also be of therapeutic value.

Cardiovascular Syphilis

LUETIC HEART

In this country syphilis and, with it, syphilitic heart disease are declining steadily in frequency. Typically syphilitic heart disease is a complication of syphilitic aortitis, which (1) causes *aneurysm* of the aortic arch; (2) extends backward to involve the aortic valve, with resulting *regurgitation;* and finally (3) causes *stenosis* of the branches of the aorta, particularly the *coronary arteries.* Men between 45 and 55 years of age are most commonly afflicted.

Luetic aortitis is due to an obliterative endarteritis of the vasa vasorum, with resultant destruction of the media and wrinkling of the intima and weakening of the wall structure. The lesion is most common in the ascending aorta. An *aneurysm* results from stretching of the thinned walls. A saccular aneurysm is less common than a diffuse dilatation of the ascending aorta with resulting aortic regurgitation. The physical findings are the same as in aortic regurgitation of the rheumatic variety. At present, the preferred treatment of syphilitic aortitis is intravenous penicillin.

Coronary Artery Disease

Atherosclerosis with narrowing of the lumen is the most common form of coronary artery disease; it is most prevalent in the fifth and sixth decades of life and is found more often in men than in women. Rarely such disorders as polyarteritis nodosa may involve the coronary vessels as well as the systemic arteries. The phenomenon of spasm of the coronary arteries (with or without atherosclerotic narrowing) is clearly recognized and of clinical significance. In the case of coronary artery narrowing but without complete occlusion, the presence or the absence of symptoms has a direct bearing on the relationship between the requirements of the myocardium for oxygen and the ability of the coronary circulation to transport that oxygen. Patients may be asymptomatic at rest, and manifestations of myocardial ischemia may develop only when the demand for an increased work load is placed upon the heart. Not only may myocardial ischemia result from the narrowing of the coronary vessels, but it may follow complete occlusion of such a vessel by thrombosis, which may follow ulceration of an atheromatous plaque or subintimal hemorrhage.

Data continue to accumulate about factors that increase risk of coronary artery disease. Hypertension, with both systolic and diastolic pressures of equal risk, hyperlipidemia, obesity, cigarette smoking, physical inactivity, Type A personality, hyperuricemia, and a strongly positive family history of coronary disease or premature cardiovascular death contribute to the increased risk.

Because the resting ECG may be normal, exercise testing may be useful; however false negatives and false positives do occur and radionuclide scintigraphy may improve the diagnostic ability of exercise testing.

ANGINA PECTORIS

This is a manifestation of coronary insufficiency characterized by paroxysmal substernal pain usually produced by exertion and relieved by rest. The pain consists of a sense of pressure in the substernal region; it is variously described as a tight pressure and squeezing or boring pains. The pain frequently radiates into the neck and along the medial aspect of the left arm and forearm; however, some patients may experience symptoms of ischemia manifested as fatigue, weakness, or dyspnea rather than chest discomfort (the so-called anginal equivalents). These episodes of stable angina usually are of short duration and, as a rule, are relieved promptly by rest. Unstable angina is defined as anginal pain that is increasing in severity, duration, and frequency. The pain may be progressively severe (crescendo angina), occurring more frequently at rest, and occurring at different times with no precipitating events. This is a high-risk group of patients for myocardial infarction. Angina pectoris often precedes coronary thrombosis. The pain in the two conditions is similar but differs in its duration. Physical examination in a patient with angina pectoris often reveals no abnormalities. Exercise testing will usually evoke conspicuous ECG changes suggestive of myocardial ischemia. The frequency of attacks of angina pectoris often can be controlled by reduction in physical activity; attacks often may be aborted or their severity decreased through the use of amyl nitrite, nitroglycerin, and long-acting nitrites. Other pharmacological agents used for the treatment of angina pectoris include the β-adrenergic receptor blocking agents and the calcium antagonists. Those patients with hyperlipidemia and angina pectoris may benefit from low-fat diets and, if indicated, pharmacological agents. Aspirin has also been reported to be beneficial in patients with unstable angina.

Some patients, especially with diabetes mellitus, may have *silent ischemia.* This condition is manifested by episodes of ischemia that may be well documented by ECG-recorded ventricular dysrhythmias without associated chest discomfort. More frequently, angina pectoris associated with severe hypertension will be ameliorated by reduction in the blood pressure toward normal. Beta-adrenergic receptor blocking agents like propranolol are widely given to patients with angina and reduce frequency of attacks by reducing cardiac work through slowing of heart rate and lowering blood pressure response to exercise. In addition, long-acting nitrates and calcium channel blockers have proved to be very useful in patients with coronary artery spasm. Although the precise indications for coronary bypass surgery are debated, some patients have marked symptomatic improvement following surgery. Patients with left main coronary disease and those who do not respond to medical therapy should especially be considered. In recent years percutaneous transluminal angioplasty (PTCA) has been used. It has been particularly effective in patients with single-vessel disease, although it has also been employed in patients with multivessel disease. Certain patients may spontaneously develop a collateral circulation with relief or at times almost complete recovery from their angina. Angina pectoris has a death rate of 3% to 5% per year.

MYOCARDIAL INFARCTION

Coronary insufficiency may result in myocardial infarction that occurs either with or without occlusion of a branch of a coronary artery. Acute myocardial infarction is caused by a coronary artery thrombosis in 85% of the cases. Not all sudden deaths in patients with coronary arteriosclerosis are the result of myocardial infarction: some of these are the results of fatal ventricular arrhythmias precipitated by an episode of myocardial ischemia. There is a circadian variation in the timing of infarction, with an increased frequency during the early morning hours when the fibrinolytic system seems to be least active and platelet aggregation increased. The clas-

sic symptoms are (1) pain, (2) shock, and (3) dyspnea. The pain is similar to that of angina pectoris in location and in quality; usually it is intense and may persist for hours. It is not caused specifically by exercise, nor is it relieved by rest; and this may be found particularly in patients with diabetes resulting in myocardial infarction (without pain). The hypotension may be of any degree and usually is associated with signs of peripheral vascular collapse; cyanosis and the signs of acute cardiac failure may be present in massive infarcts. On auscultation, the heart sounds are usually diminished in intensity and the most common extra sound is the S_4 or atrial gallop (which, obviously, is absent in atrial fibrillation). A friction rub is heard in a majority of patients at some time in the course, because of pericardial inflammation. The presence of myocardial infarction also is associated with elevation of temperature, leukocytosis, and by characteristic ECG changes. Certain enzymes are present in high concentration in cardiac muscle and are released into the blood with infarction. The level of creatinine phosphokinase (CPK) rises and falls most rapidly. The MB fraction of CPK is the most sensitive marker of myocardial necrosis (in 7% to 8%). Serum glutamic oxaloacetic transaminase (SGOT) is increased in the blood within 6 to 12 hours and reaches a peak in 2 to 3 days, then reverts to normal. Lactic dehydrogenase (LDH) and its isozymes (LDH_1, LDH_2) activity in the serum are an index of myocardial necrosis and is of greater specificity than SGOT and is elevated for a longer period.

Myocardial infarctions may be classified electrocardiographically as Q wave and non-Q wave (subendocardial). The classical electrocardiographic findings in leads overlying the infarcted muscle are (1) the presence of significant Q waves in leads that ordinarily would be expected to be dominated by R waves, (2) abnormal elevations of the S-T segments, and (3) abnormal inverted T waves. During the very early phases of myocardial infarction the characteristic electrocardiographic findings may not have evolved fully, and in such instances serial tracings are necessary. Other diagnostic tests include myocardial scintigraphy ("scans") and the echocardiogram.

Right ventricular infarction occurs in approximately 40% of patients with left ventricular inferior acute myocardial infarction. Clinical clues include elevation of jugular venous pressure; a right-sided S_3S_4 gallop rhythm; and, the most consistent ECG finding, the presence of S-T elevation of 1 mm or more in lead V_4R. Extensive right ventricular infarction causes hypotension and low cardiac output. Diagnosis can be confirmed by hemodynamic findings of elevated right atrial pressure and other findings similar to cardiac tamponade.

Treatment of acute myocardial infarction consists of:

1. Relief of pain. Morphine still is one of the drugs most widely used for this purpose, but other narcotics, such as meperidine, may be substituted if the patient has an idiosyncrasy to morphine. Because of potential for producing hypotension, the minimal effective dose should be used. Nitroglycerine and isosorbide dinitrate may be beneficial in controlling pain (the former with intravenous or paste formulations) because of their ability to increase collateral coronary blood flow and to reduce ventricular wall motion asynergy.

2. Oxygen therapy. When the pain does not respond readily to the administration of narcotics, or when cyanosis is present, oxygen therapy should be prescribed either by nasal catheter or mask.

3. Bed rest for 24 to 36 hours with progressive and individualized ambulation is always important.

4. The treatment of hypotension may be difficult. First, if possible, the cause should be determined. If there is a volume deficit, careful volume expansion should be used. If the patient is in cardiogenic shock, the choice of vasopressor drugs is controversial, as is balloon assistance and emergency bypass surgery. Under each of these circumstances hemodynamic monitoring with a Swan-Ganz catheter may be warranted.

5. Digitalis is of uncertain value in acute myocardial infarction with congestive heart failure. Evidence suggests that patients in this category are unusually sensitive to digitalis. During the acute phase diuretics are recommended to control congestive failure.

6. Adequate treatment of dysrhythmias. The sudden and unexpected occurrence of primary ventricular fibrillation (not in the context of ventricular failure) has diminished to a rate of 1% to 2% as a result of improved control of blood pressure and prompt recognition and correction of hyperkalemia. When it occurs, intravenous lidocaine may be used to treat ventricular dysrhythmias, and it may be used prophylactically in patients older than 70

years who present within 4 hours of an acute myocardial infarction without evidence of cardiac failure.

Supraventricular dysrhythmias are common and are treated with a short-acting glycoside such as digoxin and β-blockers. The calcium antagonist verapamil may also be effective. Electroshock is used if dysrhythmia persists and is refractory. In some instances, if the rhythm and rate is not normalized, cardiac failure will result.

7. Reperfusion of the myocardium can be approached therapeutically by coronary artery bypass grafts (CABG), by percutaneous transluminal coronary angioplasty (PTCA), and by thrombolytic therapy. ***Thrombolytic therapy*** comprises a variety of intravenously administered agents that have been shown to be capable of lysing a coronary thrombus. The best-studied agents are streptokinase (SK), tissue plasminogen activator (t-PA), and an isolated plasminogen-streptokinase activator complex (PSAC). Clinical trials have shown that when an agent is administered within the first 4 to 6 hours of an acute myocardial infarction, mortality will be reduced by at least 25%. If the agent is administered within the first hour, mortality may be reduced by 50%. Indications for thrombolytic therapy include chest pain typical of myocardial infarction, Q-wave infarction, and therapy administered within 6 hours after onset of chest pain. Pharmacologic interventions may be followed by percutaneous transluminal coronary angioplasty (PTCA) with consequent improved myocardial perfusion. Intracranial hemorrhage and gastrointestinal bleeding have been reported as complications of this therapy. PTCA without thrombolytic therapy should be reserved for patients with known coronary anatomy who cannot receive thrombolytic therapy or who are in cardiogenic shock. PTCA following thrombolytic therapy (either immediately or delayed) has no further advantage in reducing mortality, provided that the patient has no signs of ischemia.

8. Beta-adrenergic receptor blocking drugs. Large multicenter studies have clearly shown a reduction in overall mortality, sudden death, or reinfarction after documentation of a first myocardial infarction. This protection has not been demonstrated with those agents

possessing intrinsic sympathomimetic activity (ISA).

9. Similarly, the calcium antagonist diltiazem has shown protection, but this has been shown only with non-Q-wave myocardial infarction.

Among the more common complications of myocardial infarction are the following:

1. Cardiac failure
2. Cardiogenic shock
3. Extension of the original infarction (usually occurring around 5 days postinfarction, and in 20% of patients)
4. Pericarditis (in 7% to 15% of infarction patients)
5. Papillary muscle rupture
6. Rupture of the interventricular septum (in 1% of patients)
7. Rupture of the free wall of the left ventricle.

Other noncardiac complications include items 8 through 10, below.

8. **Shoulder–hand syndrome** (in 5% to 10% of patients) occurring any time within a year after infarction. It is characterized by pain and tenderness of the shoulder, followed by pain, redness, swelling, and stiffness of the hand and fingers, and is occasionally accompanied by atrophy of the muscles of the hand. Aspirin, physiotherapy, and an exercise program are helpful.

9. **Postmyocardial infarction (Dressler's) syndrome** may occur from 2 weeks to 2 months after the acute infarction. It is characterized by fever, leukocytosis, pleuritis, pericarditis, and pneumonitis. Pleural and pericardial exudates, which may be hemorrhagic, occur. The cause is unknown but may be due to sensitization to antigens resulting from myocardial necrosis. It is a benign disorder, which may be mistaken for recurrence of myocardial infarction. It is treated with nonsteroidal anti-inflammatory drugs.

10. **Ventricular aneurysm** occurs in about 20% of the cases within weeks or months after the acute infarct. ECG usually shows elevated ST segments. On x ray an abnormal bulge of the ventricular contour is seen, which may be evident on palpation as an abnormal area of pulsations on the chest wall. Ventricular asynergy may also be a complication. Again, the echocardiogram may also be particularly helpful.

ATHEROSCLEROSIS

Atherosclerosis is a disease in which atheroma, deposits of lipid-containing material, appear beneath the intima of arteries. Hypertension, diabetes mellitus, hyperlipidemia, obesity, and smoking are major risk factors. It is primarily a disease of the aorta and its branches, rather than of the pulmonary circuit, and is the basic etiologic factor in a high percentage of cases of coronary occlusion, cerebral thrombosis, mesenteric thrombosis, and occlusive peripheral vascular disease. The rapidity and the extent of atheromatous changes are modified to some extent by race, hereditary factors, age, sex, and previous damage to the vessel walls. The effects of diet and the cholesterol or lipid content of the blood are not fully determined. There appears to be a relationship between the amount and quality of fat consumed in the diet, the cholesterol and lipoprotein content of the blood, and the death rate from coronary artery disease. The low-density lipoprotein (LDL) fraction of cholesterol is directly related to the risk of atherosclerosis and coronary artery disease, whereas the high-density lipoprotein (HDL) fraction is inversely related. The solid saturated fats tend to elevate the blood level of lipoproteins, whereas linoleic acid and some other unsaturated fatty acids from marine and vegetable oils tend to lower it. It seems firmly established that certain dietary fats induce increased blood coagulability and decreased fibrinolysis, but the effect of these factors in coronary heart disease is not established.

Plasma Lipoprotein Abnormalities

The association of atherosclerosis and its accompanying vascular changes with alterations in the plasma cholesterol and lipoproteins has increased interest in lipoprotein abnormalities.

Hyperlipoproteinemia, not explained by other primary disease, represents metabolic problems that are difficult to classify. Lipoprotein-excess states have been classified in five categories on the basis of plasma appearance and blood cholesterol and triglyceride concentrations.

Type I hyperlipoproteinemia: Milky serum (increased chylomicrons in blood) is present with hyperchylomicronemia and absolute deficiency of lipoprotein lipase. Cholesterol concentration is normal but triglycerides are greatly increased. This disorder occurs in infancy, presents with abdominal pain and has no predisposition to coronary artery disease.

Type II hyperlipoproteinemia: Serum cholesterol is increased but triglycerides are normal. There is strong evidence of accelerated vascular disease in this category. Type II is familial and is autosomal dominant. Xanthomata are frequent. Dietary restriction of saturated fats and use of polyunsaturated fats are desirable as well as drug therapy. Type IIa is associated with elevated LDL cholesterol but normal triglycerides and VLDL. In contrast, type IIb is associated with elevated LDL, VLDL, and triglyceride levels. The most common cause of elevated cholesterol and LDL is polygenetic hypercholesterolemia; this form represents 85% of individuals with elevated cholesterol levels on routine screening.

Type III hyperlipoproteinemia: Serum cholesterol and triglycerides are increased with a broad beta band on electrophoresis. This form of hyperlipidemia is uncommon. It is characteristically associated with palmar xanthomata. Vascular disease is frequent and weight reduction with the use of polyunsaturated fats is recommended.

Type IV hyperlipoproteinemia: Serum cholesterol, VLDL, and triglyceride levels are elevated. Diabetes mellitus, hypothyroidism, lupus erythematosis, renal failure, and alcohol abuse may be associated with this type of hyperlipidemia. Premature coronary artery disease is frequent. Weight reduction and decrease in carbohydrate intake and of saturated fatty food is prescribed. Lovastatin, gemfibrozil, and other fibric acid derivatives have been effective in lowering cholesterol and triglyceride levels.

Type IV profiles are seen also with hypothyroidism, nephrotic syndrome, obstructive jaundice, dysproteinemias (multiple myeloma), and uncontrolled diabetes mellitus.

Type V hyperlipoproteinemia: Serum cholesterol and triglycerides levels are greatly elevated. Obesity and eruptive xanthomata, especially on knees, are common. This occurs in late teens and is associated with abdominal pain. Weight reduction is essential.

Hyperlipidemia demands attention when cholesterol exceeds 200 mg/100 ml and triglycerides 250 mg/100 ml. Dietary or drug treatment is indicated in patients with known coronary artery disease to reduce cholesterol and LDL cholesterol to less than 200 and 130 mg/dl, respectively. If there is no evidence of coronary artery disease, dietary treatment should be initiated if the cholesterol and LDL cholesterol are greater than 200 and 140 mg/dl, respectively. In patients with two or more risk factors (including male gender) drug

therapy should be added if the dietary measures are unsuccessful and the cholesterol and LDL cholesterol are greater than 240 and 190 mg/dl, respectively. A broad spectrum of antihyperlipidemic agents is available, including cholestyramine, colestipol, nicotinic acid, lovastatin, gemfibrozil, and probucol. Elevated triglyceride levels (>500 mg/dl) should be reduced to prevent pancreatitis. (See *Rypins' Basic Sciences Review,* 16th ed., Chap. 7, for a more detailed discussion of these agents.)

The Cardiomyopathies

The cardiomyopathies are classified clinically as follows:

Dilated: idiopathic or ischemic is manifested by poor systolic ejection function, cardiac dilatation, cardiac failure, dysrhythmias, emboli, and murmurs of mitral and tricuspid regurgitation

Hypertrophic: inappropriate left ventricular hypertrophy with preserved contractile function

Restrictive: diastolic filling of the ventricles is impaired; amyloid is the prototype; the clinical picture resembles constrictive pericarditis

Cardiomyopathies are considered primary when the heart is the chief target organ and secondary when it accompanies known systemic conditions. Primary and secondary myopathies may fall into the above clinical classification. Amyloidosis, hemochromatosis, sarcoidosis, scleroderma, lupus erythematosus, neuromuscular disease, and coronary artery disease may be both dilated and ischemic and are considered to be secondary cardiomyopathies.

Examples of primary disease are familial, alcoholic, viral myocarditis, postpartum, and endomyocardial fibrosis and endocardial fibroelastosis. These are usually manifested by dilated and low cardiac output changes.

Cor Pulmonale

Cor pulmonale is a right-sided cardiac enlargement due to disease in the pulmonary circuit, to valvular defects that increase the pulmonary pressure, or to congenital defects. Acute cor pulmonale is caused by sudden obstruction of the pulmonary artery or one of its branches, usually by an embolus from a peripheral vein. Chronic cor pulmonale is gradual in its development and may result from left ventricular failure, from mitral stenosis, or from a wide variety of pulmonary or vascular lesions resulting in increased pressure and resistance to flow through the pulmonary vascular bed.

The manifestations are cyanosis, polycythemia, clubbing of the fingers, venous engorgement, increased venous pressure, engorgement of the liver, and edema. Right ventricular dilatation and tricuspid insufficiency occur. X-ray films show enlargement of the pulmonary artery with increased pulsation. The right atrium and the right ventricle are enlarged. The ECG shows right-axis deviation and evidence of right ventricular hypertrophy. Treatment is that of cardiac failure plus treatment, when possible, of the underlying pulmonary lesion.

Congestive Heart Failure

Cardiac failure is defined as an abnormality of cardiac function in which the ventricles do not deliver adequate blood to the tissues at rest or during normal activity. The mechanism of myocardial failure is complex (Table 3-2). Even an approximate understanding of it demands knowledge of cardiac function, hemodynamics, water and electrolyte metabolism, renal, and endocrine function. Among the neurohumoral and other circulating factors that participate importantly in the progression of cardiac failure are norepinephrine, the renin–angiotensin–aldosterone system, atrial natriuretic factor, vasopressin, and other factors just being identified. In most patients, cardiac failure results from anatomic lesions of the myocardial cell, heart valves, conduction system, or pericardium. In addition there are frequently precipitating causes that lead to manifestations of cardiac failure in the presence of underlying cardiac disease. These are:

1. Pulmonary embolism
2. Infection
3. Anemia
4. Thyrotoxicosis
5. Pregnancy
6. Dysrhythmias
7. Myocarditis
8. Bacterial endocarditis
9. Physical exertion
10. Sodium excess
11. Severe hypertension

The acute onset of congestive heart failure may be due to myocarditis, and, therefore, endomyocardial biopsy might be valuable in the diagnosis of this problem. When fully developed, the syndrome is characterized by dyspnea, edema, venous hypertension, hepatomegaly, and often by pleural effusion. On further inquiry and examination, some or

TABLE 3-2. Mechanisms Underlying Congestive Heart Failure

Pressure overload
Volume overload
Impaired myocardial contractility
Restricted ventricular filling
Loss of functioning myocardium

all of the following may be found: orthopnea, paroxysmal cardiac dyspnea, pulmonary rales, enlargement of the heart, murmurs, disturbances in the cardiac mechanism, gallop (ventricular) rhythm, pulsus alternans, a positive hepatojugular reflux, and abnormal arterial pressure. There will be variation in the details, depending to some extent on the underlying type of cardiac disease, but the general pattern is consistent.

Often it is difficult (or impossible) to change the course of many types of cardiac disease, but cardiac failure sometimes may be delayed for long periods by certain prophylactic measures. As examples: the activity and the dietary habits (sodium content) of some patients may be changed. The treatment of anemia, thyrotoxicosis, obesity, and arterial hypertension, when present, is particularly helpful. Furthermore, recurrences of rheumatic fever now are largely preventable, and patients with chronic rheumatic valvular disease should be evaluated for surgery before, not after, cardiac failure appears. Lastly, prompt recognition and successful treatment of certain cardiac mechanism disturbances often will forestall cardiac failure.

The goal, once cardiac function is manifest, is to restore adequate cardiac output and to maintain it. Rest is paramount, and individual circumstances dictate the strictness of the program. Sedation may be helpful. Oxygen is indicated for the cyanotic or the severely dyspneic patient. Digitalis continues to be useful in cardiac failure, especially in patients with a ventricular (S_3) gallop having significant cardiomegaly and an ejection fraction less than 20%. Any of the active, well-standardized preparations are acceptable. Optimum digitalization and maintenance, irrespective of the preparation used, is the main point. It is seldom necessary to digitalize a patient fully by the single-dose method. Sodium restriction has become almost routine, but seldom does it need to be extremely rigid. A diet containing 800 mg (35 mEq) sodium (2.0 g salt) per day will serve for most patients. Injectable "loop" diuretics such as furosemide may be used, but oral diuretics such as the thiazide group, and furosemide are satisfactory in most cases. Spironolactone may be used in persistent therapy, primarily to avoid potassium loss. Care must be taken to guard against serum electrolyte depletion when combined sodium restriction and diuretics are used. There are selected instances when application of tourniquets to the extremities or venesection will be beneficial, and the utility of occasionally removing large collections of pleural fluid should be remembered. Specific therapy should be directed toward the particular type of underlying cardiac disease whenever possible. Therapy with peripheral vasodilating agents, particularly the angiotensin-converting enzyme inhibitors has been useful in cardiac failure refractory to more conventional measures. These agents dilate arterioles and reduce total peripheral resistance and, hence, left ventricular afterload and aortic impedance. They may also dilate the venules, reducing venous return and ventricular preload. Venodilators like nitroglycerine and long-acting nitrates also reduce cardiac preload, and as a result of these two effects a new and more effective cardiac function curve may be achieved. Anticoagulants are also important in preventing emboli, particularly in patients with left ventricular thrombi, atrial fibrillation, and peripheral venous disease.

Refractory heart failure is said to exist if symptoms of cardiac failure persist despite optimal medical therapy with digoxin, diuretics, and vasodilators. In this situation, other measures may be considered, including intravenous inotropic agents (dobatamine, amrinone). In addition, cardiac transplantation, in selected centers, has become a therapeutic option in these patients, achieving 85% survival after 1 year.

Hypertension and Hypertensive Cardiovascular Disease

The upper limits of normal atrial pressure are usually defined as 140 mmHg systolic and 90 mmHg diastolic. Recent life insurance statistics show that persistent increase in blood pressure above these figures, regardless of age, is associated with a shortened life expectancy. Patients with diastolic pressures falling between 85 and 89 mmHg have high normal pressures. Isolated systolic hypertension occurs when systolic pressure exceeds 159 mmHg and when diastolic pressure is less than 90 mmHg. Borderline isolated systolic hypertension occurs when the systolic pressure is 140 to 159 mmHg and the diastolic pressure is less than 90 mmHg. In the United States the average weight and the average blood pressure increase steadily with advancing years. Hypertension is an important risk factor underlying coronary heart disease and stroke. Systolic and diastolic levels are both major risk factors; in fact, the systolic pressure may impart an even greater risk. The higher the pressures, the greater the risk.

Over 95% of all hypertension is of unknown cause and is referred to as *"essential hypertension"*; this hypertension is primary in origin. *Secondary hypertension* (*i.e.*, when an etiology can be determined) most commonly is due to renal artery stenosis, bilateral renal parenchymal disease, or oral contraceptive agents. Less common causes of secondary hypertension include primary hyperaldosteronism, pheochromocytoma, coarctation of the aorta, Cushing's syndrome, renin-producing tumors, and excessive licorice ingestion. Recent data have emphasized exogenous obesity and alcohol as high-risk, if not causative, factors in elevating arterial pressure.

Essential hypertension is an extremely common and important disturbance after the age of 40. Plasma renin activity may be high, low, or normal depending on dietary sodium intake, severity of vascular disease, height of total peripheral resistance, plasma volume, adrenergic activity, and other physiological variables.

High blood pressure may exist for many years without symptoms. Many have associated headaches, vertigo, palpitation, rapid heart action, moderate dyspnea, or nervous tension states (for which no other cause can be found) to hypertension; but these are frequent symptoms and complaints of normotensive individuals as well. The effects of hypertension on the target organs (heart, kidney, brain) should be determined when the high blood pressure is first detected and regularly thereafter. This evaluation includes determination of renal parenchymal function (blood urea nitrogen or serum creatinine concentrations and creatinine clearance), cardiac size and rhythm, and, if necessary, vascular involvement. The earliest retinal vascular changes are tortuosity and narrowing of the arteriolar and venular lumens (the normal arteriolar-venous ratio of 3 : 4 decreases perhaps to 1 : 2). If therapy is inadequate the lesion will progress to severe arteriolar narrowing, arteriovenous (A-V) nicking, and copper or silver wire appearance of the vessel. Renal function and status should be followed by urinalysis, serum creatinine levels and, if necessary, more sophisticated studies (*e.g.*, arteriography). In the untreated patient with essential hypertension, the higher the serum uric acid level, the less the renal blood flow and the higher renal vascular resistance. Renal vessels develop arteriolar nephrosclerosis, and mild (1+) proteinuria is common and renal functional impairment may develop (particularly in black patients). Hypertensive heart disease is first manifested by left ventricular involvement; but left atrial enlargement by ECG is the first clinical indication of a less compliant left ventricle. Later, left ventricular hypertrophy is revealed by ECG, then by chest x ray. The echocardiogram is the most sensitive means of demonstrating hypertrophy (by increased left ventricular mass and wall thicknesses) and its regression. Left ventricular failure is the final stage of hypertensive heart disease; however, angina pectoris and left ventricular ischemia, cardiac dysrhythmias, and sudden death are also consequences of hypertensive heart disease. As indicated, hypertension also is a major risk factor in the development of coronary atherosclerosis. Cerebral vascular disease may be manifest as transient ischemic attacks (TIAs) or strokes.

The vast majority of untreated patients with essential hypertension die of cardiac failure and cerebral vascular accidents. Since treatment with potent antihypertensive drugs has become available, the incidence of these complications has been greatly reduced—stroke death rates by over 50%. Early, effective, and continuous treatment is critical in patients with hypertension.

Accelerated or malignant hypertension is characterized by marked blood pressure elevation in association with retinal hemorrhages, exudates, papilledema, malignant nephrosclerosis, and necrotizing arteriolitis. Other evidence of this disease is secondary hyperaldosteronism and hypokalemic alkalosis. It may also include manifestations of hypertensive encephalopathy such as headache, vomiting, visual disturbances, stupor, and coma, although acute encephalopathy may occur in the absence of malignant or accelerated hypertension. Prior to availability of effective therapy, life expectancy was less than 2 years with death due to uremia, cerebral hemorrhage, and cardiac failure. With therapy prognosis has been dramatically improved.

Cardiac disease secondary to arterial hypertension is a common cause of cardiac failure, being equally distributed in men and women but more common in blacks. The pathology of the hypertensive heart is primarily a pressure overload concentric hypertrophy that first affects the left ventricle. If untreated, this will lead to left ventricular dilatation, relative mitral and even aortic valvular regurgitation, and dilatation and hypertrophy of the left atrium and, ultimately, failure of the right ventricle as well.

The most common symptom is progressive dyspnea. Early this is manifested by increased fatigability and then reduced exercise tolerance. Paroxysmal nocturnal dyspnea is also common. Pain is unusual unless there is accompanying coronary arterial insufficiency (with or without occlusive arterial disease). The characteristic cardiac signs of left ventricular hypertrophy, associated with high blood pressure, include a loud aortic component of the second sound, a fourth heart sound (atrial gallop) before the appearance of the third (ventricular) sound of cardiac failure, rhythm disturbance, and ventricular irritability.

Hypertension with systolic pressure of over 180 mmHg may persist for many years, but even isolated systolic hypertension (*i.e.*, systolic pressure greater than 159 mmHg with diastolic pressures less than 90 mmHg) is a major risk factor. The recent (systolic hypertension in the elderly) multicenter studies demonstrate definite efficacy of treatment in preventing strokes and myocardial infarction (with diuretics alone or with metoprolol). When the heart no longer can sustain the burden of the elevated pressure, chest pain reflecting coronary arterial insufficiency and increased left ventricular tension occurs. Ultimately, cardiac failure may supervene and cardiac dysrhythmias, especially atrial fibrillation, occur. The most common associated conditions are (1) congestive heart failure, (2) stroke, (3) angina pectoris, (4) coronary thrombosis, and (5) nephrosclerosis.

Other diseases frequently associated with essential hypertension include (1) exogenous obesity, (2) carbohydrate intolerance (or diabetes mellitus), (3) hyperlipidemias, (4) hyperuricemia or gout, and, of course, (5) atherosclerosis.

As indicated, secondary causes for hypertension are not frequent (only 5%), but in the United States this may represent as many as 3 million people. Several possibilities may provide secondary causes: History of excessive alcohol intake or use of oral contraceptives, nose drops containing sympathomimetic agents, and other drugs; weight gain; history of headaches, rapid heart action, and palpitations suggesting pheochromocytoma. Clinical clues should be pursued (*e.g.*, results of discontinuing oral contraceptives should be determined); blood pressure differences between upper and lower extremities should be followed by assessment for coarctation of the aorta; hypokalemia (without diuretics) suggests hyperaldosteronism; subcostal abdominal or flank bruits of systolic timing to suggest renal arterial disease; sudden onset of hypertension or aggravation of preexisting hypertension should also suggest renovascular hypertension. Where there are no clues to cause or patients are not surgical candidates, it may be well to institute treatment directly. However, this should always follow obtaining baseline studies including hemogram, urinalysis, renal functional assessment (serum creatinine level), serum electrolytes (especially potassium concentration), fasting blood sugar, and serum lipids. If response to therapy is difficult or changing, a search for cause may be indicated.

TREATMENT

Systolic or diastolic hypertension readings (that is, above 140/90 mmHg) are indications for therapy. For any antihypertensive treatment program nonpharmacological modalities should be pursued. They include weight control, sodium restriction, alcohol moderation, and smoking cessation. Even if pressure is not controlled, they will permit use of fewer drugs and lower dosages when prescribed. Six categories of antihypertensive drugs are available: diuretics, β-adrenergic receptor blocking drugs, central and peripheral adrenergic inhibitors, direct-acting vasodilators, angiotensin-converting enzyme (ACE) inhibitors, and the calcium antagonists. The diuretics (most commonly hydrochlorothiazide) and the β-blockers are the only two classes that have demonstrated reduced mortality with treatment. This has not been tested with the other classes of drugs. For this reason the diuretics and β-blockers have been the most commonly used to begin therapy in mild and moderate hypertension. However, the ACE inhibitors, calcium antagonists, and even postsynaptic α-inhibitors have also been recommended to tailor initial therapy. If this is inadequate, an alternative agent(s) may be substituted or added.

In hypertensive crises or malignant hypertension, the ACE inhibitors and calcium antagonists have become extremely useful. If these are not effective, the addition of a diuretic or sodium nitroprusside or trimethaphan may be used.

Cardiac Dysrhythmias

The orderly and sequential contractions of the atria and the ventricles are controlled (1) by impulses that arise in the sinoatrial node, transmitted through (2) the atria to the (3) atrioventricular (A-V) node and thence through (4) the bundle of His to the ventricular musculature. As the stimulus passes from the sinoatrial node down the atria, it stimulates atrial contraction; as it passes from the A-V node down the bundle of His, it stimulates ventricular

contraction. Abnormal cardiac rhythms are caused by interferences with this mechanism.

The clinically important dysrhythmias may be divided into three major categories: (1) the atrial dysrhythmias, (2) A-V conduction defects, and (3) ventricular dysrhythmias. In some instances these dysrhythmias may be diagnosed by physical examination, but in most instances electrocardiographic study is essential, and ambulatory Holter monitoring and electrophysiologic testing may be necessary.

Sinus pauses and sinoatrial block are the result of failure of impulse formation at the sinoatrial node. This form of cardiac block may be the result of vagal or of carotid sinus stimulation, or it may follow intoxication with substances such as digitalis, potassium excess, or quinidine. Progressive disease is due to a destructive process in the sinus node and neighboring tissue.

The *"sick sinus syndrome"* is a persistent spontaneous sinus bradycardia that is not produced by drugs. It may also be manifested by apparent sinus arrest or exit block, by combinations of sinus atrial or atrioventricular conduction disturbances, or by alternation of paroxysms of rapid irregular or regular atrial tachyarrhythmias and periods of slow atrial and ventricular rates. Pacemaker installation may be required.

Premature beats may be atrial or ventricular in origin; extrasystoles are uncommon and should be referred to as interpolated beats, since they occur midway between two normal beats and are not followed by a compensatory pause. Atrial and ventricular premature beats cannot be differentiated by physical examination and should be confirmed, if warranted, by ECG. Premature beats frequently are found in patients with normal hearts and may be precipitated by nervousness or the excessive use of coffee or tobacco. In other instances they are associated with myocardial disease; they may be a manifestation of digitalis toxicity. Treatment usually is not necessary; removal of the offending agent may be indicated; in some instances administration of quinidine or procainamide will suppress the ectopic focus.

The *atrial tachycardias* may be automatic (greater than 200 beats per minute), reentry (130 to 150 beats per minute), or chaotic (with multifocal variability of P-wave morphology and irregular P-P wave intervals) and are common in patients with pulmonary disease and diabetes mellitus. *Paroxysmal supraventricular tachycardia (PSVT)* is manifested by the sudden onset of a very rapid regular atrial rhythm with similar ventricular rates. With *A-V nodal reentrant tachycardia,* the QRS complexes reflect the supraventricular origin, the dysrhythmia is sudden in onset and termination, and the atrial rate is from 150 to 250 beats per minute and regular. In PSVT the P waves may be "buried" within the QRS complex. With reentry tachycardias the mechanism originates in the A-V node and may follow slow or fast pathways. This form of PSVT may occur in more than 30% of patients. Their QRS complexes reflect the supraventricular origin, usually at a rate greater than 200 beats per minute, and the P wave occurs after the QRS complex. Significant diuresis usually follows the attack and has been associated with release of the atrial natriuretic factor. Treatment of the attack may be interrupted by vagal stimulation, such as carotid sinus pressure. The Valsalva maneuver or cholinergic drugs may be useful. The β-blockers, digitalis, verapamil, and quinidine are effective in controlling this dysrhythmia if other measures fail.

Atrial flutter is characterized by rapid contractions of the atria at rates of 250 to 350 per minute; however, the ventricular rate is slower. Varying degrees of A-V block exist. If the block is regular, such as 2 : 1, the ventricular contractions are regular at 150 beats per minute, but an irregularity in the block results in an irregular ventricular response. This dysrhythmia is more likely to develop as a complication of some organic cardiac disease; however, if it is paroxysmal, it may occur in patients without organic cardiac disease. Correct diagnosis requires electrocardiographic confirmation. Treatment consists of digitalization, β-blockers, or the calcium antagonist verapamil to slow the ventricular response and sinus rhythm. In addition, quinidine may be used to prevent recurrence. It may be necessary to employ electrical cardioversion to restore rhythm.

Atrial fibrillation (AF) is characterized by a completely irregular ventricular rhythm; the ventricles in this disorder respond irregularly and with varying force to a small portion of rapid, totally irregular, atrial impulses. AF generally is a manifestation of organic cardiac disease, but once again, if it is paroxysmal, it may occur in patients without organic cardiac disease. The more frequent organic cardiac diseases associated with AF include hypertensive heart disease, hyperthyroidism, mitral stenosis, cardiomyopathy, pulmonary emboli, coronary artery disease, and cardiac surgery. Treatment consists of slowing the ventricular rate with digitalis; this is accomplished by increasing the A-V block. The β-adrenergic receptor blockers and calcium antagonists may also be useful in certain patients. After the ventricular rate is controlled, car-

dioversion to a sinus rhythm with quinidine or electric countershock may be attempted. Prior to electric countershock the patient should be treated with anticoagulants in order to prevent potential embolic phenomena, including stroke. This is more likely to be effective in AF of recent onset than in chronic AF. In refractory cases, low doses of amiodarone have been employed to maintain sinus rhythm.

Pre-excitation syndrome, also known as the Wolff-Parkinson-White (WPW) syndrome, is produced by a premature activation through several accessory A-V pathways. With the *atrioventricular pathway* (bundle of Kent), there is a short PR interval (<0.12 second), a QRS complex ≥0.12 second, and a slowly rising delta wave that is observed on the upswing of the QRS complex. There may be a secondary delta wave in the S-T segment. With the *atriohisian (tract) pathways* the PR interval is short and the QRS complex is normal; this is the Long-Gènong-Levine syndrome. With the nodoventricular and *fasciculoventricular pathways,* the PR interval is normal but the QRS complex is abnormal. Symptoms may be associated with the tachyarrhythmias. The most common tachycardia is characterized by a normal QRS and a rapid (≥200 ventricular response. AF with a rapid ventricular response may also occur.

A-V conduction defects or block may be localized to (1) the A-V node and (2) the infranodal tissue, which consists of the bundle of His, the proximal bundle, and the distal Purkinje fibers. *A-V node block* is due to digitalis intoxication, inferior myocardial infarction, myocarditis, cardiac surgery, and congenital heart block; it is often reversible. Clinically it can be recognized by a narrow QRS complex, occasional Wenckebach periods, and an escape rate of 50 or more beats per minute with a form identical with normal beats. Permanent pacemaking is often not needed.

Infranodal block is more serious and is due to a destructive process of the bundle and its branches. Clinically the patient shows dropped beats, bundle-branch block, slow idioventricular escape beats with wide QRS. Anterior myocardial infarction may be present, and the treatment of choice is usually permanent implantation of a pacemaker.

Ventricular premature beats are the most common ventricular dysrhythmia and are essentially of the same significance as the atrial premature beats mentioned above.

Ventricular tachycardia (VT) is an ominous dysrhythmia that may terminate in ventricular fibrillation and death. The abnormal rhythm is found commonly in patients with ischemic heart disease, dilated and hypertrophic cardiomyopathies, valvular heart disease, and primary electrical disease of the conduction system. The onset may be sudden and paroxysmal or nonparoxysmal. The QRS complex during VT may be unchanging (monomorphic), may vary randomly (pleomorphic), may vary in a more or less repetitive manner (Torsades des Pointes), or may vary in alternate complexes (bidirectional). The VT may be sustained (*i.e.,* longer than 30 seconds), requiring termination because of hemodynamic collapse, or it may be nonsustained, stopping spontaneously in less than 30 seconds. The relative risk of symptoms or sudden death determines the course of therapy. Sustained VT, with or without structural heart disease, should be treated. Nonsustained VT with structural heart disease should also be treated; however, patients without structural heart disease who are asymptomatic may not require treatment. Lidocaine, quinidine, procainamide, amiodarone, β-blockers (especially in patients with coronary heart disease), electric countershock, and implantable defibrillators are useful modes of therapy. In patients with **Torsades des Points,** a severe cardiac dysrhythmia and a form of ventricular tachycardia, intravenous magnesium, isoproterenol, and temporary pacemakers are of value. Bidirectional VT is a very common manifestation of digitalis toxicity.

Pericardial Disease

Acute benign pericarditis is probably due to a viral cause and at times to an autoimmune reaction. Viral infection is poorly documented, although Coxsackie infection seems frequently implicated in pericarditis. Recurrences are frequent; effusion may occur with tamponade, and eventually constrictive disease may ensue. Glucocorticoid therapy is used to relieve symptoms but does not significantly alter the course.

Collagen vascular disease may involve the pericardium and is seen in rheumatoid arthritis, progressive systemic sclerosis, and lupus erythematosus, including the syndrome caused by procainamide.

Tuberculosis is difficult to diagnose in pericardial disease since cultures are usually negative; biopsy is needed to confirm the diagnosis. Pericardial constriction is a sequela even after appropriate and prolonged therapy.

Uremic pericarditis is often controlled through chronic dialysis; it occurs in younger patients and

does not directly relate to the level of urea nitrogen or creatinine.

Cardiac antigens appear to be involved in the immune mechanism with postpericardectomy syndrome (60%) and postmyocardial infarction syndrome (3%).

Pericardial effusion is manifested clinically by dyspnea, tachycardia, distended neck veins, and pulsus paradoxus (when pericardial tamponade is present). Pericardial tamponade is suggested clinically when there is a decline in systemic arterial pressure; an elevated venous pressure; and a small, quiet heart. The chest x ray reveals a large, water-bottle-shaped heart. The echocardiogram is definitive for diagnosis demonstrating the accumulation of fluid in the pericardial space with an inspiratory increase in right ventricular dimensions and right atrial and ventricular diastolic collapse. The ECG may be normal, but usually it demonstrates low voltage and SF and F wave changes with the S-T segment being elevated and concave in an upward direction.

Miscellaneous Vascular Diseases

THROMBOEMBOLIC DISEASE OF AORTA

This thrombotic obliteration of the bifurcation of the aorta may result from progressive thrombosis at the bifurcation, which ultimately leads to complete obliteration of the aorta. A similar clinical picture may occur with a saddle embolus lodging at this area. Intermittent claudication with pain in the low back and absence of both femoral pulses with symmetrical atrophy of the legs are the prominent symptoms with impotence being prominent in males. Aortograms make the diagnosis definite. Doppler ultrasound imaging (with color flow) has become a very useful procedure in evaluating peripheral arterial disease.

AORTIC ARCH SYNDROME (PULSELESS DISEASE, TAKAYASU SYNDROME)

Progressive atherosclerosis or inflammatory changes in the intima may lead to partial or complete obliteration of the major branches of the aortic arch. It may follow severe trauma to the upper chest that damages the media and leads to the intimal atherosclerosis. There is absence of pulses in the upper part of the body, with normal femoral pulses. The clinical features are easy fatigability of the arms and atrophy of muscles and soft tissues. Syncopal attacks may occur.

DISSECTING ANEURYSM OF THE AORTA

Dissecting aneurysm of the aorta occurs more frequently in men and usually starts from an intimal rent in the aorta. The dissection extends proximally to the aortic ring and distally, for a variable distance, into one or several of the branches of the aorta. The symptoms include pain, aortic regurgitation, interference with the blood supply through branches of the aorta, and x-ray evidence of widening of the aorta. Antihypertensive therapy with β-blocking therapy to ensure that reflexive stimulation of the heart will not aggravate the process of dissection may relieve the pain, and surgery may be indicated.

(Peripheral vascular diseases are discussed in Chap. 2, "Surgery.")

DISEASES OF THE HEMATOPOIETIC SYSTEM

Anemia

Anemia is a reduction in the number of red cells, the amount of hemoglobin, or both. It may be acute or chronic and may arise from (1) loss of blood, (2) increased destruction of blood, or (3) defective formation of blood. These mechanisms are readily distinguished by a reticulocyte count: an inappropriately low reticulocyte count suggests defective production, whereas reticulocytosis indicates hemolysis or recent blood loss. Mean cell volume (MCV), now reliably provided by the automated red cell counters, is very helpful in categorizing anemias due to defective red-cell production.

A classification based on the size of the red cells (macrocytic and microcytic anemias) or upon the hemoglobin content of the cells (hyperchromic and hypochromic) is very useful for descriptive purposes.

ANEMIAS DUE TO DECREASED OR INEFFECTIVE RED-CELL PRODUCTION

Iron Deficiency Anemias. Iron deficiency is the most common cause of anemia; in the United States in the adult this deficiency occurs through physiologic or pathologic loss of blood. Red-cell mass is maintained at the expense of iron stores as blood loss occurs. Negative iron balance induces a predictable sequence of events that develops in proportion to the severity of iron depletion: (1) depletion of bone marrow iron stores; (2) decrease in the serum ferritin level, which correlates closely with total body iron stores; (3) a fall in the concentration of serum iron and an elevation in the total iron binding capacity (TIBC, transferrin) of the serum with consequent decrease in the transferrin saturation; (4) progressive anemia, initially normocytic, then microcytic (reduced MCV, unchanged mean corpuscular hemoglobin concentration [MCHC]), and eventually microcytic–hypochromic (reduced MCV and reduced MCHC).

Loss of blood in women regularly occurs in pregnancy and from menses. In men, iron deficiency is almost always due to GI blood loss, acute or chronic. Decreased dietary iron and impaired absorption are less common causes of iron deficiency. Hypochromia and microcytosis are the morphologic findings in advanced iron deficiency but may also be found in chronic inflammatory, malignant, and other diseases, hemoglobinopathies including thalassemia, and in cases of lead poisoning.

Treatment is directed at the cause of blood loss and at correcting the iron deficit. Oral iron therapy should be maintained for 6 to 12 months to replete stores. Parenteral administration of iron is rarely indicated and may cause sensitivity reactions.

In a patient with microcytic anemia, other diagnostic considerations are anemia of chronic disorders (discussed below), lead poisoning, myelodysplastic syndromes, and hemoglobinopathies (including thalassemias). ***Thalassemic syndromes*** (α and β) are common in blacks and Southeast Asians as well as in Greeks and Italians. The diagnosis is established by normal serum iron and ferritin levels, elevated levels of hemoglobin A_2 or F, and family studies. Globin chain synthesis studies and structural analysis of hemoglobin variants may be required for unusual cases.

Homozygous β-Thalassemia (Cooley's Anemia). This is a form of congenital anemia with extremely ineffective erythropoiesis. Manifestations appear by about the sixth month of life. Patients have signs and symptoms of severe anemia (Hb < 7 g/dl) requiring repeated transfusions and show gradual enlargement of the liver and the spleen. Bony deformities such as frontal bossing and enlargement of the malar bones ("chipmunk facies") occur secondary to expansion of the erythroid marrow. The inevitable iron overload from repeated transfusions and from excessive absorption causes heart failure, liver dysfunction, and endocrine deficiencies. Death usually occurs from cardiac dysrhythmias and intractable cardiac failure. Treatment is primarily supportive with transfusions. Iron chelation therapy is indicated to minimize the long-term consequences of iron overload. Marrow transplantation is currently being investigated.

The myelodysplastic syndromes are subdivided into (1) refractory anemia; (2) refractory anemia with ringed sideroblasts (sideroblastic anemia); (3) refractory anemia with excess blasts; (4) refractory anemia in transformation to leukemia; and (5) chronic myelomonocytic leukemia. Sideroblastic anemia is characterized by normoblasts that contain iron deposits within their mitochondria. Because the latter are situated around the nucleus of the normoblast, perinuclear rings of iron deposits are seen in the bone marrow when stained for iron. The iron deposits are believed to occur because of defects in heme synthesis, which results in microcytic–hypochromic red cells. Serum levels of iron and ferritin are high, and the transferrin is almost completely saturated. Sideroblastic anemia (1) may occur as a sex-linked hereditary abnormality, which sometimes responds to large doses of pyridoxine; (2) may be caused by a variety of drugs, including alcohol, isoniazid, chloramphenicol, and cycloserine (recovery is usual upon withdrawal of the offending agent); or (3) may be idiopathic or associated with hematologic malignancies; this type is often macrocytic and may evolve into an acute leukemia. Treatment consists of red-cell transfusions, if clinically indicated.

Megaloblastic Anemias. The megaloblastic anemias are caused by impaired DNA synthesis. Most cases are due to a deficiency of vitamin B_{12} or folic acid, which in turn is caused by a variety of specific disorders. An elevated MCV is the earliest hematologic clue, often rising long before anemia sets in. A frequent and characteristic morphologic finding is the hypersegmentation of the neutrophils. Since impaired DNA synthesis affects all reproducing cells, leukopenia and thrombocytopenia commonly accompany severe anemia; the impaired renewal of mucosal cells of the mouth and the GI tract leads to glossitis, diarrhea, and malabsorption. Bone marrow shows marked hyperplasia of the red-cell precursors, which are abnormally large and have nuclei that appear much less mature than would be expected for the development of the cytoplasm (the megaloblasts). Another frequent finding is giant bands and metamyelocytes. The reticulocyte count is typically low despite the bone marrow red-cell hyperplasia (ineffective erythropoiesis). This intramedullary cell death results in an increased serum level of indirect bilirubin and lactate dehydrogenase.

Clinical manifestations usually relate to anemia, effects on the GI tract (glossitis, anorexia, diarrhea, abdominal pain, weight loss), and the causative disorder. Neurologic manifestations (peripheral neuropathy, posterolateral column degeneration, behavioral changes) occur *almost exclusively* in patients with vitamin B_{12} deficiency and, indeed, may be precipitated or worsened by erroneous treatment of such patients with folic acid.

Measurements of serum levels of the vitamins before vitamin therapy or resumption of a normal diet will reliably identify the specific deficiency. Both vitamin B_{12} and folic acid must be assayed in every patient since deficiency of either cannot be distinguished morphologically and combined deficiency is always possible.

In the Western countries *deficiency of vitamin B_{12}* is almost always due to its malabsorption. Common causes are pernicious anemia, postgastrectomy states, diseases or resection of the ileum, human immunodeficiency virus infection, and bacterial overgrowth in jejunal diverticula or blind loops. *Pernicious anemia* (PA) accounts for about 75% of the cases. Although more common in elderly whites, it also occurs quite frequently in blacks, often affecting those under the age of 40. PA is caused by an absence of intrinsic factor (IF) secretion necessary for normal vitamin B_{12} absorption. Associated gastric findings are atrophic gastritis, achlorhydria, and achylia. These abnormalities are currently thought to result from an autoimmune reaction against the gastric parietal cells. Postgastrectomy states, partial or complete (iatrogenic loss of IF secretion); various ileal disorders such as Crohn's disease, sprue, and ileal resection (loss of absorptive sites); and bacterial overgrowth in the jejunal diverticula or blind loops (destruction or consumption of the vitamin by bacteria) account for most of the remaining cases of vitamin B_{12} deficiency anemia. The Schilling test of vitamin B_{12} absorption must be employed to distinguish malabsorption due to lack of IF from that due to intestinal disorders.

Management consists of replacement of vitamin B_{12} and, when possible, correction of the causative disorder. Since nearly all cases are due to malabsorption of the vitamin, the therapy must be lifelong if the causative disorder cannot be reversed. Parenteral therapy is usually employed because it is reliable and inexpensive.

Folic acid deficiency is most often caused by dietary lack, alcohol abuse (interference with folate utilization), pregnancy, and chronic hemolytic anemias (increased requirements), chronic dialysis for renal failure (loss of folic acid), or prolonged treatment with drugs such as diphenylhydantoin (impairment of absorption and metabolism) and trimethoprim (interference with folate metabolism), and sprue syndromes (impaired absorption). A careful history is usually enough to establish the likely cause.

Treatment consists of oral administration (even in malabsorptive disorders) of folic acid for 2 to 4 weeks. Prophylactic treatment is indicated during pregnancy or with chronic dialysis and in some patients with hemolytic anemias.

Anemia of Chronic Disorders. This anemia is characterized by an impaired delivery of iron to the developing red cell. As a result, the morphologic and laboratory picture often suggests iron deficiency despite plentiful body iron stores. It occurs in association with chronic infection (*e.g.*, abscess, osteomyelitis, endocarditis, pyelonephritis), chronic inflammation (*e.g.*, rheumatoid arthritis, lupus), and cancer. Typically the hemoglobin level is between 9 g/dl and 11 g/dl. Distinction from true iron deficiency is often difficult and may require a direct assessment of bone marrow iron stores since the usual blood tests are frequently equivocal. Treatment is correction of the causative disorder.

Anemia of uremia is normocytic, roughly proportional to the degree of azotemia, and caused primarily by defective production secondary to inadequate erythropoietin secretion by the diseased kidneys. Management consists of attempts to reverse the renal failure and detection and treatment of any reversible components of the anemia (*e.g.*, bleeding, folic acid deficiency). The anemia is improved modestly by hemodialysis and peritoneal dialysis and dramatically by renal transplantation and regular parenteral administration of erythropoietin. *Anemia of liver disease* is normocytic or macrocytic and often exaggerated by the expanded plasma volume. In the alcoholic with liver disease, direct effects of alcohol on the bone marrow, dietary folate lack, and GI bleeding contribute to the anemia.

Miscellaneous Anemias. *Anemia of endocrine insufficiency* is usually normocytic but may be macrocytic in hypothyroidism and is readily corrected by adequate hormone replacement. In *aplastic anemia* the red cells are normocytic or macrocytic, and there is leukopenia and thrombocytopenia. Bone marrow is hypocellular or acellular. Causes include infections, drugs, chemicals, and radiation. Most cases, however, are idiopathic; in some of these an autoimmune suppression of the bone marrow may be present. Severe cases may be treated by bone marrow transplantation from a matched donor or with immunosuppressive agents (*e.g.*, antithymocyte globulin, cyclosporin A).

ANEMIAS DUE TO EXCESS LOSS OF RED CELLS

Acute Blood Loss Anemia. Chronic low-grade blood loss usually presents as iron deficiency anemia. Acute blood loss of more than 1,000 ml produces manifestations of volume depletion (*i.e.*, tachycardia, hypotension, shock) rather than anemia. When the blood loss is more gradual, movement of the extravascular fluid into the intravascular space restores the total blood volume by expansion of the plasma volume. This process, however, takes time and therefore a decrease in hemoglobin concentration following blood loss does not become evident for more than 12 hours. Also, the reticulocytosis does not occur until 3 to 4 days *after* the hemorrhage. Internal bleeding (*e.g.*, ruptured ectopic pregnancy) may be accompanied by an increase in unconjugated bilirubin due to breakdown of the hematoma, thus mimicking hemolysis.

Hemolytic Anemias. Hemolytic anemias comprise a diverse group in which the basic abnormality is a significantly shortened red-cell span. When the hemolysis is moderate, the bone marrow may fully compensate for the accelerated red-cell destruction and there is no anemia (compensated hemolytic state). Hemolytic anemias can be broadly classified as follows:

Hereditary (or intrinsic)

Hereditary spherocytosis
Hereditary elliptocytosis
Hemoglobinopathies (*e.g.*, sickle-cell diseases)
Homozygous thalassemias
Enzyme defects (*e.g.*, pyruvate kinase and glucose-6-phosphate dehydrogenase deficiency)

Acquired (or extrinsic)

Immune hemolytic anemias
    Autoimmune (hemolytic disease of the newborn, hemolytic transfusion reaction)
    Drug-induced
    Autoimmune
Mechanical trauma (red-cell fragmentation syndrome)
    Microangiopathic
    Cardiac (valve prosthesis, valvular disease)
Toxic effects (malaria, clostridial infection)
Membrane abnormalities
    Spur cell anemia
    Paroxysmal nocturnal hemoglobinuria

A number of clinical and laboratory features are shared by the various types of hemolytic anemias. Patients with congenital hemolysis often have lifelong anemia and a positive family history. Those with severe hemolysis are often icteric; splenomegaly is common in a variety of chronic hemolytic anemias, both congenital and acquired, as is the formation of bilirubin gallstones. The bone marrow compensation may be temporarily interrupted by erythroid hypoplasia precipitated by infections, often of a minor nature, resulting in a rapid decline in hemoglobin level, sometimes to dangerously low levels (anemic crises).

Laboratory features of hemolytic anemias include:

1. A brisk reticulocytosis, the single most useful clue for hemolysis
2. Increased serum "indirect" or unconjugated bilirubin reflecting increased heme catabolism
3. Elevated serum lactate dehydrogenase level. This derives from the excessive destruction of red cells.
4. Low or absent haptoglobin, an α-globulin that binds hemoglobin. The hemoglobin–haptoglobin complex is rapidly cleared from the plasma. However, serum haptoglobin rises in inflammation and infection and thus may be "normal" if hemolysis and inflammation coexist.
5. Methemalbuminemia. This forms when haptoglobin is depleted and free heme complexes with albumin; it is found only in severe intravascular hemolysis.
6. Hemosiderinuria. Once the hemoglobin binding capacity of the plasma is exceeded, hemoglobin dimers are filtered through the glomeruli where they are reabsorbed by the proximal tubular cells and catabolized. The iron remaining in the cells is passed in the urine with the regular shedding of the cells.

Many hemolytic disorders are associated with characteristic changes in the morphologic appearance of the red cells. Therefore, examination of a well-prepared blood smear is extremely useful in the etiologic diagnosis of hemolytic and other anemias.

Hereditary Spherocytosis (HS). This disorder is inherited as an autosomal dominant trait and is characterized by red cells that are spherical (spherocytes) rather than disc-shaped. On the blood smear, they appear as small, deeply staining cells without the central pallor. The spherocytes are less deformable and thus become trapped in the intricate circulation of the spleen and are hemolysed. They also hemolyse more readily in hypotonic saline solutions than do normal red cells; this is the basis for the osmotic fragility test. The primary red-cell lesion is in the membrane, which permits excessive sodium to enter the cell, causing it to swell into a spherocyte. The severity of anemia varies greatly, and many cases remain undetected until the sixth or seventh decade. Jaundice is common and splenomegaly is almost invariably present. Diagnostic tests include blood smear examination, osmotic fragility test, and family studies. Immunohemolytic anemia, also a cause of spherocytosis, must be excluded by a negative direct Coombs test.

Splenectomy corrects the anemia, although the red-cell defect persists. It is clearly indicated in those with symptomatic anemia but should also be considered in children and young adults with mild anemia because of the risk of anemic crises and gallstones. Splenectomy in children should be postponed until age 4 or 5 years if possible, because of the risk of infections. In patients diagnosed later in life who have had no complications, splenectomy is rarely indicated. All patients undergoing splenectomy should be immunized with pneumococcal, meningococcal, and Hemophilus influenza b vaccines, preferably several weeks before surgery.

Hemoglobinopathies. Hemoglobin A (Hb A), which accounts for approximately 95% of the normal hemoglobin, is composed of two pairs of polypeptide globin chains (two α and two β) with a heme group attached to each chain. The tetramer of globin chains with their heme groups is so arranged as to ensure stability, solubility, and maximum physiologic effectiveness of the hemoglobin. Hemoglobinopathies result from a genetically determined structural alteration in one of the globin chains. When the alteration involves a critical region of the chain, any or all of the above properties may be compromised, resulting in a variety of clinical syndromes. Structural abnormality may also alter the electrophoretic mobility of the hemoglobin with reference to Hb A; this forms the basis for the detection of abnormal hemoglobins by electrophoresis. Of the many known abnormal hemoglobins, only a few produce clinical manifestations.

Sickle-cell trait is a carrier state for hemoglobin S (Hb S). It affects about 8% of blacks in America; the incidence is much greater in parts of Africa. Hb S is the result of single amino acid substitution in the β-chain, valine for glutamic acid at position 6. When deoxygenated, it precipitates and forms cablelike structures that deform the red cell into a sickle shape, hence the name. Individuals with the trait have 35% to 45% Hb S, the rest being Hb A. Except for hyposthenuria and episodes of hematuria, the trait produces no ill effects. Rarely, thrombotic events occur, usually in the setting of physical exertion or high altitudes.

Sickle-cell anemia refers to the homozygous state for the S gene (SS). Since only sickle β-chains are synthesized, Hb S constitutes greater than 90% of the hemoglobin; there is no Hb A unless the patient has been recently transfused. Because of the high concentration of the Hb S, sickling of the red cells *in vivo* occurs more readily under hypoxic conditions and is responsible, directly or indirectly, for the major clinical manifestations. Sickled cells are fragile and lyse readily, leading to severe hemolytic anemia. Such cells are also very rigid and cause occlusion of small blood vessels, which leads to recurrent episodes of ischemic pain involving joints, bones, muscles, and the abdomen. Dyspnea, cough, pleuric pain, and fever are common symptoms of pulmonary infarctions. Virtually every organ may be affected by this process, which may ultimately lead to organ dysfunction (*e.g.,* splenic atrophy, renal failure). Hyposplenism develops early in childhood and is partly responsible for the increased incidence of and mortality from pneumococcal and *Haemophilus* infections in children under the age of 6. Adults with their immune defenses matured do not seem to be as much at risk. The treatment of sickle-cell anemia is symptomatic. Since more treatable medical disorders may precipitate or mimic pain crisis, these must be diligently sought.

Sickle-cell hemoglobin C disease (SC disease) and *sickle-cell β-thalassemia* (S β thal) are doubly heterozygous sickling disorders in which one of the abnormal genes is for C hemoglobin or β-thalassemia. Clinical and laboratory manifestations are qualitatively similar to those of SS but are generally milder.

Glucose-6-Phosphate Dehydrogenase (G6PD) Deficiency.

G6PD plays a central role in protecting the red cell from oxidant and other environmental stresses. Its gene locus is on the X chromosome. Many variants of the enzyme have been described, but only two are common in clinical practice; the most common is called G6PD A−. It decays much faster than the normal enzyme, thereby leaving the older red cell deficient in the enzyme. This variant occurs in about 11% of black males in the United States. The carrier may experience acute hemolysis within hours of exposure to an oxidant stress. Common offenders are viral infections (*e.g.,* hepatitis), bacterial infections, and certain drugs and chemicals. Drugs and chemicals that may precipitate hemolysis and should be avoided include:

Sulfonamides: Sulfamethoxazole, sulfanilamide, sulfapyridine, sulfacetamide
Other Antibiotics: Primaquine, dapsone, nitrofurantoin, nalidixic acid, furazolidone

Miscellaneous: Acetilanid, doxorubicin, methylene blue, naphthalene, phenazopyridine (hyridium), phenyltrydrazine, trinitrotoluene, toluidine blue

Hemolytic episode is often severe with hemoglobinuria but is usually self-limited even if the drug administration is continued because the remaining red cells and the reticulocytes have an adequate amount of the enzyme activity. No specific treatment is required. If hemoglobinuria develops, adequate urine output is important. Between episodes, the individuals are hematologically normal.

The Mediterranean variant primarily affects the Sephardic Jews. Because of its greater instability than that of the A− variant, it leads to a more severe deficiency of the enzyme. Consequently, some patients suffer a chronic hemolytic anemia. In addition to the drugs above, chloramphenicol, quinine, and quinidine may cause hemolysis. A minority of patients also suffer hemolysis after eating fava beans (favism).

Attention should be directed at prevention of hemolytic episodes and patient education. Any male patient of appropriate ethnic background who is about to be given an oxidant drug should be screened for G6PD deficiency. This is done reliably and simply by the fluorescent spot test.

Pyruvate kinase (PK) deficiency, an autosomal recessive defect, is associated with a chronic hemolytic anemia. The deficiency causes impaired generation of adenosine triphosphate (ATP) necessary for membrane integrity and consequently leads to lysis of cells primarily in the spleen. Splenectomy usually ameliorates the anemia and is indicated in those in whom anemia impairs normal function.

Immune Hemolytic Anemias.

Antibodies on the red cell cause its premature destruction (immune hemolysis). Their presence on the red cells is detected by the Coombs antiglobulin test. The test relies on the ability of antibodies (antisera) prepared in animals and directed against specific human serum immunoglobulins (Igs) or complement to agglutinate red cells if these serum proteins are present on the red cell surface. The ability of the antisera to agglutinate the patient's own red cells is the *direct Coombs test.* Sometimes it is advantageous to know whether there is an antibody in the serum of patients which is reactive against other human red cells. This is done by the *indirect Coombs test,* in which ABO- and Rh-compatible red cells are incubated with the patient's serum to transfer the antibody onto the red cells; subsequently, a direct Coombs test is performed on the incubated red cells. The immune hemolytic anemias fall into three major categories:

1. *Isoimmune:* **Isoantibodies** are acquired through exposure of the patient to red-cell antigens that the patient is lacking. Rh immunization of an Rh-negative mother by her Rh-positive fetus and sensitization of the recipient through mismatched red-cell transfusions are examples of isoantibody formation; such antibodies are detected by the indirect Coombs test. This type of reaction also occurs if mismatched blood is transfused.

2. *Drug-induced:* Antibodies may be produced against certain drugs. The antibody then attaches to the red cell because the drug or its metabolite is bound to the red-cell membrane. Hemolysis sometimes associated with the administration of large doses of penicillin (15 to 20 million units per day) or penicillin-type antibiotics is mediated in this manner. Alternatively, drug–antibody complexes (immune complexes) may form in the plasma and attach to the red cell. Drugs such as quinidine or quinine may complex weakly with a drug binding site on the red blood cell and antibody, leading to rapid complement mediated cell lysis. The direct Coombs test is always positive. The hemolysis ceases and the direct Coombs test becomes negative once the offending drug is withdrawn. Drugs such as methyldopa and levodopa may cause hemolysis by induction of autoantibodies to red-cell antigens.

3. *Autoimmune:* Antibodies may be formed against the patient's own red-cell antigen(s) (autoantibodies) in association with diseases that predispose to antibody production, *e.g.,* collagen vascular diseases, infections with organisms such as *Mycoplasma* or EB virus, lymphoproliferative diseases, certain chronic inflammatory diseases (ulcerative colitis), or may be of unknown cause. Failure of the mechanisms that normally permit recognition of "self" are believed to underlie such antibody production. The resultant hemolytic anemia is referred to as autoimmune hemolytic anemia (AIHA). The presence of an autoantibody on the red cell, however, does not inevitably lead to hemolysis.

The antibodies of the IgG class react best with the antigen at 37° C and hence are called **warm antibodies.** IgG-coated red cells are destroyed predominantly by the macrophages of the spleen and other reticuloendothelial organs (extravascular hemolysis). AIHA associated with lupus, lymphoid malignancies, and α-methyldopa, most idiopathic cases,

and the immune hemolysis due to penicillin are IgG mediated and therefore predominantly extravascular. IgM antibodies react best with antigen below 37° C *(cold antibodies)* and through their ability to fully activate complement on the red cell surface can cause lysis of the cells within the circulation (intravascular hemolysis). AIHA associated with *Mycoplasma* infections, infectious mononucleosis, idiopathic cold agglutinin disease (a lymphoproliferative disorder), and the immune hemolysis due to quinidine or ABO-incompatible transfusion reaction are IgM mediated.

The presentation of AIHA varies from mild to fulminant hemolysis with hemoglobinuria. Modest splenomegaly may occur in warm antibody AIHA. Signs and symptoms of the causative disorder, if present, may dominate the picture. Patients with cold agglutinin disease may experience symptoms of ischemia and cyanosis due to agglutination of red cells in the capillaries of the hands and feet which are exposed to cold temperature. Diagnosis is made by the positive direct Coombs test in a patient with hemolytic anemia. Frequently the indirect Coombs test is also positive due to excess antibody in the serum. The presence of an underlying disorder must be diligently sought since it may greatly influence the treatment and its outcome.

Treatment of warm antibody AIHA consists of corticosteroids (*e.g.,* prednisone 1 mg/kg/day). Most patients will begin to show a rise in hemoglobin after 1 week of treatment. Prednisone is continued until the hemoglobin level is normal. The primary causative disorder when present must also be treated concurrently. For nonresponders or those who relapse, splenectomy is the second line of treatment. Steroids and splenectomy are usually ineffective in cold agglutinin disease. Cytotoxic therapy with cyclophosphamide or chlorambucil is commonly used when treatment is indicated.

Red-Cell Fragmentation Syndrome. When red cells are subject to excessive physical trauma within the circulation, they may undergo fragmentation and lysis resulting in intravascular hemolysis. The hallmark of this type of hemolysis is the red-cell fragments of various shapes such as crescents, helmets, and triangles. Hemosiderinuria is regularly present. Red-cell fragmentation has been associated with fibrin deposition in the small blood vessels and may occur in disseminated intravascular coagulation, vasculitis, malignant hypertension, hemolytic uremic syndrome, thrombotic thrombocytopenic purpura, disseminated adenocarcinomas, and eclampsia (microangiopathic hemolytic anemia); the red cells are believed to be torn as they pass through the fibrin meshwork. Thrombocytopenia is frequently present in these patients. Fragmentation may also occur as a result of excessive turbulence in association with aortic valve prosthesis, severe aortic stenosis, and asymmetric septal hypertrophy. Treatment consists of correcting the underlying disorder.

Erythrocytosis

This term refers to an increase in the concentration of red cells whether measured as number of cells, hemoglobin, or hematocrit. Erythrocytosis may or may not be associated with an increase in the total number of red cells in the body. For example, a contracted plasma volume will be associated with an increase in all of the above indices without an absolute increase in the red-cell mass. This is relative or pseudoerythrocytosis, which must be distinguished from true erythrocytosis by direct measurement of the red-cell mass and the plasma volume using radioisotopic methods. The causes of true erythrocytosis are (1) chronic hypoxemia ($\downarrow$ arterial P_{O_2}), for example, chronic obstructive lung disease, cyanotic congenital heart disease, high altitude; (2) altered hemoglobin function (normal arterial P_{O_2}, $\downarrow$ O_2 delivery to tissues), for example, chronic carboxyhemoglobinemia ($>7\%$) frequently found in heavy smokers, hemoglobinopathies with increased oxygen affinity, congenital methemoglobinemia; (3) excess (inappropriate) erythropoietin production, for example, tumors of the kidney, cerebellum, liver, uterus, and renal lesions such as cysts and hydronephrosis; and (4) autonomous, for example, polycythemia vera.

Polycythemia vera is a neoplastic myeloproliferative disorder with a peak incidence between the fifth and the sixth decades. Although the red-cell proliferation predominates, a variable degree of thrombocytosis and leukocytosis is also present in the majority of the patients. Symptoms are usually due to hyperviscosity of the blood (headache, dizziness, vertigo, tinnitus, visual disturbances, vascular insufficiency) and propensity to thrombosis. A common complaint is generalized pruritus aggravated by warm showers. Peptic ulcer occurs at four to five times the normal incidence. Splenomegaly is present in the majority of cases. Laboratory findings usually include a normal arterial P_{O_2}, elevated serum B_{12} levels, elevated leukocyte alkaline phosphatase, and low serum erythropoietin levels. Repeated phlebotomies to reduce the elevated red-cell mass to normal and thus the blood viscosity are the primary treatment and should be performed even in the absence of symptoms to prevent complications. Long-term control requires regular maintenance phlebotomies. When thrombocytosis becomes severe, radioactive phosphorus or cytotoxic therapy may be needed. Surgery is associated with serious hemorrhagic and thrombotic complications unless the red-cell mass is reduced to normal preoperatively. Many patients ultimately develop myelofibrosis; some develop acute leukemia.

Bleeding Disorders

HEMOPHILIA A

Hemophilia A is a bleeding disorder due to an inherited deficiency of Factor VIII (antihemophilic factor) and is transmitted in a sex-linked recessive pattern so that only men are clinically affected. Bleeding manifestations relate directly to the degree of deficiency and may occur in any part of the body but primarily involve the joints and the muscles. Therapy with Factor VIII derived from human plasma has led to HIV infection in many hemophilia patients. Diagnosis is suspected by history and confirmed by a prolonged partial thromboplastin time (PTT) and low Factor VIII coagulant activity. Bleeding and prothrombin times are normal. Treatment consists of administration of Factor VIII and local measures. DDAVP may be adequate therapy for minor bleeding and minor surgery. Prophylactic administration is indicated prior to surgery. Patients should avoid use of aspirin and other drugs that affect platelet function.

CHRISTMAS DISEASE (HEMOPHILIA B)

The clinical manifestations and inheritance are exactly as in hemophilia A, but a different plasma coagulant protein, *viz,* Factor IX, is deficient. PTT is prolonged, and plasma level of Factor IX coagulant activity is low. Treatment consists of administration of Factor IX concentrates (Proplex or Konyne). Otherwise the same principles of treatment apply as for hemophilia A.

VON WILLEBRAND'S DISEASE

This is the most common of the hereditary bleeding disorders usually transmitted as an autosomal dominant trait (thus men and women are equally affected) and is characterized by a prolonged bleeding time (with a normal platelet count) and frequently a prolonged PTT due to reduced activity of Factor VIII. The primary defect is the deficiency of a factor in plasma called von Willebrand factor (vWF) necessary for normal adhesion of platelets to vascular endothelium in normal hemostasis. The deficiency of vWF also prevents the *in vitro* aggregation of platelets of these patients in response to ristocetin; this fact is utilized in the diagnosis of von Willebrand's disease. Most commonly the bleeding is mucosal and cutaneous. Menorrhagia and postpartum hemorrhage are common in young women. Joint bleeding is uncommon. Treatment consists of infusion of cryoprecipitates or a synthetic vasopressin (*i.e.*, desmopressin acetate) and local measures. Purified Factor VIII concentrates are generally *not* effective.

Platelet Disorders

Platelet disorders may be due to an altered number (quantitative) and/or function (qualitative). In the latter the platelet count is usually normal (150 to $450 \times 10^3/\mu l$).

Thrombocytopenia is defined as a platelet count less than $150,000/\mu l$. There is an approximate relationship between the severity of thrombocytopenia and bleeding. With platelet counts greater than $50,000/\mu l$, bleeding may occur following injury or surgery but spontaneous bleeding is uncommon. Risk of spontaneous and serious bleeding increases at platelet counts less than $20,000/\mu l$. Mucosal (mouth, gastrointestinal, and genitourinary tract) and subcutaneous bleeding (petechiae, purpura, and ecchymoses) are characteristic of thrombocytopenic bleeding. The most serious risk is intracranial bleeding. Thrombocytopenia may be due to (1) decreased production (*e.g.*, megaloblastic and aplastic anemias, alcoholism, cytotoxic drugs or radiation, acute leukemias, metastatic cancer or fibrosis in the marrow), (2) hypersplenism (excessive pooling of platelets in an enlarged spleen from any cause), (3) accelerated peripheral destruction or consumption (antibody-mediated, disseminated intravascular coagulation). *Idiopathic thrombocytopenic purpura* (ITP) is an example of (auto)antibody-mediated thrombocytopenia. It is more common in young women who present with purpura and mucosal bleeding and frequently a long history of easy bruising and menorrhagia. Splenic size is normal or mildly enlarged, and there is no evidence of an underlying disorder. Thrombocytopenia is often severe ($<10,000/\mu l$) and must be promptly treated because of the risk of intracranial bleeding. Diagnosis is made by the finding of thrombocytopenia combined with a normal or increased number of megakaryocytes in the bone marrow and exclusion of

other causes. Prednisone (1 mg/kg/day) is the initial treatment of choice. Most patients will show an increase in the platelet count within the first week. A significant proportion of patients relapse after initial response to prednisone. Danazol may also be effective. Splenectomy is indicated for these patients if platelet count remains less than $50,000/\mu l$. Thrombocytopenic purpura indistinguishable from ITP may occur in patients with HIV infection, lupus, lupus erythematosus, sarcoidosis, or chronic lymphocytic leukemia (CLL). It is important to recognize these disorders since concurrent treatment of them is essential.

Drugs are an important cause of antibody-mediated thrombocytopenia. The mechanisms are similar to those discussed under drug-induced immunohemolytic anemia. Recovery is usual upon withdrawal of the offending drug. Commonly involved drugs are quinidine, heparin, thiazide diuretics, quinine, gold salts, and sulfa drugs. Splenectomy is *not* indicated.

Qualitative platelet disorders may be congenital or acquired. Acquired disorders of platelet function are most often caused by drugs such as aspirin, indomethacin, butazolidin, ibuprofen, and the penicillins. Uremia is another frequent cause. Spontaneous bleeding is uncommon, but acquired dysfunction may aggravate or contribute to bleeding from other causes. The defect in uremia is improved by dialysis, peritoneal dialysis being more effective than hemodialysis. Examples of hereditary platelet disorders include Glanzmann's thrombesthenia and Bernard-Soulier disease.

Malignancies

CHRONIC MYELOCYTIC LEUKEMIA (CML)

CML is a myeloproliferative disorder that most frequently affects adults between 30 and 50 years of age. It is a clonal disorder of the pluripotent stem cell; thus, platelets, red cells, and granulocytes all belong to the malignant clone, although proliferation of the granulocytic series predominates. Symptoms and signs are due to greatly increased cell mass and include weight loss, fever, tachycardia (hypermetabolism), abdominal fullness and early satiety due to an often massive splenomegaly, and sternal tenderness due to hyperplastic bone marrow. Gout may occur because of hyperuricemia. Marked leukocytosis is the major laboratory abnormality; all stages of myeloid cells are present with frequently a selective increase in basophils, but myeloblasts usually account for less than 10% of the cells. Anemia and thrombocytosis or thrombocytopenia may be present. Characteristically, leukocyte alkaline phosphatase in the granulocytes is markedly decreased or absent and the serum B_{12} level is elevated. In about 90% of the patients, Philadelphia chromosome, a unique chromosomal abnormality, is demonstrable and is virtually pathognomonic for CML. The treatment consists of control of the leukocytosis by cytotoxic drugs such as hydroxyurea or busulfan and/or interferon. Marrow transplantation from an HLA-identical sibling appears to cure some patients, especially if it is carried out before acceleration of the disease. In most patients, the disease eventually enters the blastic phase, which resembles acute leukemia. This phase is usually refractory to treatment and fatal.

CHRONIC LYMPHOCYTIC LEUKEMIA (CLL)

CLL is a clonal disorder characterized by production and accumulation of functionally defective B lymphocytes. It is predominantly a disease of older adults. Laboratory findings are a variable degree of leukocytosis and, in advanced cases, anemia, granulocytopenia, and thrombocytopenia. The majority of the leukocytes are mature-appearing small lymphocytes. About a quarter of the patients are diagnosed incidentally during routine blood counts. Others may present with lymphadenopathy and splenomegaly. Bacterial pneumonia may be the presenting manifestation because of hypogammaglobulinemia, which frequently occurs. About a quarter of the patients may develop AIHA sometime during the course of the disease; a few may present with this complication. Those with early-stage disease and no symptoms should not be treated. Indications for treatment are anemia, thrombocytopenia, progressive disease, and AIHA. Most commonly used cytotoxic agents are chlorambucil and cyclophosphamide with or without corticosteroids.

ACUTE LEUKEMIAS

These are relatively uncommon but frequently fatal disorders. The main morphologic types are acute myeloblastic (AML) and acute lymphoblastic (ALL) leukemias. Since therapy and prognosis are quite different for the two types, differentiation is important and is made on the basis of morphology, histochemical stains, and immune phenotyping. The leukemic cell grows in the marrow at the expense of the normal clones, resulting in neutropenia, anemia, and thrombocytopenia. Clinical manifestations usually relate to these abnormalities; thus, the patient may present with infection, bleeding, and symptoms of anemia in any combination. Modest splenic enlargement is common. Leukocyte count may be low, normal, or elevated, but in all cases there is predominance of blast forms. The bone marrow usually shows infiltration with blast cells and a paucity of normal hematopoietic cells. Treatment consists of support with blood products and multidrug chemotherapy. Bone marrow transplantation is under intense investigation in this disease.

PLASMA CELL DISORDERS

With few exceptions, a monoclonal immunoglobulin (Ig) or portion of an immunoglobulin molecule is found in the serum, urine, or both. The most common plasma cell disorders are myeloma, Waldenström's macroglobulinemia, and monoclonal gammopathies of undetermined significance.

Myeloma is a malignant clonal proliferation of plasma cells that primarily affects those over 40. It manifests primarily by widespread bony destruction with consequent fractures and hypercalcemia, anemia, renal failure, and recurrent infections, usually bacterial pneumonias, the latter because of suppression of normal Ig synthesis. The bone lesions are characteristically lytic or "punched out" and are most often found in the skull, vertebrae, and pelvis. High levels of monoclonal Ig (usually IgG or IgA) lead to an elevated sedimentation rate and rouleaux formation on blood smear and occasionally symptoms of hyperviscosity. A firm diagnosis of myeloma requires (1) marrow plasmocytosis of greater than 25% and (2) monoclonal immunoglobulin or light chain in the serum or κ or λ light chains in the urine (Bence Jones protein). Initial treatment consists of chemotherapy with an alkylating agent such as malphalan and prednisone and treatment of complications. Painful bone lesions should be radiated for pain relief and prevention of fractures.

In Waldenström's macroglobulinemia, the monoclonal Ig secreted is IgM. As a result, manifestations of hyperviscosity (headache, dizziness, confusion, impaired vision, stupor, coma) often dominate the clinical picture. Lymphadenopathy and hepatosplenomegaly are common, but bone involvement is rare. Treatment consists of plasmapheresis for relief of hyperviscosity and chlorambucil or cyclophosphamide to control IgM production.

In the general population, about 1% of those over 30 years of age are found to have a monoclonal serum Ig without the evidence for myeloma or macroglobulinemia; the incidence rises to 3% for those over 70. About 20% of these will progress to develop myeloma or macroglobulinemia in 10 years. All patients with a monoclonal Ig must be followed for this progression by serial measurement of the Ig and observation for other signs of neoplasia. Rising concentration of Ig is a clue to malignant transformation.

HODGKIN'S DISEASE (HD)

HD has a bimodal age distribution with a peak in the late 20s, a decline to age 45, and then a gradual increase with age. Typical presentation is painless lymph node enlargement with or without fever, weight loss, and severe night sweats. In most cases the cervical nodes are the first site of involvement, but any lymphoid organ including the spleen and extranodal sites may be involved. The diagnosis is established by a lymph node biopsy showing the Reed-Sternberg (R-S) cell, the malignant cell of HD, in the appropriate cellular milieu. The choice and outcome of treatment are largely determined by the extent of the disease at the time of diagnosis. An accurate assessment of the extent, referred to as staging, is, therefore, the most crucial step after the diagnosis. This may require the use of lymphangiography, computerized tomography (CT) scanning, bone scan, bone marrow and liver biopsies, and, in selected cases, laparotomy:

Stage I: Single node region
Stage II: Two or more node regions on the same side of the diaphragm
Stage III: Node regions on both sides of the diaphragm ± spleen
Stage IV: Diffuse involvement of one or more extralymphatic organs
All stages: (A) Without weight loss/fever/night sweats (B) With weight loss/fever/night sweats

There are many nuances to the selection of proper treatment for a patient with HD: for some stages (IIB and IIIA), the treatment strategy is still evolving. In general, patients with stages IIIB and IV are treated with chemotherapy; patients with stages IA, IB, and IIA usually receive radiotherapy, with chemotherapy often given to those with balky mediastinal disease or localized extralymphatic involvement. Currently the 10-year survival rate for all patients with HD is 70%.

NON-HODGKIN'S LYMPHOMA (NHL)

These are malignant disorders of T- or B-lymphocytes and are the lymphomas most commonly associated with HIV infection. Extralymphatic disease is more common than in HD. Also, autoimmune hemolytic anemia (AIHA) and thrombocytopenia may occur. Diagnosis is by a lymph node biopsy. Staging is similar to HD but laparotomy is rarely employed. Unlike HD, the prognosis and treatment are dependent more on the nodal architecture and the morphology of the malignant tissue than on the stage of the disease. Therapy of indolent lymphomas (nodular, small cleared-cell, and nodular mixed) is very controversial; choices range from observation until symptoms mandate therapy to initial intensive chemotherapy. Intermediate and high-grade lymphomas usually require treatment, which consists primarily of chemotherapy, since a sizable proportion of patients are cured and most symptomatic patients are palliated. Radiation may be given after chemotherapy in patients with stage I or stage II disease or for palliation of symptoms if the disease is unresponsive to chemotherapy.

DISEASES OF THE LUNGS

Respiratory Failure

Respiratory failure is defined as failure of the respiratory system resulting in life-threatening hypoxemia and/or hypercapnia. It may be caused by dysfunction of the lungs, respiratory pump, or both. The respiratory pump, which is responsible for moving gas in and out of the lungs, consists of the respiratory muscles, the chest wall, and the respiratory center in the brain stem with its connections to the muscles. Failure of the respiratory pump (respiratory muscle fatigue, respiratory center depression, chest wall defects) results in hypoxemia with hypercapnia, whereas failure of gas exchange (pneumonia, adult respiratory distress syndrome) does not usually lead to hypercapnia. In some diseases [chronic obstructive pulmonary disease (COPD), acute pulmonary edema] abnormal gas exchange may coexist with pump failure due to respiratory muscle fatigue. The obvious consequences of respiratory failure are inadequate oxygenation of organs and respiratory acidosis due to the CO_2 retention. Respiratory failure may be either acute or chronic, and in the latter situation the patient may tolerate a level of hypoxemia or hypercapnia that in the acute situation would not be tolerable.

The immediate goal of therapy in respiratory failure is to correct the hypoxemia. This is accomplished by controlled administration of supplemental oxygen in some instances, but mechanical ventilation and positive end-expiratory pressure

(PEEP) may be required in others. Therapy should also be directed toward the underlying cause of the respiratory failure and include measures directed toward improving oxygen transport to the tissues, such as transfusion and treatment of coexistent circulatory failure.

PULMONARY FUNCTION TESTS

A number of tests to determine pulmonary function may be performed. In addition to the measurements of blood gases—Po_2, Pco_2, and pH—specific functions of the lung can be measured. Gas flow is tested by measuring the amount of air moved by voluntary effort in 1 minute (the maximal voluntary ventilation or MVV) or by a maximal forced expiratory maneuver. The maximal amount of air that can be expelled from the lung by forced exhalation is the forced vital capacity (FVC), and the amount of air expelled in the first second of this maneuver (the forced expiratory volume in 1 second or FEV_1) and the flow rate across the middle portion of the FVC (the maximal midexpiratory flow or MMEF) are also measured. The total volume of gas in the lungs (total lung capacity or TLC) may be assessed from the chest x ray, by gas dilution methods, and by plethysmography. Two general types of functional abnormalities are recognized. An obstructive ventilatory defect (asthma, COPD) is characterized by normal or increased TLC and reduced MVV, MMEF, FEV_1, and FEV_1:FVC ratio. The FVC is normal in early obstructive disease and falls with more advanced disease. A restrictive pattern (obesity, interstitial lung disease, neuromuscular disorders) is characterized by reduction of total lung capacity as well as the FVC; the FEV_1 is also decreased, with the result that the FEV_1:FVC ratio is normal or even slightly increased. The MVV is usually decreased in proportion to the reduction in FEV in obstructive lung disorders, but may be disproportionately decreased in the presence of neuromuscular disorders or central airway obstruction.

Chronic Obstructive Pulmonary Disease (COPD)

COPD is usually a combination of chronic bronchitis and pulmonary emphysema, although one or the other may predominate. COPD is usually related to smoking cigarettes, although there may be other causes, such as hereditary α_1-antitrypsin deficiency. The disease becomes apparent after age 40 with chronic cough and sputum production accompanied by dyspnea and wheezing. These symptoms progress as the disease advances. Physical examination reveals diminished breath sounds, rhonchi, wheezes, and if the disease is advanced, the use of accessory muscles of respiration, cyanosis, and right ventricular enlargement. There may be secondary polycythemia, a low Po_2, elevated Pco_2 and a partially compensated respiratory acidosis. Pulmonary function tests are those of an obstructive defect. Episodes of bronchopulmonary infection are common. Patients with COPD should receive yearly influenza vaccinations and a single pneumococcal vaccine.

Treatment includes stopping smoking, β-adrenergic agonist bronchodilator therapy, and the early use of antibiotics for infection. Corticosteroids and anticholinergic bronchodilators may be useful adjuncts for those patients with moderate to severe disease. Continuous low-flow oxygen is of proven benefit for patients with chronic, severe hypoxemia.

Bronchial Asthma

Asthma is characterized by the presence of "hyper-irritable" airways such that the airways respond to a variety of stimuli by smooth muscle constriction, mucosal edema and inflammation, and mucous hypersecretion. The result is a syndrome of episodic, generalized airway narrowing that produces dyspnea, wheezing, prolonged expiration, hyperinflation, and arterial hypoxemia and hypocapnia. In some patients chronic cough may be the only manifestation of asthma, or the patient may be normal by physical examination and laboratory testing at presentation. Common stimuli to airway narrowing include environmental irritants (cigarette smoke, air pollution), specific antigens (grass, pollens), drugs (aspirin, β-adrenergic blockers), occupational inhalants (cotton dust, chemicals), physical agents (cold air), and respiratory infections.

Asthmatics are often characterized as either extrinsic or intrinsic types, although many patients do not fit easily into one group. The *intrinsic asthmatic* tends to have no known allergens, negative skin tests, and nonseasonal attacks, whereas subjects with *extrinsic asthma* are usually children with readily identifiable allergens, seasonal attacks, skin test reactivity, high levels of IgE, and a family history of asthma or other allergic disease. Asthma tends to be an episodic disorder, but in some patients the symptoms become chronic and continuous. The diagnosis is made by the typical history and physical findings, and confirmatory evidence is provided by an obstructive pattern on spirometry that normalizes or is strikingly improved by an inhaled bronchodilator.

Usually the acute attacks can be controlled by administration of inhaled β-adrenergic receptor agonist bronchodilators. Patients not responding to these measures should receive systemic corticosteroids early in the management of the acute attack. Other important measures include fluids to ensure hydration and antibiotics for associated infection. Controversy now exists over the role of theophylline. Inhaled corticosteroids and cromalyn sodium are important for long-term management of patients with more severe disease to avoid prolonged or frequent need for systemic steroids.

Children sensitive to food may be cured by elimination of the offending substances. Alternatively, desensitization by increasing inoculations with the specific proteins is of value in some cases. In cases in which the causal allergen cannot be discovered or removed, bronchodilator drugs or steroid maintenance therapy or both often provide complete control of the symptoms. The antihistamine drugs usually are disappointing.

Pulmonary Emboli

The most common sources of pulmonary emboli are thrombi from the veins of the lower extremities, pelvis, or from the right atrium. These may obstruct a branch of the pulmonary artery and cause a wedge-shaped infarct with its base toward the pleura. These emboli vary in size from a few millimeters to many centimeters and are often multiple. They most frequently involve the lower lobe. The incidence of pulmonary embolism is 25% to 30% in autopsied patients. Most of these were not detected before death.

The symptoms of pulmonary embolism are (1) acute unexplained dyspnea and tachycardia, (2) acute cardiovascular collapse with evidence of elevated right atrial pressure, (3) acute development of pleuritic pain with or without a pleural friction rub, and (4) fever. The acute onset is characteristic and may cause death immediately, but in many cases the symptoms are much less evident. An ECG may give evidence of right-axis deviation and is an aid in the diagnosis. Chest x ray and blood gases may be useful but not diagnostic. A normal radioisotope lung scan is strong evidence against pulmonary embolus. A venogram of the lower extremities or pulmonary angiogram may be used in selected instances in establishing the diagnosis.

Treatment is designed to sustain life and prevent recurrence. Immediate anticoagulation with intravenous administration of heparin is advised. Surgical placement of vena caval filters is reserved for anticoagulant failures and when coexisting conditions contraindicate anticoagulant use. Embolectomy and use of thrombolytic agents are reserved for extreme circumstances.

Pleural Effusions

History, physical examination, and examination of the pleural fluid usually allow for a diagnosis of the cause of pleural effusion. Although large effusions may cause dyspnea, many effusions do not directly cause symptoms. Physical examination varies, depending on amount of fluid and the condition of the underlying lung. Characteristic findings include decreased expansion, decreased fremitus, flat percussion note, reduced breath sounds, and sometimes tracheal deviation to the contralateral side. Examination of the fluid should include gross appearance, cells, and analysis of transudate versus exudate. The latter is often critical, and an exudate is usually present if the pleural fluid to serum total protein ratio exceeds 0.5; pleural fluid LDH exceeds 200 IU/liter; or the pleural fluid to serum LDH ratio exceeds 0.6. Additional studies often aiding in diagnosis of exudative effusions include stains and cultures for infectious agents, cytologic studies, pH, glucose concentrations, and pleural biopsy.

Interstitial Lung Disease

A variety of diseases afflict primarily the interstitial tissues of the lung. These include inorganic dusts (silica, asbestos), organic dusts (fungal antigens, animal proteins), fumes and gases, drugs (antibiotics, gold, antineoplastic agents), radiation, infectious agents, or any one of a variety of diseases of unknown etiology (sarcoidosis, rheumatoid arthritis, idiopathic pulmonary fibrosis). Whatever the initial cause of injury, interstitial fibrosis may be the outcome. The most common manifestation is dyspnea, which is progressive. Physical examination may be normal except for dry ("Velcro") basilar rales; later there may be tachypnea, clubbing, and cor pulmonale. The laboratory may show secondary polycythemia and evidence of an autoimmune process (i.e., antinuclear antibodies, rheumatoid factor). Chest x ray is either normal or shows a nodular infiltrate at the bases. Pulmonary function tests reveal a restrictive ventilatory defect, decreased diffusing capacity and reduced lung compliance. Physical examinations, x-ray studies, and pulmonary function studies are often of little help in defining the cause of fibrosis. Special laboratory tests and history of occupational exposure are vitally important in establishing a specific etiology. The treatment depends on cause. In patients in whom no etiology is identified, that is, idiopathic interstitial fibrosis, steroids, or immunosuppressive agents may be tried, although the results are questionable. The prognosis varies with cause and the effectiveness of therapy. Lung transplantation is a consideration in those patients for whom medical therapy has not been of help.

Carcinoma of the Lung

Cigarette smoking plays a major etiologic role in the most common varieties of lung cancer, the squamous and poorly differentiated small-cell ("oat cell") types, and is less related to adenocarcinoma. Patients may have no symptoms or may have cough, hemoptysis, pneumonia, or wheeze. Local thoracic invasion and metastases to local nodes cause superior vena caval obstruction, hoarseness, and pleural effusion. Distant metastases involve virtually all organs. Remote manifestations include neuromuscular syndrome, clubbing, ectopic endocrine disorders (ADH, hyperparathyroidism, Cushing's syndrome), and thrombophlebitis. In addition to the clinical picture and the x-ray findings, bronchoscopy, mediastinoscopy, or thoracotomy are usually required for diagnosis. Surgery remains the preferred treatment in resectable non-oat-cell tumors. The role of chemotherapy is established in oat-cell and non-oat-cell types with advanced disease. Overall, long-term results remain poor, although the outlook is considerably better for the patient with a solitary "coin" lesion.

The Pneumonias

(See discussion in *Rypins' Basic Sciences Review*, Chap. 5, "General Microbiology and Immunology," and Chap. 6, "Pathology.")

Acute bacterial pneumonia in the adult is classically designated as either **lobar pneumonia** or **bronchopneumonia**. The former term applies when the infection is localized primarily to alveoli and the chest x ray demonstrates a large, localized consolidation. If the pneumonia is untreated, it extends to involve the entire lobe (hence the term *lobar*), but this occurs much less commonly when antibiotics are used early in the course. *Bronchopneumonia* is the result of bacterial invasion of terminal and respiratory bronchioles with extension into the surrounding alveoli, and the chest x ray reveals multiple, usually bilateral foci of pneumonia that coalesce into large consolidations if the infection progresses. From a practical point of view, the distinction between bronchopneumonia and lobar pneumonia is far less important than establishing the etiologic agent. The radiographic appearance is never diagnostic of a particular microorganism, and other methods such as sputum examination and culture of blood, sputum, or pleural fluid are imprecise or require several days to provide an answer. Since antibiotic therapy must be initiated as early as possible, choice of antimicrobials is often empiric and based on the most likely etiologic agent(s).

STREPTOCOCCAL PNEUMONIA

Most community-acquired pneumonia is due to *Streptococcus pneumoniae*. It accounts for some pneumonia in young, previously healthy adults but is the most common cause of pneumonia in elderly or debilitated subjects. The patient typically presents with sudden onset of shaking chill, fever, cough productive of rusty or bloody sputum, and pleuritic pain. The physical findings are those of consolidation: local dullness, "bronchial" breath sounds, and fine, inspiratory rales. The x ray may be normal early in the disease, but evidence of lobar pneumonia and pleural effusions are common. Leukocytosis is typically present, and abnormalities of liver function tests may also be found. Since the organism is an inhabitant of the upper airway in about 50% of normal persons, its presence on Gram stain of a coughed sputum specimen is not necessarily diagnostic unless the organism is present in overwhelming numbers. Because the organism is very fastidious, false-negative sputum cultures occur, but culture of *Streptococcus pneumoniae* from blood or pleural fluid is virtually diagnostic. Complications of pneumococcal pneumonia include empyema, meningitis, endocarditis, and arthritis. Bacteremia is accompanied by a substantial increase in mortality. Acquired deficiency of the IgG subtype, as well as multiple myeloma and splenectomy, predispose these patients to pneumococcal sepsis. Treatment with penicillin usually results in a prompt defervescence and an improvement in the patient's sense of well-being, but in patients with serious underlying disease, fever may persist for as long as 4 days after penicillin is begun. Erythromycin or vancomycin should be used in penicillin-allergic patients. The 23 polyvalent pneumococcal vaccine is useful for patients over the age of 50 years as well as for younger patients with chronic illnesses.

AEROBIC GRAM-NEGATIVE PNEUMONIA

Aerobic gram-negative bacilli such as *Klebsiella pneumoniae, Pseudomonas aeruginosa, Proteus,* and *Escherichia coli* are common causes of hospital-acquired pneumonia and cause community-acquired pneumonia in immunocompromised hosts with alcoholism, diabetes mellitus, renal failure, and malignancy and in persons from chronic care facilities. The clinical findings are similar to those described for *Streptococcus pneumoniae*. The chest radiograph typically shows a bronchopneumonia, although lobar pneumonia is the rule with *K. pneumoniae*. Bulging of a fissure adjacent to the consolidation is also characteristic of infection with *K. pneumoniae*. There is a tendency for early empyema formation and tissue destruction with development of one or more abscesses with gram-negative bacillary infection. Broad-spectrum penicillin or cephalosporins plus aminoglycosides are the treatment for pneumonia due to these agents, but the illness is usually protracted and mortality high despite appropriate treatment.

HEMOPHILUS PNEUMONIA

Hemophilus influenza b is another cause of gram-negative pneumonia. It may occur in healthy adults but appears to be more common in patients with chronic lung disease or chronic alcoholism. These organisms appear as small, pleomorphic bacilli on Gram stain, and treatment is with ceftriaxone or ticarcillin/clavulanate potassium.

STAPHYLOCOCCAL PNEUMONIA

Pneumonia due to *Staphylococcus aureus* occurs most commonly (1) following influenza, (2) in hospitalized patients, and (3) in intravenous drug users with tricuspid endocarditis. In the form that follows influenza there is frequently an asymptomatic interval between recovery from the influenza and onset of the pneumonia. The onset is typically abrupt and not different from acute pneumonia of other causes. The chest x ray reveals diffuse, patchy infiltrates, and empyema and multiple small abscesses are common. Pneumatoceles (rounded, subpleural cystic structures) are common in children but rare in adults. Staphylococcal pneumonia in drug users is often due to septic embolization from tricuspid valve endocarditis and tends to have a more subacute onset with ill-defined nodular, cavitating lesions on chest x ray. When staphylococcal pneumonia is accompanied by bacteremia, distant foci of infection may be established and prognosis is considerably worsened. Treatment is with penicillinase-resistant penicillins or cefazolin. Vancomycin is used in the patient with penicillin allergy or for methicillin-resistant staphylococcal pneumonia.

MYCOPLASMA PNEUMONIA

Mycoplasma pneumoniae is a primary respiratory pathogen in humans that is transmitted person to person. Infection is most prevalent in school-age children and young adults, and the vast majority of illnesses due to this agent range from a minor febrile upper respiratory illness with or without pharyngitis to severe bronchitis. Clinically apparent pneumonia develops in less than 10% of those infected. The pneumonia typically presents as fever, chills, headache, nonproductive cough, and malaise. Hemoptysis and pleuritic pain are rare. Examination of the chest usually does not reveal evidence of consolidation, and the roentgenographic manifestations vary from a fine reticular pattern to patchy airspace consolidation. Pleural disease and abscess formation are extremely rare. Bullous myringitis may be seen. Culture of *Mycoplasma pneumoniae* may take from 2 weeks to 3 months and serves only to confirm the diagnosis after the illness has resolved. The diagnosis can be suspected from a rise in the titer of cold agglutinins and confirmed with specific serologic tests. Treatment is with tetracycline or erythromycin.

LEGIONELLA PNEUMONIA

Infection by *Legionella* species is recognized as an important cause of pneumonia both in the community and among hospitalized patients. The organism is not usually seen on Gram stain of sputum or of infected tissue. Diagnosis is made by demonstration of the bacteria by direct immunofluorescent staining of sputum. Clinically patients may be severely ill with the radiographic pattern of either bronchopneumonia or lobar pneumonia. Treatment of choice is parenteral erythromycin or doxycycline. Rifampin may be added when patients do not respond.

Since the bacterial etiology cannot always be identified with certainty at the time of presentation, the choice of antibiotics is usually empiric. Community-acquired pneumonia in a previously healthy individual should be treated with penicillin or, if *Mycoplasma* or *Legionella* is suspected, erythromycin or doxycycline. Community-acquired pneumonia in a debilitated or immunocompromised host is frequently due to *Streptococcus pneumoniae*, but the incidence of gram-negative bacillary pneumonia is increased in these individuals. These patients should be treated with an aminoglycoside as well as a broad spectrum penicillin or cephalosporin to cover this possibility. If the sputum Gram stain suggests infection due to *Haemophilus influenzae,* ceftriaxone may be used. Since pneumococcal pneumonia frequently responds to antibiotics within 2 to 3 days but gram-negative bacillary pneumonia is more protracted, one may correlate the patient's clinical course with culture results after 48 to 72 hours of treatment, and inappropriate antimicrobials may be discontinued. Empiric antibiotic coverage for hospital-acquired pneumonia should include antistaphylococcal and gram-negative coverage.

Tuberculosis

The present concept of the common pattern of pulmonary tuberculosis of the adult type is that it has the following pathogenesis:

1. Childhood infection, usually brief, benign, and undiagnosed, leaving a calcified Ghon tubercle or hilar node
2. A long-lasting sensitivity to the tubercle bacillus, manifested by a positive tuberculin test
3. A reinfection in youth or adult life, with entirely different features, that is the result of the sensitization to the organism and progresses to a chronic phase

Chronic pulmonary tuberculosis may follow the primary infection after a short or long period of dormancy. Features are (1) absence of recent exposure, (2) tendency to chronicity and cavitation, and (3) production of fibrous tissue of repair. The most common site is the apical portion of the lung and posterior portions of the upper lobes with spread downward and medially because of endobronchial spread of bacillus-laden liquid caseum.

Onset may be insidious; the patient may be asymptomatic and the disease diagnosed only by chest roentgenogram. Early constitutional symptoms are due to absorption of tuberculoprotein in the hypersensitive host. Fever is often present in late evening, leading to night sweats. General malaise, weight loss, and cough productive of morning sputum may be noted.

Since tuberculosis causes nonspecific symptoms and may involve the pleura, mediastinum, or almost any part of the lung, it should be included in the differential diagnosis in most patients with pulmonary disease. A presumptive diagnosis is made by demonstrating acid-fast bacilli in sputum smears or tissue, but positive identification of *Mycobacterium tuberculosis* is made by culture. When the suspicion is high for tuberculosis, treatment should be initiated even if smears are negative. Rarely, treatment may be indicated even in the presence of negative cultures.

Activity is indicated by (1) fever, (2) night sweats, (3) rapid pulse, (4) loss of weight and strength, (5) increased sedimentation rate, (6) hemoptysis, (7) less significantly, cough, and (8) expectoration. Increase of physical signs or x-ray findings at intervals of about 2 months may be the only evidence of progression but indicates what has taken place, as contrasted with symptoms, which indicate present activity. A positive tuberculin reaction does not indicate present activity, but a negative reaction is highly significant in excluding the diagnosis of tuberculosis except in an anergic patient.

Complications include cavitation, making the patient highly infectious: hemoptysis; pleurisy with effusion; tuberculous pneumonia; and bronchopleural fistula with empyema. Patients may continue with these symptoms for many years before presenting for treatment.

Extrapulmonary complications of pulmonary tuberculosis include involvement of the middle ear, the larynx, the intestines, the lymph nodes, the bones, the peritoneum, the meninges, the kidneys, and the genital area.

Treatment of chronic pulmonary tuberculosis may be summarized under (1) specific drug treatment, (2) surgical treatment, and (3) nonspecific measures.

1. Standard treatment of active disease is with a "short-course" regimen of 6 or 9 months' duration. The initial phase of the 6-month regimen consists of 2 months of daily INH, rifampin, and pyrazinamide. This is supplemented with ethambutol or striptomyan. If INH resistance is suspected, or extensive disease is present, the final 4 months consist of INH and rifampin daily or twice weekly.
2. Only rarely is surgery needed in cases where response to medical treatment seems incomplete.
3. Included under nonspecific measures are rest, diet, occupational therapy, and rehabilitation. Hospitalization usually is not required.

Acute miliary tuberculosis is a blood-borne infection in which the organisms are seeded throughout the body from a primary focus. The lungs are affected principally when the bacilli come through the thoracic duct or systemic veins, while a pulmonary focus that breaks into the veins of the lungs results in a generalized distribution.

Miliary tuberculosis without treatment is uniformly fatal. Lesions are found not only in lung but liver, spleen, bone marrow, and meninges. Diagnosis is best made by biopsy of liver, node or marrow, searching for caseating granulomas. The clinical picture is similar to chronic infection due to other causes such as histoplasmosis, coccidioidomycosis, or cryptococcosis, or to the picture of diffuse carcinomatosis. Prompt treatment with isoniazid and rifampin has improved survival rate. The tuberculin test may be negative.

Tuberculous meningitis usually occurs as part of acute miliary tuberculosis. It is found most often in young children. The diagnosis is suggested by the history and the physical condition and is established by a positive spinal fluid test or by the finding of tubercles in the choroid. The spinal fluid reveals from 25 to 1,000 or more white cells mm^3, predominantly lymphocytes. Spinal fluid protein is elevated. Tubercle bacilli may be found in the cobweblike clot of fibrin. In young children a positive tuberculin skin test is significant. With the several drugs now available, survival rates are high, with some incidence of permanent brain injury but relatively little recurrence of the meningitis.

Other Pulmonary Infections

BRONCHIECTASIS

Seen far less often than in years past, bronchiectasis is characterized by cylindrical, fusiform, or sacculated dilatation of the bronchi. The condition is the result of destruction of the cartilage and elastin that support the brachial walls. The lesion may be unilateral or bilateral. The bases are involved more frequently than the apices, except that tuberculous bronchiectases are usually in the upper lobes.

The symptoms are (1) paroxysmal cough; (2) large amounts of sputum, which on standing separates into three layers; (3) dyspnea on exertion; and (4) sometimes hemoptysis. Constitutional symptoms are absent as long as drainage is maintained.

Physical signs are absent in mild cases but there may be rales. Signs of coexisting bronchitis, emphysema, and fibrosis may be present. There is often some enlargement of the right heart. Clubbing of fingers is common.

Diagnosis depends on the history, the physical signs, the characteristic foul sputum, and bronchograms. A bronchogram has been the standard way to establish the diagnosis; however, high-resolution CT scanning now provides a more easily tolerated means of diagnosis.

Treatment is directed toward improving the patient's general condition and diminishing the amount of sputum by postural drainage. The medical treatment is that of chronic bronchitis and in some cases includes frequent intermittent use of antibiotics on a long-term basis. Rarely, patients with localized bronchiectasis are cured or improved by resection of segments or lobes or combinations of segments and lobes. The prompt diagnosis and treatment of bacterial infections of the lower respiratory tract is the best way of avoiding a chronic complication such as bronchiectasis.

LUNG ABSCESS

Suppuration in the lung may result (1) following pneumonia, particularly aspiration forms of bronchopneumonia; (2) from wounds or operations of the throat, particularly tonsillectomy or dental manipulation in patients with periodontal disease; (3) from infective embolism; (4) from perforating carcinoma; or (5) from perforation of the lung. If abscess occurs during the course of another disease, the symptoms are greatly aggravated at once. If it occurs in a patient previously well, the onset may be insidious, and the first characteristic sign may be the appearance of a large amount of foul sputum when the abscess ruptures into a bronchus. The odor is offensive but at first is not fetid. The sputum contains fragments of elastic tissue from the lung.

Fever, cyanosis, dyspnea, and clubbing of the fingers are frequent manifestations.

Except when lung abscess occurs following surgery or chest trauma, the history usually reveals an episode of altered mental status or presence of a swallowing disorder. Physical examination usually reveals periodontal disease. On chest x ray one or more infiltrates with air fluid levels may be present.

Intensive antibiotic therapy is the most important factor in treatment. With the exception of some bacteroides and staphylococci, most pathogens found are sensitive to penicillin. Clindamycin should be considered in penicillin-allergic patients, patients not responding to initial treatment with penicillin, or when infection is believed to be life-threatening. Antibiotics should be given parenterally until constitutional symptoms have resolved (usually 2 to 3 weeks) and continued orally until the chest x ray abnormalities clear completely or reach a stable residual. Chest percussion and postural drainage will promote drainage of the abscess. Surgical resection is rarely necessary. Bronchoscopy is indicated to exclude abscess behind an obstructing endobronchial malignancy in patients who fail to respond to medical management, when the location is atypical for aspiration, and when no predisposing factors for aspiration are present.

Farmer's lung is a condition caused by inhalation of spoiled or moldy hay that is characterized by the sudden onset of dyspnea some hours after exposure to this or other vegetable material. It is the prototype of "hypersensitivity pneumonitis." There may be fever, chills, and cyanosis, and a roentgenogram of the chest suggests diffuse interstitial pneumonia. Histologically there are numerous granulomas involving the pulmonary interstitium, and there may be obliterative bronchitis. The cause of the condition is apparently a hypersensitivity reaction to moldy hay. The disease usually lasts for several days and is followed by complete recovery.

Silo-filler's disease results from inhalation of oxides of nitrogen that are formed within a silo soon after it is filled. The disease is limited to individuals who enter silos within a day or two after filling, and the clinical picture consists of cough and dyspnea immediately after exposure, relative remission of symptoms during the next 2 or 3 weeks, followed by a second phase of the illness with fever, chills and progressive dyspnea and cyanosis. Numerous bubbling rales are heard over the lungs, and there is wheezing respiration during the third phase of the illness. An x-ray examination reveals generalized infiltration of the lungs with innumerable discrete densities. Adrenal steroids are valuable in the treatment of the acute phase of the disease.

Cystic fibrosis or mucoviscidosis is a familial systemic disease characterized by abnormal secretory products of a number of exocrine glands. Involvement of the bronchial glands leads to production of thick viscid pulmonary secretion; consequently, radicals of the tracheobronchial tree become plugged, and recurrent pulmonary infections and destruction of lung tissue result. Pulmonary infection is most commonly caused by staphylococci, and *Pseudomonas* is another important bacterial cause. A history of repeated attacks of pneumonia throughout life is characteristic of this disease. The pancreatic secretions are similarly affected, producing pancreatic insufficiency with malnutrition and steatorrhea. The mucous glands of the entire GI tract may be involved. The sweat and saliva contain unusually high concentrations of sodium and chloride, and detection of the increase in sweat electrolytes is the simplest means of diagnosis.

Sarcoidosis is a granulomatous disease of unknown etiology. It may involve any organ system, but it commonly affects the lungs and thoracic lymph nodes, liver, eyes, bones, and skin. Pulmonary involvement ranges from asymptomatic hilar and paratrachial node enlargement, which usually resolves spontaneously, to diffuse pulmonary fibrosis, which may cause progressive restrictive lung disease and cor pulmonale. Diagnosis requires demonstration of granulomas in biopsy material from the involved organ and exclusion of other granulomatous diseases such as tuberculosis. Treatment is with corticosteroids and is reserved for pulmonary involvement for the minority of patients with restrictive impairment. Other manifestations that may require aggressive treatment include hypercalcemia, uveitis, and cardiac or central nervous system (CNS) involvement.

Spontaneous pneumothorax is collapse of the lung in the absence of trauma. This may result from a superficial bulla that ruptures through the pleura with the escape of air directly into the pleural space. This is typically seen in young adults of tall, thin stature. Spontaneous pneumothorax is rarely observed in association with menstruation (*i.e.,* catamenial pneumothorax).

Respiratory Disturbances During Sleep

It is now recognized that a variety of symptoms and disorders in adults result from recurrent periods of apnea during sleep. Apnea, defined as the cessation of airflow at the nose and mouth for more than 15 seconds, is generally classified as being central, obstructive, or mixed. *Central apneas* occur because respiratory drive ceases, as evidenced by a lack of respiratory muscle activity and movement of the chest and abdomen. In the more common *obstructive apnea,* respiratory drive is present and often increases during the apneic episode, but airflow is absent because of upper airway obstruction. The *mixed apneas* usually begin as a central apnea followed by an obstructive apnea. Apneic episodes lasting from 15 to 120 seconds may recur throughout the night and result in progressive hypercapnia, hypoxemia, increased systemic and pulmonary artery pressure, and sinus bradycardia or ventricular dysrhythmias. The apnea is finally terminated by an arousal response (transient lightening of sleep stage or outright awakening), ventilation resumes, and the patient falls asleep again, only to repeat the sequence.

The nature and severity of the clinical symptoms depend to some extent on the type and frequency of apneic episodes and the severity of the associated blood gas and hemodynamic disturbances. In patients with predominantly obstructive apnea loud snoring is invariable. The patient may complain only of excessive daytime somnolence. Other characteristic symptoms reported by the patient or a spouse include abnormal motor activity during sleep, intellectual or personality changes, sexual impotence, and morning headache. Daytime systemic and pulmonary arterial hypertension are common, and in severe cases polycythemia and cor pulmonale may result. The majority of patients have obstructive sleep apnea and are males between the ages of 40 and 60. Obesity is the most common predisposing factor in patients with obstructive sleep apnea, but several other disorders may predispose to its development: acromegaly, myxedema, adenotonsillar hypertrophy, micrognathia, myotonic dystrophy, and temporomandibular joint disease. CNS abnormalities, especially those affecting the brain stem or spinal cord, are associated with central apneas, or there may be no associated disorders. Diagnosis and assessment of the severity of sleep apnea can be made by monitoring the patient while asleep.

Treatment depends on the type of apnea that predominates as well as the severity of desaturation, daytime symptoms, and dysrhythmias. In the case of central apneas, a variety of medications have been used to increase respiratory drive. When obstructive apneas predominate, administration of continuous positive airway pressure (nasal CPAP) to stint open the upper airway is often successful. Weight loss is beneficial. Tracheostomy is reliably corrective and may be indicated in severe disease. Surgery to correct the anatomic abnormalities of the upper airway may also be helpful in selected cases. Medical treatment includes avoidance of alcohol and sedative medications.

DISEASES OF THE KIDNEYS

The kidneys perform two vital functions. The normal *excretory* control of water, electrolytes, and metabolic products maintains the volume and composition of body fluids. The *regulatory* (nonexcretory) functions of the kidney play roles in determining red-cell formation (erythropoietin), bone metabolism (through generation of 1,25-dihydroxycholecalciferol), and regulation of arterial pressure (renin, prostaglandins). When renal function fails, there are abnormalities secondary to failure of both the excretory and nonexcretory functions.

The methods of evaluation of a patient includes those that diagnose disease and those that measure function. In addition to history and physical examination, the urinalysis is critical. Other major tests include 24-hour urine for protein and determination of creatinine clearance as a measure of glomerular filtration rate (GFR), urine culture, serum creatinine, blood urea nitrogen (BUN), serum electrolytes, x rays, ultrasound, and radiorenograms.

Renal Failure

Renal failure is defined as the stage of renal function when the kidney cannot maintain the integrity of the internal environment. It may be divided into chronic (CRF) and acute (ARF) forms. The *uremic syndrome* may occur in either CRF or ARF and is a clinical constellation including (1) CNS manifestations (lassitude, memory loss, insomnia, anxiety, stupor, coma, peripheral neuropathy); (2) cardiopulmonary abnormalities including pericarditis and adult respiratory distress; and (3) GI symptoms of anorexia, nausea, vomiting, and gastrointestinal bleeding. Uremia is due to retained metabolic waste products and reverses with dialysis.

CHRONIC RENAL FAILURE

CRF is the result of a host of chronic renal diseases of diverse cause that have in common the progressive destruction of the kidney. The manifestations may be divided into the following categories:

1. Fluid and electrolyte abnormalities. This includes extracellular fluid excess or deficit, hyponatremia, hypocalcemia, hyperphosphatemia, metabolic acidosis, and hypermagnesemia. Hyperkalemia is uncommon in CRF unless excess potassium is administered or oliguria occurs.
2. Abnormalities of nonexcretory function. Anemia due to marrow failure (relative erythropoietin deficiency), osteomalacia due to vitamin D deficiency, and occasionally hypertension due to increased renin production.
3. Metabolic abnormalities. Those such as glucose intolerance and hyperlipidemia may occur.
4. The uremic syndrome.
5. Social and emotional problems of chronic illness.

Treatment consists of (1) searching for treatable disease, for example, obstruction; (2) searching for reversible factors that might make renal function worse, for example, volume depletion, heart failure, hypertension (especially bilateral occlusive renal arterial disease), infection, superimposed obstruction, nephrotoxic drugs; (3) use of appropriate diet and salt and water intake; (4) maintaining normal serum phosphorus by use of calcium carbonate or aluminum-containing antacids to minimize hyperparathyroidism; (5) being careful about dosage of medications excreted by the kidney. (6) Finally, chronic intermittent dialysis and transplantation may be needed. Clinical guides are primary indicators for dialysis but generally when serum creatinine reaches 10 mg to 12 mg/100 ml and GFR is less than 7 ml to 10 ml/minute, dialysis should be given serious consideration.

ACUTE RENAL FAILURE

Acute renal failure may be divided into three clinical settings: (1) prerenal failure (heart failure, hypovolemia); (2) intrarenal failure; and (3) postrenal failure (obstruction). The most common cause of intrarenal failure is *acute tubular necrosis* (ATN). ATN is caused by ischemia or nephrotoxic agents and may or may not be associated with oliguria. Other causes of acute intrarenal failure are acute glomerular diseases, acute interstitial nephritis, and acute vascular disease (vasculitis, malignant hypertension, bilateral arterial occlusion). These various causes can usually be distinguished by clinical examination, urinalysis, and the determination in a random urine sample of sodium concentration and osmolality. In prerenal azotemia, urine sodium is less than 20 mEq/liter and urine osmolality over 500 mOsm/kg while in ATN urine sodium is greater than 40 mEq/liter while urine osmolality is less than 400 mOsm/kg. It may be helpful to determine fractional excretion of sodium (FE_{Na}): values less than 1 indicate prerenal cause; values greater than 1 are more indicative of ATN (or obstruction).

Treatment depends on cause. In ATN the goal is to maintain life and nutrition while hoping for spontaneous recovery. In particular, this means careful monitoring of fluid balance to avoid volume overload and hyperkalemia, and dialysis to prevent uremic symptoms and to permit adequate nutrition. Mortality in "surgical" ATN is 60%, in "medical" ATN 30%, and in "obstetrical" ATN 15%.

Glomerular Diseases

Glomerular diseases may be divided according to pathogenesis as follows: (1) immunologic; (2) vascular (polyarteritis, malignant nephrosclerosis); (3) coagulation (disseminated intravascular coagulation [DIC], hemolytic-uremic); (4) metabolic defects (diabetes, amyloid); (5) hereditary (Alport's syndrome); and (6) unknown (lipoid nephrosis). Diagnosis may require renal biopsy with histological and other techniques (including electron microscopy) to provide a specific cause. The immunologic mechanism is further divided into the more common immune-complex variety where a circulating antigen–antibody complex damages the glomerulus and an antiglomerular basement membrane antibody disease (anti-GBM) in which an antibody reacts with antigen fixed to basement membrane.

Glomerular diseases of diverse cause produce certain *glomerular syndromes:* acute glomerulonephritis; rapidly progressive glomerulonephritis, chronic progressive glomerular disease; asymptomatic proteinuria/hematuria; and the nephrotic syndrome. All glomerular syndromes are characterized by proteinuria and many have hematuria and red blood cell (RBC) casts as well. The particular diseases causing the glomerular syndromes may be *primary* renal diseases or *secondary* to some systemic illness.

Acute glomerulonephritis is characterized by oliguria, edema, hypertension, hematuria, proteinuria, and RBC casts. The clinical prototype is acute poststreptococcal glomerulonephritis (immune complex). Multisystem diseases may cause the same syndrome, for example, systemic lupus erythematosus (SLE), vasculitis, and infective endocarditis.

Rapidly progressive glomerulonephritis (RPGN) has a similar clinical picture as acute glomerulonephritis, but it develops more insidiously and generally results in end-stage renal failure within 1 to 3 months. Pathologically there is epithelial proliferation in the form of crescents. Goodpasture's syndrome (*i.e.,* anti-GBM disease with associated lung hemorrhage) is the prototype. There is also an idiopathic form as well as multisystem disease production of RPGN (*e.g.,* SLE, Henoch-Schonlein purpura, vasculitis, Wegener's granulomatosis).

Chronic progressive glomerular disease is the result of many glomerular illnesses of varied causes. It is generally characterized by hypertension, proteinuria, microscopic hematuria, and progressive reduction in GFR.

Asymptomatic proteinuria or hematuria without reduced GFR may occur as an early manifestation of diffuse disease or may represent focal illnesses such as IgA (Berger's) nephropathy. The overall outlook is relatively good.

Nephrotic syndrome is defined as the renal excretion of 3.5 g or more of protein in 24 hours. There are usually edema and hypoalbuminemia, and often hyperlipidemia. About 60% to 75% of patients have idiopathic nephrotic syndrome; that is, the disease is of unknown origin and is restricted to the kidney. In children the most common variety of idiopathic nephrotic syndrome is lipoid nephrosis ("minimal" or "nil" lesion). It has a good prognosis. In adults the most common lesion is membranous nephropathy (immune complex) with a 20% spontaneous remission rate. Other types of lesions are membranoproliferative, and focal sclerosis. Only the lipoid lesion is responsive to steroid. For the other lesions, debate persists. Causes of secondary nephrotic syndrome include diabetes, SLE, tumors, AIDS, amyloid, malaria, drugs, and pregnancy.

SELECTED GLOMERULOPATHIES

Diabetes mellitus produces a nodular as well as diffuse lesion. The nodular lesion of Kimmelstiel and Wilson is diagnostic of diabetes. The nephrotic syndrome and chronic progressive syndromes are common clinical expressions. When renal failure develops progression is expected. Contrast material may produce acute renal failure especially if renal failure is present. Recent reports suggest that angiotensin-converting enzyme (ACE) inhibitors and some calcium antagonists may reduce proteinuria and retard progression; however, more definitive conclusions await large, controlled clinical trials. Dialysis is associated with greater morbidity and mortality than in nondiabetics. Kidney or kidney/pancreas transplantation has been effective in selected patients when used with cyclosporine immunosuppressive therapy.

SLE (immune complex) produces all the glomerular syndromes described. There is a focal lesion that is more benign but may progress into the more destructive diffuse membranoproliferative disease. Treatment with steroids and immunosuppressives may be followed by arrest of the disease or improvement.

Hepatitis B antigenemia may result in immune-complex glomerular disease producing all the glomerular syndromes.

AIDS is associated with focal or diffuse (more rarely) mesangial proliferation and proteinuria (in approximately one half of these patients), which may progress to the nephrotic syndrome range. Renal failure due to focal sclerosis is occasionally a terminal event.

Interstitial Disease

Diseases that involve primarily the interstitium of the kidney are characterized by mild proteinuria (less than 1,500 mg per day), pyuria, and variable reduction of GFR. Acute interstitial nephritis includes bacterial pyelonephritis and drug-induced nephritis. The prototype is methicillin-induced nephritis, and in addition to acute renal failure patients may have skin rash and eosinophilia. Nonsteroidal anti-inflammatory drugs (NSAIDs) may also cause acute interstitial nephritis. Discontinuing the drug is usually sufficient therapy. Chronic interstitial nephritis can be due to chronic pyelonephritis, analgesic abuse nephropathy, papillary necrosis, gout, sarcoid, or heavy metals. In all cases of pyelonephritis in children, vesicoureteral reflux should be considered.

Analgesic abuse nephropathy is not rare. It is most often caused by combination analgesics that include phenacetin. Most patients have pain, indigestion, anemia, pyuria, and azotemia. They may have renal calculi, papillary necrosis, and ureteral tumors. Discontinuing the drugs often results in arrest or improvement.

Vascular Diseases

Vascular diseases include (1) "benign" nephrosclerosis, (2) "malignant" nephrosclerosis (see hypertension), (3) renal artery occlusion due to embolism or clot that results in renal infarction, (4) atherosclerotic or fibrosing renal arterial disease with hypertension, and (5) bilateral renal vein thrombosis associated with the nephrotic syndrome.

Polycystic Kidneys

This is a congenital and familial disease, in which the normal renal tissue is gradually replaced and encroached upon by multiple cysts of the renal parenchyma. The kidneys are enlarged and filled with grapelike clusters of cysts containing clear or hemorrhagic fluid. In some patients this may be associated with hepatic cysts, aneurysmal disease of cerebral vessels, or polycythemia. Ultrasound and intravenous pyelograms reveal the enlarged kidneys with deformed pelvis and flattening of the calyces. Hypertension and renal insufficiency develop later. Puncture of the cysts does not prolong life.

Obstructive Nephropathy

Urinary tract obstruction results in dilatation of the system proximal to the obstruction and ultimately leads to renal atrophy, possible infection, and renal failure. Obstruction may occur at any point in the urinary system and common causes include benign prostatic hypertrophy, cancer of the prostate, bladder, or ureters, neurogenic bladder, pelvic tumors, retroperitoneal fibrosis, stones, and ureteropelvic narrowing. Early diagnosis and surgical treatment are needed. After relief of obstruction there may be a period of postobstructive diuresis; in some instances, this is massive enough to cause volume depletion and electrolyte abnormalities.

Renal-Cell Carcinoma (Hypernephroma)

Although this condition is discussed more fully in the urology section, the triad of hematuria, flank pain, and a mass occurs in only a small number of patients. However, renal-cell carcinoma is especially known for its many systemic manifestations, including fever or hormonal abnormalities such as hypercalcemia, hypertension, polycythemia, and Cushing's syndrome. IVP, CT scanning, and selective renal arteriography are the basic diagnostic tools.

Renal Stones

Calcium stones are most common and occur most often in hypercalcemic states (hyperparathyroidism, sarcoidosis) and hypercalciuric conditions (idiopathic hypercalciuria, renal tubular acidosis). Uric acid stones are next most common and are radiolucent; they occur in gout and chronic diarrhea. Struvitz stones are associated with unremitting infections produced by urease-producing bacteria (*e.g.*, *Pseudomonas aeruginosa*). Other types of stones are cystine and triple phosphate stones. To prevent calculi, hydration and therapy of the underlying cause should be done wherever possible. Idiopathic hypercalciuria can be treated with thiazide diuretics, phosphates, and uric acid stones with allopurinol and alkalinization.

Selected Electrolyte Abnormalities

Hyponatremia is divided into three categories: (1) extracellular volume (ECFV) deficit due to renal or extrarenal losses of sodium, (2) excess ECFV (edema), and (3) syndrome of inappropriate ADH. In the first category, isotonic saline may be used; for categories two and three, water restriction is the appropriate treatment. Serious CNS symptoms including coma generally develop with serum levels below 120 mEq/liter.

Hypokalemia is a result of urinary loss as in diuretic therapy or of gastrointestinal loss of potassium. Treatment of the underlying cause and potassium replacement are the basis of therapy.

Hyperkalemia usually results from acute oliguric renal failure. Treatment consists of reduced intake, GI ion exchange, resins, and dialysis.

Hypercalcemia is seen in primary hyperparathyroidism, neoplasm, vitamin D excess, sarcoid, vitamin A excess, and thiazide therapy. Malignancy and hyperparathyroidism are the most common causes. Treatment in selected patients consists of saline, loop diuretics, and dialysis.

Hypophosphatemia is noted in alcoholics, diabetics receiving insulin, and in patients receiving sucralfate or parenteral alimentation. Levels less than 1 mg/100 ml cause rhabdomyolysis, hemolysis, bone pain, and encephalopathy. Oral or intravenous replacement is indicated.

Metabolic acidosis is characterized by a reduction in serum HCO_3^- leading to a reduction in pH and Pco_2. There are two types according to whether the anion gap is increased or normal. In the former acid is added (*e.g.*, diabetic ketoacidosis, lactic acidosis), toxic substances are ingested that generate acids (*e.g.*, salicylates, methyl alcohol, ethylene glycol) or there is a failure to excrete acids (renal failure). In normal anion gap (hyperchloremic) acidosis, there is a loss of HCO_3^- as in diarrhea, ostomies, renal tubular acidosis, or dilutional acidosis. Acidosis can produce Kussmaul's breathing, cardiac malfunction, and shock. The treatment is directed at the underlying condition and may include the administration of alkali.

Metabolic alkalosis is characterized by increased serum HCO_3 leading to increased pH and Pco_2. It is due either to ECF volume depletion (responds to saline) or to excess mineralocorticoid activity (resistant to saline).

Respiratory acidosis is characterized by reduced pH, increased Pco_2 and increased HCO_3^-. It is due to impaired ventilation. The treatment must be directed at improving air exchange.

Respiratory alkalosis is characterized by increased pH, decreased Pco_2 and decreased HCO_3^-. It is due to overventilation and treatment is directed at its cause.

DISEASES OF THE ESOPHAGUS, STOMACH, AND INTESTINES

Esophagus

The esophagus is responsible for the transit of food from the mouth to the gastrointestinal tract. This is not a passive action, but rather a complex, orchestrated sequence of events. The bolus of food or liquid is passed from the pharynx to the proximal esophagus. A peristaltic wave carries the bolus distally to the lower esophageal sphincter (LES), which is in a constant tonic state. With LES relaxation, the food then passes into the stomach. The two most important symptoms referable to the esophagus are heartburn and dysphagia.

GASTROESOPHAGEAL REFLUX

Gastroesophageal reflux (GER) is the passage of gastric contents inappropriately into the esophagus. This should be prevented by a competent LES. However, ambulatory pH recordings have revealed that normal, asymptomatic individuals will experience very brief episodes of reflux daily. This is probably due to brief relaxation of the LES.

Heartburn is the chief symptom associated with GER. This is retrosternal burning that may occur in the postprandial period or when the individual stoops or becomes supine. It is estimated that 40% of the adult population experiences heartburn at least monthly. For most of these persons, the symptoms are merely inconvenient and require the occasional use of antacids. Some have frequent symptoms and seek medical care.

Diagnosis of GER is based usually on history. A barium swallow x ray may reveal a hiatal hernia, demonstration of the reflux, or irregularity of the distal esophagus associated with esophagitis. Presence of the hiatal hernia is not essential for the diagnosis of GER. Upper endoscopy more accurately assesses the degree of gross esophagitis but is not needed in most patients with reflux symptoms. Symptoms may not correspond to the degree of endoscopic esophagitis.

Complications of GER include esophageal ulceration with possible hemorrhage or stricture formation, development of *Barrett's esophagus,* and pulmonary complications (*e.g.,* aspiration, asthma, chronic cough). Barrett's esophagus is the change of the normal squamous that lines the distal esophagus to a columnar mucosa type in response to longstanding GER. The patient is typically a white male in the sixth or seventh decade. The clinical significance of Barrett's esophagus lies in its predisposition toward malignant change. There is an approximate 10% prevalence of adenocarcinoma of the esophagus in patients with Barrett's esophagus; and those without cancer may expect a slight risk of developing this in future years.

Therapy of GER is directed at improving symptoms and reducing the risk of complications. The most important aspects of treatment are conservative measures. The patient should eat small meals and an early dinner. The diet should be low in fatty foods and should restrict caffeine, chocolate, and alcohol. Cigarette smokers should quit smoking and obese patients should lose weight. The head of the bed should be elevated and antacids can be taken when needed.

The next step in the therapy of GER is the use of H_2 receptor antagonists, which reduce gastric acid. Patients who still do not respond should undergo endoscopy to exclude complications. Formerly, the next step employed metoclopramide. This is a prokinetic agent that promotes gastric motility and therefore gastric emptying. However, CNS side effects (*e.g.,* anxiety, sedation, and rare cases of dystonia and tardive dyskinesia) were frequent. For patients with ulcerative esophagitis, the third step of treatment might now be considered the substitution of omeprazole for the H_2 antagonist. This potent new drug is dramatically effective in eliminating acid secretion by inhibiting gastric H-K ATPase (*i.e.,* the "proton pump"). The resultant achlorhydria induces hypergastrinemia, which many fear may have long-term disadvantages. Therefore, omeprazole is not approved for prolonged use at this time (except for patients with Zollinger-Ellison syndrome).

Not all cases of esophagitis result from GER. Infectious causes include candidiasos, cytomegalic virus (CMV), and herpes, which generally occur in patients with an immune deficiency. These patients typically experience odynophagia (pain with swallowing). Medications such as doxycycline may cause esophageal ulcers. Radiation treatment and lye ingestion produce esophagitis that leads to esophageal strictures.

DYSPHAGIA

The sensation of food or liquid sticking in the esophagus is known as dysphagia. The cause of dysphagia is considered organic, until proven otherwise, and the medical history is vitally important in making a specific diagnosis.

The most common cause of dysphagia is a lower esophageal ring that is associated with hiatal hernia and intermittent solid-food dysphagia. The diagnosis is easily made with a barium-swallow x ray, and treatment is generally esophageal dilation. Esophagitis or esophageal strictures secondary to GER may cause progressively severe solid-food dysphagia. Esophageal cancer generally presents as dysphagia. There are several disturbances of esophageal motility that also produce dysphagia (*e.g.,* achalasia, diffuse esophageal spasm).

Oropharyngeal dysphagia occurs when the patient has difficulty with the initial transfer of the food bolus from the mouth into the esophagus. Characteristic symptoms include nasal regurgitation, aspiration, and cough. Cerebrovascular accidents are the single most common cause of this type of dysphagia. Other causes include Parkinson's disease, amyotrophic lateral sclerosis, myasthenia gravis, multiple sclerosis, and muscular dystrophy. Obstructive lesions such as pharyngeal tumors must be excluded.

MOTILITY DISORDERS OF THE ESOPHAGUS

Achalasia is characterized by a lack of esophageal peristalsis with incomplete relaxation of the LES. The patient presents with dysphagia or, occasionally, with chest pain or a complication such as aspiration. The patient with achalasia may regurgitate undigested food, especially at night. Diagnosis may be suspected by a barium swallow that demonstrates a dilated esophagus with few uncoordinated contractions. The distal esophagus may have a tapered or "bird beak" deformity. Confirmation of diagnosis requires esophageal manometry, and all patients with suspected achalasia should undergo endoscopy, as distal esophageal or proximal gastric tumors can present similarly. Treatment of achalasia involves pneumatic balloon dilation or a surgical myotomy.

Scleroderma should be discussed in the context of the esophageal abnormalities associated with this multisystem disease. These patients demonstrate a lack of esophageal peristalsis, a greatly reduced LES pressure, and a resulting persistent and severe gastroesophageal reflux. If dysphagia occurs, it results from stricture formation. Patients with scleroderma should be instructed early on conservative antireflux measures and may require lifelong acid suppression.

There are a number of esophageal motility disorders that may present as noncardiac chest pain. These include patients with atypical chest pain for which cardiac causes have been excluded. Approximately 50% of these patients will demonstrate an esophageal cause (e.g., GER) for which dysphagia may be associated with chest pain. This may occur in the absence of typical pyrosis. The diagnosis can be confirmed by 24-hour ambulatory esophageal pH recording or by the Bernstein test (reproduction of chest pain with installation of acid in the esophagus).

Other diagnoses may be found by esophageal manometry. Diffuse esophageal spasm is characterized by intermittent simultaneous esophageal contractions rather than normal peristalsis. Contrac-

tions of very high-pressure amplitude have been termed "nutcracker esophagus." Nonspecific tertiary contractions can be seen on barium swallow or with manometry. The exact mechanism of these motility chest-pain-producing disorders is unknown; controversy exists on its relevance as they are generally benign and nonprogressive. The anxiety of chest pain can be assuaged by reassurance. Pharmacological treatment with anticholinergic agents or calcium channel antagonists can be used in selected cases, although their value over placebo has not been demonstrated.

ESOPHAGEAL CANCER

Cancer of the esophagus is relatively uncommon in the United States. The patient presents with dysphagia, initially for solids and progressing to involve liquids. Weight loss may occur and chest pain portends a poor prognosis. Cigarette smoking and alcohol abuse appear to be risk factors; lye stricture is another major risk. Diagnosis of esophageal cancer can be suspected by a barium-swallow x ray but requires endoscopy with biopsies for confirmation.

There are two histological types of esophageal cancer: squamous-cell and adenocarcinoma. The latter occurs in association with Barrett's esophagus. CT scanning is the single most useful tool in staging esophageal cancer. Surgical resection should be performed on patients without evidence of metastasis. Radiation may provide benefit in patients with squamous-cell carcinoma. The prognosis is generally poor because the tumor is usually discovered late. Palliative techniques (esophageal stents, laser tumor ablation, gastrostomy tubes) are helpful in the advanced cases to provide some calorie intake and to avoid dehydration.

Stomach

The stomach is responsible for the temporary storage of ingested liquids and solids. Facilitated by adaptive relaxation, the proximal stomach becomes more compliant after a meal. This action is mediated via the vagus nerve. After a vagotomy, there is a rapid emptying of liquids. The stomach is also responsible for the secretion of intrinsic factor and gastric acid. Acid-secreting parietal cells have the following receptors: gastrin, histamine-2, and cholinergic. The ultimate secretion of H^+ ion involves the H-K ATPase (the "proton pump"), which can be blocked by omeprazole. The mechanical actions of mixing and grinding occur in the gastric antrum. The migrating motor complex (MMC) is a forceful peristaltic wave that clears the stomach and intestines during the fasting state. The final function of the stomach is the delivery of gastric contents to the duodenum. Disorders of gastric function are best studied by the nuclear medicine gastric emptying scan. Abnormal gastric emptying occurs in diabetes, scleroderma, postvagotomy, and as a side effect of certain medications.

PEPTIC ULCER DISEASE

Peptic ulcer disease (PUD) is the most important disease involving the stomach. Duodenal as well as gastric ulcers (GU) will be discussed in this section, with the pertinent differences highlighted. The incidence of duodenal ulcer (DU) is decreasing, while the incidence of GU remains approximately the same. The incidence of severe complications such as hemorrhage and perforation is unchanged. Many attribute this latter statistic to the widespread use of NSAIDs among the elderly.

The precise pathogenesis of PUD is probably multifactorial, involving a precarious balance between the potentially injurious gastric acid and the gastric defense mechanisms (bicarbonate and mucus secretion, endogenous prostaglandins, and mucosal blood flow). The pathogenesis of ulcer formation is more complicated than simple excess acid secretion. Some DU patients do indeed secrete above-average amounts of acid, but most have normal secretion, and GU patients often have decreased amounts of acid. Other factors appear to play a role, too. Aspirin and NSAIDs are an important cause of PUD and its complications. The exact role of *Helicobacter pylori* is controversial, although many aspects of this bacterium have been well documented. This bacterium may be found in the stomach of almost all DU and most GU patients (it is also found in many asymptomatic individuals, which confuses the issue). *H. pylori* is the cause of the type B antral gastritis. The organism is able to survive in the harsh gastric environment by the elaboration of urease and its ability to colonize beneath the mucosal gel layer. *H. pylori* is unaffected by the usual antiulcer medications and requires antimicrobial therapy. Limited studies have demonstrated that eradication of this bacterium leads to fewer recurrences of ulcer disease.

PUD may be associated with the typical description of gnawing or burning epigastric pain that is relieved by antacids. However, many patients have atypical symptoms, and some may present with a complication (such as hemorrhage) without warning.

Diagnosis of PUD allows for some variability. A young patient with a typical history may appropriately be managed with a therapeutic trial of H_2 antagonists. Although endoscopy is the most accurate diagnostic tool, its expense is considered a disadvantage that favors the upper GI series.

When an ulcer is diagnosed, there are several options for treatment. Antacids are effective, but compliance is poor. The histamine-2 receptor antagonists (cimetidine, ranitidine, famotidine, and nizatidine) have equal efficiency, healing 90% of ulcers within 8 weeks. A single nighttime dose is the preferred dosing schedule. Sucralfate heals ulcers through unknown mechanisms. Misoprostol is a prostaglandin agonist that is indicated for the concomitant use with ASA/NSAID to prevent ulceration. The most important reasons for nonhealing of ulcers are noncompliance and cigarette smoking. After treatment of the acute ulcer, remember that gastric ulcers require follow-up study to document healing; by its very nature, PUD is a recurrent disease. Some patients may be candidates for long-term maintenance therapy with H_2 blockers to reduce this risk (the elderly, previous hemorrhage, frequent recurrences, severe underlying medical problems).

No text designed for review would be complete without mention of the Zollinger-Ellison syndrome. Z-E syndrome occurs when a nonbeta islet cell tumor of the pancreas, a gastrinoma, causes a marked increase in gastric acid secretion that results in ulcer disease of the upper GI tract (some patients will experience diarrhea as well). Suspicion of this disease should prompt the physician to order a serum gastrin level. A greatly elevated gastrin level is associated with Z-E syndrome; the secretin test can be confirmatory. This tumor is usually metastatic at the time of diagnosis. Remember that 20% of these patients will have MEA type I. If the tumor is not resectable, omeprazole has replaced palliative gastric resection as the treatment of choice.

UPPER GASTROINTESTINAL HEMORRHAGE

Upper gastrointestinal (UGI) hemorrhage is a relatively common medical emergency. Despite technological and therapeutic advances, the mortality of this complication has not improved, remaining at 10%. There are many potential causes of UGI hemorrhage. PUD is the most common, accounting for about half of all cases. Gastritis is a common cause in the ICU patient or in one who takes aspirin (or NSAIDs). A Mallory-Weiss tear of the distal esophagus is often encountered in alcoholics. Any patient may have portal hypertension and esophageal varices with bleeding, which has the highest mortality of any cause.

The initial management of a patient with suspected upper gastrointestinal hemorrhage requires stabilization of hemodynamic status as the primary goal. Control of intravascular volume must precede any diagnostic procedures. Endoscopy, the diagnostic method of choice, should correctly identify the bleeding source in most patients. There are therapeutic aspects of endoscopy as well. Endoscopic cautery devices can be used for bleeding ulcers, and **sclerotherapy** is the treatment of choice for variceal hemorrhage. If endoscopy reveals an ulcer that is not bleeding but contains a mound within the ulcer crater known as a visible vessel, there is great risk for rebleeding.

The patient should be started on an H_2 antagonist. This probably has no benefit on the actively bleeding ulcer but may reduce risk of rebleeding. Most ulcer bleeding will cease spontaneously. Hemorrhage that is severe and persistent (or recurrent) is an indication for emergency surgery. Patients with variceal hemorrhage from cirrhosis may be candidates for a portocaval shunt. The high initial mortality associated with this surgery must be considered in light of the fact that this is the best protection from subsequent bleeding episodes.

GASTRITIS

Gastritis may cause symptoms similar to peptic ulcer disease, but on endoscopic examination no ulcer is visible. It may be of unknown cause, although it may be produced by aspirin, bile, alcohol, or NSAIDs. Recent studies have shown the presence of *Campylobacter* to be more prevalent in patients with gastritis, although at this time a cause–effect relationship has not been established. Treatment includes removal of the offending agent, correction of the underlying condition, or use of H_2 blockers or antacids.

GASTRIC CANCER

Cancer of the stomach has declined in incidence in the 20th century for unknown reasons. However, the diagnosis is usually made late and the prognosis is poor. The symptoms are nonspecific: anorexia, nausea, vomiting, and abdominal discomfort. The patient may lose weight and be anemic from either occult or overt bleeding. Most cases of gastric cancer appear spontaneously, but there are a few patients with recognized high-risk conditions: pernicious anemia, adenomatous gastric polyps, and Ménétrier's disease all have an increased risk. All of these conditions share a common denominator with gastric cancer: achlorhydria.

If cancer of the stomach is suspected, endoscopy is the diagnostic method of choice, as it allows inspection and biopsy of the lesion. The most common types of cancer are adenocarcinoma and lymphoma. These have similar clinical presentations, but lymphoma has a slightly better prognosis. Other gastric tumors include leiomyosarcoma and carcinoid. Surgical resection should be considered, but many cases will be too advanced. Chemotherapy is believed to prolong survival slightly.

Small Intestine

The small intestine is responsible for electrolyte, water, and nutritional absorption. Approximately 9 liters of fluid enter the duodenum each day (2 liters of ingested liquid and 7 liters of endogenous secretions: salivary, gastric, biliary, and pancreatic). Absorption of this liquid is very effective, as the normal fecal output of water is about 100 ml/d.

MALABSORPTION

Failure of the small intestine to appropriately absorb nutrients is known as malabsorption. This may result from small-intestinal or pancreatic disorders (see Table 3-3). If malabsorption is not severe, no nutritional deficits or symptoms may be evident.

TABLE 3-3. Causes of Malabsorption

Deficient Pancreatic Enzymes
Chronic pancreatitis
Pancreatic cancer
Cystic fibrosis

Deficient Intraluminal Bile Acids
Biliary obstruction
Ileal disease (resection, Crohn's disease)

Small-Intestinal Disease
Massive resection
Radiation enteritis
Intestinal ischemia
Celiac sprue
Tropical sprue
Whipple's disease
Primary intestinal lymphoma
Lymphangiectasia

Multisystem Disorders
Diabetes mellitus
Scleroderma (often with bacterial overgrowth)
Endocrinopathies

However, chronic diarrhea with weight loss, edema, or evidence of vitamin deficiency states (hypoprothrombinemia, hypocalcemia, or anemia) should prompt an evaluation for possible malabsorption.

If one suspects malabsorption, a fat stain of fecal material can be a useful screening test. The most accurate test is the cumbersome 72-hour fecal fat. Normally, less than 8 g of fat should be found in the stool each day. A variety of other tests can be useful after the diagnosis of malabsorption is made. The D-xylose test measures small intestine function. The upper GI series with small-bowel follow-through may show mucosal irregularity or abnormality. A small-bowel biopsy is useful in confirming several diagnoses—e.g., sprue, Whipple's disease. Routine lab tests may reveal anemia, hypocalcemia, hypoalbuminemia, and low serum carotene levels.

Celiac sprue is characterized by gluten-induced damage to the mucosa of the small intestine. Gluten is the protein moiety of wheat, barley, rye, and oats. The mechanism of this damage is not fully understood but appears to involve genetic, immunologic, and possibly environmental factors. Diagnosis is established by a small-bowel biopsy demonstrating the shortening or absence of intestinal villi and the infiltration of the lamina propria with lymphocytes and plasma cells. Adherence to a gluten-free diet will allow for resolution of symptoms and nutritional deficiencies as well as histologic normalization of the small-bowel mucosa.

Whipple's disease is an uncommon cause of malabsorption that can affect virtually any part of the body. The patient may have various symptoms: malaise, weakness, weight loss, fever, arthritis. The physical exam may reveal pigmentation and lymphadenopathy. Complications may include pericarditis, pleuritis, and CNS symptoms. Involved tissues are infiltrated by large glycoprotein-containing macrophages and unidentified small rod-shaped bacilli. These findings are readily apparent on small-bowel biopsy. Although the bacterium has not been identified, it can be successfully treated. One recommended treatment regimen is penicillin and streptomycin for 2 weeks, followed by trimethoprim-sulfamethoxazole for a year. The patient should be followed closely in subsequent years for possible central nervous system relapse.

DISACCHARIDASE DEFICIENCY

The mucosal deficiency of disaccharidase leads to impaired absorption of carbohydrates. The most common type of this disorder would be lactose intolerance. Primary lactase deficiency is so widely prevalent that it cannot be considered abnormal, affecting 20% of Caucasians and most blacks and Asians. Affected persons lack or have low levels of the enzyme lactase in the brush border of intestinal absorptive cells. The ingestion of food items with lactose leads to bloating, flatulence, abdominal cramps, and diarrhea. Diagnosis can be confirmed by a lactose tolerance test, and treatment involves either avoidance of lactose products altogether or by ingesting commercially available lactose products. Lactase deficiency can be a secondary and transient phenomenon with other small-bowel diseases, most commonly being associated with viral gastroenteritis.

TUMORS OF THE SMALL INTESTINE

Tumors of the small intestines are rare, being the least frequent neoplasms of the entire GI tract. The patient may present with small-bowel obstruction, or perhaps occult GI bleeding and vague abdominal pain. Rarely is an abdominal mass present; usually the physical examination is unremarkable. Adenocarcinoma is the most common tumor of the small bowel, usually proximal in location (duodenum or proximal jejunum). Several conditions are associated with an increased risk of this tumor: familial polyposis coli; Gardner's syndrome; Peutz-Jeghers syndrome; and, possibly, Crohn's disease.

Lymphoma of the small bowel can present as above or as malabsorption. Patients who have been previously diagnosed and treated for celiac sprue appear to have a slight risk of developing this tumor in subsequent years for unknown reasons. Leiomyosarcoma of the small intestine is noted for its large bulky size (often with a palpable mass on exam) and its tendency for recurrent hemorrhage.

CARCINOID

Malignant carcinoid tumor can arise in various sites within and outside the GI tract but most commonly develops from a primary lesion in the ileum. Other GI sites include the stomach, appendix, and rectum. Large amounts of serotonin are present in the tumor cells. Metastatic disease to the liver can be associated with the carcinoid syndrome. The patient may experience paroxysmal flushing of the face and neck, periorbital edema, tachycardia, hypotension, and respiratory distress. Diarrhea and abdominal pain may occur. Advanced disease may result in pulmonary and cardiac valvular complications. The diagnosis may be confirmed by finding elevated levels of 5HIAA in a 24-hour urine collection. The tumor should be resected if possible, but unfortunately it is often widely metastatic when discovered. This is a slow-growing tumor and persistent symptoms may be ameliorated by somatostatin.

Colon

The colon functions in conjunction with the small intestine, allowing more complete absorption of water and electrolytes and thereby converting the fecal stream from liquid to solid form.

DIARRHEA

Diarrhea is a common problem encountered by the physician. A useful definition of diarrhea is the passage of more than 250 g of feces per day. The stool may vary from slightly loose to watery. Remember that to the patient diarrhea is subjective, and many who complain of this will not actually have diarrhea as strictly defined. Diarrhea may be classified as being osmotic or secretory. *Osmotic* diarrhea occurs when there is malabsorption of nutrients or electrolytes. Diarrhea resulting from increased secretion of electrolytes and fluids is termed *secretory*. This initial classification can be helpful in the evaluation and can be easily accomplished by measuring fecal Na^+ and K^+. In osmotic diarrhea the sum of fecal Na^+ and K^+ will be less than half of the stool osmolality.

The initial approach to diarrhea depends on duration, type of diarrhea, and associated conditions. Acute diarrhea is usually infectious or toxic in origin, whereas various conditions may lead to chronic diarrhea. The most common cause of acute diarrhea is viral gastroenteritis, a self-limited illness that can be complicated by volume depletion. Traveler's diarrhea is usually caused by the acquisition of a toxigenic *E. coli*. Bismuth subsalicylate and various antibiotics can shorten the duration of this form of diarrhea. A number of invasive organisms can cause acute diarrhea (*e.g., Shigella, Salmonella,* and *Campylobacter*). This may be suspected if fecal leukocytes are found on stool exam, and confirmation is achieved with stool cultures. Parasites such as *Giardia* and *Entamoeba histolytica* may cause diarrhea.

Clostridium difficile is an important cause of diarrhea to consider. The patient with this diarrhea will have taken antibiotics previously, often while in a medical facility for another problem. Virtually every antibiotic has been associated with this infection. The patient presents with diarrhea that contains fecal leukocytes. Complications include fulminant colitis or toxic megacolon. Proctosigmoidoscopy may reveal the presence of pseudomembranes, yellowish plaque covering the colon wall, although this is not mandatory for the diagnosis that is established by finding the toxin of *C. difficile* in the stool or by culturing the organism. This infection can be treated by vancomycin or metronidazole, although recurrence can be a problem.

If diarrhea persists for more than 3 weeks, other causes must be considered, including inflammatory bowel disease and malabsorption. The initial evaluation includes a complete history and physical examination, proctosigmoidoscopy, and stool examinations.

One should be familiar with the various GI aspects of AIDS. Homosexual men have an increased incidence of infectious diarrhea, with common pathogens being *Giardia, N. gonorrhea, Salmonella,* and *Campylobacter. Cryptosporidium,* cytomegalic virus, and *M. avium-intracellulae* have all been associated with chronic and debilitating GI infection.

IRRITABLE BOWEL SYNDROME

Irritable bowel syndrome is characterized by altered bowel function (constipation, diarrhea, or both) and abdominal pain that is often in the left lower quadrant. Although the patient complains of diarrhea, the daily stool volume is less than 250 g and therefore not technically so. The patient may describe symptoms that began years earlier, with exacerbations often coinciding with stressful life events. The diagnosis is made by excluding other diseases, such as inflammatory bowel disease. The treatment is supportive and symptomatic.

DIVERTICULOSIS COLI

Colonic diverticula are herniations of mucosa and submucosa through the colon muscle. This is a commonly encountered condition that usually produces no symptoms and is rarely complicated. The diverticulae are most frequently found in the sigmoid colon but can be present throughout the colon (multiple small-bowel diverticulae can be found in scleroderma). The pathogenesis of colonic diverticular disease is unknown but may be related to the relative lack of dietary fiber. Although most patients are asymptomatic, complications can occur. Diverticulitis occurs when a diverticulum perforates. This leads to inflammation and even abscess formation. The patient experiences localized lower abdominal pain and fever. The examining physician may find a mass, tenderness, and peritoneal signs. The mass can be defined by imaging studies such as ultrasound or CT scan. Treatment consists of bowel rest and parenteral antibiotics, which will be successful on most occasions. Abscess formation, fistulae, persistent inflammation, and bowel obstruction are indications for surgery.

Another complication of diverticular disease is hemorrhage. This is the most common cause of massive lower GI bleeding. The patient has maroon or bright-red stools. Initial treatment involves blood replacement and volume stabilization. The bleeding usually ceases spontaneously. Useful diagnostic studies are colonoscopy, angiography, and tagged RBC studies. Recurrent or massive bleeding necessitates surgery.

INFLAMMATORY BOWEL DISEASE

Chronic ulcerative colitis and Crohn's disease will be considered together as idiopathic inflammatory bowel disease (IFBD). These disorders share clinical features, but there are sufficient differences to allow distinction. The pathogenesis of IFBD is unknown. There is a familial tendency (15% risk in the immediate family or first-degree relatives). Both disorders demonstrate abnormalities of cell-mediated and humoral immunity.

Chronic ulcerative colitis (CUC) is characterized by rectal bleeding, diarrhea, and lower abdominal discomfort. The amount of colon affected is variable—from distal disease or proctitis to total colonic involvement or pancolitis. Although the extent is variable, the mucosal abnormalities are always continuous from the rectum. The mucosa is edematous, friable, and granular with superficial ulcers. The small bowel is never involved.

Crohn's disease may involve any part of the gastrointestinal tract. It commonly presents as abdominal pain, weight loss, fever, and diarrhea. Bloody diarrhea is unusual (unlike CUC). Several other features allow the distinction from CUC: (1) fistula formation; (2) perirectal abscess; (3) abdominal mass; (4) "skip areas" (which refers to areas of normal mucosa between areas of disease involvement); (5) small-bowel, particularly ileal, involvement; (6) large, deep ulcers in the colon; and (7) small-bowel obstruction. The differential diagnosis of IFBD includes tuberculosis, lymphoma, ischemic colitis, diverticulitis, and cancer. Both CUC and Crohn's disease are associated with disorders outside the GI tract (Table 3-4).

TABLE 3-4. Extraintestinal Manifestations of Inflammatory Bowel Disease

Skin	Pyoderma gangrenosum
	Erythema nodosum
Musculoskeletal	Arthritis—peripheral, nondeforming
	Sacroileitis—associated with HLA-B27
Ocular	Episcleritis, uveitis
Hepatobiliary	Pericholangitis
	Sclerosing cholangitis

The treatment of CUC is determined by the extent and severity of the disease (see Table 3-5). Sulfasalazine is the mainstay for treating mild to moderate disease. Corticosteroids, given orally or topically in the form of enemas, can be used. Complications of CUC include (1) disease refractory to treatment, (2) fulminant colitis or toxic megacolon, and (3) adenocarcinoma of the colon. The risk of cancer is greatest for those patients with total colon involvement, and this risk increases as the disease duration increases.

Treatment of Crohn's disease is also determined by severity and disease extent. Sulfasalazine and corticosteroids are the usual drugs employed. Immunosuppressants such as 6-mercaptopurine have been successfully used for severe and refractory disease. Metronidazole is a helpful adjunctive treatment for perianal disease and fistula. Hospitalization and total parenteral nutrition can likewise be helpful in severe cases. Crohn's disease is commonly associated with severe protein malnutrition. Surgery is often needed, but the approximate 75% disease recurrence rate after surgery is well known (Table 3-6).

ISCHEMIC COLITIS

Ischemic colitis is the most common form of intestinal ischemia. This usually occurs in elderly patients, often with a history of atherosclerotic cardiovascular disease. The patient presents with abdominal pain and acute rectal bleeding. The initial

TABLE 3-5. Indications for Colectomy in Ulcerative Colitis

1. Disease refractory to appropriate medical treatment
2. Severe complications such as toxic megacolon, hemorrhage, and perforation
3. Development of adenocarcinoma or the demonstration of dysplasia of the colonic mucosa
4. Colonic stricture with fear of possible malignancy

TABLE 3-6. Indications for Surgery in Crohn's Disease

1. Fistula not responding to medical treatment
2. Bowel obstruction not responding to medical treatment
3. Intra-abdominal abscess—some can now be treated by percutaneous drainage by radiologist
4. Severe perianal disease or abscess
5. Toxic megacolon or severe hemorrhage

management consists of bowel rest and IV fluids. The cautious use of a barium enema may reveal the characteristic "thumb printing" due to submucosal edema or hemorrhage. A likewise cautious colonoscopy will reveal nonspecific mucosal changes, but the biopsy may provide confirmation. Angiography is usually not indicated. The blood vessels are usually patent, indicating a low flow state rather than an occlusive cause. Most cases resolve and recurrence is unusual. Complications include severe colitis and stricture formation.

COLON CANCER

Colorectal cancer is the second most frequent cause of death from cancer in the United States. The risk of colon cancer is highest in countries with a diet high in animal fat and low in dietary fiber. Most colon cancers develop in an adenomatous polyp, but only a small percentage of adenomas will develop into cancer. There are several well-recognized risk factors for colon cancer (see Table 3-7).

Symptoms of colon carcinoma are usually vague and nonspecific. Weight loss and malaise are common. The patient may note a change in stool caliber or bowel habits. Overt rectal bleeding is uncommon, but occult bleeding is commonly found. Cancer may involve any part of the colon. For unknown reasons, there has been a recent shift to more cancers being found in the right colon. The diagnosis can be suspected by barium enema and confirmed by colonoscopy with biopsies. Curative therapy for

TABLE 3-7. Risk Factors for Colon Cancer

1. Adenomatous polyps—the risk is highest for large polyps and those with a villous component
2. Chronic ulcerative colitis—based on disease extent and duration
3. *Familial polyposis coli*—this would also include Gardner's syndrome
4. Family cancer syndrome—multiple family members with not only colon cancer but also cancer of the breast, the ovary, and/or uterus

colon cancer relies on surgical resection. If the tumor is not entirely resectable, chemotherapy has recently been shown to improve survival. Radiation treatment is helpful for cancers that arise in the rectum. The patient with successfully resected colon cancer should be followed with periodic colonoscopy and carcinoembryonic antigen (CEA). An elevation of the latter is associated with recurrent cancer. Again, CEA has no role in the primary diagnostic process or initial screening strategy.

The current techniques for colon cancer prevention are imperfect, but screening strategies for occult blood have been developed and should be employed in the routine health management of patients. Asymptomatic patients begin to have an increased risk of developing colorectal cancer at 50 years of age; the risk doubles with each succeeding decade. The patient without increased risk (see Table 3-7) should have a yearly digital rectal exam and fecal occult blood test (FOBT) starting at age 40. Of these patients, 1% to 3% can be expected to have a positive FOBT, and, of these, 20% to 40% will have a colon adenoma or cancer. FOBT has its limitations, and unfortunately, the test misses 30% to 50% of asymptomatic cancers. Flexible sigmoidoscopy should be used as a screening test for asymptomatic patients greater than 45 to 50 years of age, with repeat exam every 3 to 5 years. The discovery of an adematous polyp is an indication for total colonoscopy with removal or destruction of the polyp. The commonly found hyperplastic polyp (indistinguishable grossly from an adenoma) does not have malignant potential.

LOWER GASTROINTESTINAL HEMORRHAGE

Hemorrhage from a colonic source is characterized by the passage of bright-red or maroon blood from the rectum. It is important to remember that on occasion a massively bleeding upper source, like a duodenal ulcer, may present as hematochezia. (See Table 3-8.)

As with upper GI hemorrhage, initial management is supportive and based on volume stabilization and blood replacement. Colonoscopy is the

TABLE 3-8. Common Causes of Acute Lower GI Bleeding

1. *Diverticulosis coli*
2. Arteriovenous malformations (AVMs)
3. Colon cancer
4. Ischemic colitis
5. Inflammatory bowel disease

most accurate diagnostic tool and can be used after stabilization of the patient.

Arteriovenous malformations (AVMs), also known as angiodysplasia, occur most commonly in the right colon but may also occur in the stomach or small intestine. These lesions may be responsible for either overt or occult bleeding, which can vary in severity from persistent and life-threatening to minor. Patients with isolated AVMs are often elderly, and many have concurrent heart disease. Chronic renal failure is a risk factor for symptomatic AVMs. A familial syndrome is also associated with AVMs: Rendu-Osler-Weber syndrome, or hereditary hemorrhagic telangiectasia. These patients often have recurrent epistaxis as a youth and GI bleeding in adulthood. Physical examination may reveal telangiectasia of the fingers and the nasal and oral mucosa. The treatment of AVMs is dictated by the severity of bleeding. Minor bleeding can often be managed by simple iron supplementation. Severe bleeding can be treated by surgical resection or endoscopic cauterization.

There are other rare causes of lower GI bleeding. Peutz-Jeghers syndrome is a familial condition characterized by the development of harmartomas throughout the GI tract. The patient may have the characteristic perioral hyperpigmentation. Meckel's diverticulum is a developmental defect of the distal small bowel that may also cause GI bleeding.

DISEASES OF THE SPLEEN, PANCREAS, GALLBLADDER, AND LIVER

Splenomegaly

Enlargement of the spleen may be understood best in terms of its physiology and pathologic physiology.

The spleen is a part of the reticuloendothelial system and removes abnormal elements from the bloodstream whether they are infectious organisms or otherwise. In this process it enlarges. The infections that most often cause splenic enlargement are typhoid fever, malaria, infectious mononucleosis, subacute bacterial endocarditis, brucellosis, and septicemia.

The splenic vein drains into the portal system; hence it enlarges for mechanical reasons when there is back pressure in the portal system, as in cirrhosis of the liver. This syndrome of chronic congestive splenomegaly is characterized by portal hypertension, hemorrhage from the GI tract, leukopenia, anemia, and thrombocytopenia.

The spleen is a repository for all cellular elements in the blood and removes abnormal cells. The convenient but not universally accepted concept of hypersplenism refers to the theory that the spleen may become overactive and remove cellular elements that are much needed and even apparently normal. In this condition there is (1) an enlarged spleen, (2) a deficiency of one or all of the formed elements in the circulating blood, (3) normal or hyperplastic bone marrow demonstrated by biopsy or aspiration, and (4) the possibility of cure by splenectomy. A secondary form of hypersplenism may occur in lymphocytic leukemia, lymphomas, and other diseases associated with splenomegaly and results in a hemolytic type of anemia complicating the primary disease.

Splenectomy

Removal may be required as an emergency operation in case of rupture of the spleen—a condition that can result from even mild trauma to an enlarged spleen. Splenectomy may be necessary only on rare occasions for purely mechanical reasons of extreme degree. Splenectomy should be of specific value in hypersplenism, and it has an established value in two conditions that might fall into this classification: (1) congenital hemolytic jaundice or congenital spherocytosis and (2) ITP. Also, idiopathic splenic neutropenia and splenic pancytopenia may be improved by splenectomy. In one other condition, thrombosis of the splenic vein, splenectomy may be required because of bleeding from distended collateral veins in the stomach. If possible, vaccination against pneumococci, *Haemophilus influenzae* type b, and meningococci should be done prior to splenectomy.

Cholelithiasis

Cholelithiasis occurs in 10% of the general population. More than 90% of gallstones are cholesterol stones. The remainder are primarily pigment stones. Cholesterol stones may result from either increased cholesterol or decreased bile acid secretion by the liver. Women (particularly those taking oral contraceptives), American Indians, and obese patients are at increased risk of developing cholelithiasis.

Approximately 50% of patients with cholelithiasis are asymptomatic, but when symptoms occur, they are usually initiated when the stone enters the cystic duct. These symptoms include right upper quadrant or epigastric pain, nausea, and vomiting. Acute cholelithiasis is accompanied by the foregoing symptoms with fever, leukocytosis, and hepatic function tests (especially the alkaline phosphatase) that may be normal or mildly elevated.

The diagnosis of cholelithiasis is primarily by ultrasound, a test that has replaced oral cholecystography in many major centers.

Most patients with symptomatic gallstones should undergo cholecystectomy. Oral dissolution of gallstones can be achieved with ursodeoxycholic acid. However, this requires a prolonged period of treatment and is associated with high recurrence rates. The best success rates are approximately 30%. Management of the asymptomatic patient with gallstones is controversial since most who respond will develop symptoms. Traditionally, patients with diabetes mellitus have been said to have an increased risk of complications, and cholecystectomy has been advocated for those who are asymptomatic. However, this concept has been challenged recently.

Pancreatitis

ACUTE PANCREATITIS

The primary events that initiate acute pancreatitis are unknown. These events lead to activated pancreatic enzymes entering the pancreatic parenchyma. The result is acute inflammation, edema, cell injury and death, fat necrosis, vascular damage, and occasionally hemorrhagic necrosis.

Alcohol abuse and gallstones are responsible for most cases of acute pancreatitis. Most patients with acute alcoholic pancreatitis have already established chronic pancreatitis. Gallstones cause pancreatitis by partial obstruction of the pancreatic duct. There are other less common causes of acute pancreatitis (see Table 3-9).

The patient with acute pancreatitis describes epigastric pain that may radiate to the back. Vomiting may occur with volume depletion. Serum amylase

TABLE 3-9. Etiologies of Acute Pancreatitis

1. Alcohol abuse
2. Gallstones
3. Hypertriglyceridemia (values usually >1,000)
4. Hypercalcemia
5. Trauma, includes iatrogenic causes, such as postoperative or post-ERCP
6. Pancreatic cancer
7. Drug-induced pancreatitis: thiazide diuretics, furosemide, estrogens, azathioprine, L-asparaginase, 6-mercaptopurine, methyldopa, sulfonamides, tetracycline, pentamidine

TABLE 3-10. Complications of Acute Pancreatitis

1. Volume depletion
2. Hypocalcemia
3. Ileus
4. Pancreatic pseudocyst
5. Pancreatic abscess
6. Hemorrhagic pancreatitis
7. Obstructive jaundice

and lipase are usually elevated. Abdominal ultrasound and CT scans are helpful in assessing the disease; the former may also demonstrate the presence of gallstones. Acute pancreatitis may be severe with a high mortality rate and numerous complications (see Table 3-10). The treatment of acute pancreatitis includes hydration, bowel rest, nasogastric suction, pain control, and careful attention to electrolyte and calcium levels and volume status.

CHRONIC PANCREATITIS

Chronic pancreatitis is characterized by a recurrent or persistent abdominal pain or evidence of pancreatic insufficiency (steatorrhea or diabetes). The most important cause of chronic pancreatitis is long-standing alcohol abuse. Other causes include trauma and cystic fibrosis, familial and idiopathic. Evaluation may reveal significant steatorrhea or calcification of the pancreas on plain films of the abdomen. CT scan is helpful and endoscopic pancreatography will reveal dilated and abnormal pancreatic ducts. Treatment is supportive. Diabetes requires insulin and the steatorrhea can usually be well controlled with supplemental pancreatic enzymes. Management of chronic pain is difficult in this patient population, and addiction to narcotics is frequently encountered.

PANCREATIC CARCINOMA

Pancreatic carcinoma is the second most common GI cancer after colon cancer and seems to be increasing in incidence. The most common tumor type is adenocarcinoma. The tumor is usually discovered late and the prognosis is poor. The patient may present with back or epigastric pain, weight loss, and jaundice. The diagnosis can be made by CT scan or ultrasound. Confirmation can often be obtained by needle biopsy or aspiration by the radiologist. Treatment involves surgical removal, when possible. Jaundice in the unresectable patient can be successfully managed by endoscopically placed biliary stents.

Endocrine tumors of the pancreas are a less common type of pancreatic tumor. The gastrinoma responsible for Zollinger-Ellison syndrome has been discussed. Insulinoma is characterized by symptoms of excess insulin with fasting, a fasting blood sugar being usually less than 40 mg/dl. Diagnosis involves the measurement of insulin and c-peptide levels concurrently with glucose determinations. Most insulinomas can be resected. Another unusual pancreatic endocrine tumor is the VIPoma, so called by its elaboration of VIP (vasoactive intestinal polypeptide). Through the actions of VIP, this tumor is characterized by prolonged and severe secretory diarrhea, with hypokalemia and dehydration. This tumor is also known as Verner-Morrison syndrome. The diagnosis is made by an elevated level of VIP. Surgical resection should be performed if the tumor is resectable. Somatostatin appears to be of benefit in treating the diarrhea. In patients with metastatic disease, 5FU and streptozotocin may be rewarding.

Other unusual endocrine tumors include the glucagonoma (diabetes and necrolytic migratory erythema) and somatostatin (diabetes, gallstones, and diarrhea) and carcinoid tumors (already discussed).

Jaundice

Jaundice, a yellowish discoloration of skin, mucous membranes, and body fluids, is due to an excess of bile pigments. *Bilirubinemia*—total bilirubin levels of 1.5 mg/dl or total higher—is present before the tissues become discolored, and bilirubinuria often precedes the appearance of jaundice. Bilirubin is a derivative of the iron-free porphyrin of hemoglobin and is formed in the reticuloendothelial system where the erythrocytes are destroyed. When liberated to the bloodstream, bilirubin gives an indirect van den Bergh reaction because of its insolubility in water and its nonpolar structure. This portion is known as "indirect bilirubin." Ordinarily it is not excreted by the kidney but is taken up by liver cells. In the liver, bilirubin is conjugated with glucuronic acid to water-soluble bilirubin glucuronide, which gives a direct van den Bergh reaction. Elevation of this direct reacting fraction indicates disease of the liver parenchyma or of the biliary tract.

Jaundice is of three types: (1) obstructive (cholestatic), in which excretion of bile pigments is hampered by blocking of the bile ducts; (2) hemolytic, whereby excretion of bile pigments is incomplete

because of their too rapid formation by hemolysis of RBCs; and (3) hepatic, in which excretion of bile pigments is impaired by damage or destruction of the hepatic cells.

Cholestatic (obstructive) jaundice comprises about 85% of all cases and may be caused by (1) internal obstruction of the bile ducts by gallstones (the most common cause); (2) obstruction due to changes in the walls of the ducts by inflammation, neoplasm, or stricture; and (3) obstruction by pressure on the ducts from tumors, cysts, enlarged nodes, or adhesions.

Hemolytic jaundice may be due to congenital and acquired hemolytic anemia, malaria, chemicals that produce hemolysis, erythroblastosis fetalis, transfusion with incompatible blood, and so forth. It is caused by excessive destruction of erythrocytes and liberation of their pigments. Unless there is associated liver damage, it is characterized by an absence of bile in the urine, increased urobilinogen in the urine and the stools, and an indirect van den Bergh reaction in the serum.

There are familial disorders of bilirubin metabolism associated with jaundice, the most common of which is *Gilbert's syndrome.* This patient may have a history of recurrent brief episodes of mild jaundice associated with stress, fasting, or viral illnesses. The other hepatic function tests are normal, except for the indirect bilirubin, and no further evaluation is usually indicated.

Hepatic jaundice is due primarily to liver parenchymal disease. This may be seen in cirrhosis of any etiology; inflammatory disease of the liver, which includes infectious hepatitis, chronic active hepatitis, and toxic and drug-induced hepatitis; carcinoma; or abscess of the liver. Adverse drug reactions of the liver may be caused by such agents as halothane, isoniazid, PAS, rifampin chlorpromazine, and oral contraceptives.

No single test can be relied upon to distinguish these three types of jaundice. Many tests have been proposed to distinguish the three mechanisms of jaundice. Bile pigments are never absent from the stools in pure hemolytic jaundice, whereas clay-colored stools are characteristic of complete obstructive jaundice and even may be found in the acute phase of hepatic jaundice. The hepatic enzymes, SGOT and serum glutamic pyruvic transaminase (SGPT) (or AST and ALT, respectively, for the aspartate and alanine aminotransferases) and serum proteins, including albumin, globulin, prothrombin, and fibrinogen, are abnormal from the onset of hepatic jaundice. They are not abnormal in hemolytic jaundice and are not abnormal in obstructive jaundice until long-standing biliary obstruction has produced secondary liver damage. Alkaline phosphatase is a good indicator of obstructive hepatobiliary disease. However, an isolated alkaline phosphatase elevation may also be generated from other sites (bone, placenta, intestinal). In this situation, a GGT (γ-glutamyl transpeptidase) elevation indicates the liver as the origin. Ultrasonography may be useful in detecting dilated ducts in extrahepatic obstruction. In some patients percutaneous cholangiography and ERCP are needed to localize the cause of obstruction.

Acute Viral Hepatitis

Acute viral hepatitis is a systemic infection involving primarily the liver; it occurs in three immunologically different but clinically similar forms: *hepatitis A* (infectious hepatitis); *hepatitis B* (serum hepatitis) and *hepatitis C*. All are characterized by hepatic cell necrosis; the usual picture is that of an anicteric period followed by jaundice and then total recovery. Many cases are mild and recognized only by abnormal liver function tests. The delta antigen is a RNA virus that is infectious only in persons with hepatitis B, because it needs the hepatitis B virus (HBV) as a viral envelope protein. The delta antigen can cause fulminant hepatitis in patients previously infected with the HBV and should be suspected when a carrier of the HBV suddenly becomes ill.

The incubation period for hepatitis A is 15 to 50 days and for hepatitis B is 50 to 180 days. Transfusion hepatitis is more frequently due to hepatitis C, with an incubation period of 30 to 180 days. Serologic tests are presently available for all three types of hepatitis.

The first symptom is usually painless jaundice, associated with a variable fever, malaise, and often a mild GI upset. The liver and spleen may be enlarged and tender. In hepatitis B disease there may also be urticaria, arthritis, and arthralgia due to immune complexes. The disease ordinarily resolves in about 4 weeks. Transaminases are markedly elevated (> 500) although this degree of elevation can be seen in other entities such as drug-induced or ischemic hepatic damage. The diagnosis may not be established conclusively until the patient recovers. Some tests of liver function may not return to normal for several months after symptomatic recovery. Patients should rest in bed until acute symptoms have subsided. Hospitalization is indicated for patients unable to eat or drink because of vomiting and those with prolongation of the prothrombin time.

Patients with acute viral hepatitis usually recover completely. Cytomegalovirus, Epstein-Barr virus, *Toxoplasma, Histoplasma,* and *Candida* may cause a clinically similar hepatitis. Chronic liver disease may occur in 10% of hepatitis B and notably a greater percentage of hepatitis C patients. It probably does not occur after type A. Two forms of chronic hepatitis are identified by liver biopsy. Chronic persistent hepatitis is benign and self-limited but may cause mild symptoms. Chronic active hepatitis on the other hand often progresses to cirrhosis.

Cirrhosis of the Liver

Chronic disease of the liver may ultimately lead to cirrhosis, a scarring of the liver with subsequent loss of functioning hepatocytes. Three major pathways lead to cirrhosis: (1) chronic active hepatitis, (2) alcoholic hepatitis, and (3) progressive fibrosis. The major etiologies of cirrhosis are listed in Table 3-11.

Alcohol is the predominant cause of hepatic disease. Hepatocellular injury is a direct toxic effect of alcohol, and it may occur independently of any associated vitamin or nutritional deficiencies. There is a variety in severity of alcoholic liver disease. The main histopathologic types are fatty metamorphosis, alcoholic hepatitis, and cirrhosis.

Patients with alcoholic hepatitis may be totally asymptomatic; in contrast, they may present with fever, jaundice, abdominal pain, or hepatomegaly. Hepatic function tests may all become abnormal, especially γ-glutamyl transpeptidase. The transaminases are not elevated to the degree seen in viral hepatitis; values are less than 250 even in severe cases. The ratio of SGOT to SGPT is usually greater than 1:1. Alkaline phosphatase is usually mildly elevated. On the other hand, all hepatic function tests may be normal because of previous hepatic necrosis.

TABLE 3-11. Etiologies of Cirrhosis

1. Alcoholic liver disease
2. Primary biliary sclerosis
3. Chronic active hepatitis
   a. Autoimmune idiopathic
   b. Hepatitis B
   c. Hepatitis C
   d. Drug-induced
4. Primary sclerosing cholangitis
5. Wilson's disease
6. Hemochromatosis
7. Alpha-1-antitrypsin deficiency
8. Budd-Chiari syndrome

Biliary Cirrhosis

Primary biliary cirrhosis (PBC) is a chronic cholestatic disease seen primarily in women. The pathogenesis is unknown but may involve T-cell dysfunction leading to destruction of small bile ductules. The patient presents with pruritus, jaundice, and hyperpigmentation. Evaluation reveals markedly elevated alkaline phosphatase, positive antimitochondrial antibody and elevated IgM levels. Treatment involves use of fat-soluble vitamins and calcium supplements to prevent often debilitating osteoporosis.

Autoimmune chronic active hepatitis is also a disease that primarily affects women. Other autoimmune diseases are often present. Evaluation reveals a positive anti–smooth muscle antibody, and the diagnosis is confirmed by liver biopsy. Treatment with azathioprine and corticosteroids is beneficial in most patients.

Primary sclerosis cholangitis is another entity that appears to have an autoimmune pathogenesis. This disease process is uniquely tied to chronic ulcerative colitis; more than half of the patients have a history of CUC. The patient presents with weakness, fever, lethargy, and elevated alkaline phosphatase. Endoscopic cholangiography reveals multiple strictures of the intra- and extrahepatic bile ducts. There is no effective medical treatment, although dominant strictures may be dilated endoscopically. The patient may ultimately require liver transplantation for end-stage disease.

Wilson's disease or *hepatolentricular degeneration* is an autosomal recessive disease marked by the accumulation of copper in the liver, basal ganglia, kidneys, and erythrocytes. It may therefore present as dysfunction of several organ systems (see Table 3-12).

Hemochromatosis is also an autosomal recessive disease that can affect multiple organ systems. Inappropriate iron absorption leads to iron deposition in the liver and other organs. (See Table 3-13.)

TABLE 3-12. Wilson's Disease: Clinical Characteristics

1. Kayser-Fleischer rings seen on slit-lamp ophthalmic exam
2. Neurologic findings: tremor, dysarthria
3. Variable liver findings: asymptomatic, chronic active hepatitis, and fulminant hepatitis
4. Renal tubular acidosis
5. Hemolytic anemia
6. Diagnosis by laboratory results
   a. Low ceruloplasmin level
   b. High urinary copper
7. Treatment: Penicillamine

TABLE 3-13. Hemochromatosis: Clinical Characteristics

1. Diabetes mellitus
2. Cardiomyopathy
3. Hyperpigmentation
4. Diagnosis
   a. Serum iron >150 mg/dl
   b. Iron saturation >75%
   c. Serum ferritin >1,000
   d. Liver biopsy demonstrating iron in liver parenchyma
6. Treatment: Phlebotomy, desferoxamine

Alpha-1-antitrypsin deficiency can be associated with several forms of liver disease: neonatal jaundice, childhood cirrhosis, and adult cirrhosis. A low blood level makes the diagnosis, and there is no available medical treatment. Liver transplantation is available for advanced cases.

Postnecrotic cirrhosis is the most common form of cirrhosis on a worldwide basis. It represents the sequela of viral hepatitis (HBV or HCV). The liver is usually small on physical exam. It is believed that HBV is uniquely related to hepatocellular cancer (HCC) in the cirrhotic liver. However, all forms of cirrhosis have been associated with HCC, and recent studies have found this to be true for HCV.

Regardless of the cause or type of cirrhosis, the clinical characteristics are similar. The patient may be asymptomatic or exhibit symptoms that are nonspecific: lethargy, fatigue, anorexia, nausea, pruritus. The patient may also present with a complication of cirrhosis (see Table 3-14). The physical exam may reveal muscle wasting, spider angiomas, ascites, splenomegaly, or hepatomegaly. Liver function tests are variable: the albumin may be depressed and the serum bilirubin elevated.

TABLE 3-14. Cirrhoses: Complications

1. Variceal hemorrhage
2. Ascites
   a. If hepatic in origin; low ascitic albumin level
   b. Spontaneous bacterial peritonitis
      (1) Usually a single, gram-negative bacteria
      (2) Ascitic PMN count >250 cells
3. Portosystemic encephalopathy
   a. Exact cause unknown: ammonia, GABA
   b. Can be precipitated by diuretics, sedatives, infection, GI bleeding
   c. Treatment with lactulose; neomycin
4. Hepatorenal syndrome
   a. Renal failure
   b. Oliguria
   c. Urinary Na < 10 mg/l
5. Hepatocellular carcinoma
   a. Can occur in any type of cirrhosis
   b. Elevated alpha-fetoprotein level

Drug Hepatotoxicity

The liver is particularly susceptible to drug-induced injury because a large number of drugs may be affected by the cytochrome P-450 enzyme of the liver. Some drugs form toxic metabolites, especially isoniazid, acetaminophen, and chlorpromazaine. Drug toxicity may also be directly toxic (*e.g.*, carbon tetrachloride). Other toxic hepatic reactions include hypersensitivity reactions to methyldopa, sulfonamides, or chlorpromazine. Drug-induced liver disease may produce acute hepatocellular responses varying from a cholestatic type of hepatic dysfunction to obvious cirrhosis.

METABOLIC AND ENDOCRINE DISEASES

Tests of Thyroid Function

Thyroxine (T_4) and triodothyronine (T_3) are the two active thyroid hormones circulating in the blood. Most of these thyroid hormones are bound to thyroid-binding globulin (TBG); only the unbound hormone is active. Free T_4 and free T_3 can be measured by radioimmunoassay, but generally free T_4 is estimated as the free thyroid index (FTI). This calculation is based on the T_3 resin uptake (T_3RU), which is a number inversely proportional to the TBG. (FTI = $T_4 \times T_3RU$.) Thyroid-stimulating hormone (TSH) is secreted by the pituitary gland and stimulates the thyroid gland to secret T_4 and T_3. A new radioimmunoassay called sensitive TSH (sTSH) can now distinguish low from normal TSH levels. Thyrotrophin-releasing hormone (TRH) is secreted by the hypothalamus into the hypophyseal portal circulation to stimulate release of TSH.

During assessment of thyroid function, it is important to determine whether the patient has hyperthyroidism or hypothyroidism and whether the patient has primary thyroidal dysfunction or secondary dysfunction due to pituitary dysfunction. T_4, T_3RU, FTI, and sTSH are usually measured. If the FTI and sTSH are low, this suggests secondary hypothyroidism; if sTSH is high and the FTI is low, primary hypothyroidism is indicated. If the sTSH is normal or high and the FTI is high, this suggests secondary hyperthyroidism [TSH-secreting pituitary (rare)]; but, if TSH is low and FTI is high, primary hyperthyroidism is likely. If the sTSH is low and FTI is normal, the patient may have T_3-toxicosis, which can be confirmed by measurement of T_3 by radioimmunoassay. If hyperthyroidism is suspected but the above tests do not clearly show hyperthyroidism, a TRH stimulation test can be performed. TRH tests are performed by measuring TSH at the baseline and 30 minutes after TRH injection. This response is suppressed in patients with primary hyperthyroidism, but it will be exaggerated in patients with primary hypothyroidism.

If primary hyperthyroidism is diagnosed in a nonpregnant patient, ^{131}I uptake of the thyroid should be determined 24 hours after administration. If uptake is elevated, this suggests a diagnosis of toxic multinodular goiter (or Graves' disease), and if suppressed diagnosis of subacute thyroiditis, painless thyroiditis, or surreptitious thyroid hormone ingestion is suggested. If a nodule is palpated in the thyroid of a hyperthyroid patient, a thyroid scan should be performed to determine whether the patient has a toxic nodule that will be "hot" on the thyroid scan with suppression of iodine uptake in the rest of the gland.

Microsomal antibodies and thyroglobulin antibodies are present (*i.e.*, positive) in Hashimoto's disease. Thyroid-stimulating Igs are positive in patients with Graves' disease (hyperthyroidism).

Simple Colloid Goiter

The simple colloid goiter usually starts at the age of puberty. It is characterized by slow, painless, diffuse enlargement of the thyroid gland without any symptoms except occasional sensations of pressure. There is a normal metabolic state, and hypothyroidism or hyperthyroidism rarely develops. The condition is due to a low iodine content in the drinking water and the soil of the endemic area. The condition has become much less frequent in the United States since the commercial introduction of iodized salt.

In the presence of an enlarged gland, thyroid hormone often will reduce the goiter size by suppressing TSH secretion. Surgery is necessary for pressure symptoms only and therefore is rarely needed.

Thyroiditis

Subacute thyroiditis is an inflammatory condition of the thyroid of unknown etiology associated with swelling and tenderness of the gland with accompanying malaise and fever. The iodine uptake is usually depressed to a very low level. There is transient elevation in T_3 and T_4 levels initially, followed by a period of hypothyroidism. The condition is usually self-limited and resolves within a few months. Analgesics and thyroid hormone are used; in severe instances, prednisone may be employed.

Hashimoto's thyroiditis, struma lymphomatosa,

is a chronic autoimmune disease manifested by progressive enlargement of the thyroid associated with atrophy of the parenchyma and lymphocytic infiltration. It may now be the most common cause of goiter in the adult. In advanced disease, hypothyroidism supervenes. There is an increased incidence of lymphomas of the thyroid in these patients.

Thyroid Nodules

The evaluation of the patient with thyroid nodules has undergone changes in recent years because of the introduction of ultrasound and fine-needle aspiration techniques in addition to the classic approach of thyroid scan. Classically, a solitary nodule was scanned and divided into functioning or nonfunctioning (cold) groups. Since patients with hypofunctioning nodules are at increased risk for developing thyroid cancer, surgery or thyroid suppression was frequently recommended. Radiation history and family history of thyroid cancer further influenced the clinician to surgery.

However, in recent years the fine-needle aspiration technique in the hands of an excellent cytopathologist has removed some of this guesswork. And, at the present time, ultrasound can differentiate solid tumors from cysts. Therefore, clinicians at some institutions are performing the fine-needle aspiration as the first diagnostic modality. Recommendations as to the evaluation of the thyroid nodule must be based on the expertise available in the community. Presently there is a debate whether thyroid suppression is or is not indicated.

The multinodular goiter has a lower risk of later malignancy, but may go on to Plummer's disease (*e.g.*, toxic multinodular goiter). If thyroid functional suppression is to be undertaken on a multinodular gland, this should be done starting with a low dose of thyroid hormone since there are frequently autonomous regions of thyroid hormone secretion.

Thyroid Cancer

Thyroid cancers are more often differentiated than anaplastic. The most common of all are the differentiated papillary and papillary–follicular carcinomas. They have a relatively low-order malignancy, and patients may live for many years even with metastases.

The primary treatment of thyroid carcinoma is surgical; and, in the hands of experienced thyroid surgeons, a near-total thyroidectomy is recom-

mended because many of these tumors are multifocal. The prognostic factors are age, size of tumor, and invasion of the capsule. In the poorer prognosis groups radioactive iodine (^{131}I) therapy is given. All patients are given suppressive therapy with T_4.

Follicular carcinomas may be small and are more likely to metastasize widely to bone and lung. These tumors may be very sensitive to ^{131}I therapy. Medullary thyroid carcinomas may be sporadic or familial and associated with multiple endocrine adenomatosis type II or type III. These tumors secrete calcitonin and are treated surgically, and they may also be associated with pheochromatocytoma. Anaplastic tumors are associated with an extremely poor prognosis and surgery is rarely curative.

Hyperthyroidism

Hyperthyroidism is the symptom complex associated with excessive thyroid hormone. T_3 is the more active hormone and may be preferentially secreted. The causes include exogenous thyroid intake, Graves' disease, solitary hyperfunctioning nodule, toxic multinodular goiter, iodine-induced hyperthyroidism, subacute thyroiditis, struma ovarii, and tumors that secrete β human chorionic gonadotropin (HCG). Graves' disease is associated with a diffusely enlarged thyroid, Graves' ophthalmopathy, and rarely pretibial myxedema. The disease is most commonly found in young women and is familial. Thyroid-stimulating Igs bind to the TSH receptor to produce the thyroid stimulation. There is associated hyperactivity of the sympathetic nervous system.

The classic signs and symptoms are (1) goiter; (2) exophthalmos; (3) tachycardia; (4) fine tremor; (5) nervousness; (6) loss of weight; (7) excessive sweating and sensitivity to heat; (8) muscular weakness; (9) emotional lability; and (10) frequently, vomiting and diarrhea.

Most of the symptoms are referable to an increased thyroid secretion that causes an increased metabolic rate with excessive oxidation in the tissue cells, resulting in the loss of weight despite increased appetite. The uptake of ^{131}I by the thyroid gland is generally increased. Cardiovascular findings include a wide pulse pressure, atrial dysrhythmias, systolic murmurs, and at times cardiac failure.

There are three available options in treatment: (1) surgery, (2) medication, and (3) ^{131}I therapy. Each modality is effective, and debate continues about which is the most effective. ^{131}I will successfully control the manifestations of most patients with exophthalmic goiter. It is less satisfactory in toxic adenoma. It is especially valuable in those with complicating cardiac disease, which makes operation hazardous, and also in those in whom there is recurrence of the disease after surgery. There is a high and cumulative incidence of permanent myxedema. The long-continued use of antithyroid drugs requires careful and close supervision, but it may control the disease successfully. Antithyroid drugs are also useful in hyperthyroidism in pregnancy. Surgical treatment may be useful in patients with toxic adenoma. To reduce the sympathomimetic activity of Graves' disease and in thyrotoxic crisis, adrenergic blocking agents such as propranolol are used. The solitary hyperfunctioning nodule is most commonly associated with T_3 toxicosis and may be treated with either surgical ablation or, more recently, with ^{131}I therapy. The toxic multinodular goiter is more common in the elderly, and it may present primarily with cardiac toxicities. When surgery is too dangerous because of their underlying cardiac situation, high dosages of ^{131}I are required. Iodine most commonly causes hyperthyroidism in a multinodular goiter. Subacute thyroiditis may present with systemic symptoms of malaise, fever, and pain over the thyroid region. It may be associated with hyperthyroidism, but the thyroid uptake is less than 2%. This entity frequently progresses to a hypothyroid phase, but in 95% of patients the euthyroid state returns. Treatment with NSAIDs (and occasionally glucocorticoids) is frequently very helpful.

Hypothyroidism

Hypothyroidism occurs as (1) endemic *cretinism* originating from thyroid deficiency during fetal life and infancy and characterized by stunted mental and physical development and (2) *myxedema,* which occurs sporadically in adults and in the elderly as the result of thyroidectomy, thyroiditis, or atrophy. Both conditions are due to thyroid deficiency. With improved ability to measure thyroid hormone and TSH, and with improved clinical and diagnostic skills, diagnosis of hyperthyroidism is made much earlier.

The symptoms of cretinism are usually noticed after the first year of life because of slow development in stature, intelligence, and activity. In addition to retarded development, there is dry skin, imperfect dentition, flaring nostrils and sunken nasal bridge, potbelly, fatty pads on the shoulders and buttocks, and thickening of the tongue.

Prophylactic treatment is all-important. In goiter areas iodine should be given to pregnant women.

Thyroid hormone replacement will produce an amazing physical improvement in a cretin. Unfortunately, however, the condition is often not diagnosed early enough to save the child from permanent mental impairment. Thyroid tests are performed on neonates to avoid cretinism.

The most common cause of hypothyroidism is Hashimoto's disease, an autoimmune disease, manifested by antibodies against the thyroid tissue. These antibodies block the binding of TSH to the TSH receptor.

Other causes of primary hypothyroidism include thyroid surgery, thyroid ablation, subacute thyroiditis, iodine, and goitrogens. The circulating TSH level should be elevated in all patients with primary hypothyroidism. Secondary hypothyroidism generally occurs with a large tumor in the hypothalamus or pituitary and causes deficiencies of other hormones in addition to the thyroid hormone.

The symptoms of hypothyroidism usually develop slowly between the ages of 30 and 60 years. They are usually the opposite of hyperthyroidism and include the slowing of most bodily and mental activities. Fatigue, dry skin, coarse hair, decreased appetite, constipation, food retention, muscular cramps, arthralgias, bradycardia, low cardiac output, hypertension, edema, mental slowing, and weight gain are frequent features.

Thyroid replacement therapy is generally safe and inexpensive; however, patients with heart disease need to be observed closely. In those patients with severe coronary (or other surgically remediable) cardiac disease, cardiac surgery may have to be performed prior to thyroid replacement therapy. It is common medical practice to replace thyroid in elderly patients with low dosages of T_4, gradually increasing the thyroid hormone dose over weeks to months until the TSH is in the normal range. In younger healthy patients a full replacement dose may be given initially. Recent data suggest that the average dosages of l-thyroxine required for replacement are generally in the range of 0.1 mg to 0.125 mg/day.

Addison's Disease

Chronic primary adrenal cortical insufficiency may result from tuberculous fibrocaseous destruction of the adrenal cortex or from idiopathic bilateral adrenal cortical atrophy. The symptoms consist of weakness, fatigability, weight loss, pigmentation of the skin and mucous membranes, and GI manifestations. The pigmentation is a diffuse tanning with accentuation in scars, over pressure areas, and dark freckles. Blood pressure is low and the heart small. The serum sodium and chloride levels are low, and the potassium elevated. Serum cortisol levels are low while ACTH levels are increased. Administration of ACTH does not stimulate the adrenal to increase the secretion of plasma cortisol; however, in secondary adrenal insufficiency there is a subnormal increase. Treatment consists of administration of cortisone. The addition of NaCl to the diet may be helpful, or the administration of 9-α-fluorocortisol may be necessary at the beginning of treatment.

Acute adrenal cortical insufficiency may occur at the beginning or during the course of the chronic form as a result of infection, operation, or other stress. It is manifest by anorexia, nausea, vomiting, diarrhea, abdominal pain, and collapse. It requires immediate intravenous infusion of isotonic saline, glucose, and hydrocortisone.

Cushing's Syndrome

This condition is caused by excessive secretion of glucocorticoids by the adrenal cortex. An identical syndrome is produced by excessive amounts of corticosteroids administered to patients for therapeutic purposes. There is decrease of protein matrix in the bone, causing osteoporosis; muscle weakness; alterations in the skin, causing stria; decreased carbohydrate tolerance, causing mild diabetes; retention of sodium; hypertension; and excessive loss of potassium. There is weight gain, alteration or cessation of the menses in women, muscle weakness, and rounding of the face. Fat pads appear over the upper dorsal vertebra causing a buffalo hump and in the superclavicular fossae. Depressed purple striae appear over the abdomen and hips.

The most common form is bilateral adrenocortical hyperfunction due to excessive and unremitting secretion of pituitary ACTH. This is termed *Cushing's disease.* The best screening tests are elevated plasma or urine cortisol levels, which are not diminished by dexamethasone. Simultaneous measurement of ACTH in the petrosal sinuses following corticotrophin-releasing hormone (CRH) administration can be used to diagnose central Cushing's disease and to locate the tumor in difficult cases. Treatment is with transsphenoidal resection of a pituitary tumor, pituitary irradiation, or bilateral total adrenalectomy with long-term replacement as given in Addison's disease. Adrenal adenoma is much more common in women, onset is more rapid than in the pituitary-dependent form, and virilism is more common than in pituitary Cushing's syndrome. Treatment is removal of the adenoma with recovery occurring through normal function of the remaining gland on the other side. Adrenal carcinoma causes severe Cushing's syndrome; steroid values are high and are not suppressed by dexamethasone. The treatment is similar to that for adenoma. In addition, hypercortisolism can be caused by cancers of nonendocrine organs such as the lungs (oat-cell carcinoma), thymus, and pancreas.

Primary Aldosteronism

This results from an increase in the secretion of aldosterone by an adrenal tumor or bilateral hyperplasia leading to hypertension and increased sodium retention without edema but with varying degrees of potassium wasting and hypokalemic alkalosis. The result is a state of hyperaldosteronism that is associated with reduced plasma renin activity. Elevated aldosterone and reduced plasma renin activity that does not increase appropriately with volume depletion are diagnostic. In later stages potassium depletion and alkalosis may provoke characteristic attacks of muscle weakness or tetany, polyuria, nocturia, and cardiac dysrhythmias.

Pheochromocytoma

This is a catecholamine-producing tumor arising from chromaffin cells of the sympathoadrenal system. It is a rare condition but must be considered in the differential diagnosis of patients with hypertension. About 80% of pheochromocytomas originate in the adrenal glands. More than 95% of the tumors are located in the abdominal cavity, with the remainder in the paravertebral areas of the thorax and neck. The manifestations result from increased secretion of norepinephrine and epinephrine. Excessive dopamine secretion may be associated with postural hypotension in a normotensive patient. Hypertension is the principal sign and may be either persistent or paroxysmal in nature. Attacks are characterized by severe headache, sweating, palpitation, tremor, pallor, nausea, vomiting, pain in the chest, and hypertension. Pheochromocytoma may be associated with medullary carcinoma of the thyroid and hyperparathyroidism (MEA-II).

Hypopituitarism

Resulting from destruction of the anterior lobe of the pituitary, hypopituitarism is accompanied by secondary atrophy of the gonads, thyroid, and adrenal cortex together or individually. Sheehan's disease is hypopituitarism caused by postpartum necrosis of the gland. If tumor (*e.g.,* chromaphobe adenoma) is the cause, transsphenoidal resection or pituitary radiation may be indicated. Hormonal replacement therapy is indicated.

Acromegaly

This is a chronic disease characterized by overgrowth of bone and connective tissue in response to excessive secretion of growth hormone by a pituitary tumor, usually an eosinophilic adenoma. It is a disease of adult life, characterized by enlargement of the hands, feet, face, and head. *Gigantism* is a childhood counterpart of acromegaly resulting from oversecretion of growth hormone in a child before closure of the epiphyses. Prolonged active acromegaly leads to increased incidence of cardiovascular disease and hypertension and should be treated if possible. Surgery or high-voltage radiation to the anterior pituitary is used. Recently, octreotide, a somatostatin analogue, has been used to treat acromegaly not cured by transphenoidal surgery.

Prolactin-Producing Tumors

Many anterior pituitary tumors that, in the past, would have been labelled as "nonfunctional" are now known to produce prolactin. Prolactin hypersecretion is the most common abnormality due to hypothalamic-pituitary disorders and the hormone most commonly secreted by pituitary adenomas. On routine histologic exam these tumors appear to be chromophobe adenomas as the secretory granules are not visible with ordinary stains. The excess prolactin may be associated with decreased libido and impotence in men and is now recognized as the cause of amenorrhea, with or without galactorrhea, characteristic of several syndromes in clinical gynecology. At the time of diagnosis, most of these tumors are small and still confined within the sella turcica. Treatment with bromocriptine is effective in controlling prolactin secretion and tumor growth. When bromocriptine is unsuccessful in reducing prolactin tumor size, or when it is not tolerated, transphenoidal adenomectomy may be indicated. Normal reproductive function may be achieved with this therapy. Large tumors with extrasellar extension will get smaller with bromocriptine therapy. However, regrowth is possible if drug therapy is discontinued. Often, a combined medical–surgical approach is used to treat larger prolactin-secreting tumors.

Secondary hyperprolactinemia is associated with certain drug therapy including reserpine, methyldopa, clonidine, phenothiazines, metoclopramide, opiates, and cimetidine.

Elevated values are also found in hypothyroidism, chronic renal failure, and severe liver disease.

Primary Hyperparathyroidism

This results from overproduction of the parathyroid hormone caused by an adenoma or hyperplastic glands. Osteitis fibrosa cystica may result, as well as hypertension. Elevated serum calcium, increased urinary calcium, and lowered serum phosphorus levels are present. There are anorexia, weakness, fatigability, difficulty in swallowing, nausea, vomiting, and hypotonicity of muscles. *Hypoparathyroidism* usually results from inadvertent removal of the parathyroid glands during an operation for thyroid disease. There is decreased serum calcium with low urinary calcium excretion and increased serum phosphorus. The lowered serum calcium results in increased excitability of the peripheral nerves, and tetany results.

Osteoporosis

Osteoporosis is defined as a proportionate decrease in the matrix and mineral of bone. Minimal trauma leads to fractures, the most debilitating of which are hip fractures. Vertebral fractures tend to occur at a younger age and more frequently than hip fractures. Bone density measurements performed by single photon, dual photon absorptiometry, and CT scan have demonstrated that the lower the bone density the more likely a bone fracture. It is still unproved but thought that the bone density is primarily determined by the maximal bone density achieved at approximately age 25 minus the bone loss that occurs thereafter. The most important factors related to bone density are (1) age, (2) menopausal status, and (3) weight. The older the patient the less the bone density; the earlier the menopause the less the bone density; and the greater the body weight the greater the bone density. Other factors that are important include the use of exogenously administered glucocorticoids, immobilization, diseases that affect calcium and vitamin D absorption, and chronic alcoholism.

It now appears that prevention of bone loss is preferable to treatment of severe osteoporosis. At the present time estrogen therapy in women has been clearly demonstrated to be associated with fewer fractures and greater bone density. Calcium administration is seldom harmful. It is argued that the typical American diet is reduced in calcium; but this is controversial. Multiple therapeutic modalities have been advocated including estrogens, calcium, vitamin D, calcitonin, and fluoride. Recent studies have found that fluoride does not decrease fracture risk. However, there is no clear strategy for the treatment of severe osteoporosis. Thus, prevention of calcium depletion is being stressed and estrogen therapy at the menopause is suggested, particularly for women with decreased bone mass. It is also important to exclude other causes of osteopenia including such diseases as Cushing's disease, osteomalacia, hyperparathyroidism, and multiple myeloma. Finally, weight-bearing exercise also seems to be of some benefit.

Diabetes Insipidus

This disorder results from a deficiency of antidiuretic hormone from the posterior pituitary and causes persistent excretion of large volumes of urine of low specific gravity, which produces extreme thirst and secondary polydipsia. There is no renal disease, and replacement therapy relieves the symptoms promptly. Radioimmunoassay of arginine vasopressin will confirm the diagnosis.

There is also a form of nephrogenic diabetes insipidus in which the kidney fails to respond to vasopressin.

Diabetes Mellitus

Diabetes mellitus is a syndrome characterized by certain abnormalities of carbohydrate, fat, and protein metabolism and associated with both acute and chronic complications. There are undoubtedly many causes of the diabetic syndrome, most of them unknown at the present time. In general, abnormal glucose tolerance can be classified as: (1) *overt diabetes mellitus* (see below); (2) *impaired glucose tolerance,* in which the fasting plasma glucose or oral glucose tolerance test is not normal but is not abnormal enough to diagnose diabetes—people in this group do not develop retinopathy or nephropathy, but are at increased risk to develop atherosclerotic vascular disease; (3) *gestational diabetes,* in which diabetes is present only during the pregnancy—special diagnostic criteria and therapeutic objectives apply to this group of patients; (4) *previous abnormalities of glucose tolerance;* and (5) *potential abnormalities of glucose tolerance.* The last two groups have epidemiologic importance but little immediate clinical utility.

Overt diabetes mellitus is divided into *insulin-dependent* (IDDM, Type I), *non-insulin-dependent* (NIDDM, Type II), and other or secondary forms. IDDM includes the former category of juvenile-onset or brittle diabetes. Although the onset is usually prior to age 40 years, it may occur at any age. Patients in this category are *dependent* upon the administration of exogenous insulin for life. Under basal conditions, that is, no exogenous insulin and no physiologic stresses, they have a tendency to develop ketosis. Serum insulin concentrations are low, and the pancreas does not secrete insulin normally in response to stimulation. This type of diabetes is more often diagnosed in the fall and winter months. Frequently, an association can be made with a preceding viral infection. The symptoms of polyuria, polydipsia, polyphagia, weight loss, and weakness usually develop abruptly. People with IDDM have an increased frequency of histocompatibility antigens HLA-B8, B15, D3, and D4. For a variable period after diagnosis 70% of IDDM patients have detectable serum antibodies against the B cell of the pancreas. Histologic examination of the pancreas early after diagnosis reveals lymphocytic infiltration of the islets of Langerhans.

NIDDM includes the former category of adult (maturity)-onset or stable diabetes. Classically the onset is after the age of 40 years; however, this type of diabetes may be diagnosed at any age. These patients do not depend upon the administration of exogenous insulin for life, but they may require insulin administration for acceptable metabolic control. Under basal conditions they do not develop ketosis; however, if under a physiologic stress some of them may develop ketoacidosis. Serum insulin concentrations may be low, normal, or high. In addition to abnormal insulin secretion, insulin resistance at target tissues is thought to play a major pathophysiologic role. There is no association of NIDDM with viral infections, histocompatibility antigens, antibodies against the B cells, or lymphocytic infiltration of the islets. The disorder is diagnosed with equal frequency throughout the year. Symptoms usually develop insidiously. Many patients are unaware they are actually having symptoms. From 60% to 90% of patients with NIDDM are obese.

There are three generally accepted ways to make the diagnosis of overt diabetes mellitus. (1) Any patient who has classic symptoms of polyuria (including nocturia), polydipsia, polyphagia, and weight loss with an unequivocal elevation of the blood sugar (*e.g.,* random serum glucose greater than 200 mg/dl) has overt diabetes mellitus. Further diagnostic procedures are not necessary. (2) A person with a fasting serum glucose of 140 mg/dl or greater on two separate occasions has diabetes mellitus. (3) The demonstration of sustained hyperglycemia during a standardized oral glucose tolerance test is also diagnostic of diabetes.

Acute complications of diabetes mellitus include (1) ketoacidosis and coma; (2) hypoglycemia; (3) nonketotic, hyperglycemic, hyperosmolar coma; (4) recurrent infections; (5) muscle weakness; (6) lethargy; and (7) poor wound healing. The major chronic complications are (1) microvascular (involving the small blood vessels), frequently involving vessels in the eye and kidney, leading to retinopathy and nephropathy; (2) macrovascular (involving medium to large vessels), with accelerated atherosclerosis; (3) neuropathic (involving motor, sensory, and autonomic nerves), and multiple neurologic syndromes can be produced by diabetes, the most classic being a stocking-glove distribution of paresthesias; (4) cataract formation. The combined effects of macrovascular and neuropathic complications lead to diabetic foot disease, a devastating problem, which may result in lower extremity amputation.

The goals of treatment of diabetes mellitus are to (1) correct underlying metabolic abnormalities to as normal as possible (i.e., normalize blood glucose levels); (2) prevent acute complications and eliminate symptoms; (3) maintain ideal body weight; and (4) prevent or minimize the chronic complications. Frequently, self-monitoring of blood glucose is very helpful. This new approach has been said to represent the most significant change in diabetic care since the introduction of insulin. Patient education and involvement of the patient in therapeutic decisions are crucial to successful therapy. Appropriate diet prescription and counseling by a dietitian are the cornerstones upon which all other therapeutic maneuvers are built. For patients with NIDDM, diet is often the only form of therapy necessary. Should diet therapy fail to achieve acceptable metabolic control, sulfonylurea drugs or insulin may be added to the therapy. Patients with IDDM must receive insulin from the time of diagnosis.

HYPOGLYCEMIA

The sulfonylurea drugs and insulin are given to lower blood glucose concentrations. If there is not a proper balance between these agents and diet and exercise, hypoglycemia may result. Symptoms include weakness, sweating, mental confusion, incoordination, trembling, and sometimes loss of con-

sciousness and convulsions. The symptoms begin when the serum glucose falls below the 50 mg/dl to 70 mg/dl range and become severe when the level falls below 40 mg/dl. Any rapidly absorbable carbohydrate given orally will reverse mild symptoms. Severe symptoms may require the intravenous injection of 10 ml to 50 ml of 50% glucose or the subcutaneous injection of glucagon. Recovery is usually dramatic. Patients experiencing severe hypoglycemia should be observed for relapse for a period of time equal to the duration of action of the agent producing the hypoglycemia.

DIABETIC KETOACIDOSIS

Acute ketoacidosis occurs when the CO_2-combining power of the plasma falls below 15 mEq/liter and the pH below 7.35. The symptoms are (1) nausea, (2) vomiting, (3) epigastric pain and distress, (4) hyperpnea (Kussmaul breathing), (5) dry skin and oral mucosa, and (6) drowsiness or coma. The mucous membranes are bright red. The breath has a fruity odor of acetone bodies, and the breathing is very labored. Omission of insulin, infection, vascular accidents, and alcoholic pancreatitis are prime precipitating causes of ketoacidosis. Beta-hydroxybutyrate and acetoacetate are the ketone bodies responsible for the acidosis. Hypokalemia may result from too vigorous therapy of ketoacidosis.

Hemochromatosis

Hemochromatosis is an iron-storage disease characterized by deposition of iron in the tissues and organs with resultant fibrosis and interference with the function of the organs involved. Hemosiderin is deposited in the tissues, giving a bronze pigmentation at autopsy and giving the skin either a bronze or a blue-gray discoloration. The deposition is greatest in the liver but involves other organs and tissues. Fibrosis is thought to result from the accumulation of iron. Clinically the disease is characterized by skin pigmentation, diabetes, hepatomegaly with evidence of liver insufficiency, cardiac irregularities, and cardiac failure. Hemochromatosis may result from an idiopathic metabolic error, from repeated blood transfusions, or from excessive iron administration.

INFECTIOUS DISEASES

Numerous infectious diseases are not described here because all essentials of these diseases are included in other chapters (see Index).

Measles

Measles is a communicable disease of viral etiology, usually epidemic during the winter and the spring. Most cases occur in inadequately vaccinated adolescents and young adults.

The disease has an incubation period of about 12 days and a prodromal period of 2 days. Infectivity is highest late in the prodromal period and diminishes rapidly after the rash appears.

The prodrome consists of catarrhal symptoms, classically conjunctivitis, cough, coryza, fever, and Koplik's spots. Koplik's spots are seen on the buccal mucosa as bluish white spots of pinpoint size surrounded by a bright red areola. Leukopenia with relative lymphopenia usually is present in the preeruptive stage. Later there is leukopenia with relative lymphocytosis.

The eruption first appears about 2 days after the temperature has risen. It is noticed first behind the ears or on the forehead and spreads rapidly over the face and the neck and downward, covering the entire body in 2 or 3 days and lasting for 4 or 5 days. The lesions first appear as dusky red maculopapules, which form blotches and may become confluent. The fever and the respiratory symptoms increase with the rash, which after running its course leaves a fine, branlike desquamation. Atypical measles occurs in partially immune persons with the rash having a vesicular or hemorrhagic character.

Complications include measles pneumonia, acute or chronic encephalitis, subacute sclerosing panencephalitis, and bacterial superinfection of the upper or lower respiratory tract. Measles may activate latent tuberculosis and render the patient anergic for tuberculin skin tests. Complications are particularly hazardous in children.

Active immunization with attenuated live virus vaccine (two doses) is effective in preventing measles. A killed virus vaccine is available for immunocompromised patients. Gamma globulin in doses of 0.25 ml/kg should be given intramuscularly to prevent measles in a susceptible person within 6 days of exposure. A susceptible person is one who has not been vaccinated or has not had measles previously.

Treatment is largely symptomatic. Careful attention should be given to pulmonary and ear complications. Antibiotics should be reserved for bacterial superinfection.

Rubella

Rubella (German measles) is an acute contagious viral infection usually affecting children and young adults that is characterized by a skin rash and lymphadenopathy, especially posterior cervical. It occurs in epidemics. The usual course is mild and of short duration. Immunity is lasting, so that second attacks are rare. The importance of rubella lies not in the course of the disease itself but the frequency with which fetal abnormalities appear when the mother is infected in the early months of pregnancy. Maternal infection may lead to intrauterine death (stillbirth) or to delivery of a viable fetus with mental retardation or variable degrees of congenital abnormalities.

The key to prevention of the congenital rubella syndrome is vaccination of all children with the live attenuated virus vaccine. Women who have not been vaccinated and are planning to bear children should be serologically tested, and vaccinated if not immune, several months prior to conception. The vaccine should not be administered to women who are pregnant or might become pregnant within 2 months of immunization. A susceptible pregnant woman exposed to rubella during the first trimester should consider abortion.

Prophylactic use of immune serum globulin in susceptible pregnant women may prevent disease without suppressing viremia and the risk to the fetus. Arthralgia may occur with rubella and following rubella vaccination.

Influenza

Influenza type A or *influenza type B* virus infection results in an acute, usually self-limited respiratory infection that occurs in epidemics worldwide and almost always during the winter. Epidemics occur as a result of minor changes in the antigenic structure of certain viral envelope-associated proteins known as hemagglutinin and neuramidase. These changes, known as *antigen drift,* result in mutant viruses that are more easily transmitted. The antigen change is only minor, and previously established antibody responses provide some immunity. Pandemics occur about every 10 years as a result of major changes in these same antigens. Since no partial immunity is present, the incidence of clinical infection is much higher. Transmission is thought to be by inhalation of aerosolized, virus-containing respiratory secretions from infected patients. Immunity may be complete, partial, or absent depending on prior exposure, ability to mount an antibody response, levels of antibody, and degree of antigen shift or drift.

Following an incubation of 1 to 2 weeks, clinical illness is characterized by abrupt onset of fever, chills, headache, myalgia, and anorexia. Photophobia, tearing, burning, and pain with eye movement are common. In most cases the systemic symptoms resolve after 3 days. Nasal obstruction, dry cough, hoarseness, and sore throat may develop as the systemic symptoms subside. Examination early reveals a clear nasal discharge and injection of conjunctival vessels and mucous membranes of the throat and nose. Mild cervical adenopathy and rhonchi may be present.

Complications include primary viral pneumonia, secondary bacterial pneumonia, myositis with myoglobinuria, pericarditis, myocarditis and rarely encephalitis, transverse myelitis, and Reye's syndrome (if aspirin has been taken).

Amantadine has been shown to decrease the duration of type A illness and is approved for treatment and prophylaxis. Vaccination is effective in preventing or modulating the disease. Based on yearly worldwide surveillance a new vaccine containing the most prevalent strains is made each year. Vaccination is indicated for certain high-risk groups including patients with chronic cardiac, pulmonary, or renal diseases, diabetes mellitus, or asthma; nursing home residents; persons older than age 65; and physicians, nurses, and health care workers who are in contact with these high-risk groups.

Epstein-Barr Viral Infections

Epstein-Barr virus is a deoxyribonucleic acid (DNA) virus of the herpes group. It is transmitted among humans by intimate contact between susceptible and asymptomatic viral shedders. Epstein-Barr virus has been cultured from the oropharynx of 10% to 20% of normal, healthy adults. Acute infection after an incubation period of 30 to 60 days results in a spectrum of clinical manifestations. Minimal or nonspecific symptoms occur in childhood infections, while the characteristic syndrome of fever, sore throat, and lymphadenopathy is seen most often when primary infection occurs in adolescence or young adulthood.

Clinical manifestations include fever peaking in the afternoon, tonsillar enlargement with exudate in one third of cases, skin rash, palatal petechiae, cervical adenopathy (most commonly posterior), arthralgia, and generalized lymphadenopathy. Less common findings include erythema multiforme, hepatitis, splenomegaly, arthritis, pericarditis, myocarditis, aseptic meningitis, cranial nerve palsies (especially VII), and meningoencephalitis. Ampicillin administration should be avoided because it causes a pruritic, idiosyncratic maculopapular skin rash. Splenic rupture may occur. Hematologic find-ings include a white blood cell differential with greater than 50% mononuclear cells; greater than 10% of these are atypical lymphocytes. Hemolytic anemia and thrombocytopenia may occur. Serologic features include the development of nonspecific heterophile antibodies and specific antibodies to viral components. Diseases to be considered in the differential diagnosis include Group A streptococcal pharyngitis, viral tonsillitis, hepatitis A and B, viral meningitis, leukemia, and lymphoproliferative diseases. A heterophile-negative mononucleosis syndrome can be caused by infection with cytomegalovirus, HSV, rubella, adenovirus, *Listeria, Toxoplasma,* and certain drugs such as isoniazid and dilantin. Epstein-Barr virus infection can occur with a negative heterophile response. Most cases resolve spontaneously within 2 to 3 weeks. There is no specific treatment. Epstein-Barr virus has been isolated in malignant cells in Burkitt's lymphoma and nasopharyngeal carcinoma, and may play an etiologic role. Recently, attempts have been made to correlate elevation of Epstein-Barr virus specific antibody titers with a clinical syndrome characterized by fever, malaise, fatigue, myalgia, sore throat, and depression. This has been designated the chronic mononucleosis, or fatigue, syndrome by some. Whether this actually represents illness due to reactivation of latent Epstein-Barr viral infection remains to be determined, but more serious treatable diseases should be excluded.

Diphtheria

Diphtheria is caused by *Corynebacterium diphtheriae* and is still common in parts of the world. The lesions of diphtheria are (1) local, due to the action of toxin at the site of infection and (2) systemic, due to the action of the exotoxin absorbed through the blood and the lymphatics, which affects primarily the heart (myocarditis), peripheral and cranial nerves (paralysis), and kidneys.

Diphtheria occurs in unvaccinated children and young adults. Fever is relatively slight, and there is usually little pain on swallowing. The typical greyish white pseudomembrane may be found in the larynx, nasopharynx, tonsils, trachea, epiglottis, nose, and bronchi.

Clinical diagnosis is confirmed by culture of the nose and throat on Loeffler's medium. A single negative culture does not rule out the diagnosis.

In any suspected case of diphtheria, antitoxin should be administered without waiting for culture reports. Patients should be tested for hypersensitivity to horse serum before treatment with the antitoxin. Penicillin or erythromycin should be given to eradicate the carrier state. Fortunately, immunization with toxoid is rapidly making the disease a curiosity.

Acute Streptococcal Tonsillopharyngitis and Scarlet Fever

These diseases are caused by Group A β-hemolytic streptococci. Most cases occur in children, with peak incidence during the first few years of school. Epidemics are more common in the fall and winter.

The incubation period is usually 2 to 5 days. Acutely infected individuals are more likely to transmit the disease than those in the incubation period or those with convalescent or asymptomatic carriage of the organism.

In older children and adults a characteristic clinical picture of abrupt onset of sore throat, fever, malaise, and headache may occur. Prominent physical findings include redness, edema, and lymphoid hyperplasia of the posterior pharynx; follicular tonsillitis; enlarged and tender lymph nodes at the angles of one or both mandibles. However, a wide spectrum of illness occurs, with many cases clinically indistinguishable from common viral upper respiratory tract infections. Therefore, antibiotic therapy should be reserved for those patients with a positive rapid identification test for Group A streptococci. Within 12 to 24 hours after onset of illness, patients with scarlet fever develop a finely punctate rash on the neck and chest, which spreads gradually over the entire body and remains 4 to 5 days. Concurrent with rash these patients develop strawberry tongue. The skin desquamates, beginning on the chest, 3 to 10 days after disappearance of the rash. The rash may be limited to the groins, the axillae, and the elbows.

The common suppurative complications are peritonsillar abscess, otitis media, sinusitis, and cervical lymphadenitis. The nonsuppurative complications are acute rheumatic fever and acute glomerulonephritis. A urinalysis should be performed on all patients. Glomerulonephritis but not rheumatic fever is a complication of skin infection caused by Group A streptococci.

All patients with documented Group A streptococcal tonsillopharyngitis should receive antibiotic therapy to reduce the risk of suppurative complications and rheumatic fever. The treatment of choice is penicillin V for 10 days. Alternatively, a single intramuscular injection of benzathine penicillin can be administered. Treatment of choice for penicillin-allergic patients is erythromycin.

Erysipelas

Erysipelas is an acute inflammation of the skin (*i.e.*, cellulitis) caused by Group A streptococci or *Staphylococcus aureus*. It is most common on the face but occasionally occurs on the umbilicus of the newborn, the vulva during the puerperium, or around wounds or injuries.

It begins as a small area of red, swollen, and tender skin with margins that are sharply marked, elevated, and indurated. It extends by contiguity, with involution of the central portion. The onset is abrupt with chills, fever, malaise, headache, and anorexia. On the face there is often the symmetrical butterfly pattern.

Complications include subcutaneous abscesses, gangrene of the skin, orbital abscess, and septicemia with disseminated infection. Treatment with a β-lactamase-resistant β-lactam or vancomycin is generally dramatically effective in uncomplicated cases.

Rheumatic Fever

Rheumatic fever is a late complication of Group A streptococcal infection of the upper respiratory tract and is preventable by early treatment of these infections. It is most common between the ages of 5 and 30 and is characterized by (1) focal proliferative and (2) diffuse exudative lesions. The focal lesions are typified by Aschoff bodies in the myocardium and periarticular nodules and foci in the endocardium and the central nervous system. The exudative lesions involve the joints, the pericardium, and the pleura.

The latent period between streptococcal infection and the onset of rheumatic fever is approximately 3 weeks. The mode of onset of rheumatic fever is quite variable. The disease may have abrupt onset with fever, prostration, and migratory large-joint polyarthritis.

The diagnosis of rheumatic fever requires the presence of two major manifestations (carditis, polyarthritis, chorea, erythema marginatum, subcutaneous nodules), or one major manifestation and two minor manifestations (fever, arthralgia, prior rheumatic fever or rheumatic heart disease, acute phase reactants, prolonged PR interval on ECG), and serologic evidence of recent Group A streptococcal disease.

Carditis is the only manifestation of rheumatic fever that has the potential to cause long-term disability or death. The manifestations of rheumatic pancarditis include tachycardia, dysrhythmia, development of organic cardiac murmurs not previously heard, congestive cardiac failure, pericardial friction rub, and signs of pericardial effusion.

Bed rest and a nourishing diet are indicated. Practically all the acute symptoms *except those of the heart* are relieved by salicylates—these should be begun at high dosage to achieve serum salicylate levels of 20 mg/ml or more. Cardiac failure should be treated in the usual fashion. Group A streptococci should be eradicated from the throat with a 10-day course of penicillin.

Lyme Disease

Lyme disease is caused by the bite of a tick carrying the spirochete *Borrelia burgdorferi.* It was first recognized in 1975 when a cluster of cases occurred in an area around Old Lyme, Connecticut. An early manifestation is the pathognomonic skin lesion, erythema chronicum migrans (ECM); however, this is present in only 50% of patients. ECM usually begins as a small macule or papule that widens over 2 to 3 weeks to form an erythematously bordered, circular lesion with a central area of clearing. The patient may also experience flulike symptoms including malaise, chills, headache, arthralgia, and fever. Four to six weeks after the initial exposure aseptic meningitis, encephalitis, myocarditis, or arthritis may develop and persist. Diagnosis is made on clinical grounds and confirmed with specific IgM and IgG antibodies. The treatment of choice is doxycycline for 21 days, with intravenous penicillin G or ceftriaxone administered for chronic manifestations.

Listerial Infections

Listeria monocytogenes infections are recognized more frequently in patients with compromised host defenses. *Listeria* infect infants and the elderly as well as patients with neoplastic disease and transplant recipients who are receiving immunosuppressive therapy. These infections are the leading cause of bacterial meningitis in patients with neoplasms. *Listeria* are intracellular, gram-positive coccobacillary bacteria that may be confused with diphtheroids on Gram stain and culture. They are widespread in nature, and up to 5% of asymptomatic persons may harbor the organism in the GI tract.

Listeria cause a variety of clinical syndromes including granulomatosis infantiseptica, neonatal meningitis, sepsis, meningoencephalitis, cerebritis, conjunctivitis, endophthalmitis, endocarditis, osteomyelitis, and a mock "mononucleosislike" syndrome. Ampicillin is the treatment of choice, but trimethoprim/sulfamethoxazole may be used in penicillin-allergic patients. Cephalosporins are inactive against *Listeria* and should not be used.

Leprosy

Leprosy (Hansen's disease) is caused by *Mycobacterium leprae,* an acid-fast bacillus. The organism cannot be cultured on artificial media. Disease occurs as a spectrum from **tuberculoid leprosy,** characterized by large, erythromatous, anesthetic, sharply demarcated plaques, to **lepromatous leprosy,** characterized by extensive, bilaterally symmetrical macules, papules, or nodules. The sulfone drug dapsone is the mainstay of therapy, with rifampin and clofazimine added to therapy for patients with a large bacillary burden (lepromatous leprosy).

Typhoid Fever

Typhoid fever is an acute infection with *Salmonella typhi,* characterized by involvement of the lymphoid tissues, usually with marked hyperplasia and ulceration of Peyer's patches and enlargement of the spleen. A very similar illness is occasionally caused by other *Salmonella* species. Typhoid fever most commonly occurs in epidemics which result from human fecal contamination of food or water. In the United States, typhoid fever was very common a half century ago but is rare at present.

The incubation period averages 10 days, usually followed by 5 to 7 days of prodromal malaise, anorexia, and drowsiness. Typhoid fever is clinically characterized by (1) protracted fever, (2) headache, (3) mental confusion or stupor, (4) a variety of intestinal symptoms, (5) cough, (6) leukopenia, and (7) a slow pulse rate that is out of proportion to the amount of fever.

Many patients develop a characteristic skin rash, rose spots, which appear in crops over the abdomen toward the end of the first week.

Diagnosis depends on the entire clinical picture and isolation of the organism from cultures of blood, urine, stool, or bone marrow aspirate. Serodiagnosis is not reliable.

Complications of typhoid cause three fourths of the deaths. Hemorrhage is most frequent during the third week. It is manifested by (1) tarry stool, (2) chills, (3) marked fall in temperature, (4) pallor, and (5) rapid rise in pulse rate and leukocytosis. Abdominal pain is rare but when present suggests perforation. Perforation is most common in the second or third week; its most frequent site is the lower 18 inches of the ileum. As a rule, there is sudden and severe pain involving the entire abdomen, followed by the signs of general peritonitis.

Treatment includes (1) enteric isolation precautions; (2) antimicrobial chemotherapy; and (3) observation for signs of hemorrhage, perforation, or other complications. Pending *in vitro* sensitivity data, ciprofloxacin is the preferred antimicrobial therapy. Ceftriaxone, chloramphenicol, or trimethoprim sulfamethoxazole may also be used, but *in vitro* susceptibility to these agents should be documented. Treatment should be continued for up to 3 weeks. After treatment, patients should be evaluated for the presence of a fecal (or rarely urinary) carrier state. Chronic fecal carriers should be treated with cholecystectomy if cholelithiasis is present; otherwise a course of ciprofloxacin should be administered. At present, an effective oral vaccine is available for travelers to an endemic area.

Rickettsial Diseases

Rickettsia are obligate intracellular microorganisms with a reservoir in mammalian hosts such as rats, dogs, mice, and flying squirrels. Except for the agent of Q fever, *Rickettsia* are transmitted to humans exclusively by insect vectors—fleas, lice, and ticks. **Q fever** is usually transmitted to humans by the inhalation of aerosols from infected cattle, sheep, or goats. During spring and summer the triad of fever and headache followed in 3 to 5 days by a rash should lead to considerations of rickettsial disease. In the United States the most common of these are Rocky Mountain spotted fever caused by *Rickettsia rickettsii* and Q fever caused by *Coxiella burnetii*. The pathogenesis of rickettsial disease involves a vasculitis of arterioles, venules, and capillaries caused by endothelial proliferation of the organism. A spectrum of clinical illness occurs from asymptomatic to fulminant and life-threatening with disseminated intravascular coagulation. The clinical manifestations of Rocky Mountain spotted fever include fever, chills, severe headaches, myalgia, photophobia, and a rose-colored, fine, macular rash first appearing on the distal extremities, including the palms and soles, and spreading centripetally. In Q fever the clinical presentation is that of an atypical pneumonia. Hepatitis and endocarditis also occur. Diagnosis of rickettsial disease is by measurement of acute and convalescent antibody titers. Immunofluorescent techniques have recently been developed that can detect the organisms in tissue. Therapy with doxacycline or chloramphenicol is initiated on the basis of clinical and epidemiologic

grounds since serologic confirmation may be delayed by several weeks.

Nosocomial Infections

A nosocomial infection is defined as an infection that occurs in an institutional setting, which the patient did not have nor was incubating at the time of admission. Predisposing factors include alteration of normal flora with broad-spectrum antibiotics, use of invasive procedures and devices, extensive surgical procedures, and the use of immunosuppressive therapy. A major risk factor is inadequate attention of medical personnel to hand washing between patient examinations. Approximately 40% of all nosocomial infections involve the urinary tract with up to 2.5% of all hospitalized patients developing nosocomial **urinary tract infection.** *Escherichia coli* is the usual offending pathogen; however, other common bacteria include enterococci, *Pseudomonas aeruginosa, Proteus, Providencia, Enterobacter,* and *Staphylococci.* Urinary catheterization is the single most important risk factor. Failure to use strict sterile technique during catheter insertion and failure to maintain the closed drainage system with indwelling catheters are major predisposing factors. After 2 weeks, virtually all patients become infected in spite of an appropriately maintained, closed indwelling catheter system. The pathogenesis of urinary tract infections involves ascending extraluminal migration of bacteria or yeast along the periurethral mucous sheath of the catheter.

The incidence of nosocomial **surgical wound infections** varies with the type of procedure from less than 2% in clean operations to as much as 20% in contaminated procedures where the GI, respiratory, or genital tracts of women patients are entered. The majority are skin and subcutaneous tissue infections that manifest more than 3 days after surgery. Staphylococci (*Staphylococcus aureaus* and *Staphylococcus epidermidis*) are frequent pathogens, but enterococci and gram-negative bacilli occur as well. Major factors associated with an increased risk of postoperative infections include serious underlying diseases and prolonged hospitalization prior to surgery.

Pneumonias represent about 15% of all nosocomial infections but are most significant in that they are associated with the highest mortality rate (up to 50%). Gram-negative bacilli cause the majority, with *Pseudomonas aeruginosa, K. pneumoniae, Enterobacter,* and *Legionella* being most important. Gram-positive cocci (especially *S. aureus*) cause about 20% of cases. Precise etiologic diagnosis is often difficult because of the contamination of respiratory secretions by organisms colonizing the upper respiratory tract. Replacement of the normal, nonpathogenic, upper respiratory tract bacteria with more pathogenic, hospital-acquired varieties allows for aspiration of the latter into the lower respiratory tract. Risk factors for colonization and subsequent development of nosocomial pneumonia include the use of broad-spectrum antibiotics, trauma to the upper respiratory tract mucosa by nasogastric and endotracheal tubes, decreased level of consciousness, and decreased cough and gag reflexes. The use of agents that inhibit normal gastric acidity and motility may allow colonization of the stomach with large numbers of these bacteria, and this may serve as a reservoir for organisms subsequently causing pneumonia. Gram-negative bacillary pneumonia frequently requires prolonged antimicrobial therapy (up to 6 weeks).

Bacteremia represents about 7% of nosocomial infections. Bacteria may gain entrance to the blood stream through a percutaneous catheter at the site of skin penetration. In addition to colonization of the skin with pathogenic bacteria secondary to the use of broad-spectrum antibiotics and the failure of hand washing by medical personnel, other important predisposing factors include location of the catheter in the lower extremity, emergency placement, frequent manipulations, prolonged placement, and use of hypertonic, high-glucose-containing fluids. Host factors predisposing to bacteremia include neutropenia, immunosuppression, burns, and other skin diseases. The diagnosis of intravascular device-related sepsis can be difficult. Signs of local inflammation at the site of insertion are present in only about half of cases. Culture of the removed catheter tip by innoculation into broth is less reliable than a semiquantitative method of rolling it over an agar plate, yielding 15 or more colonies. Important, potentially fatal complications include suppurative thrombophlebitis of the great veins and endocarditis. Therapy consists of appropriate antibiotics and the removal of the catheter or other foreign body source of bacteremia (if possible).

Infections in Compromised Hosts

An increasing number of patients are encountered whose host defense systems are compromised by virtue of disease (diabetes, alcoholism, hematologic or lymphoreticular malignancy, etc.) or immunosuppressive therapy (administered for treatment of immunologic or malignant disease or to minimize organ transplant rejection). Such patients have increased susceptibility to infections due to common pathogens and additionally are susceptible to infections caused by organisms that are only rarely the cause of disease in normal hosts. Such opportunistic pathogens include certain bacteria, fungi, viruses, protozoa, and metazoa.

The most common opportunistic *fungal infection* is candidiasis. Predisposing factors include urinary catheters, intravascular catheters, prosthetic heart valves, broad-spectrum antibacterials, glucocorticoids, and hyperalimentation. Candidiasis may occur as urinary tract infection, oral thrush, esophagitis, suppurative phlebitis, and candidemia, which may result in widely disseminated infection including endocarditis and endophthalmitis. Cryptococcal infection is seen most commonly in patients with impaired cell-mediated immune systems, such as those with Hodgkin's disease, AIDS, or sarcoidosis. *Mucor* species cause a usually fatal rhinocerebral infection in patients with diabetic ketoacidosis or with leukemia. *Aspergillus* and *Mucor* species cause pulmonary infection in patients with protracted neutropenia. Disseminated histoplasmosis occurs more commonly in immunocompromised hosts. The mainstay of treatment for the mycoses remains amphotericin B (which is fungicidal), Flucytosine, ketoconazole, and fluconazole have more limited roles in selected patients.

The members of the herpesvirus family cause the most common serious opportunistic *viral infections.* HSV can cause severe mucocutaneous or disseminated infection in immunocompromised hosts. Varicella zoster virus causes shingles and disseminated infection in these patients. Serious infections with these two organisms are treated with intravenous acyclovir. Particularly in organ transplant recipients, cytomegalovirus infections manifest as protracted febrile illnesses often accompanied by hepatitis and pneumonitis. Ganciclovir and/or hyperimmune globulin has been used with some success experimentally for cytomegalovirus infections.

Three *protozoa* can cause serious infections in immunocompromised hosts. *Pneumocystis carinii* causes pneumonitis in patients with neutropenia or human immunodeficiency virus (HIV) infection. Treatment of choice for this infection is high-dose therapy with trimethoprim-sulfamethoxazole or intravenous pentamidine. *Toxoplasma gondii* can cause serious pulmonary and intracerebral infections in such patients; treatment for this infection is the combination of pyrimethamine and a sulfonamide with folic acid to prevent bone marrow suppression. Protracted diarrhea can be caused by *Cryptosporidium* for which no effective therapy is available.

Disseminated strongyloidiasis is usually associated with eosinophilia and occurs most frequently in patients receiving glucocorticoids. Treatment is with thiabendazole.

(Smallpox and malaria are discussed in Chap. 6, "Public Health and Community Medicine.")

SEXUALLY TRANSMITTED DISEASES

It is estimated that in excess of 10 million people each year contract a sexually transmitted disease (STD). In addition to the short-term morbidity, many STDs are now associated with long-term sequelae. For example, human papilloma virus (HPV) has been linked to cervical cancer; pelvic inflammatory disease (PID) may result in infertility; and infection with HIV may result in the development of AIDS. Far from being benign, easily eradicated infections, STDs are on the way to becoming the leading cause of death in urban 20- to 35-year-olds.

Certainly the best method of avoiding the sequelae of these infections is to prevent the STD in the first place. Beyond that, however, early recognition and therapy continues to be the mainstay of optimal management. What follows in the text and in Table 3-15 is a summary of the essential points of diagnosis and treatment of the most commonly encountered STDs.

Viral STDs

The prevalence of viral STDs seems to be rising (especially HIV and HPV) and effective antiviral therapies are being developed. Improved diagnosis of viral disease has been facilitated by rapid methods utilizing antigen or antibody detection techniques.

HERPES SIMPLEX VIRUS (HSV) INFECTION

HSV infections may be due to HSV-I or HSV-II. They are distinctly different double-stranded DNA viruses in the Herpesviridae family. Recent estimates indicate that there are as many as 500,000 new cases per year of these infections. HSV is the most common cause of genital ulcers in the United States.

Transmission occurs by exposure of skin or mucous membranes to secretions containing HSV. Asymptomatic shedding of virus may occur even

TABLE 3-15. Etiologic Agents of Common STDs and Associated Disease States

	DISEASE(S)
Virus	
Herpes simplex virus, types I and II (HSV-I, HSV-II)	Genital herpes, "cold" sores
Hepatitis A virus (HAV)	Hepatitis A
Hepatitis B virus (HBV)	Hepatitis B
Human immunodeficiency virus (HIV)	AIDS-related complex (ARC), AIDS
Human papilloma virus (HPV)	Genital warts
Chlamydia	
Chlamydia trachomatis	Urethritis, cervicitis, PID, perihepatitis, proctitis, lymphogranuloma venereum, etc.
Bacteria	
Neisseria gonorrhoeae	Gonorrhea (urethritis, cervicitis), PID, perihepatitis, proctitis, etc.
Haemophilus ducreyi	Chancroid
Treponemes	
Treponema pallidum	Syphilis
Parasites	
Entamoeba histolytica	Amebiasis
Trichomonas vaginalis	Trichomoniasis
Insects	
Phthirus pubis	Pubic (crab) lice
Sarcoptes scabi	Scabies

when there are no active herpetic lesions. At the time of the skin or mucous membrane infection, the virus also enters peripheral sensory nerves and is transported to the dorsal root ganglion and back to the site of contact. It is this phenomenon that is responsible for the characteristic recurrence of herpetic lesions.

Clinical manifestations depend on the patient's history of exposure, the site involved, gender, viral type, immunocompetence, and other unidentified virus–host interactions. Either virus may cause primary genital herpes, but recurrent episodes are more likely due to HSV-II. The incubation period of the primary infection is variable and is probably dependent on the inoculum size; it ranges from 1 to 30 days, averaging 4 to 7 days. A 24- to 48-hour prodrome of headache, malaise, and fever occurs in 40% to 70% of patients. Genital disease consists of rapidly developing, widely spaced, pustular or ulcerative lesions. These lesions are frequently accompanied by painful, unilateral or bilateral lymphadenopathy. The lesions slowly heal with crusting over a 2- to 3-week period. In heterosexual men, the lesions most commonly occur on the glans penis and penile shaft; in gay men perianal or rectal lesions are common. In women the lesions are seen most frequently in the perineal area, vulva, vagina, and cervix. Recurrent disease is typically more focal, milder in intensity, and shorter in duration. The only prodrome may be sensations of tingling, burning, or itching at the site of recurrence.

Diagnosis can be established on a clinical basis in the majority of cases. The best and most sensitive method of confirming the diagnosis is by culturing the lesions. Used in conjunction with an indirect fluorescent antibody-staining method, virus may be detectable within 24 to 48 hours of inoculation. HSV may also be detected by cytologic techniques such as the Tzanck prep. But, whereas these methods are simple, quick, and inexpensive, they are also insensitive and nonspecific. Serologic studies are generally less useful; the presence of IgM antibodies to HSV or a fourfold increase in IgG antibodies may be seen with the first episode of infection.

Treatment for the first episode with oral acyclovir has been shown to reduce the pain, duration of viral shedding, and time for healing. If the primary episode is unusually severe, intravenous acyclovir may be given. The efficacy of acyclovir for recurrent episodes is less certain and generally it is not required. If recurrences occur frequently (three episodes per 6 months) a prophylactic regimen of acyclovir may be instituted.

VIRAL HEPATITIS

Hepatitis A, hepatitis C, and especially hepatitis B may be transmitted sexually. Diagnosis is confirmed by serologic testing. There is no proven antiviral therapy.

Prophylaxis for recent sexual contacts of persons with hepatitis A consists of immune globulin. Susceptible contacts of patients with hepatitis B should receive hepatitis B immune globulin and a full series of hepatitis B vaccine series. All sexually active adults should be tested for hepatitis B core antibody and if negative, given hepatitis B vaccine.

HUMAN IMMUNODEFICIENCY VIRUS INFECTION AND AIDS

The etiologic agent of AIDS has been identified as a retrovirus, now known as HIV. This virus is especially infectious for cells bearing the cluster designation-4 (CD4) receptor including T-helper/inducer lymphocytes, monocytes/macrophages, and certain neuronal cells.

Transmission of the virus occurs through intimate sexual contact, needle sharing by intravenous drug abusers, blood transfusions received prior to April 1985, and from an infected pregnant mother to her fetus or newborn. Receptive anal intercourse is probably the most efficient method of transmission, but infection through vaginal intercourse has been repeatedly documented. There are anecdotal reports of transmission during exclusive oral intercourse in homosexual men. Saliva and tears may harbor infectious particles, but their contribution to transmission remains unclear. Transmission by blood products received since April 1985 is not likely because of testing of donated blood for HIV antibodies.

Clinical manifestations of HIV infection vary widely. Probably the largest number of infected patients are asymptomatic or nearly so. A small proportion of patients may present with an acute mononucleosislike syndrome consisting of fever, lymphadenopathy, fatigue, and malaise at the time of their acute HIV infection. AIDS-related complex (ARC) describes the syndrome of chronic fatigue, weight loss, oral candidiasis, diarrhea, fever, and persistent generalized lymphadenopathy with which many of these patients present. Other recently identified clinical presentations include hairy leukoplakia of the tongue, acute and chronic meningitis or encephalitis, peripheral neuropathies, and nephropathies. In many cases the patient will present with full-blown AIDS, which is strictly defined by the Centers for Disease Control (CDC). However, for practical purposes, the demonstration of antibodies to HIV and evidence of an opportunistic infection such as *Pneumocystis carinii* pneumonia or certain neoplasms such as Kaposi's sarcoma or non-Hodgkin's lymphoma will make the diagnosis of AIDS. ***Chronic wasting disease ("slim disease")*** and dementia are also recognized as AIDS-defining illnesses.

Diagnosis of HIV infection currently relies on the demonstration of antibodies to HIV by way of enzyme-linked immunosorbant assay (ELISA). All positive tests should be repeated immediately, and all negative tests should be repeated at 6 weeks, 3 months, and 6 months, especially for patients with risk factors for HIV infection. Recent data indicate that the time from infection to seroconversion may exceed 3 years in a very small subset of patients. Western blot testing should be reserved for patients with positive HIV antibody tests who do not have identifiable risk factors for HIV infection. Many assays with improved sensitivity and specificity for HIV infection are under development including a polymerase chain reaction for HIV DNA as well as one for HIV antigen (p24). These tests are useful in identifying persons infected with HIV who have not yet developed antibodies. In addition, detectable levels of antigen late in the course of HIV infection indicate a poorer prognosis. HIV antigen levels may fall with therapy.

Management of the patient with HIV infection includes counseling, evaluation of the immune status, consideration of drug therapy, and psychological/psychiatric referral when appropriate. Counseling is provided to inform the patient of the results of HIV testing regardless of that result. If the testing is negative, the patient should be informed of the following: (1) blood testing, although negative at that time, should be repeated periodically, especially if there has been recent possible exposure; (2) the patient is not immune to HIV infection; and (3) safer sex practices should be instituted or maintained. If HIV antibody testing is positive, the patient should be informed of the following: (1) the test does not mean that the patient has AIDS, although infection with the virus that causes AIDS is present; (2) all body secretions should be considered infectious, especially blood and semen; and, therefore, (3) unprotected sexual intercourse (including "deep kissing"), sharing needles with others, and the donation of any body tissues including blood are forbidden. Evaluation of the patient includes examinations for opportunistic infections as well as measurement of T4-helper and T8-suppressor lymphocytes. Skin testing with a Merieux panel to assess cell-mediated immunity and with intermediate-strength purified protein derivative (IPPD) to assess for exposure to tuberculosis is useful. Therapeutic considerations include antimicrobial agents to eradicate or suppress opportunistic infections as well as antiviral agents active against HIV. At this time zidovudine is the only antiretroviral compound approved by the FDA for use in patients with AIDS or symptomatic HIV infections, and while proven effective in reducing mortality as well as the frequency and severity of opportunistic infections, zidovudine is fairly toxic. Its use in patients who are less ill or asymptomatic is based on the CD4 lymphocyte count <500 or the presence of HIV antigen. There are many potentially effective drugs and vaccines undergoing evaluation at this time. Specific therapy for the management of opportunistic infections is complex or not available; therefore, prevention is of major importance. For example, *Pneumocystis carinii* pneumonia can be effectively controlled by monthly inhaled pentamidine or daily oral trimethaprim sulfamethoxazole.

HUMAN PAPILLOMA VIRUS (HPV) INFECTION

Genital warts or condyloma accuminata are caused by HPV, of which there are at least 40 different types. Integration of certain types of HPV into the host genome has been associated with malignancy.

Transmission of HPV through sexual contact was reported in the mid-1950s. Studies on the rate of transmission of HPV from one partner to another have reported rates varying to 95%.

Clinical manifestations of HPV infection are variable, ranging from large fungating warts to subclinical cytologic findings. In heterosexual men the most common location is the surface and base of the penis, but meatal, urethral, scrotal, and perianal lesions may be seen. Homosexual men clearly have an increased incidence of anal warts. Women may have warts in the posterior introitus, labia, vagina, cervix, rectum, and urethra. Malignant degeneration of warts is rare, but the locally invasive giant condyloma has features of both wart and carcinoma. Evidence is accumulating of a link between HPV and cervical cancer.

Diagnosis of HPV infection is usually made clinically; however, colposcopy combined with cytologic or histologic studies may be required to recognize cervical lesions. HPV antigens may be detected in tissue by immunoperoxidase staining.

Treatment presently depends on destruction of all visible warty tissue. Cryotherapy with liquid nitrogen may be slightly more effective than podophyllin.

Chlamydial STDs

MUCOPURULENT CERVICITIS AND URETHRAL SYNDROME

Mucopurulent cervicitis and the urethral syndrome may be caused by *Chlamydia trachomatis*. Chlamydiae are thought to contribute to up to 50% of the 1 million cases of PID diagnosed annually. Subclinical PID caused by these organisms is a major factor in the increasing incidence of ectopic pregnancies and in involuntary infertility. Neonates may become infected at birth, which results in inclusion conjunctivitis or pneumonia.

Clinical manifestations are highly variable, ranging from subclinical infection to acute dysuria or purulent cervicitis. Chlamydial urethritis should be suspected in any sexually active woman who complains of acute dysuria and has pyuria, but the Gram stain of unspun urine is negative for bacteria. According to the CDC, mucopurulent cervicitis due to

Chlamydia trachomatis should be suspected in the following setting: (1) yellow or green mucus or purulent material on a swab of endocervical secretions; (2) more than 10 polymorphonuclear leukocytes per oil-immersion field of a Gram stain of endocervical secretions free of intracellular bacteria; or (3) evidence of tissue friability, erythema, or edema within a zone of cervical ectopy. Patients with PID (which may be due to a variety of pathogens in addition to *Chlamydia trachomatis*) may present with lower abdominal pain, dyspareunia, cervical/uterine hemorrhage, or fever.

Diagnosis of chlamydial infection is based on clinical findings. Currently confirmation of the diagnosis of chlamydial infection is a research and epidemiologic endeavor that is undertaken almost exclusively by referral centers. Accurate and cheap antigen detection techniques are under development. Serial serologic testing may be useful in excluding active infection. Culture may be helpful in special circumstances as a test of cure in patients remaining symptomatic after empiric treatment.

Doxycycline (100 mg every 12 hours) administered for a minimum of 7 days is the treatment of choice for chlamydial infections in men and nonpregnant women. Erythromycin (500 mg every 6 hours) for 7 days is an alternative. Sexual partners of infected persons should also be treated. Any person treated for gonorrhea should receive a course of therapy for possible chlamydia infection, and all women with PID should receive doxycycline for 14 days in combination with an appropriate β-lactam, such as ceftriaxone or cefoxitin.

LYMPHOGRANULOMA VENEREUM (LGV)

LGV is caused by certain serotypes of *Chlamydia trachomatis,* and it is transmitted through intimate contact, probably through small abrasions. This infection is relatively uncommon in the United States, occuring at a rate of about 500 to 600 cases per year.

Bacterial STDs

GONOCOCCAL INFECTIONS

The most frequently reported communicable disease is gonorrhea. It is largely a disease of young people with a peak incidence in 20- to 24-year-old men and 18- to 24-year-old women. Other risk factors include low socioeconomic status, residence in a city, unmarried status, minority status, male ho-

mosexuality, and prostitution. The risk of acquiring gonorrhea is higher for uninfected women exposed to infected men than the reverse. This is probably explained on the basis of anatomic factors.

Clinical manifestations in men range from an asymptomatic carriage state to full-blown urethritis, epididymitis, or prostatitis. An incubation period of 2 to 7 days is commonly observed. Acute urethritis is the most common manifestation in heterosexual men and is characterized by a purulent urethral discharge and dysuria. Proctitis due to *Neisseria gonorrhoeae* may be the only site of infection in homosexual men who engage in receptive anal intercourse. Other sites of primary infection include the conjunctiva, pharynx, and skin.

Clinical manifestations in women are less specific than those in men. Dysuria and urinary frequency may signal gonococcal urethritis, while increased vaginal discharge may indicate gonococcal cervicitis. Labial tenderness and swelling may be due to infection of the Bartholin's gland. Pharyngitis or proctitis also is seen.

Diagnosis may be made on clinical or laboratory grounds. A Gram stain of urethral exudate showing polymorphonuclear leukocytes with intracellular gram-negative diplococci is highly sensitive and specific in symptomatic heterosexual men. The Gram stain is less useful in the diagnosis of gonococcal cervicitis, pharyngitis, and proctitis. Culture on selective media and assay for β-lactamase production are recommended for the evaluation of any potentially infected site. The gonococcus is rather fragile; therefore, appropriate swabs of secretions should be inoculated on media at the site of patient care, and the media should be incubated as soon as possible. Gonococcal antigen detection procedures are also available, but they seem to be flawed by low positive predictive value.

Clinical manifestations of gonococcal PID include lower abdominal pain, dyspareunia, uterine hemorrhage, and fever. On exam there may be uterine and adnexal tenderness and a mucopurulent cervicitis. Patients with the Fitz-Hugh–Curtis perihepatitis syndrome usually present with clinical evidence of PID and right upper quadrant pain or tenderness.

Treatment of gonococcal infection should always be accompanied by a course of antichlamydial medication. The rapid emergence of penicillinase-producing *Neisseria gonorrhoeae* (PPNG) has led to a single IM injection of ceftriaxone being the treatment of choice for gonococcal urethritis, cervicitis, pharyngitis, proctitis, or dissemination.

PELVIC INFLAMMATORY DISEASE (PID)

Neisseria gonorrhoeae and *Chlamydia trachomatis* are the two organisms most frequently isolated from the pelvic organs of women with PID. Both organisms can cause similar symptoms and may be the cause of the **Fitz-Hugh–Curtis syndrome** (perihepatitis). The gonococcus may disseminate from any mucosal surface and cause skin lesions, arthritis, or tenosynovitis. The skin lesion most often associated with disseminated gonococcal infection is a pustule with an erythematous base. A mono- or oligoarticular arthritis may involve any joint but most commonly affects the knees, elbows, ankles, wrists, or joints of the hands or feet. Rarely disseminated gonococcal infection may involve the liver, myocardium, cardiac valves, or meninges.

Diagnosis of PID rests on clinical or laparoscopic findings. The total white blood cell count, erythrocyte sedimentation rate, and C-reactive protein may all be increased. Diagnosis of disseminated gonococcal infection relies on the isolation of the gonococcus from blood, skin lesions, cerebrospinal fluid (CSF), or joint fluid. Blood cultures may be positive in up to 30% of cases; skin lesions and synovial fluid cultures are positive up to 10% and 30% of the time, respectively. Diagnosis of disseminated gonococcal infection often is made in the appropriate clinical setting with the isolation of *Neisseria gonorrhoeae* from a mucosal surface or from a sexual partner. Therefore all possible sites of infection should be cultured in any patient with suspected disseminated gonococcal infection.

Treatment of PID usually consists of broad-spectrum antibiotic combinations designed to eliminate the gonococcus, Chlamydiae, and opportunistic pathogens from the lower genital tract of women. Ceftriaxone or cefoxitin plus doxycycline are usually employed.

CHANCROID

Chancroid is one of the most common causes of genital ulceration outside of the United States. Approximately 1,000 cases of chancroid are reported each year to the CDC, but in 1985 that number doubled. This disease may achieve new significance if the link between genital ulceration and transmission of HIV is confirmed.

Clinical manifestations of chancroid relate to the genital ulcer and the associated lymphadenopathy. As with other forms of genital lesions the disease is more frequently recognized in men. The incubation period is 3 to 10 days. There may be a prodrome of low-grade fever and malaise. The ulceration begins as an erythematous tender papule that rapidly becomes pustular and ulcerated over 24 to 48 hours. There may be one or more deep, tender ulcers with uneven edges and a purulent base that bleeds easily. Swelling and phymosis may obscure coronal ulcers, and exudate may be so profuse as to mimic gonococcal urethritis. Enlarged inguinal lymph nodes occur in about half of the cases, and they are usually unilateral, painful, and tender. Lymph nodes may enlarge, and the overlying skin may be thin and erythematous in untreated patients. Lymph nodes greater than 5 cm in diameter may spontaneously rupture and form an inguinal ulceration or bubo. Chancroid is suggested by ulcers on the legs or abdomen caused by autoinoculation of *Hemophilus ducreyi* from genital lesions.

Diagnosis of chancroid rests on isolation of *Hemophilus ducreyi* on selective media. Gram stain of the ulcer material is neither sensitive or specific. All suspected chancroid lesions should be evaluated for HSV and syphilis.

Treatment options include cephriaxone, erythromycin, amoxicillin/clavulanate, and ciprofloxacin. Ulcers heal within 2 weeks, but lymph nodes take up to 3 weeks to resolve. Lymph nodes may require aspiration (not directly, but through normal adjacent skin) but never should be incised as this may delay healing. All sexual contacts should be treated, even if they are asymptomatic.

Treponemal STDs

Despite increasing awareness of HIV infection the annual number of cases of **syphilis** reported to the CDC, which remained nearly constant for the period 1980 to 1986, has shown a rise. The causative organism, *Treponema pallidum*, is thought to enter the body through small inapparent abrasions that may occur during sexual intercourse. Replication of the spirochete occurs at the site of entry, and then wide dissemination occurs if untreated.

PRIMARY SYPHILIS

Following an incubation period of 2 to 3 weeks a small erythematous papule appears at the site of infection. The characteristic chancre of primary syphilis develops as the papule ulcerates; the chancre is a red, ulcerative lesion surrounded by an indurated margin. The lesion is usually painless, and it may have a gray or yellowish exudate covering the base. There may be multiple chancres, and bilateral enlargement of inguineal lymph nodes is seen frequently. Chancres are usually located on the penis in men, and on the labia, fourchette, or cervix in women, although they may be found in any genital or extragenital location. In homosexual men they are frequently found in the anal area. They frequently go undiscovered because of the paucity of associated symptoms. Secondarily infected chancres may be painful and resemble herpes simplex lesions.

Diagnosis of primary syphilis is made by darkfield examination of material scraped from the suspected chancre. Nonspecific serologic tests such as the Veneral Disease Research Laboratory (VDRL) and rapid plasma reagin (RPR) are positive in about 80% of patients at the time they seek medical attention for primary syphilis. Serologic tests for specific antigens of *Treponema pallidum* such as the fluorescent treponemal antibody absorption test (FTA-ABS) and microhemoglutination assay for antibodies to treponema pallidum (MHA-TP) may be positive in about 90% of these patients. Therefore a negative serologic test does not exclude the diagnosis, and a positive test may reflect previous treated disease.

Treatment consists of benzathine penicillin G 2.4 million units IM. For patients allergic to penicillin, doxycycline and erythromycin are alternatives.

SECONDARY SYPHILIS

The lesions of secondary syphilis are due to dissemination of the spirochetes and are highly infectious. If left untreated, the syphilitic chancre will heal spontaneously within 1 to 3 months, and secondary lesions are seen 4 to 10 weeks after the primary lesion appears. Skin manifestations are variable, and syphilis should be in the differential diagnosis of any skin lesions without a clear etiology. A transient erythematous macular rash may appear, followed closely by a symmetrical papular eruption involving the entire skin surface, including the palms and soles. The papules are red or red brown and may have a variety of morphologies: scaly, smooth, pustular, vesicular, or hyperkeratotic. Mucosal lesions may be seen, and they consist of small painless ulcers or gray plaques. Condylomata lata are large, pale, warty growths that are found in warm, moist areas near the genitalia and perineum. Symptoms such as low-grade fever, tinnitus, hearing loss, malaise, diffuse lymphadenopathy, sore throat, headache, and arthralgias may be seen.

Signs of bone, visceral organ, and CNS involvement are rarely observed, but hepatic enzymes may be abnormal. Frank iritis, uveitis, and arthritis are uncommonly part of the picture.

Diagnosis of secondary syphilis may also be made by way of darkfield examination of material from papules, vesicles, pustules, or condylomata lata. Nonspecific serologic testing (VDRL, RPR) is positive virtually 100% of the time in disseminated disease, and usually in high titers ($\geq 1 : 32$). Biologic false-positive tests are not as high titered. In the case of apparently negative serology the test should be performed on diluted serum to negate the prozone effect. Specific antitreponemal serologic testing (FTA-ABS, MHA-TP, etc.) is uniformly positive.

Treatment of secondary syphilis involves 2 weekly injections of benzathine penicillin G (2.4 million units).

LATENT SYPHILIS

The lesions of secondary syphilis will heal spontaneously in 1 to 3 months. Following this, the patient may remain asymptomatic for a prolonged period until the development of tertiary syphilis. Patients are said to have early latent syphilis if they are within 1 year of their manifestations of secondary syphilis; late latent syphilis is arbitrarily assigned to patients who are more than a year out from the manifestations of disseminated disease. Any patient with a reactive specific and nonspecific serologic test who has no signs of disease is said to have latent syphilis. Unfortunately many of these patients are those who retain serologic evidence of past infection despite adequate treatment.

Diagnosis of latent syphilis is established by positive specific and nonspecific serologic testing and a clinical assessment of no active disease. Lumbar puncture to assess for the presence of asymptomatic neurosyphilis is indicated for all patients with latent syphilis.

Treatment consists of three weekly injections of 2.4 million units of benzathine penicillin G.

TERTIARY SYPHILIS

The clinical manifestations of tertiary syphilis develop after a highly variable period. ***Benign late syphilis*** is characterized by the presence of gummas, which are granulomas. These may involve skin and soft tissues of the face, neck, and extremities and present as indurated or nodular lesions that describe an arc or oval shape. Lesions may occur at the sites of minor trauma such as the elbows or knees. Bone or cartilage involvement is signaled by the presence of pain and swelling. Gummas may involve visceral organs such as the liver and testes. *Cardiovascular syphilis* implies involvement of the aortic vasa vasorum with resultant medial necrosis. While most patients remain asymptomatic, some develop aortic insufficiency, left ventricular hypertrophy, congestive cardiac failure, and aortic aneurysms. Symptoms of coronary artery disease may occur if the ostia of the coronary arteries are affected. *Neurosyphilis* may present in a variable way depending on the site(s) of involvement in the CNS. Meningitis, transverse myelitis, blindness, psychosis, dementia, tabes dorsalis, paresis, or a mixed picture may be present. The workup of a cerebrovascular accident as well as loss of sight or hearing should always include evaluation for syphilis.

Diagnosis of tertiary syphilis is made on clinical and serologic grounds. The FTA-ABS is the most sensitive serologic method. While CNS involvement in secondary syphilis is usually manifest by abnormalities in the CSF (increased polymorphonuclear leukocytes, especially lymphocytes and increased protein), the diagnosis of neurosyphilis may be very difficult. In late neurosyphilis the serum RPR or VDRL may be reactive at low titers, weakly reactive, or nonreactive. Lumbar puncture may reveal a lymphocytic pleocytosis, an elevated protein level, and a positive VDRL; however, CSF studies may be entirely normal.

Treatment of tertiary syphilis is the same as for the latent disease except intravenous penicillin is used for patients with neurosyphilis.

Parasitic STDs

AMEBIASIS

Amebiasis as well as other intestinal protozoan infections such as giardiasis occur as STDs in sexually active homosexual men between 20 and 40 years of age. Analingus is a major risk factor for these pathogens.

Clinical manifestations range from asymptomatic cyst excretion to acute rectocolitis, chronic nondysenteric intestinal disease (which may mimic inflammatory bowel disease), appendicitis, or toxic megacolon. Extraintestinal amebiasis usually presents with liver abscesses. Pleuritis, pericarditis, peritonitis, cutaneous genital lesions, and brain abscesses have been reported.

Diagnosis of amebiasis is usually made by stool examination. Three stool specimens or one purged stool should be examined prior to the administration of any interfering substances such as barium, antacids, enemas, antimicrobial agents, and so forth. Stool specimens should be refrigerated if they cannot be examined immediately. A saline wet mount is used first to look for amebic trophozoites or cysts. Permanent stains are required to differentiate *Entamoeba* species. The stool exam is positive in approximately 90% of patients with invasive amebic colitis. If the stool exam is negative where there is a high index of suspicion, proctoscopy or colonoscopy is indicated. There is a high yield of trophozoites from material scraped from the margins of colonic ulcers. Serologic testing may be useful in excluding amebiasis as a cause of invasive colitis or hepatic abscess.

Treatment for intestinal amebiasis is best accomplished with metronidazole 750 mg every 8 hours for 10 days. Patients should be cautioned not to consume any alcohol during or immediately after treatment with metronidazole to avoid a disulfiram reaction.

TRICHOMONIASIS

Trichomoniasis is caused by a flagellated protozoan. An estimated 2.5 to 3 million American women contract this disease annually. The prevalence of trichomoniasis in certain groups correlates with the general level of sexual activity. Spermicidal contraceptives such as nonoxylol-9 have antitrichomonas activity.

Clinical manifestations include vaginal itching and discharge, dyspareunia, and mild dysuria. The vaginal discharge is frequently copious, malodorous, frothy, or bubbly yellow green. Examination may reveal erythema and edema of the vulva, labia, and vaginal mucosa. Most men with trichomoniasis are asymptomatic and come to treatment because they are sexual contacts of women with symptomatic disease. Trichomonads have been associated with nongonococcal urethritis (NGU) and should be strongly considered in the differential diagnosis of doxycycline unresponsive NGU.

Treatment of choice for men and women consists of metronidazole as a single 2 g oral dose. The sexual partners of infected women should be treated whether or not they have symptoms.

Insect STDs

PHTHIRUS PUBIS: PUBIC (CRAB) LICE

Any form of pediculosis may be transmitted through intimate sexual contact. Those populations with the highest risk of gonorrhea and syphilis also have the highest incidence of pubic lice ("crabs").

Clinical manifestations probably relate to the development of hypersensitivity to the bite of the louse. The main symptom is itching. The groin or pudendal areas are most commonly affected, but any hairy area may be infested. Scratching may lead to excoriation, erythema, irritation, and inflammation. Bacterial superinfection may occur in this setting.

Diagnosis is made by close examination of the affected area with a magnifying lens. Adult lice may be seen on the skin surface. Eggs or nits may be seen on hair shafts. Sometimes groups of adult lice may be mistaken for scabs.

Treatment is with lindane (gamma benzene hexachloride). Lindane is available in a variety of formulations, but the shampoo is the easiest to use.

SARCOPTES SCABIEI: SCABIES

As with the pubic louse, disease produced by scabies is probably a result of hypersensitivity to the mite. Transmission of mites occurs during sexual intercourse, but scabies may also be transmitted within families, nursing homes, mental institutions, and hospitals.

Clinical manifestations are variable depending on host response. Classic scabies produce nocturnal itching and involve the wrists and hands as well as the genital area, breasts, and buttocks. Hand lesions usually involve the finger web spaces and the sides of the fingers. Insect burrows produce small, wavy lines that cross skin lines. Papules may be the site of larval development. Scratching may produce excoriation and secondary infection. Manifestations but not transmissibility may be suppressed by the administration of topical or systemic corticosteroids.

Diagnosis is made by demonstrating the presence of mites within burrows and treatment usually consists of one application of lindane lotion or cream (not shampoo) for 8 to 12 hours, and then the medication is washed off.

RHEUMATIC DISEASES, CONNECTIVE TISSUE DISEASES, VASCULITIDES, AND RELATED DISORDERS

Systemic Lupus Erythematosus (SLE)

Systemic lupus erythematosus (SLE) is a multisystem disease of unknown etiology associated with an unregulated production of antibodies against self-antigens. The various clinical manifestations are produced either by vascular inflammation (vasculitis or glomerulitis), which occurs when immune complexes are deposited in the blood vessel wall, or by antitissue antibodies damaging cells or cell products (AIHA, thrombocytopenic purpura, lymphocytopenia, lupus anticoagulants, and anticardiolipin antibodies). The latter has been associated with recurrent abortions, thrombocytopenia, thromboembolism, and possibly CNS lupus.

SLE primarily affects women in the childbearing age, but preadolescents and older persons, both men and women, may be affected. Malaise, arthralgias and arthritis, and skin rash are the most common complaints, but oral and nasal mucosal ulcerations, alopecia, fever, nephritis, pleurisy, pericarditis, peritonitis, Raynaud's phenomenon, cutaneous vasculitis, psychiatric and neurologic disorders (including convulsions), hemolytic anemia, thrombocytopenia, and leukopenia are all frequently encountered. Many patients develop a rash or constitutional symptoms on sun exposure. The disease may flare during pregnancy or in the postpartum period. The clinical course is that of chronicity; symptoms may remit and recur or may persist without remissions. Severity of involvement may vary greatly. Death occurs because of neurologic involvement (cerebritis or cerebrovascular accident), renal failure, infections or, rarely, following myocardial infarction secondary to premature atherosclerosis or coronary arteritis.

Laboratory findings helpful in making the diagnosis are antinuclear antibodies (ANAs), elevated sedimentation rate, low serum complements (C3, C4, CH_{50}), a biologic false-positive reaction for syphilis, direct Coombs positive hemolytic anemia, thrombocytopenia, lymphopenia, and urinary findings of protein and casts. Almost all SLE patients will give a positive ANA test. ANAs may be directed against various nuclear antigens. The antinative DNA (anti-double-stranded DNA) is elevated in "active" lupus, and it and the anti-Sm antibodies are specific markers for SLE. Antihistone antibodies are seen in over 90% of drug-induced lupus cases (e.g., due to procainamide or hydralazine). Antibodies to nuclear ribonuclear protein (RNP) may be seen in SLE and in high-titer, mixed connective tissue disease (MCTD). SS-A antibody is a marker for neonatal lupus and increased risk of congenital complete heart block in the offspring of pregnant connective tissue disease patients. SS-A and SS-B antibodies are most commonly seen in SLE, Sjögren's syndrome, and occasionally in rheumatoid arthritis.

Therapy depends on the extent of involvement. Salicylates or NSAIDs are useful for arthritis, mild disease, and serositis. Topical corticosteroids and sunscreens are used for the rash. If these involvements are severe or unresponsive, hydroxychloroquine may produce relief. Systemic corticosteroids are used for persistent serositis (pleuritis, pericarditis, peritonitis), active or severe nephritis, cerebritis, cutaneous vasculitis, and hematologic autoimmune complications. Cytotoxic drugs (azathioprine, cyclophosphamide) have been used in patients resistant to other therapies, and monthly intravenous bolus cyclophosphamide may have benefit in severe lupus nephritis. Pulse high-dose intravenous corticosteroids may be considered to treat rapidly deteriorating lupus nephritis or progressive CNS lupus. Apheresis has been tried in refractory, life-threatening disease but is of unproven efficacy.

Progressive Systemic Sclerosis (Scleroderma)

Progressive systemic sclerosis (PSS) may take a mild form with only sclerodactyly and Raynaud's phenomenon for many years. This is most commonly known as the CREST syndrome, which stands for *c*alcinosis, *R*aynaud's phenomenon, *e*sophageal dysmotility, *s*clerodactyly, and *t*elangiectasia. This subtype is associated with anticentromere antibody and has a more benign prognosis than generalized scleroderma. The disease may be slowly progressive with masklike facies and waxy, smooth fingers. In some cases there is rapid progression with esophageal disease, cardiopulmonary involvement, arthralgias, and renal disease. Scleroderma-70 (Scl-70) antibody correlates with severe systemic sclerosis and is also known as topoisonevase antibody. Many patients demonstrate ANA, and some have positive rheumatoid factor. No drug therapy has proven efficacy. Steroids have improved symptomatic myositis and may improve the early "edematous" phase of active dermal lymphocytic infiltration.

Treatment with D-penicillamine may, after several years of continuous use, result in fewer sites of sclerodermatous involvement, decrease in skin "weight," and possibly improved pulmonary function. Captopril is effective for renal involvement and hypertension. Nifedipine, diltiazem, or prazosin may be helpful for the Raynaud's phenomenon.

Polyarteritis Nodosa and Other Vasculitides

Necrotizing arteritis of small and medium arteries almost anywhere in the body is the hallmark of polyarteritis nodosa. The lungs are usually spared in polyarteritis but are involved in Churg-Strauss (allergic angiitis and granulomatosis). Symptoms derive from the pattern of involved vessels and resulting ischemia. A triad of renal involvement, hypertension, and mononeuritis multiplex is highly suggestive of polyarteritis, but coronary arteritis and involvement of GI vessels (stomach, intestine, gallbladder, pancreas, and appendix) are also common. Fever, weakness, and weight loss, an elevated erythrocyte sedimentation rate, and increased serum Igs are noted. HBV infection, illicit use of intravenous amphetamines, and drug reactions have been implicated in the etiology of polyarteritis. Diagnosis is by biopsy of affected organs, particularly sural nerve and symptomatic muscle, or by celiac and renal angiography. High-dose corticosteroids may control the disease manifestations, but cyclophosphamide is often necessary for successful remission, especially if there is renal involvement.

Hypersensitivity angiitis involves smaller vessels, especially postcapillary venules in the skin. The pathologic lesion is described as leukocytoclastic vasculitis because of the presence of nuclear fragments of infiltrating polymorphonuclear leukocytes. Treatment includes removing the patient from contact with potentially pathogenic antigens by treating any infection, discontinuing offending drugs, avoiding chemicals or toxins, and treating any underlying connective tissue disease. Oral colchicine may help the skin involvement, but associated disease (*e.g.,* SLE) or significant renal, GI, or neurologic involvement may warrant the use of corticosteroids. In refractory severe cases, immunosuppression with or without plasmapheresis can be considered but is rarely warranted or necessary.

Wegener's granulomatosis presents as a necrotizing and granulomatous vasculitis of the upper airway (nose, sinuses, and middle ear), lungs, and kidneys. Giant cells are present in these lesions. Fever, malaise, and arthralgias are common. Death formerly occurred from uremia, but frequent remissions and cures are routinely achieved with cyclophosphamide.

Giant-cell arteritis (temporal arteritis) is common in the elderly and associated with malaise, weakness, headache, acute visual symptoms, fever, and other constitutional symptoms. Anemia and an elevated erythrocytic sedimentation rate are usually present. Treatment is with immediate high-dose corticosteroids to prevent blindness. Confirmation of the diagnosis is accomplished with an urgent temporal artery biopsy.

Polymyalgia Rheumatica

This disease is related to giant-cell arteritis (15% of persons with polymyalgia rheumatica will have biopsy evidence of temporal arteritis; 50% of persons with temporal arteritis will have the symptom complex of polymyalgia rheumatica). Polymyalgia rheumatic also has elements of synovitis of the proximal joints of the extremities. The symptoms may begin gradually or abruptly and consist of neck, shoulder, and pelvic girdle aching pain and stiffness with exacerbation after periods of rest, but especially upon arising in the morning. Systemic involvement with weight loss and low-grade fever is seen. The erythrocyte sedimentation rate is almost always elevated. Low-dose daily oral corticosteroids produce prompt remission of this disease.

Dermatomyositis–Polymyositis

This disease involves the skin and the underlying muscles. Early in the disease there may be pain in the muscles, but, more commonly, painless proximal muscle weakness is present. The skin may (dermatomyositis) or may not (polymyositis) be involved; the muscle disease is nearly identical in the two illnesses. Diagnosis is by the finding of elevated muscle enzymes (CPK, SGOT, LDH, aldolase), electromyogram (EMG) and muscle biopsy. The skeletal muscles may be weak and atrophied. The upper eyelids may have a purplish (heliotrope B) discoloration. Other skin manifestations include characteristic Gottron's papules over the metacarpophalangeal (MCP) and proximal interphalangeal (PIP) joints, elbows, and extensor knees.

Malignant neoplasm may be associated with a significant number of cases, perhaps 8%. Other subtypes of myositis include a childhood form and the type associated with another connective tissue disease such as SLE. High-dose corticosteroids, with or without methotrexate or azothioprine, is the treatment of choice. Usually, immunosuppressive agents are reserved and added to steroid-resistant cases or used in those patients with major contraindications to long-term steroid use, for example, IDDM.

Sjögren's Syndrome

This syndrome consists of dryness of the eyes and mouth as well as chronic arthritis. It is seen commonly in middle-aged to older women and recently in male patients with HIV. The dryness of the eyes and mouth results from lymphocytic infiltration of the lacrimal and salivary glands. This disease should be differentiated from malignant lymphocytic infiltration or sarcoidosis involving the same areas. The treatment is symptomatic (i.e., artificial tears, ocular and oral lubricants, and assiduous dental hygiene). The secondary form of Sjögren's occurs in conjunction with another connective tissue disease, most commonly SLE or rheumatoid arthritis. The primary form may evolve over time from an initially benign to an ultimately malignant lymphoproliferative process. The primary form of Sjögren's may be diagnosed with a minor salivary gland biopsy of the inner lip and by careful ophthalmologic evaluation.

Mixed Connective Tissue Disease

Some patients, mostly women, have an overlapping of features of SLE, scleroderma, and polymyositis, with ANA to RNP in high titer. Patients have joint pain, swollen hands, Raynaud's phenomenon, myositis, impaired esophageal motility, pulmonary disease, and splenomegaly. Renal and CNS disease is less common than in SLE. Many patients will respond to low to moderate doses of corticosteroids.

Arthritis

Strictly speaking, arthritis should be restricted to inflammatory diseases of the synovial membrane, joint space, and articular cartilage. However, the term has been expanded to involve disease of joint capsules, ligaments, tendinous insertions, and bone-adjoining joints.

The following classification includes the major forms of arthritis:

1. Rheumatoid arthritis
2. Osteoarthritis [degenerative joint disease (DJD)]
3. Arthritis seen in connective tissue disease (SLE, Sjögren's syndrome)
4. Crystal-induced arthritis [gout, calcium pyrophosphate dihydrate (CPPD), hydroxyapatite, calcium oxalate]

5. Seronegative spondyloarthropathies (ankylosing spondylitis, Reiter's disease, psoriatic arthritis, arthritis associated with inflammatory bowel disease, and reactive arthritis)
6. Arthritis seen with vasculitis
7. Infectious or septic arthritis (staphylococci, streptococci, gonococci, gram-negative rods, anaerobic bacteria, mycobacteria, fungi, and viruses, including HBV, Lyme disease (*Borrelia burgdorferi*)
8. Arthritis associated with metabolic disorders and endocrinopathies (hemochromatosis, acromegaly, thyroid disease)
9. Arthritis seen in hemorrhagic diseases (hemophilia)
10. Traumatic arthritis
11. Neuropathic arthritis (diabetic neuropathy, tabes dorsalis)

RHEUMATOID ARTHRITIS

Rheumatoid arthritis is a common inflammatory disease of joints, occasionally remitting but usually chronic and progressing to joint destruction and deformity. The disease is more common in women than in men (2:1). Although generally believed to be an autoimmune disorder, an infectious etiology has long been sought. A genetic basis for the disease is suggested by the high frequency of the presence of histocompatibility antigens DR4 and DW4 in persons with adult rheumatoid arthritis.

It is a multisystem disease, with constitutional symptoms of anemia, weakness, aching and generalized stiffness, and weight loss. Extra-articular organ involvement includes scleritis and episcleritis, the sicca syndrome of xerophthalmia and xerostomia, subcutaneous rheumatoid nodules, pleuritis, pulmonary nodules and pulmonary fibrosis, pulmonary arteritis, pericarditis, myocarditis, coronary arteritis, Felty's syndrome consisting of neutropenia and splenomegaly, and nerve entrapment syndromes such as the carpal tunnel syndrome involving the medial nerve. Many of these organ manifestations are due to a vasculitis.

The essential pathologic lesion is an inflammation of the synovial membrane, leading to destruction of the articular cartilage, invasion of the capsule and periarticular structures by granulation tissue and ultimately to fibrous or bony ankylosis. The synovitis is the primary change, and the cartilage destruction is secondary.

Clinically, the arthritis presents as a symmetrical involvement of small and medium joints, especially of the hands and wrists. There is pain, especially on movement; joint stiffness; joint swelling; and limitation of motion. Generalized morning stiffness is characteristic, typically lasting more than 1 hour. Later, as capsular fibrosis, fibrous or bony ankylosis, muscle weakness, or ligament or tendon damage occur, impairment of function and deformity become more marked. The classic chronic appearance of the fingers is called the "swan neck" and "boutonniere deformity" of the PIP joints, and ulnar deviation at the MCP joints is common. The joints of the hands, wrists, knees, and feet are usually involved early. Later, almost any joint may be involved, but the spine (except for the upper cervical spine) and the sacroiliac joints are usually spared. The atlantoaxial joint of the cervical spine, the temporomandibular joints, and the cricoarytenoid joints may be involved and present special problems.

In the early stages, x-ray findings may be negative but may show early periarticular osteopenia and marginal erosions. Later, they may show diminished intra-articular space with atrophy and rarefaction of the ends of the involved bones.

Secondary anemia, mild leukocytosis, and increased sedimentation rate are common. Cardiac and renal disturbances are unusual.

Present in the serum of these patients is the rheumatoid factor, noted in 70% of cases. Inert particles, such as latex and bentonite or tanned sheep erythrocytes, when coated with human gamma globulin, are agglutinated by rheumatoid serums as a result of this rheumatoid factor.

Treatment includes the following:

1. Rest, especially in early acute stages. However, excessive quiet and immobility lead to stiffness and muscle atrophy so that a combination of rest and exercise should be adapted to the individual patient.
2. Analgesics. High-dose (enteric coated) salicylates to achieve a therapeutic blood level of 15 mg/dl to 30 mg/dl are started initially in the absence of contraindications. Other NSAIDs may be better tolerated in certain individuals but are no more effective than salicylates.
3. Physiotherapy. Moist heat and therapeutic exercise are important in all stages of the disease.
4. Orthopedic measures to correct deformities in advanced stages.
5. Surgical removal of synovium (synovectomy) particularly of the knee, or surgical fusion of selected joints (*e.g.*, the ankles) is sometimes of temporary benefit.
6. General health. A nutritious diet, especially for

those who are overweight, and correction of anemia when due to iron deficiency or with better control of the rheumatoid arthritis is important.

7. Supportive psychotherapy to counteract the emotional factors inherent in this crippling disease.

8. DMARDs (disease-modifying antirheumatoid drugs) are used for cases not adequately controlled with aspirin or NSAIDs. These include hydroxychloroquine, sulfasalazine, or auranofin for mild cases; and methotrexate, IM gold or D-penicillamine for aggressive disease. All patients with clinically important rheumatoid arthritis should receive a DMARD, and these should generally be started within 6 to 12 months of onset. These may produce satisfactory remissions in many patients. Toxic reactions are common and include rash, oral ulcers, cytopenias, and proteinuria.

9. Corticosteroids are restricted to cases not adequately controlled by aspirin or NSAIDs, and are used only with DMARD initiation.

OSTEOARTHRITIS

The differential diagnosis of the two principal types of chronic arthritis is illustrated in Table 3-16.

Osteoarthritis is most common in elderly people and appears not to be infectious or immunologic in origin. It is characterized by degenerative changes in the bone and the cartilage, with late thickening of the synovial membrane. There are simultaneous bone absorption and production. Most frequently affected are the hip, knee, spine, and finger joints.

Age, trauma (particularly prior fracture), congenital dysplasia, familial factors, and overweight are contributing factors.

An x-ray examination shows characteristic joint space narrowing, subchondral sclerosis, and subchondral cyst formation as well as osteophytosis ("spurs").

Treatment includes (1) rest for the affected joint and avoidance of overuse; (2) therapeutic exercise to strengthen adjacent muscles and maintain range of motion of the affected joint; (3) moderate doses of salicylates or NSAIDs, which are also helpful, including appropriate analgesics of nonnarcotic variety; (4) weight reduction in the obese patient for lower extremity joints; and (5) local corticosteroid injections, which may be used judiciously.

SERONEGATIVE SPONDYLOARTHROPATHIES

Ankylosing spondylitis is the prototype of a group of diseases characterized by inflammatory involvement of the axial skeleton as well as peripheral joints and in which studies for rheumatoid factor and ANAs are negative. Besides ankylosing spondylitis, other diseases in this group are Reiter's syndrome, psoriatic arthritis, intestinal or enterocolitic arthropathy, reactive arthropathy, and a juvenile-onset chronic arthropathy. These diseases should not be considered variants of rheumatoid arthritis. A genetic pattern is seen in these conditions, and the HLA-B27 antigen is seen in 90% of whites with ankylosing spondylitis and 50% of black Americans with the disease. A similar high incidence of the B27 marker is seen in Reiter's syndrome; however, only 30% of persons with psoriatic arthritis are B27 posi-

TABLE 3-16. Differential Diagnosis: Rheumatoid Arthritis and Osteoarthritis

	RHEUMATOID ARTHRITIS	OSTEOARTHRITIS
Average age at onset	Any age (30–50)	Sixth decade and older
Weight	Normal	Overweight (knees only)
Condition of bones	Rarefaction near joints (osteopenia)	Condensation of articular margins, with spurs and osteophyte formation
Joints involved	Any joint in body (especially of small fingers, wrists, knees, and toes)	Chiefly knees, spine, fingers, 1st MTP, and hips
Appearance of joints	Articular swelling	Little swelling
Type	Primarily an inflammation of its soft tissue around the joint with later rarefaction of bone adjoining the joint	Primarily an irregular overgrowth of bone at the joint margin
Special signs	Fusiform finger joints	Heberden's nodes (DIPs). Bouchard's nodes (PIPs)
Blood count	Secondary anemia and slight leukocytosis	Normal blood count
Sedimentation rate	Considerably accelerated	Normal
Course	Usually progressive	Stationary or slowly progressive
Termination	Ankylosis and deformity (15%)	No ankylosis

tive. Reiter's syndrome has followed arthritis due to *Chlamydia* and also after *Shigella, Salmonella, Campylobacter,* and *Yersinia* enteritis.

Ankylosing spondylitis presents usually in young men as morning stiffness and pain in the sacroiliac and lumbar spine. Onset is insidious, without preceding trauma, and symptoms improve with movement or activity. Nocturnal stiffness and discomfort may be significant. This may progress to fibrous and then bony fusion of the spine ("poker spine"). Other joints (cervical spine, shoulders, hips and, rarely, knees) may be involved, and acute iritis, upper lobe pulmonary fibrosis, and, rarely, cardiac involvement may be present (aortic insufficiency, conduction system disease).

The disease is predominantly an inflammatory and fibrosing–ossifying process in cartilaginous joints such as the sacroiliac joint and at sites of insertion of ligaments on bone (entheses). Radiographs will show the diagnostic changes of sacroiliitis, loss of the anterior concavity of vertebrae, the "bamboo spine," plantar spurs, and periostitis at the insertion of the Achilles tendon. Anemia and an elevated erythrocyte sedimentation rate are seen in the inflammatory stage of the disease. Therapy is postural support, exercise to maintain flexibility, and indomethacin, or other NSAIDs.

Reiter's syndrome is a triad of urethritis, conjunctivitis, and arthritis. The syndrome may be incomplete. Other findings are painless oral ulcers, balanitis, and a hypertrophic dermatitis on the soles and palms called keratoderma blennorrhagicum and resembling pustular psoriasis. The arthritis of Reiter's syndrome is treated with indomethacin or the newer nonsteroidal anti-inflammatory agents. The urethritis should be evaluated by stain and culture of the discharge and treated with appropriate antibiotics. Although the disease may be acute and self-limited, a chronic relapsing course is to be expected.

Arthritis is seen in 7% of persons with *psoriasis.* The various forms of the arthritis include asymmetric involvement of the PIP and DIP joints, a rheumatoid arthritislike involvement, involvement of the DIP joints only, arthritis mutilans, and spondylitis. If treatment of the psoriasis and the use of indomethacin or other NSAIDs do not produce relief, therapy with methotrexate may remit the arthritis.

GOUT AND CRYSTAL-INDUCED ARTHRITIS

Gout is the prototype of crystal-induced arthritis. Excess levels of uric acid in blood lead to accumulation of monosodium urate monohydrate crystals in tissues with resultant tissue inflammation in the synovial spaces (synovitis); deposition in bursae, tendons, bones, and subcutaneous sites (tophi); and deposition in the interstitium of the kidneys. Excessive excretion of uric acid leads to uric acid calculi and perhaps to renal tubular obstruction. Elevated serum uric acid is the hallmark of gout. However, many persons have mild to moderate hyperuricemia without symptoms of gout or renal stones and do not require drug treatment. The diagnosis of gouty arthritis should be confirmed by finding the needle-shaped negatively birefringent crystals in synovial aspirate.

Primary hyperuricemia is due either to a metabolic defect in the purine biosynthetic pathway leading to increased uric acid production or to decreased renal excretion of uric acid. Increased turnover of nucleic acids resulting in *secondary hyperuricemia* is seen in myeloproliferative diseases, polycythemia vera, multiple myeloma, pernicious anemia, certain hemoglobinopathies, and some hemolytic anemias. Chemotherapy of leukemia can cause dramatic increase in blood uric acid levels and requires the use of prophylactic allopurinol. Secondary hyperuricemia due to decreased renal excretion is noted in renal insufficiency, organic acidosis, ethanol-induced lactic acidosis, chronic lead poisoning, low doses of aspirin, and with the use of most diuretics.

Gout is primarily a disease of middle-aged men, but more recently it is becoming a disease of elderly women treated with diuretics. Obesity and hyperlipidemia are associated with the disease, and ethanol overindulgence can significantly increase blood uric acid. The classic pattern of symptomatology is that of a very painful monoarticular arthritis involving joints of the feet (first metatarsophalangeal joint, tarsal joints, and ankles) and the knees. Later the hands, wrists, and elbows are involved. Soft tissues overlying the joints share in the inflammation, with edema and dusky erythema being seen. The painful attack, if untreated, may persist for several days to several weeks. Early in the course of the disease, joints will return to a normal appearance between attacks. However, as the disease becomes chronic and tophi become more prominent in the synovia, erosion of cartilage and subchondral bone occurs and joint deformities develop.

The inflammatory process in the joint is produced by the monosodium urate monohydrate crystals being released into the joint space. Here they are phagocytized by polymorphonuclear leukocytes leading to (1) generation of chemotactic factors and (2) release of hydrolytic lysosomal and cytoplasmic enzymes. Monosodium urate crystals also may stimulate macrophages in the inflammatory exudate to release prostaglandins and synovial fibroblasts to liberate collagenase.

Treatment of the acute gouty attack is directed at interrupting the inflammatory response. NSAIDs or ACTH gel, IM (40–80 U) can produce rapid relief. After the acute inflammation is controlled and, while the patient still remains on anti-inflammatory medication or colchicine, a long-term program of reducing blood and tissue stores of urates is begun. Uricosuric agents such as probenecid are utilized in the absence of pre-existing hyperuricosuria. Allopurinol, a structural analogue of hypoxanthine, blocks uric acid synthesis, offering another modality for reducing the body pool of urates.

Weight reduction, avoidance of foods high in purine content, temperance in ethanol use, and avoidance of thiazide diuretics are recommended.

Other Causes of Crystal-Induced Arthritis. Calcium pyrophosphate dihydrate may deposit in cartilage, tendons, ligaments, joint capsules, and synovia and be an asymptomatic finding on radiography or necropsy (chondrocalcinosis). However, these deposits may cause acute episodes of pseudogout, more chronic disease mimicking rheumatoid arthritis, or progressive degeneration of knees and hips (as well as large and small joints of the upper extremities), leading to confusion with osteoarthritis. Apatite deposits may present as periarthritis, but acute goutlike oligoarthritis is also seen. Calcium oxalate may deposit in joint cartilage, leading to chondrocalcinosis, especially in CRF patients undergoing hemodialysis. Treatment includes NSAIDs or intra-articular corticosteroids.

DISEASES OF THE NERVOUS SYSTEM

Cerebrovascular Disease

Cerebrovascular disease or stroke is divided into two major groups: ischemic infarction and intracranial hemorrhage. Both ischemic infarction and intracranial hemorrhage can produce varying neurologic deficit based on the size and location of the event. This may include asymptomatic events, focal weakness, numbness, immediate coma, or death.

ISCHEMIC INFARCTION

Ischemic infarction produces symptoms that vary with the severity and duration of ischemia. Clinically, these are categorized according to the dura-

tion of symptoms as either TIAs (transient ischemic attacks) that by definition are completely resolved within 24 hours, or ischemic stroke, which results in neurologic deficit at 24 hours. The maximum severity of a TIA or stroke may vary from subtle symptoms (amaurosis fugax, mild numbness) to severe symptoms (complete hemiplegia with global aphasia, coma). Strokes may recover completely over a few days to weeks or may persist without improvement from the maximum severity.

The major causes of stroke include (1) embolism from the heart or from the extracranial carotid or vertebral arteries; (2) occlusion of large arteries (carotid, middle cerebral) or occlusion of small arteries (lacunar infarction); (3) arteritis; and (4) arterial injury (trauma, radiation therapy, iatrogenic). The risk factors for stroke include age, hypertension, smoking, diabetes mellitus, hyperlipidemia, hypercoagulable disease states (*e.g.,* polycythemia, macroglobulinemia), cardiac valvular disease, and chronic atrial fibrillation.

Evaluation of the patient with cerebrovascular ischemia includes an immediate CT of the brain to exclude the possibilities of a hemorrhage or mass lesion that can mimic ischemic symptoms. A follow-up CT scan after 7 to 10 days to visualize any permanent damage is useful to help determine the size and location of the stroke. Magnetic resonance imaging (MRI) is a more sensitive than CT scanning. MRI is used if the CT scan is inconclusive and for imaging the posterior fossa (brain stem and cerebellum).

Evaluation of the vasculature may include carotid arterial ultrasound. This is an accurate screening test for disease at the carotid artery bifurcation. Oculoplethysmography (OPG) can add sensitivity to this test by assessing the distal perfusion pressure of the internal carotid artery.

A cardiac evaluation including the echocardiogram to explore for an embolic source (valvular disease, enlarged left atrium with fibrillation or other atrial dysrhythmias, endocarditis, atrial myxoma) and 24-hour cardiac rhythm (Holter) monitoring in order to document episodic cardiac dysrhythmias are both important. Demonstration of a cardiac source of embolism is important for long-term prevention of recurrent stroke. Cerebral angiography is indicated to determine the mechanism of stroke (embolus, occlusion, stenosis, arteritis, dissection) when noninvasive evaluation is inconclusive.

Treatment is best directed toward the basic mechanism of a stroke. Anticoagulation is indicated for long-term prophylaxis of emboli from a cardiac source and is useful for the short-term treatment of artery-to-artery emboli after carotid artery dissection or acute vessel occlusion. Aspirin is indicated for prophylaxis of stroke for carotid artery disease or small-vessel infarction. All patients should have aggressive risk factor management. Patients with arteritis require treatment of their underlying disorder.

Carotid endarterectomy is indicated in addition to aspirin therapy in symptomatic (ischemic symptoms ipsilateral to the diseased carotid artery) and reasonably healthy patient with greater than 70% carotid artery stenosis. The intracranial/extracranial bypass procedure (EC/IC bypass) has been demonstrated to be ineffective as a treatment for stroke prophylaxis.

INTRACRANIAL HEMORRHAGE

Intracranial hemorrhage may occur in the subarachnoid space, the subdural space, the epidural space, or intraparenchymally.

Subarachnoid Hemorrhage. A nontraumatic subarachnoid hemorrhage is most commonly (80%) caused by intracranial saccular (berry) aneurysm. These are small (usually 3 mm to 15 mm) outpouchings at arterial bifurcations located around the circle of Willis. There is a defect in the muscular layer or internal elastic membrane of the blood vessels that allows this outpouching to occur. Aneurysmal rupture results in a 50% mortality. Many patients who do survive are left with significant brain damage. Occasionally an unruptured intercranial aneurysm will present with a cranial nerve compression (usually CN III). Most often, rupture is the first presentation with an explosive headache and sometimes with focal signs or coma. Polycystic kidney disease, fibromuscular arterial dysplasias, coarctation of the aorta, and Ehlers-Danlos syndrome are associated with saccular aneurysms. About 5% of all aneurysms are mycotic aneurysms from bacterial endocarditis (BE). Diagnosis of subarachnoid hemorrhage is based on demonstration of blood by CT scan or lumbar puncture. Cerebral arteriography is necessary to determine the location of the aneurysm(s). Approximately 20% of patients have multiple aneurysms. Definitive treatment involves surgical clipping of the aneurysm.

Arteriovenous malformations (AVMs) cause subarachnoid hemorrhage in approximately 20% of nontraumatic cases. They are more common in children than aneurysms and prior to rupture they may cause seizures or focal deficits. Diagnosis can be made prior to rupture by contrast-enhanced CT scanning. Cerebral angiography is necessary to define the extent of the AVM. Treatment may be medical or surgical depending on location of the AVM and history of previous hemorrhage.

Subdural Hemorrhage. *Subdural hematomas* are caused by rupture of the bridging veins between the dura and the brain surface. Although most cases involve trauma, in the elderly population minimal or no trauma may produce a subdural hematoma. Blood dyscrasia and anticoagulant therapy may also produce spontaneous subdural hematomas. The diagnosis of subdural hematoma is made by CT or MRI demonstrating a crescent-shaped or concave hematoma that follows the contour of the skull and surface of the brain. Lumbar puncture is contraindicated. Treatment of subdural hematoma is surgical drainage of the hematoma.

Epidural Hemorrhage. *Epidural hematomas* are caused by traumatic injury to the middle meningeal artery as it crosses on the inner surface of the skull. This typically causes reduction in consciousness after a lucid interval following the head injury. The diagnosis is made by CT or MRI. Similar to subdural hematoma, lumbar puncture is contraindicated. The CT scanning appearance of an epidural hematoma is a convex or lens-shaped hematoma. Treatment for epidural hematoma is surgical drainage.

Intraparenchymal Hemorrhage. Nontraumatic intraparenchymal hemorrhage is commonly the result of systemic arterial hypertension, which induces a lipohyalinoid degeneration of small penetrating arteries in the putamen, thalamus, pons, and cerebellum. These deep hemorrhages may be small, medium, or large. Diagnosis is by CT or MRI scanning. Treatment involves supportive measures, with emergency surgery indicated only in cerebellar hematomas. Treatment is otherwise directed at maintaining intracranial pressure in the normal range. Other causes of intraparenchymal hemorrhage include trauma, AVM, blood dyscrasias, anticoagulant therapy, arteritis, hemorrhage into a tumor (melanoma, choriocarcinoma), and cerebral amyloid angiopathy (CAA, congophilic angiopathy). CAA is not related to systemic amyloidosis and is caused by amyloid deposition in blood vessels of elderly patients. CAA can cause recurrent intracerebral hemorrhages that are located peripherally in the various lobes of the brain. The diagnosis is usually based on clinical factors, and there is no known treatment beyond supportive measures.

Epilepsy

Epilepsy is a disorder of the nervous system characterized by recurrent unprovoked seizures. Seizures may be of many types and are classified according to the International Classification (Table 3-17).

Simple partial seizures may be focal motor or focal sensory seizures. *Complex partial seizures* (previously called temporal lobe seizures or psychomotor seizures) are nonconvulsive seizures that cause a change in consciousness. Any partial seizure may secondarily generalize and cause a *generalized seizure,* such as a tonic–clonic seizure. This is fairly common in complex partial epilepsy, when an aura (complex partial seizure) precedes a generalized tonic–clonic seizure.

Myoclonus is a rapid single jerk. Repetitive unprovoked myoclonus, with or without generalized tonic–clonic seizures, is called myoclonic epilepsy.

Generalized seizures can be of the *absence* type, with a brief (seconds) suspension of consciousness. These typically begin in childhood and are described as "staring spells." Absence seizures are occasionally accompanied by generalized tonic-clonic seizures.

Generalized *tonic–clonic seizures* (grand mal seizures) can occur in isolation or in association with other types of epilepsy. Some epileptics have no warning that they will have a spell. Others have an aura (this is actually a complex partial seizure that secondarily generalizes) or have a focal initiation of the seizure indicated by head or eye turning in the early phase of the seizure. The tonic–clonic seizure is named because of the tendency for the extremities to stiffen (tonic) and then jerk in a rhythmic pattern (clonic) during the first seconds or minute of the seizure. After this phase stops, there is a period of simple unconsciousness that resolves over a few minutes. Postictal symptoms include headache, fatigue, confusion, incontinence, and trauma (tongue laceration, lumbar compression fracture).

TABLE 3-17. International Classification of Epileptic Seizures

I. Partial Seizures
  A. Simple partial seizures (Jacksonian seizures)
  B. Complex partial seizures (temporal lobe seizures)
    1. With impairment of consciousness
    2. With secondary generalized tonic–clonic convulsion
II. Generalized Seizure
  A. Absence (petit mal)
  B. Myoclonic seizure
  C. Tonic–clonic (grand mal)

TABLE 3-18. Epilepsy: Treatment Guidelines

SEIZURE TYPE	MAJOR ANTIEPILEPTIC DRUG CHOICES	ALTERNATIVE
Partial Seizures	Carbamazepine Phenytoin Phenobarbital Primidone	Valproic acid
Generalized Seizures		
Absence	Valproic acid	Ethsux
Myoclonic	Valproic acid	Clonazepam
Tonic–clonic	Carbamazepine Phenytoin Phenobarbital Primidone Valproic acid	
Status Epilepticus		
Tonic–clonic	Phenytoin 20 mg/kg IV or	Pentobarbital
	Phenobarbital 20 mg/kg IV and	Diazepam
	Diazepam 10–20 mg IV or	
	Lorazepam 4–8 mg IV	Lidocaine

The diagnosis of epilepsy is based on a clear pattern of unprovoked seizures. The exclusion of medication, alcohol, and metabolic effects is necessary before labelling recurrent seizures as due to epilepsy. The electroencephalogram is very helpful in determining what type of epilepsy is causing the seizures. Some types of epilepsy, most notably complex partial epilepsy, can have normal electroencephalograms. A brain imaging study with CT or preferably MRI scanning is necessary to exclude a structural lesions as the cause of the epilepsy (mesial temporal sclerosis, tumor, AVM, stroke).

The treatment of epilepsy is dependent on the type of epilepsy and the type of seizures manifested in the individual. Treatment guidelines are outlined in Table 3-18.

Status epilepticus describes a state in which recurrent seizures continue without a return to normalcy. This can occur in both nonconvulsive seizures (such as absence or complex partial seizures) or convulsive seizures (generalized tonic–clonic seizures). Generalized tonic–clonic status epilepticus is a life-threatening condition that should be treated by intravenous anticonvulsants. Treatment must be individualized to the patient and seizure type. Phenytoin or phenobarbital is the drug of choice to stop and prevent recurrence of the seizures. Intravenous benzodiazepines (lorazepam 4–8 mg, diazepam 10–20 mg IV) are useful adjunctive agents that may work quicker than phenytoin and phenobarbital but have a much shorter duration of action, making them unsuitable as a single agent for most patients.

Brain Tumors

Brain tumors can arise from the parenchymal brain (glioma) or the coverings of the brain.

Astrocytomas are the most common glioma. These are not completely resectable but do respond to radiation therapy. Prognosis for lower-grade astrocytomas is quite good, but higher grades (glioblastoma multiforma) do poorly even with surgery, radiation, and chemotherapy. Other intrinsic brain tumors are ependymoma, oligodendroglioma, and ganglioglioma.

The coverings of the brain and tissues extrinsic to the brain produce tumors that are often completely resectable (depending on location). This includes meningioma, pituitary adenoma, and nerve sheath tumors (also called schwannoma, neuroma).

Brain tumors present with a variety of symptoms. Seizures, behavioral disturbances, and headaches are common and nonspecific symptoms that any brain tumor can produce. Some tumors produce fairly specific symptoms that are extremely diagnostic. This includes the bitemporal hemianopsia of pituitary adenoma, the progressive unilateral hearing loss and dizziness from VIIIth nerve acoustic neuroma, and complex partial seizures from a low-grade temporal lobe glioma.

Headache

Migraine is a very common disorder that refers to a variety of different headache types that vary from periodic, occasional, hemicranial, throbbing headaches to chronic daily headaches. Associated symptoms include nausea, vomiting, paresthesias, visual disturbance, and behavioral changes. Some migraines are precipitated by an aura. This is most commonly a visual phenomenon that may be homonymous, monocular, or binocular. Other auras include hemiparesis, aphasia, or other neurological disturbances. This is followed by headache (usually within 20 to 30 minutes). Some patients may have an aura without a headache. The headaches often last a few hours, a day, or a few days.

Treatment of migraines includes the removal of clear migraine triggering factors (sleep loss, stress, oral contraceptives, foods and medications). Prophylactic medication to prevent migraines include propranolol, amitryptyline (low dose), calcium channel blockers, methysergide (Sansert), and nonsteroidal anti-inflammatory drugs.

Once a headache has been initiated, medication treatment is often disappointing. Ergot alkaloids and intravenous dihydroergotamine are able to abort certain migraines. Analgesics and antiemetics are helpful. Any intravenous medication that heavily sedates the migraine sufferer (narcotic, benzodiazepine, phenothiazine) will usually stop the headache.

Chronic daily headaches (often called muscle contraction headaches or stress headaches) are common headaches that are on the far end of the migraine spectrum. There are typically few associated symptoms aside from pain in the musculature around the head and neck, but many patients with these headaches will also suffer from occasional migraines. Often the cause is chronic analgesic abuse. This occurs with acetaminophen, aspirin, and Ibuprofen, but is more severe with medications containing barbiturates or narcotics. Treatment includes withdrawal of analgesics, institution of good health practices (sleep, diet, exercise), and use of small doses of prophylactic headache agents such as amitryptyline (or other tricyclic) or propranolol.

Cluster headaches are an unusual variant of migraine that tends to occur in men who are smokers. These are brief, stabbing, unilateral, retro-orbital pains that come on and last for a few minutes. They may recur through the day, and in some people occur only nocturnally. During a headache there is nasal stuffiness, tearing, and an ipsilateral Horner's syndrome. Treatment for the acute attack is oxygen. Medications are difficult to administer quickly enough to have any effect. Occasionally inhaled ergotamines or lidocaine nose drops can break the headache once it has begun. Prophylactic medications include ergotamines, calcium channel blockers, prednisone, or medications used for migraine. In severe refractory cases surgical destruction of the first division of the Vth cranial nerve can be effective.

Trigeminal neuralgia (tic douloureux) is a sudden lancinating pain that follows a division of the Vth cranial nerve. These last only seconds but can recur many times a day. They are often triggered by eating, toothbrushing, or any stimulus to the affected area. The cause is a disordered sensory transmission close to the origin of the Vth cranial nerve in the brain stem or proximal nerve. Treatment with carbamazepine, phenytoin, and/or baclofen typically stops the pain. If necessary, surgical ablation of the affected trigeminal branch or retromastoid microvascular decompression of the Vth cranial nerve is effective.

Giant-cell arteritis (temporal arteritis, cranial arteritis) is a unilateral headache in the elderly associated with jaw claudication, scalp tenderness, polymyalgia rheumatica, and elevated erythrocyte sedimentation rate or C-reactive protein. Diagnosis is based on clinical grounds and confirmed by temporal artery biopsy. Because this disorder can progress to blindness (monocular or binocular), diagnoses or exclusion of this diagnosis is necessary. Steroid treatment is highly effective.

Demyelinating and Degenerating Diseases

MULTIPLE SCLEROSIS

Multiple sclerosis (MS) is a disease of the CNS characterized by recurrent or progressive patchy demyelination in multiple areas. Widely diversified symptoms are experienced involving the sensory, motor, visual, and cognitive systems.

Symptoms may include virtually any dysfunctions of the nervous system. Among the common symptoms are diplopia, disturbed urinary bladder control, numbness in the extremities, disturbed equilibrium, unilateral visual loss (optic neuritis), spasticity, nystagmus, loss of abdominal reflexes, ataxia, dementia, and emotional disturbances.

The spinal fluid usually demonstrates a mild pleocytosis, increased γ-globulin, and oligoclonal bands. The MRI scan may show areas of demyelination, and evoked responses may be abnormal. An autoimmune mechanism is the etiologic factor in multiple sclerosis. A viral "trigger" has been postulated.

The diagnosis of multiple sclerosis should be made with the greatest caution. Spinal cord tumors, platybasia, cerebellar tumors, porphyria, hysteria, and many others usually masquerade as early multiple sclerosis. The diagnosis is based on the demonstration of two episodes of demyelination separated by both time and location. MRI, evoked potential, and lumbar puncture are helpful to confirm the diagnosis and exclude other disorders. Corticosteroids reduce the length and severity of exacerbations. Immunosuppression can slow rapid MS progression.

AMYOTROPHIC LATERAL SCLEROSIS (LOU GEHRIG'S DISEASE)

The cause of the amyotrophic lateral sclerosis is entirely unknown; the principal complaints are weakness and wasting of muscles. The involved muscles show fasciculations, which are spontaneous contractions of groups of muscle fibers that can be felt by the patient and observed as sudden ripples under the skin. The anterior horn cells in the spinal cord are usually first affected and lead to wasting and fasciculations in the upper extremities, particularly in the small muscles in the hand. Swallowing can be affected. There is preservation of the reflexes in the atrophied muscles or spasticity (increased reflexes). The characteristic picture of the disease is a combination of diffuse muscle atrophy, fasciculation, and retained reflexes in the muscles, with spastic paraparesis of the lower extremities. Sensory changes are absent. The course is progressive, and death usually occurs within 5 years of the onset.

ALZHEIMER'S DISEASE

Senile dementia of the Alzheimer type is the most common dementia. The disease increases in frequency with age and may have as high as 10% to 15% prevalence by age 85 years. The etiology is unknown. Some cases are familial. The earliest symptoms are recent memory loss and subtle emotional changes. With time, language, abstract thinking, ability to cope socially, and many other cognitive and adaptive functions are lost in a slowly progressive fashion. Neurofibrillary tangles and senile plaques are found pathologically.

The differential diagnosis includes multi-infarct dementia, mass lesions, hydrocephalus, slow virus infection, hypothyroidism, alcoholism, Pick's disease, Huntington's disease, tertiary syphilis, pernicious anemia, chronic meningitis, AIDS, and a variety of metabolic and degenerative diseases.

PARKINSONISM

Parkinson's disease, or parkinsonism, is a degenerative disease that is more common with advanced age. Some cases are familial. The etiology is not well understood. It is characterized by (1) muscular hypertonia—"cogwheel rigidity"—without hyperreflexia or other evidence of corticospinal tract involvement, (2) resting tremor, (3) slowness (bradykinesia), (4) abnormal gait (stooped, shuffling, and unsteady), (5) soft speech, and (6) motionless (masked) facies.

Patients with parkinsonism have very small amounts of dopamine in the basal ganglia. Present management, therefore, utilizes L-dopa and carbidopa (a circulating peripheral inhibitor of L-dopa degradation). Other medication of use includes Amantadine, bromocriptine, pergolide, selegiline (deprenyl), and anticholinergic drugs.

CREUTZFELDT-JAKOB DISEASE

Creutzfeldt-Jakob disease is a rapidly progressive dementia with myoclonus and a characteristic periodic EEG pattern. There is no therapy. The etiology is a subviral particle called a prion. The disease can be transmitted by contaminated neurosurgical instruments.

MUSCLE DISEASES

Muscle disease typically presents with proximal weakness or pain in the muscles. Reflexes and sensation are typically preserved unless there is an associated neuropathy. Main categories of muscle disease include the following.

Inflammatory Myopathies. Inflammatory myopathies include *polymyositis,* which is an inflammation of the muscles causing weakness and pain. This can be associated with connective tissue disorders. A similar entity, dermatomyositis, is indistinguishable from polymyositis but is by definition associated with a rash. *Dermatomyositis* is considered a paraneoplastic syndrome because of the common association with cancer. The diagnosis is made on clinical findings, elevated CPK, and electromyographic abnormalities. Muscle biopsies confirm the diagnosis. Treatment is directed at any underlying disorder (collagen vascular disease, cancer) and corticosteroids. Other immunosuppressive agents probably work as well and are under investigation.

Noninflammatory Myopathies. Noninflammatory myopathies are not painful but cause progressive proximal weakness. Metabolic disorders, or endocrinopathies (corticosteroid use, hypothyroidism), present in this manner. Differential diagnosis includes nutritional myopathies, alcoholic myopathies, and disuse weakness. The diagnosis of a true myopathy from disuse weakness is based on clinical findings, electromyography, CPK elevations, and family history and often requires muscle biopsy.

Muscular Dystrophy. Muscular dystrophy is any of a number of genetic diseases in which muscles slowly deteriorate. *Duchenne's* sex-linked, recessive muscular dystrophy strikes young males and is usually fatal by adolescence. Other types can be adult-onset autosomal dominant and affect specific muscle groups (limb girdle, facioscopulohumeral).

Myotonic Dystrophy. Myotonic dystrophy is also an autosomal-dominant inherited disease causing muscle stiffness. It is associated with heart block, testicular atrophy, premature balding, and cataract development.

Myasthenia Gravis. Myasthenia gravis is a disease in which antibodies are produced against the acetylcholine receptor. Typical symptoms fluctuate with fatigue on effort, prominent double vision, swallowing difficulties, and general muscle weakness. Diagnosis is by antibody levels, typical decay pattern on repetitive nerve stimulation, and clinical improvement noted on injection of an anticholinesterase drug (edrophonium). Treatment is with thymectomy, anticholinesterase drugs, prednisone, and plasmapheresis.

PERIPHERAL NEUROPATHY

Peripheral neuropathies are a heterogeneous group of conditions that affect the peripheral nerves after they leave the spinal cord but before they affect the muscle. These can affect both motor (weakness) and sensory (numbness and paresthesias) nerves. Reduced sensation and decreased reflexes are common.

Diabetes mellitus, alcohol, nutrition, drugs (especially chemotherapeutic agents), uremia, paraproteinemias, and immunological disorders all can be the cause. Certain inherited neuropathies may present identically to those caused by other factors. Evaluation requires electromyography with nerve conduction velocities, serum chemistries for diabetes, B_{12}, abnormal proteins, urinary functions, and in selected cases porphyria. Urinalysis for toxins is occasionally of use when there is a history of exposure to heavy metals. Cerebral spinal fluid examination to demonstrate an elevated protein is necessary to identify the inflammatory neuropathies such as acute inflammatory demyelinating polyneuropathy (AIDP or Guillain-Barré syndrome) or chronic inflammatory demyelinating polyneuropathy (CIDP, "chronic" Guillain-Barré).

Treatment is focused on removing the underlying cause if possible. If no treatment is available, then amitriptyline is helpful to reduce the painful burning of sensory neuropathies, and bracing or physical therapy is useful in motor neuropathies. Topical creams such as capsaicin are helpful in refractory painful neuropathies.

Infectious Disorders of the Nervous System

MENINGITIS

Bacterial meningitis is a life-threatening medical emergency. Morbidity includes hearing loss, seizure activity, and learning disorders. *Haemophilus influenzae* meningitis in children is a leading cause of acquired mental retardation. The pathophysiology of meningitis involves hematogenous seeding of the meninges from local or distant sites of infection, direct extension of a parameningeal suppurative focus, or direct innoculation of micro-organisms following skull fracture or neurosurgery. The inflammatory response that occurs in the subarachnoid space may cause blockage of drainage pathways of the CSF, increased intracranial pressure, and necrosis of nerve roots. Glucocorticoids can diminish this host-damaging, nonspecific inflammatory response.

The common causes of bacterial meningitis are age-specific, and some are associated with predisposing conditions. The most common organisms found in infants younger than 2 months of age are Group B streptococci, *Listeria monocytogenes*, and *Escherichia coli*. In children younger than 10 years of age, *Haemophilus influenzae*, *Neisseria meningitis*, and *Streptococcus pneumoniae* are most common. In adults *Neisseria meningitidis, Haemophilus, Streptococcus pneumoniae*, gram-negative rods, and *Listeria* are most frequent.

The initial evaluation of patients with meningitis is directed toward determining whether or not the patient has bacterial meningitis. Most patients with bacterial meningitis have an acute onset of fever, headache, and stiff neck rapidly evolving over 24 hours. In these cases, provided no contraindications exist, lumbar puncture should be performed and the patient should begin receiving empiric therapy immediately. Choice of antibiotic treatment depends on the patient's age and associated predisposing factors. CSF findings characteristic of bacterial meningitis include a white blood cell count greater than 1,000, a differential count showing greater than 50% polymorphonuclear neutrophil leukocytes (PMNs), a glucose level of less than 30 mg/dl, and a protein level greater than 150 mg/dl. A Gram stain of centrifuged CSF sediment is positive in 80% to 90% of patients with cultures positive for bacteria. This may allow changing therapy to less broad-spectrum agents. Ten percent of patients

with bacterial meningitis have an initial cell differential showing a predominance of lymphocytes.

Penicillin G is the treatment of choice for *Streptococcus pneumoniae* and *Neisseria meningitidis meningitis*. Chloramphenicol is the best alternative in penicillin-allergic patients. *Neisseria meningitidis meningitis* is primarily seen in adolescents and young adults; petechiae and purpura occur in about 50% of patients. Gram-negative bacterial meningitis may follow head trauma, neurosurgical procedures, or gram-negative bacteremia. Most patients respond to a third-generation cephalosporin (ceftriaxone). *Pseudomonas aeruginosa*, *Enterobacter*, and *Acinetobacter* may be relatively resistant and require additional intrathecal or intraventricular administration of an aminoglycoside. *Listeria* most often is seen in the immunosuppressed. It may be mistaken for diphtheroids on a CSF Gram stain and considered a skin contaminate. Treatment of choice is ampicillin or trimethoprim/sulfamethoxazole. *Staphylococcus aureus meningitis* is seen with brain abscess, sinusitis, endocarditis, and infected burns. Treatment is with a pencillinase-resistant penicillin such as nafcillin and vancomycin.

Aseptic meningitis is defined as the absence of a positive culture for bacteria in the CSF of patients with meningitis. These are assumed to be viral meningitis. The differential diagnosis includes partially treated bacterial meningitis, parameningeal suppurative infections such as brain abscess, sinusitis, epidural abscess, mycobacteria, fungi, protozoa, *Treponema pallidum*, carcinomatous or lymphomatous meningitis, chemical meningitis, Behçet's syndrome, Molleret's syndrome, sarcoidosis, and meningitis due to SLE. Antibacterial therapy may be begun empirically while awaiting results of cultures and evaluating for other etiologies. Patients with viral meningitis are more likely to have a subacute presentation with symptoms developing over a period of up to 7 days; however, some cases may develop acutely. Characteristic CSF findings include a white blood cell count less than 1,000, predominance of lymphocytes, normal glucose, and increased protein.

Patients with ***mycobacterial*** or ***fungal infections*** are more likely to have chronic presentation of symptoms for weeks to months. In addition to increased CSF lymphocytes and protein, a low CSF glucose is common.

Tuberculous meningitis may occur in the course of miliary tuberculosis or as the result of rupture of a subependymal tubercle. Treatment is with rifampin, isoniazid, and dexamethazone. ***Cryptococcal meningitis*** is seen most often with immunosuppression or AIDS. India ink of the spun CSF sediment or latex agglutination studies for cryptococcal antigen in CSF and serum have a sensitivity of about 90%. Treatment is with amphotericin B plus 5-flucytosine or fluconazole alone.

Free-living **amoebae** of the genus *Naegleria* can cause meningitis in swimmers in nonchlorinated, freshwater lakes and pools. Spirochetal causes of meningitis include **syphilis, leptospirosis,** and **Lyme disease.** In patients with AIDS or immunosuppression, meningitis can be seen from cytomegalovirus, histoplasmosis, atypical mycobacterium, and toxoplasmosis.

Prevention of meningitis is accomplished by antimicrobial therapy and vaccination. In cases of meningococcal and *Haemophilus influenzae* meningitis, prophylaxis with rifampin should be administered to intimate contacts of the patient. Vaccinations are available for protection against selected strains of *Streptococcus pneumoniae*, *Neisseria meningitidis*, and *Haemophilus influenzae* type B.

BRAIN ABSCESS

A brain abscess develops when the parenchyma of the brain is seeded with microorganisms arising from the following: (1) contiguous sites of infection such as paranasal sinusitis, otitis media, mastoiditis, and facial and dental infection; (2) direct innoculation such as may occur with skull fracture, fracture of the cribiform plate, and neurosurgery; or (3) distant sites by hemotogenous spread such as with endocarditis, pneumonia, empyema, and congenital heart disease with right-to-left shunts. Multiple abscesses would be characteristic of a hematogenous source.

The most common organisms are aerobic and anaerobic streptococci, *Staphylococcus aureus,* the *Enterobacteriaceae,* and *Bacteroides* species. Mixed aerobic and anaerobic infections are common and may occur in more than 50% of cases. In patients with AIDS or immunosuppression, brain abscesses may develop due to *Listeria, Nocardia, Cryptococcus, Candida, Aspergillus,* and *Toxoplasma.*

Symptoms may be nonspecific but, in general, include altered levels of consciousness, headache, lethargy, nausea, vomiting, seizures, and focal neurologic deficits. The duration of symptoms in most cases is over a 2-week period. A minority of patients manifest fever or nuchal rigidity. Lumbar puncture is contraindicated in a patient with sus-

pected brain abscess. The diagnostic procedure of choice is CT or MRI scan of the brain, which shows a rounded mass lesion with a central area of hypolucency, contrast enhancement, and edema of the surrounding tissue.

Empiric antibiotic therapy for brain abscesses includes penicillin G plus metronidazole or chloramphenical. A third-generation cephalosporin (ceftriaxone) can be added if gram-negative rods are suspected and a penicillinase-resistant penicillin substituted for penicillin G if *Staphylococcus aureus* is a consideration. In a penicillin-allergic patient, chloramphenicol plus metronidazole are the drugs of choice. Decisions regarding surgical therapy must be made on an individual basis and depend on the location of the abscess(es), the neurologic condition of the patient, and the response to antibiotic therapy as determined by serial CT or MRI.

ENCEPHALITIS

Encephalitis results either from direct invasion of the brain by microorganisms or from post- or parainfectious processes that activate an inflammatory response within the CNS. Most organisms reach the brain by the hematogenous route, but some such as herpes simplex, poliomyelitis, and rabies viruses travel along peripheral nerves to invade the brain.

Postinfectious encephalitis may follow primary infection with measles, mumps, rubella, and varicella. Reye's syndrome of fatty liver infiltration and encephalopathy in children has been associated with acetylsalicyclic acid treatment of influenzae type B or varicella.

Clinical findings vary with the organism and area of the brain affected. These include headache, fever, altered mental status with depressed consciousness progressing to coma, focal neurologic deficits, seizures, motor weakness, increased reflexes, a positive extensor–plantar reflex, involuntary movements, diabetes insipidus, syndrome of inappropriate antidiuretic hormone, and dysregulation of the autonomic control of temperature and blood pressure.

Tissue tropism results in localization of most herpes simplex infections to the temporal lobes, arbovirus infections to the gray matter, and the papovirus to the white matter. Temporal lobe involvement in herpes simplex encephalitis may be manifested by auditory and olfactory hallucinations and bizarre behavior. Spinal fluid examination in viral encephalitis usually shows pleocytosis with 10 to 2,000 white blood cells, predominantly mononuclear cells. Glucose is usually within normal limits, and RBCs protein may be normal to slightly increased. Increased CSF is found with herpes simplex encephalitis. Diagnosis of herpes encephalitis is suggested by the EEG, nuclear brain scan, CT, or MRI scans demonstrating involvement of the temporal lobes. The diagnosis should be confirmed by brain biopsy. Herpes simplex encephalitis is treatable with acyclovir, but therapy of other types of viral encephalitis is only supportive.

Common viral etiologies of encephalitis have characteristics such as seasonal variation and geographic distribution, which aid in their differential diagnosis. Eastern, Western, Venezuelan, and St. Louis equine encephalitides, and California encephalitis, are transmitted by arthropod vectors and are therefore most active in the spring and summer. Enterovirus infection such as poliomyelitis, Coxsackie virus, and echovirus occurs most often in the late summer and fall. Mumps infection occurs in the winter and spring. HSV encephalitis has no seasonal variation and occurs at any time of the year.

Diagnosis of the specific virus is made by the demonstration of a rise in antibody titer between acute and convalescent sera.

NEUROSYPHILIS

Neurosyphilis is a late manifestation of infection with *Treponema pallidum*, occurring many years after the primary infection. It is thought that the spirochetemia that accompanies primary infection results in meningeal seeding.

Meningovascular syphilis usually occurs 5 to 10 years after the primary infection. Primary brain involvement, called *general paresis*, occurs after 15 to 40 years. Often these two manifestations overlap. In some patients neurosyphilis may be asymptomatic, and the diagnosis is established only by the abnormal spinal fluid. Clinical manifestations of meningovascular syphilis include a presentation of subacute or chronic meningitis along with multiple focal neurologic deficits secondary to vasculitis and infarctions. Hemiparesis and seizure disorder are common. General paresis causes progressive dementia, change in personality, delusions, hallucinations, Argyll Robertson pupil, hyperreflexia, optic atrophy, and hearing deficits.

Tabes dorsalis is a late effect of syphilis on the spinal cord. Demyelination of the posterior columns and dorsal nerve roots causes ataxia, paresthesias, lancinating pain in the extremities, decreased position and vibration sensation, bladder dysfunction, loss of pain and temperature sensation, and Charcot joints.

Diagnosis of neurosyphilis is made with positive serum fluorescent treponemal antibody test showing previous infection with *Treponema pallidum* and a compatible clinical illness with unexplained abnormal spinal fluid showing pleocytosis and elevated protein. A positive VDRL serologic test and the spinal fluid confirms the diagnosis. Treatment is with intravenous penicillin G. Follow-up CSF studies should be repeated every 3 months for the first year, then every 6 months for 2 years to document clearing of the pleocytosis and decrease in the protein and VDRL titers.

GUILLAIN-BARRÉ SYNDROME

The Guillain-Barré syndrome is described as an ascending, predominantly motor polyneuritis of unknown etiology. In about half of cases, it is preceded by a mild respiratory or GI infection. In most patients it results in varying degrees of motor weakness affecting both proximal and distal extremity muscles. Pain is uncommon but paraesthesias are frequently seen. Cranial nerves may be affected. Pathologically, it is characterized by foci of demyelination of peripheral nerves and perivascular lymphocyte infiltration. It is thought to result from cell-mediated immunity directed against myelin, but systemic involvement is also seen with lymphocyte infiltration of the lymph nodes, spleen, liver, and other organs. In most patients the CSF is within normal limits or has mildly elevated protein. In 10% of cases there may be pleocytosis with 10 to 200 cells, predominantly lymphocytes and monocytes. Respiratory muscle weakness may progress to the point that tracheostomy and ventilatory support are necessary. Autonomic neuropathy with cardiac dysrhythmias and hypotension is a most serious feature of the disease. Although some may have a prolonged course, 75% of patients recover completely within a few weeks.

SLOW VIRUS INFECTIONS

Slow and chronic virus infections are rare but are associated with syndromes of dementia, myoclonus, and death in adults (Jakob-Creutzfeldt disease), and a similar picture is seen in children (subacute sclerosing panencephalitis), with high titers of measles antibody and myxovirus found in the brain. No treatment is known for these disorders.

QUESTIONS IN INTERNAL MEDICINE

Both essay and multiple-choice questions are presented in this section. The answers to the multiple-choice questions are at the end of this chapter. The answers to the rhetorical questions are in the text.

Cardiology

Describe the most common forms of congenital cardiac disease and their treatment.

Name the common extracardiac lesions of rheumatic heart disease.

Give the principal signs and symptoms of congestive cardiac failure.

Name the frequent precipitating causes of congestive cardiac failure.

Outline the treatment of congestive cardiac failure.

Describe the murmur of mitral insufficiency and the mechanism of its production; describe the same for mitral stenosis.

What happens to the presystolic murmur of mitral stenosis if atrial fibrillation intervenes?

Give the etiology, signs, symptoms, prognosis, and treatment of subacute bacterial endocarditis.

Describe the symptoms, diagnosis, and treatment of angina pectoris and contrast them with those of acute myocardial infarction.

Review the diagnosis and treatment of HCM and contrast with other cardiomyopathies.

Describe clinical manifestations of cor pulmonale.

What causes are known for hypertension?

What pathologic changes are found in the heart and the arterioles in hypertension?

Describe accelerated hypertension.

Classify the cardiac arrhythmias and describe the treatment of each.

Name the causes of pericarditis.

Hematology

Name the common causes of anemia.

Name and describe an example of each major class of anemia.

Contrast the hereditary hemolytic anemias with acquired hemolytic anemias.

Name the causes of secondary aplastic anemia.

Give the clinical picture and the outstanding pathology of pernicious anemia; describe the gastric contents and the blood picture; outline the treatment of pernicious anemia; explain how the blood picture indicates the response.

Give the clinical picture and the blood findings of chronic myelocytic leukemia; chronic lymphatic leukemia. How are the two differentiated by blood examination; what are their therapy and results?

Describe acute leukemia.

Differentiate infectious mononucleosis from leukemia.

Give the clinical picture, pathology, diagnosis, and treatment of Hodgkin's disease.

How is hemophilia transmitted? Give the blood findings and treatment for each syndrome.

Classify the purpuras and their blood pictures. What is the value of splenectomy?

Describe the causation, clinical picture, and treatment of agranulocytosis.

Describe the clinical picture of multiple myeloma.

Pulmonology

Describe the clinical picture of chronic tuberculosis of the lungs.

Discuss the therapy of tuberculosis.

Discuss the etiology of lobar pneumonia.

Describe the onset and typical symptoms of pneumococcal pneumonia.

What are the common complications of pneumococcal pneumonia?

Describe the viral pneumonias.

Discuss the etiology, symptomatology, and diagnosis of pulmonary infarct.

Describe chronic obstructive pulmonary disease.

What is the characteristic respiration of bronchial asthma? Discuss the etiology and treatment.

Name the most common form of pneumoconiosis.

Nephrology

How do you measure GFR clinically?

List the glomerular diseases.

What is the nephrotic syndrome?

Describe idiopathic membranous nephropathy.

Discuss lupus nephritis.

What is the natural history of diabetic nephropathy?

Contrast the etiology and course of acute renal failure with chronic renal failure.

Describe the uremic syndrome and outline available treatment.

Gastroenterology

Describe the major diseases of the esophagus.

Discuss the etiology, location, pathology, symptomatology, diagnosis, and complications of peptic ulcer.

How is peptic ulcer treated medically?

What are the indications for surgery of peptic ulcer?

Name the causes of the malabsorption syndrome.

Differentiate the two types of chronic inflammatory bowel disease.

Describe the type of viral hepatitis and discuss the clinical picture of each.

Differentiate three types of jaundice.

Discuss the etiology, pathology, and differential diagnosis of cirrhosis.

Endocrinology

Describe the thyroid nodules and give reasons for their surgical removal.

Describe the classic symptoms, pathologic physiology, differential diagnosis, laboratory findings, and treatment of exophthalmic goiter.

Classify diabetes mellitus.

What are the early symptoms of diabetes mellitus?

Discuss the etiologic factors and the pathology of diabetes mellitus and give the common complications.

Discuss the treatment of diabetes mellitus.

Describe the clinical picture, laboratory findings, and treatment of diabetic acidosis.

Describe hypothyroidism and its treatment.

Classify hyperadrenalism and the diagnosis and treatment of each category.

What is a prolactinoma?

Infectious Diseases

Discuss the incubation period and the infectivity of measles.

List the common complications of measles.

Describe the pathology and clinical manifestations of rheumatic fever.

Discuss the diagnosis of diphtheria. What are the principal complications? How is antitoxin used? Discuss prophylactic immunization.

Discuss the etiology, incubation period, infectivity, and clinical picture of Group A streptococcus infections. What are the common sequelae?

Discuss the treatment of hemolytic streptococcal infection.

What are the complications of streptococcal infections?

Discuss the etiology, clinical picture, complications, and treatment of erysipelas and wound infections.

Give three examples of opportunistic infections; that is, infections that may develop in a compromised host.

Define *retrovirus* and describe the pathophysiology of AIDS, including its complications.

Rheumatology

Distinguish rheumatoid arthritis from osteoarthritis pathologically and clinically.

Which laboratory procedures assist in differentiation of rheumatoid and osteoarthritis? How is each condition treated, and what is the prognosis for each?

Describe the immunologic process of systemic lupus erythematosus (SLE).

Name the clinical manifestations of SLE.

What drugs induce SLE?

What is the treatment of SLE?

What signs and symptoms characterize polyarteritis?

What is current therapy for gout?

Neurology

Describe three types of neurosyphilis.

Discuss the pathology and clinical picture of multiple sclerosis.

Describe the clinical picture of amyotrophic lateral sclerosis.

Describe parkinsonism and discuss its pathology.

Describe epilepsy.

Describe a grand mal epileptic seizure and differentiate it from a hysterical attack.

Differentiate cerebral hemorrhage from cerebral thrombosis and describe the clinical picture of each; give the prognosis and treatment.

What are the etiology and course of transient ischemic attacks?

Contrast the treatment of evolving stroke with completed stroke.

Describe a migraine syndrome.

Describe the clinical picture and diagnosis of cranial arteritis.

Name the causes of bacterial meningitis and review treatment of each.

List the causes of viral encephalitis.

Discuss the clinical picture, laboratory findings, and prognosis of tuberculous meningitis.

Multiple-Choice Questions

1. Mitral valve prolapse:
   (a) Occurs equally in men and women
   (b) Occurs mostly in women
   (c) Is a disease of the aged
   (d) Is the end of rheumatic mitral insufficiency
   (e) Is one manifestation of Libman-Sacks disease

2. High blood pressure
   (a) Always needs a thorough search for all possible causes
   (b) Never needs a thorough search for all possible causes
   (c) Must be treated unless the patient is asymptomatic and is over 40 years of age
   (d) Must be treated
   (e) Should not be lowered to normal because it may result in renal failure

3. Which one of the following statements is true with regard to the syndrome of relapsing idiopathic acute pericarditis?
   (a) Cardiac tamponade usually develops.
   (b) Constrictive pericarditis usually develops.
   (c) Cardiac arrhythmia is a frequent complication.
   (d) Chest pain is usually the only major disabling feature.
   (e) Pericardiectomy consistently provides long-term relief.

4. Patients with which of the following cardiac disorders have the highest risks of developing bacterial endocarditis?
   (a) Congenital aortic stenosis
   (b) Mitral valve prolapse without a murmur
   (c) Secundum atrial septal defect
   (d) Aortocoronary bypass

5. Which of the following is/are the best treatment of "Torsades des Pointes"?
   (a) Discontinued quinidine
   (b) Magnesium (intravenously)
   (c) Isoproterenol
   (d) Temporary pacemaker
   (e) All of the above

6. Which of the following is true of the angiotensin-converting enzyme (ACE) inhibitors in the treatment of heart failure?
   (a) Increase the incidence of arrhythmias
   (b) Hypokalemia
   (c) Increase contractility
   (d) Improve long-term survival

7. Which of the following is a feature/are features of hypertrophic cardiomyopathy?
   (a) Normal systolic function
   (b) Impaired ventricular relaxation
   (c) Asymmetric septal hypertrophy
   (d) All of the above

8. Which of the following is a feature/are features of the aging process?
   (a) Mitral stenosis
   (b) Aortic stenosis
   (c) Aortic regurgitation
   (d) Tricuspid stenosis
   (e) Mitral regurgitation

9. Which of the following is a feature/are features of myocardial infarction?
   (a) Mitral stenosis
   (b) Aortic stenosis
   (c) Aortic regurgitation
   (d) Tricuspid stenosis
   (e) Mitral regurgitation

10. Which of the following is a feature/are features of carcinoid tumors?
    (a) Mitral stenosis
    (b) Aortic stenosis
    (c) Aortic regurgitation
    (d) Tricuspid stenosis
    (e) Mitral regurgitation

11. Which of the following is a feature/are features of Marfan's syndrome?
    (a) Mitral stenosis
    (b) Aortic stenosis
    (c) Aortic regurgitation
    (d) Tricuspid stenosis
    (e) Mitral regurgitation

12. Which of the following is a feature/are features of brisk carotid pulse?
    (a) Aortic stenosis
    (b) Hypertrophic cardiomyopathy
    (c) Both
    (d) Neither

13. Which of the following is a feature/are features of systolic murmur?
    (a) Aortic stenosis
    (b) Hypertrophic cardiomyopathy
    (c) Both
    (d) Neither

14. Which of the following is a feature/are features of S_4 gallop?
    (a) Aortic stenosis
    (b) Hypertrophic cardiomyopathy
    (c) Both
    (d) Neither

15. Which of the following is a feature/are features of absent second sound?
    (a) Aortic stenosis
    (b) Hypertrophic cardiomyopathy

(c) Both

(d) Neither

16. Which of the following is a feature/are features of sustained apical impulse?
    (a) Aortic stenosis
    (b) Hypertrophic cardiomyopathy
    (c) Both
    (d) Neither

17. Which of the following conditions contribute to altered cardiac function in congestive heart failure?
    (a) Decreased contractility
    (b) Pressure overload
    (c) Volume overload
    (d) Restricted ventricular filling
    (e) All of the above

18. Echocardiographic thickened and redundant mitral valve leaflets in patients with MVP are associated with increased risk of:
    (a) Cerebral ischemic event
    (b) Infective endocarditis
    (c) Sudden death
    (d) All of the above
    (e) None of the above

19. Atrial flutter can be treated with which of the following?
    (a) Digoxin
    (b) β-blockers
    (c) Verapamil
    (d) Quinidine
    (e) All of the above

20. Anemia in women:
    (a) Is treated with iron
    (b) Is treated with iron and if unresponsive vitamin B_{12} and folic acid are added
    (c) Is the autoimmune hemolytic anemia of lupus until proved otherwise
    (d) Requires a search for cause
    (e) Should not be treated unless the hemoglobin is below 11.5 g/100 ml.

21. A 50-year-old man complains of fatigue. History is otherwise negative as is the physical examination. CBC is entirely normal. Urinalysis is normal. The only abnormal finding is a monoclonal IgG gammopathy in the serum. Which statement is correct?
    (a) Bone x rays and a bone marrow biopsy are indicated.
    (b) The patient has multiple myeloma.
    (c) The patient has a benign monoclonal gammopathy.
    (d) Cytoxan or Alkeran should be started.
    (e) He probably has leukemia and should be followed.

22. A 50-year-old patient previously in good health had sudden onset of right anterior chest pain without chills, fever, or cough. On physical examination he was tachypneic and had a temperature of 99.4° F. Over the right lower rib cage there was an inspiratory rub. Chest x ray was negative. Which statement is correct?
    (a) Viral pneumonia is the most likely diagnosis.
    (b) Pneumococcal pneumonia is most likely and penicillin should be given.
    (c) Pulmonary embolus must be considered promptly.
    (d) Bronchoscopy needs to be done promptly.
    (e) Bronchogenic carcinoma is most likely.

23. Bronchogenic carcinoma:
    (a) May be a largely preventable disease
    (b) Has a 50% cure rate
    (c) Responds to cytoxan
    (d) Is synonymous with "coin" lesion
    (e) Responds well to x rays

24. A 28-year-old woman has the acute onset of oliguria, gross hematuria, nausea, and vomiting. On physical examination she has 1+ edema, blood pressure of 180/110. Urinalysis was 3+ protein, red blood cells, and red cell casts. BUN is 40 mg/100 ml. Which statement is correct?
    (a) She has the nephrotic syndrome.
    (b) She has lupus nephritis.
    (c) She has pyelonephritis.
    (d) She has acute tubular necrosis.
    (e) She has the acute glomerular syndrome.

25. A 50-year-old woman begins to experience fatigue and weakness. Her only past history is severe headache for 20 years. Physical examination reveals a sallow, chronically ill-appearing woman; the remainder of the physical is negative. She is found to have a hemoglobin of 9 g/100 ml. Urine reveals a trace of protein, 10 to 12 white cells and a rare white cell cast. Urine culture is sterile. BUN is 40 mg/100 ml. Which statement is correct?
    (a) She has chronic glomerulonephritis.
    (b) She has lupus.
    (c) She has interstitial nephritis, for example, analgesic abuse, tuberculosis, obstruction.
    (d) She has inactive pyelonephritis.
    (e) She has multiple myeloma.

26. Which statement is correct?
    (a) With cimetadine's availability, antacids

have no place in managing peptic ulcer (except in the patient who is allergic to cimetadine).

(b) The indications for peptic ulcer surgery are obstruction, perforation, uncontrolled or recurrent hemorrhage, and intractability.

(c) Everyone with peptic ulcer should have a serum gastrin determination.

(d) Everyone with peptic ulcer should have a parathyroid hormone assay done.

(e) With cimetadine, smoking and alcohol in moderation are less harmful in patients with a peptic ulcer.

27. Which statement is correct?
(a) Crohn's disease never involves the colon.
(b) Ulcerative colitis never involves the small bowel.
(c) Colectomy is good treatment for Crohn's disease.
(d) Cancer of the colon is rare.
(e) Many cancers of the colon can be diagnosed by proctoscopy.

28. Which of the following laboratory values would *not* be expected in iron deficiency anemia?
(a) Low ferritin level
(b) Low haptoglobin level
(c) Elevated total iron-binding capacity
(d) Normal MCV

29. Which study is the most accurate in differentiating iron deficiency anemia from the anemia of chronic disease?
(a) MCV
(b) Multiphasic blood chemistry profile
(c) Bone marrow iron stain
(d) Ferritin level

30. A 30-year-old black female complains of an unsteady gait and a sore tongue. A CBC includes WBC 3,600; hemoglobin 9.6 g/dl; and MCV 124. Which of the following is most appropriate as the *next* step in her laboratory evaluation?
(a) B$_{12}$ and folate levels
(b) Bone marrow exam
(c) Schilling test
(d) LDH level

31. A 30-year-old white male is found to have moderate splenomegaly at the time of a pre-employment physical exam. To evaluate this finding, the *initial* approach should be which of the following?
(a) CBC

(b) Bone marrow exam
(c) Additional history
(d) CT scan of the abdomen

32. Which of the following results would *not* be expected in a patient with chronic hemolytic anemia?
(a) Elevated reticulocyte count
(b) Elevated haptoglobin
(c) Elevated "indirect" bilirubin
(d) Elevated LDH

33. Hemolytic anemia with red-cell fragments (schistocytes) is associated with which of the following disorders?
(a) Thrombotic thrombocytopenia purpura
(b) DIC
(c) Severe aortic valvular stenosis
(d) All of the above

34. A 20-year-old black female was found to have sickle-cell trait at a "health fair." Which of the following is appropriate advice?
(a) Avoid airline travel
(b) Have genetic counseling before pregnancy
(c) Have yearly retinal exams by an ophthalmologist
(d) Take folic acid 1 mg daily

35. Which of the following medications is most frequently associated with a positive direct Coombs test?
(a) Cimetidine
(b) Diazepam
(c) Methyldopa
(d) Chloramphenicol

36. A 60-year-old male with peptic ulcer disease and hypertension is found to have a hematocrit of 59%. He has no history of tobacco use or pulmonary symptoms. His WBC is 8,900 and his platelet count is 495,000. The next study to investigate the elevated hematocrit should be:
(a) Erythropoietin level
(b) Measurement of red-cell mass
(c) LAP (leukocyte alkaline phosphatase)
(d) IVP

37. Which of the following hematologic diseases has a sex (x-) -linked pattern of inheritance?
(a) Hereditary spherocytosis
(b) Thalassemia
(c) Von Willebrand's disease
(d) Glucose-6-phosphate dehydrogenase deficiency

38. Which of the following findings would *not* be expected in a patient with multiple myeloma?

(a) Lymphadenopathy
(b) Bone pain
(c) Pneumonia
(d) Anemia

39. Which statement is correct?
    (a) An elevated T_4 means hyperthyroidism.
    (b) Antithyroid drugs have no place in treatment of hyperthyroidism.
    (c) Inorganic iodine should be given to all patients with hyperthyroidism.
    (d) Elevation of both T_3 and T_4 geneally indicates hyperthyroidism.
    (e) Abortion is indicated if hyperthyroidism develops during early pregnancy.

40. Which statement is correct?
    (a) Primary hypothyroidism may reverse spontaneously.
    (b) Propranolol controls the symptoms in 40% of patients with myxedema.
    (c) Myxedema coma is an emergency.
    (d) Myxedema is uncommon in an affluent society.
    (e) Myxedema is never associated with goiter.

41. Which statement is correct?
    (a) SLE is very rare.
    (b) Antinuclear antibodies are an almost consistent feature of SLE.
    (c) There is no satisfactory treatment of SLE.
    (d) Renal involvement with SLE does not respond to treatment.
    (e) Arthritis is against true lupus.

42. Which statement is correct?
    (a) Gout is rare without hyperuricemia.
    (b) Gouty arthritis does not result in crippling.
    (c) Gout never occurs in women.
    (d) Allopurinol is indicated only after the first uric acid stone is passed.
    (e) Hyperuricemia in malignancy does not require treatment.

43. Anticardiolipin antibodies have been associated with all but which one of the following conditions:
    (a) Recurrent spontaneous abortions
    (b) Thromboembolism
    (c) Hypertension
    (d) Thrombocytopenia

44. Which of the following is a *specific* marker for SLE?
    (a) ANA
    (b) Anti-Sin
    (c) SS-A, SS-B
    (d) LE prep

45. The drug of choice for renal scleroderma with hypertension is:
    (a) Thiazide diuretic
    (b) Methyldopa
    (c) β-blocker
    (d) ACE inhibitor

46. Effective therapy for Raynaud's phenomenon includes all of the following except:
    (a) Propranolol
    (b) Prazosin
    (c) Diltiazem
    (d) Nifedipine

47. Wegener's Granulomatosis is best treated with:
    (a) Prednisone
    (b) Salicylates
    (c) Plasmapheresis
    (d) Cyclophosphamide

48. All of the following are helpful in diagnosing polymyositis except for:
    (a) Westergren sedimentation rate
    (b) Electromyogram
    (c) CPK, SGOT, LDH, aldolase
    (d) Muscle biopsy

49. The diagnosis of primary Sjögren's syndrome is *best* made by:
    (a) Minor salivary gland biopsy (lip biopsy)
    (b) Sialogram
    (c) ANA
    (d) Joint x rays

50. *Borrelia burgdorferi* is the etiologic agent of:
    (a) Rheumatoid arthritis
    (b) Sjögren's syndrome
    (c) Systemic lupus erythematosus
    (d) Lyme disease

51. The radiographic findings of rheumatoid arthritis include all of the following except:
    (a) Juxta-articular osteopenia
    (b) Joint space narrowing
    (c) Osteophytes
    (d) Bony erosions

52. Which of the following *best* supports the diagnosis of ankylosing spondylitis?
    (a) Radiographic sacroiliitis
    (b) Elevated sedimentation rate
    (c) HLA-B27 positivity
    (d) Elevated C-reactive protein

53. A 70-year-old man undergoes a sigmoid colon resection for diverticulitis. Gentamicin and ampicillin are given for one week. Two weeks after surgery he develops fever (39.5° C), ab-

dominal pain, and tenderness. The incision appears normal. The most likely bacterial etiology of his symptoms is:
(a) *Staphylococcus aureus*
(b) *Escherichia coli*
(c) *Clostridium perfringens*
(d) *Bacteroides fragilis*
(e) *Proteus mirabilis*

54. A 64-year-old white male is admitted to the hospital with a history of recurrent intermittent episodes of maroon-colored stools. X rays of the stomach and small bowel are negative. Colonoscopy reveals no bleeding site. The procedure most likely to reveal the diagnosis is:
(a) Abdominal ultrasound
(b) Gallium scan
(c) Exploratory laparatomy
(d) Angiography
(e) A string test

55. A 60-year-old man with a bicuspid aortic valve presents with fever, tachycardia, and dyspnea on exertion. Five blood cultures grow *Streptococcus bovis*. Following response to penicillin G therapy, which of the following should be performed?
(a) Intravenous pyelogram
(b) Colonoscopy
(c) 24-hour urinary protein excretion
(d) Indium scan
(e) Antinuclear factor

56. An asymptomatic 22-year-old woman (nonsmoker) has a chest x ray as part of her pre-employment evaluation. A 1.5 cm non-calcified nodule is seen in the left lower lobe. An IPPD skin test is negative. The next step is:
(a) Thoracotomy
(b) Histoplasmin skin test
(c) Second strength PPD skin test
(d) Fungal immunodiffusion screen
(e) Observation

57. All but which of the following are major risk factors for coronary artery disease?
(a) Obesity
(b) Hyperlipidemia
(c) Cigarette smoking
(d) Hyperuricemia
(e) Hypertension

58. Isolated aortic insufficiency:
(a) Is one clinical manifestation of a congenitally bicuspid aortic valve
(b) Is seen in most cases of dissection of the abdominal aorta

(c) May complicate long-standing arterial hypertension
(d) Is often due to rheumatic fever
(e) All of the above

59. A 30-year-old female presents with diarrhea of 1-week duration and a 2-day history of tender, red nodules over the anterior lower legs. Diagnostic possibilities include all of the following except:
(a) Ulcerative colitis
(b) Yersinia infection
(c) Sarcoidosis
(d) Regional enteritis
(e) Gluten-sensitive enteropathy

60. A 27-year-old male homosexual comes to you for evaluation to rule out sexually transmitted diseases. He has discovered a maculopapular rash on his trunk and palms. It is appropriate after counseling to initially obtain:
(a) HIV antibody
(b) Rapid plasma reagin
(c) Fluorescent treponemal antibody absorption
(d) Hepatitis B core antibody
(e) Antichlamydial antibody test

61. Pneumococcal vaccine is indicated for patients with:
(a) Chronic bronchitis
(b) Splenectomy
(c) Valvular heart disease
(d) Chronic renal disease
(e) All of the above

62. Pericardial tamponade:
(a) Develops when more than 150 ml of fluid collects in the pericardial space
(b) Is characterized by clear lung fields and an elevated central venous pressure
(c) Is frequently associated with acute myocardial infarction
(d) Is an indication for surgical removal of the pericardium
(e) All of the above

63. High serum amylase levels may be seen in all of the following except:
(a) Ruptured pancreatic cyst
(b) Chronic congestive heart failure
(c) Ruptured ectopic pregnancy
(d) Mumps
(e) Acute pancreatitis

64. A screening endoscopy shows multiple duodenal ulcers in a patient who has not responded to antacids. The most likely diagnosis is:
(a) Duodenal carcinoma

(b) Gastrinoma

(c) Pernicious anemia

(d) Carcinoid syndrome

(e) Cushing's syndrome

65. A 45-year-old woman comes to the emergency room because of nausea, vomiting, and abdominal pain. Differential diagnoses include:

(a) Acute intermittent porphyria

(b) Familial hyperlipemia

(c) Diabetic ketoacidosis

(d) Adrenal insufficiency crises

(e) All of the above

66. Factors that suggest a need for admission to the hospital of a 24-year-old female having an asthmatic attack include:

(a) Tachycardia of 115 beats per minute

(b) Arterial PaO_2 of 68 mmHg

(c) Hemoglobin of 16 g/dl

(d) Eosinophilia

(e) All of the above

67. Increased alveolar ventilation is characteristic of:

(a) Acute airway obstruction

(b) Pulmonary embolus

(c) Hepatic failure

(d) Lactic acidosis

(e) None of the above

68. Carcinoma of the lung is likely nonresectable with which of the following:

(a) Malignant cells in the pleural fluid

(b) Mediastinal node metastasis

(c) Preoperative arterial $pO_2 = 85$

(d) Paralysis of a vocal cord

(e) None of the above

69. A 34-year-old woman with disseminated lupus erythematosus being treated for nephritis with prednisone develops a cough. Chest x rays show an infiltrate. Cryptococci are seen in bronchoalveolar lavage fluid. Appropriate evaluation includes each of the following *except:*

(a) Skin testing for fungi

(b) Serologic testing for cryptococcal antigen

(c) Lumbar puncture

(d) Bone marrow culture for fungi

(e) Urine culture for fungi

70. A dyspneic 28-year-old black woman has symmetrical bilateral hilar lymphadenopathy without parenchymal infiltrates on chest roentgenograms. Which of the following is most likely to be diagnostically useful?

(a) Transbronchial biopsy

(b) Mediastinoscopy

(c) Serum angiotensin converting enzyme

(d) Sputum culture

(e) Diffusion pulmonary function tests

71. A 36-year-old woman with tigtening facial skin and dysphagia has gradually become dyspneic. Further evaluation is likely to reveal which of the following?

(a) Hypoxemia

(b) Raynaud's phenomenon

(c) Decreased total lung capacity and diffusing capacity

(d) A decrease in $FEV_1 : FVC$ ratio with administration of a bronchodilator

(e) All of the above

72. Empyema fluid is characterized by which of the following:

(a) Spontaneous clotting

(b) Elevated protein concentration

(c) $pH \leq 7.2$

(d) Elevated glucose concentration

(e) Decreased lactic dehydrogenase concentration

73. Predisposing factors associated with the development of acute respiratory disease syndrome (ARDS) include:

(a) Bacteremia

(b) Acute pancreatitis

(c) Multiple organ trauma

(d) Diabetic ketoacidosis

(e) All of the above

74. Physical examination reveals a blood pressure of 200/110 mmHg, thin extremities, and ecchymoses in a 39-year-old man who complains of a gradual increase in weight and emotional instability. The most useful initial screening test is:

(a) A CT scan of the adrenal glands

(b) 24-hour urinary excretion of 17 ketosteroids

(c) 24-hour urinary excretion of catecholamines

(d) Dexamethasone suppression test

(e) Measurment of serum potassium concentration

75. Secondary polycythemia in a 68-year-old man with chronic obstructive pulmonary disease is *not* associated with:

(a) Splenomegaly

(b) Leukocytosis

(c) Decreased erythrocyte survival time

(d) Arterial $pO_2 = 90$

(e) Any of the above

76. A 46-year-old man has nontrauma-associated ecchymoses on his arms and legs. Laboratory

evaluation shows a prothrombin time of 17 seconds (control = 11 sec). After administration of vitamin K, the prothrombin time returns to normal. Possible causes of his prolonged prothrombin time include:
(a) Carcinoma of the pancreas
(b) Viral hepatitis
(c) Celiac disease
(d) A calculus in the common bile duct
(e) All of the above

Matching Questions

Match the diagnoses with the blood concentrations and pH (a–e).

pH	Arterial PaO_2	Arterial $PaCO_2$
(a) 7.45	105	30
(b) 7.20	115	21
(c) 7.53	80	50
(d) 7.26	64	64
(e) 7.47	60	25

77. Status asthmaticus
78. Pulmonary embolism
79. Diabetic ketoacidosis
80. Prolonged vomiting
81. Hyperventilation

ANSWERS TO MULTIPLE-CHOICE AND MATCHING QUESTIONS

1. (b)	**28.** (b)	**55.** (b)
2. (d)	**29.** (c)	**56.** (b)
3. (d)	**30.** (a)	**57.** (d)
4. (a)	**31.** (c)	**58.** (a), (c)
5. (e)	**32.** (b)	**59.** (e)
6. (d)	**33.** (d)	**60.** (a), (b), (c)
7. (d)	**34.** (b)	**61.** (e)
8. (b)	**35.** (c)	**62.** (b)
9. (e)	**36.** (b)	**63.** (b)
10. (d)	**37.** (d)	**64.** (b)
11. (c)	**38.** (a)	**65.** (e)
12. (b)	**39.** (d)	**66.** (b)
13. (c)	**40.** (c)	**67.** (b), (c), (d)
14. (c)	**41.** (b)	**68.** (a), (b), (d)
15. (a)	**42.** (a)	**69.** (a), (d)
16. (c)	**43.** (c)	**70.** (b)
17. (e)	**44.** (b)	**71.** (e)
18. (d)	**45.** (d)	**72.** (b), (c)
19. (e)	**46.** (a)	**73.** (e)
20. (d)	**47.** (d)	**74.** (d)
21. (a)	**48.** (a)	**75.** (e)
22. (c)	**49.** (a)	**76.** (a), (c), (d)
23. (a)	**50.** (d)	**77.** (d)
24. (e)	**51.** (c)	**78.** (e)
25. (c)	**52.** (a)	**79.** (b)
26. (b)	**53.** (d)	**80.** (c)
27. (e)	**54.** (d)	**81.** (a)

Rypins' Clinical Sciences Review, 16th Edition, edited by Edward D. Frohlich. J. B. Lippincott Company, Philadelphia © 1993.

4

Obstetrics and Gynecology

Martin L. Pernoll, M.D., F.A.C.O.G., F.A.C.S.
Clinical Professor,
University of Kansas Medical School,
Kansas City, Kansas
Hermann Hospital
Houston, Texas

OBSTETRICS

Obstetrics is that branch of medicine dealing with parturition, its antecedents, and its sequelae. The objectives of maternity care set forth by the World Health Organization (WHO) are to ensure that every expectant and nursing mother maintains good health, learns the art of child care, has a normal delivery, and bears healthy children. In the narrower sense maternity care consists of care of the pregnant woman, her safe delivery, her postnatal examination, the care of her newborn infant, and the maintenance of lactation. In the wider sense it begins much earlier in measures aimed to promote the health and well-being of the young people who are potential parents, and to help them to develop the right approach to family life and to the place of the family in the community.

The reduction in maternal mortality over the past half-century has been one of the most dramatic and gratifying trends in medicine. Except for two brief periods, the rate has fallen steadily in that time span; maternal mortality has declined from rates of 668.6/100,000 live births during the period 1925

to 1929, from rates of 245.2 down to 116.6 in the mid-1940s, to the current rate of less than 8.5/100,000. The maternal mortality rate reflects the quality of obstetric care since studies have shown that up to two thirds of maternal and between one third and one half of perinatal (sum of fetal and neonatal) death rates might have been prevented with modern-day management practices. These same considerations bear upon the likelihood of permanent damage among surviving infants born under adverse circumstances. In addition, these several parameters provide an index of the overall socioeconomic status of the population under study. Despite great overall reduction in maternal mortality in the United States in recent decades, nonwhite populations are still disadvantaged when compared with whites. Currently, maternal mortality rate in the nonwhite population is approximately three times that of the white. The former rate recorded for nonwhite women was achieved in the white population during the mid-1960s.

The many variables relating to higher risks of maternal mortality include such cultural variables as age at marriage, age at first pregnancy, number of children, state of nutrition, degree of health abuse involving adverse drinking, drug and smoking habits, as well as knowledge and cooperation in participating in health care delivery. Despite the considerable progress in reducing maternal mortality rates, the specific causes of death have remained the same: toxemia, hemorrhage, and sepsis, followed by ectopic pregnancy and abortion, which of course may be associated with both hemorrhage and infection. All other causes, classified under miscellaneous complications, account for an increasing proportion of total cases, representing more than one third. In individual health care institutions, notably tertiary care centers, certain causes of death, such as heart disease and anesthesia-related deaths, may loom relatively larger. The factor of maternal age in relation to the risk of childbearing is particularly noteworthy because older women tend to be more vulnerable to toxemia (which may be superimposed upon preexisting chronic hypertension), heart disease, chronic cardiovascular disease, placenta previa and ruptured uterus and postpartal hemorrhage; this is particularly true among those of advanced years who are also highly parous. Past obstetric history, reflecting on the quality of the reproductive performance in prior pregnancies, is a particularly important prognostic variable for both mother and infant. Traditionally, maternal mortality is lowest at ages 20 to 24, is slightly higher under 20 years, and rises dramatically after age 30. Maternal mortality rates triple in women aged 35 to 39 and rise five to ten times higher in the decade of the 40s (ten times after age 45).

Traditionally, it has been customary to attribute the dramatic decreases in maternal mortality to delivery in the hospital and avoidance of traumatic operative procedures, availability of blood, antibiotics, more qualified obstetricians, and effective reviews of maternal deaths at local and state levels. Since 1957, more than 95% of all deliveries in the United States have occurred in hospitals, in contrast to only 37% in 1935. Currently, over 98% of births occur in hospitals. At the same time, the concept of high-risk pregnancy calls for identification of women at risk and provision of increased care, usually by transporting vulnerable mothers to tertiary care centers where there are highly trained personnel and sophisticated resources to manage complex medical problems. Undoubtedly, improved socioeconomic and nutritional health over the years, achieved through efforts to reduce poverty and to expand education, has had some impact in lowering maternal mortality rates. Obviously, some societal groups have benefited more than others, and much more is required to make lower maternal risks equal among all women. Responsible family planning practice is one of the key preventative measures.

Throughout the 1970s there were rapid developments and changing concepts in medicine generally and in the field of obstetrics and perinatal medicine in particular. Since 1974 the American Board of Obstetrics and Gynecology has awarded a certification signifying special competence in the subspeciality of maternal and fetal medicine. These individuals, with 2 years of postresidency training become closely associated with neonatologists and other health professionals who together form the perinatal health care team at regional centers. These combined efforts by professionals with special knowledge of perinatal medicine have brought about the recent reductions in fetal and neonatal death rates that had tended to level off in the 1960s (Fig. 4-1). Several striking alterations have occurred in perinatal care; for example, the capability to sustain the life of immature infants in the nursery, the close liaison between the obstetrician and

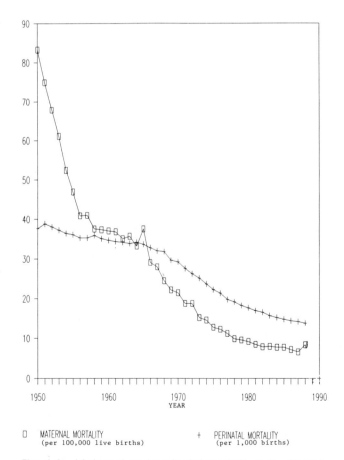

□ MATERNAL MORTALITY
(per 100,000 live births)

+ PERINATAL MORTALITY
(per 1,000 births)

Fig. 4-1. Maternal and perinatal mortality in the United States from 1950 to 1988.

pediatrician in decision making, and a great increase (four- to fivefold) in abdominal delivery since the 1970s. Avoidance of trauma, intervention on a timely planned basis, and extirpation of the fetus from its hostile environment based on objective data gained through continuous fetal monitoring and biometric testing constitute the foundations for these changing attitudes about methods of delivery. Improvement of perinatal and maternal health as a major medical priority has created a sense of direction and a focus for greater effort and prospect for progress. Moreover, recognition that the solution of these health problems necessitates a joint effort of multiple health and health-related agencies, as well as representation by multiple disciplines, has broadened the base of programs directed toward vulnerable groups on a regional basis.

The availability and liberal use of blood and blood products probably transcends all other advances in management of hemorrhage and reduction of the risk of maternal death. By the same token, the routine use of oxytocic agents and ergot preparations to improve uterine tone and to minimize postpartal hemorrhage during the past 5 decades or more has been a significant advance. The availability of an increasing variety of antibiotic agents for specific as well as prophylactic use has made it possible to prevent or control intrapartal or postpartal infections to a large extent. This advance, coupled with strict rules and regulations to establish and maintain appropriate infection-control measures for maternity and newborn services, has caused major reductions in maternal death from infection. A reduction in traumatic obstetrics has resulted in a reduction of maternal and prenatal death from injuries, hemorrhage, and sepsis. Increasing safety of cesarean section, so that this operation now can be performed at the optimal time in a variety of medical and obstetric conditions in the best interests of the fetus as well as the mother, has made it possible to spare most women long complicated labors and difficult vaginal deliveries. The status of obstetric anesthesia has improved with respect to choices, techniques, and qualified personnel. Moreover, the increasing emphasis on the education of the patient, her emotional support, the use of minimal analgesia and on "physiologic" or "natural" childbirth has minimized the necessity for deep narcosis and general anesthesia and acceptance of the potential risks of such management. The advance of conduction anesthesia, including saddle block, lumbar epidural, caudal, and pudendal blocks, has added a significant dimension of safety in the conduct of labor and delivery.

The WHO has encouraged uniform reporting practices and the use of standard definitions that can be universally applied. *Maternal death* is defined as "a woman dying of any cause whatsoever while pregnant or within 90 days of termination of the pregnancy, irrespective of duration of the pregnancy at the time of termination or the method by which it was terminated." When the death results from complications of pregnancy itself, from intervention that is elected or required, or from the chain of events initiated by the complication or the intervention, it is classified as a direct obstetric cause. A death resulting from disease present before or developing during pregnancy that is not a direct effect of the pregnancy, although it may be aggravated by its physiologic effects, is classified as an *indirect obstetric cause.* There may be a nonrelated cause classification applied to any maternal death in which the fatal condition is totally unrelated to pregnancy, its complications or management. Proper classification is dependent upon accurate and complete record keeping. Traditionally almost one third of all maternal deaths are reported as deaths due to nonobstetric causes. It is customary to group maternal deaths into six major categories as follows: (1) sepsis of pregnancy, childbirth, and the puerperium; (2) toxemias of pregnancy and the puerperium; (3) hemorrhage of pregnancy, childbirth, and the puerperium; (4) abortion without mention of sepsis or toxemia; (5) abortion with sepsis; and (6) other complications of pregnancy, childbirth, and the puerperium. Of course, additional subgroup classifications, based on specific nature of the disorder, underlying conditions, and stage of pregnancy when death occurred, are applied to provide more clarification.

Unfortunately, vital statistics of the United States are somewhat misleading because maternal deaths associated with maternal heart disease and other coincidental conditions are not included. Moreover, deaths listed by cause based on data derived from certificates are unclassifiable since no specific complication is mentioned in over 40% of the cases. Nevertheless, hemorrhage, toxemias of pregnancy, and infection still account for almost 60% of reported maternal deaths in the United States. A direct cause of death such as infection may have a significant predisposing factor such as hemorrhage.

As the mortality rates from toxemia, hemorrhage, and infection have decreased, other conditions resulting in maternal deaths have attracted increased clinical attention. Cardiac disease seems destined to become one of the foremost causes of maternal mortality. In some hospitals heart disease already accounts for as much as one quarter of all maternal deaths. Currently, between 10% and 20% of all maternal deaths are considered secondary to vascular catastrophes that may take the form of embolism, hemorrhage, or thrombosis. Maternal deaths directly or indirectly related to complications of anesthesia, notably aspiration of vomitus or overdosage of spinal anesthetics, make up a small but important proportion of all deaths related to pregnancy. Acute infectious hepatitis, pulmonary complications, nonobstetric hypertension, renal diseases, and a variety of other medical disorders loom relatively larger as causes of maternal death as the more traditional obstetric causes are curtailed.

The unfavorable position of the nonwhite group is more marked in maternal mortality than in all but a few nonmaternal causes of death. Moreover, within each geographic division of the United States maternal mortality among nonwhite women is three or four times the rate among white mothers. With respect to cause, the differential between nonwhite and white maternal deaths is fivefold for toxemia, fourfold to fivefold for abortion (sixfold with sepsis), and eightfold to ninefold for ectopic pregnancies. The great increase in pelvic inflammatory disease among white women in all levels of social strata, relating to infections, may be reducing the discrepancy between the races with respect to ectopic gestation.

It is appropriate to consider reproductive losses rather broadly and to recognize that in addition to deaths there will be remote sequelae reflecting damage among surviving infants. The consequences to the mother may be either immediate or remote, depending on the nature and severity of the obstetric problem. In the United States there are approximately 4 million live births a year, representing an annual "fertility rate" of 68.0 live births/1,000 women of reproductive age (15 to 44 years) and a "birth rate" of 15.5/1,000 population. Effective family planning practices and methods in the 1970s resulted in a decline in the United States birth rate, but the trend has favored white women whose fertility rate is 62.4 compared with 83.2 for nonwhites.

Worldwide, it is estimated that perhaps only about one third of all conceptions will terminate in a live birth at term by a normal delivery. A pregnancy terminated before 20 weeks of gestational age or passage of a fetus weighing less than 500 g is designated an **abortion.** These may be either spontaneous or induced. Roughly, 15% of all identified pregnancies are known to terminate by spontaneous abortion. Estimates of the true incidence may be placed much higher, perhaps up to 40% since many early abortions go unrecognized. The general incidence of chromosomal defects in spontaneous abortion is above 50%, but the earlier the abortion, the higher will be the incidence of cytogenetic anomalies. The distribution of errors shows that up to one half take the form of autosomal trisomy, whereas about one quarter exhibit a chromosomal polyploidy and about one eighth demonstrate a monosomy for the X chromosome.

A death *in utero* of a fetus of 20 weeks' gestational age or older or 500 g or over in weight is a *"fetal" death* and the rate is expressed per 1,000 births. The death of a live-born infant of any weight within the first 28 days of life is a *"neonatal" death* and the rate is expressed per 1,000 live births. Some will qualify the definition to exclude any infants of less than 20 weeks of gestational age or weighing less than 500 g (abortions), regardless of any evidence of life at birth. The "perinatal" mortality rate is the sum of the neonatal and fetal death rates. A special designation is the "immature" birth, which represents a pregnancy terminated between 20 weeks and the end of the 27th week or the delivery of an infant weighing between 500 g and 999 g. Infants of 28 weeks' gestational age (up to 36 weeks) or weighing between 1,000 g and 2,500 g are referred as *"prematures"* by the traditional definition. However, these distinctions have less importance at the 28th gestational week since perinatal survival during the immature period is now a realistic potential justifying planned delivery under certain circumstances. Approximately 70% of the neonatal deaths occur in low-birth-weight (for length of gestation) infants, which constitutes a rate 20 times higher than in newborns of normal weight. More infant deaths occur in the first 3 days of life than in the remainder of the entire first year. The special vulnerability lies in the risk, first, of respiratory distress, which is the largest cause of concern, but also of importance are hypoxia, intracranial hemorrhage, malformation, and sepsis. Multiple gestation results in a 50% premature birth rate when traditional definitions are applied. In addition to perinatal deaths, there are morbidity aftermaths of the birth process, including anomalies, neurologic deficits, mental retardation, functional disorders, epilepsy, behavioral problems, etc. For example, roughly 4 or 5 newborns/1,000 will exhibit cerebral palsy. Moreover, perhaps sublethal perinatal insults causing not only cerebral palsy but also epilepsy, mental retardation, learning disabilities, and so forth, occur in about 2% or more of newborns.

Perinatal outcomes reflect more sensitively upon quality of obstetric care than maternal mortality now that the latter rates have been so dramatically reduced. Some studies show that up to about one third of all pregnancies end in abortion, fetal death, or in the death of an infant during the neonatal period, or the infant has a significant anomaly that requires medical care or will interfere with normal functioning, or a low birth weight that imposes its own special hazards and influences the pattern of growth and development. Women whose last prior pregnancy had a poor outcome are subject to relatively high reproductive loss or damage in subsequent pregnancies, and there is a tendency for the same untoward event to occur.

In recent years the neonatal mortality rate, fetal death rate, and perinatal mortality rate have fallen substantially. Currently, perinatal mortality rates of about 14.0/1,000 live births are being achieved, and the neonatal segment is approximately 7.0/1,000 live births. There has been more than a 40% reduction in these rates in the past decade, which reflects favorably upon perinatal care. The postneonatal mortality rate up to 1 year of life is approximately 3.2/1,000 live births. Thus, independent of unrecognized spontaneous abortions, total pregnancy wastage from conception to 1 year of life may be conservatively estimated at about 250/1,000 known conceptions. Significant anomalies, morbidities, and learning disabilities add even more casualties to this public health problem, probably exceeding 5%.

The proportion of fetal deaths among perinatal deaths has remained consistently higher in the nonwhite population than among whites—that is, 11.5 versus 7.4/1,000 live births. Interestingly, advanced maternal age seems to favor fetal mortality, while young mothers tend to have greater risk of neonatal mortality. In addition to the maternal age factor, many other variables influence outcome, among them, birth order, legitimacy, prior reproductive experience, gestational age, socioeconomic level, birth weight, medical–obstetric conditions, health care, and nutrition.

Unfortunately, even the most recent studies show that the cause of perinatal death cannot be determined by examination of the mother, infant or placenta in about one quarter of cases. In another 15% there will be no pathognomonic histologic changes in the infant, but the mother's pregnancy will have been complicated by toxemia, diabetes mellitus, or other diseases. The overall incidence of respiratory distress syndrome now tends to exceed that of placental disease in most studies and so does fetal malformation. Placental disease, complica-

tions of labor, and infection are each responsible for 6% to 8% of perinatal deaths. Birth injuries due to trauma are responsible for less than 1% of the deaths. The incidence of erythroblastosis fetalis as a cause of death is similarly low. Meconium aspiration, cord compression, and other conditions give rise to only about 5% of the perinatal deaths as a group. Widespread use of surfactant replacement appears to be substantially decreasing neonatal mortality; as a result, the relatively fixed numbers of each of the other aforementioned causes of death now account for larger percentages of the smaller total.

Hemorrhagic vasculitis is an interesting placental finding that has been noted by Sander (1980) in association with fetal hypoxia and perinatal brain damage. Pathologically, there is fragmentation of erythrocytes and destruction of vessel walls along with a villitis. These findings are similar to changes associated with the TORCH group of viruses that are implicated in many perinatal disorders (*e.g.*, toxoplasmosis, rubella, cytomegalovirus, herpes). However, at this time this link has not been established for this particular pathologic lesion of the placenta. Recently, there has been renewed interest in the placenta to help clarify some of the perinatal deaths that either are unexplained or are attributed, perhaps unjustifiably, to injuries arising out of obstetric procedures or practices.

The infants of young primigravidas are at a greater risk of toxemia; however, in supervised cases, the traditional concerns for the fetus have been minimized by use of updated monitoring techniques. The modern trend of liberalizing abdominal delivery in cases of breech presentation and other malpresentations has likewise reduced the significance of trauma as a cause of perinatal death.

The current practice of evaluating risk factors at the initial and each subsequent prenatal visit, of utilizing broadly based laboratory screening, and implementation of indicated biometric monitoring should suffice to identify the patient who is vulnerable during pregnancy. Intrapartal screening and supervision is also crucial, since up to one third of fetal losses occur during labor and delivery. However, despite many advances, a number of critical studies show that as many as one third of all perinatal deaths may have been preventable.

It is important for the physician to check for and correct significant medical, endocrinologic, metabolic, and emotional disorders in women prior to and during their reproductive years, because perinatal problems arise disproportionately and recurrently among vulnerable groups. By so doing, the physician is practicing preventive medicine and at the same time providing a basis for a continuum of care and supervision throughout the adolescent period and the years of reproduction.

ANATOMY AND PHYSIOLOGY OF FEMALE SEX ORGANS

Bony Pelvis

The linea terminalis forms the boundary between the false pelvis above and the true pelvis below. The *true, lower* or *small, pelvis* is intimately concerned in childbirth and defines the shape of the parturient canal. It is tubular and curves slightly anteriorly. The walls of the true pelvis are partly ligamentous and partly bony. The four bones making up the pelvis are the sacrum, the coccyx, and two innominate bones. The innominate bones articulate strongly with the sacrum (sacroiliac synchondroses) and with each other at the symphysis pubis. Anteriorly the pelvis is bounded by the symphysis pubis and posteriorly by the length of the sacrum.

The clinical evaluation of the bony pelvis is based on estimation of the inlet, the midpelvis, and the outlet. The diagonal conjugate of the inlet (normal exceeds 11.5 cm) is from the inner inferior border of the symphysis to the midpoint of the sacral promontory (or false promontory, whichever is shorter). The true conjugate (conjugata vera) is the distance from the anterior midpoint of the sacral or false promontory to the superior margin of the symphysis in the midline and is calculated to be 1.5 cm shorter than the diagonal conjugate; this is the available anteroposterior space at the inlet. A diagonal conjugate of less than 11.5 cm or a conjugate vera of less than 10 cm indicates contracture of the pelvic inlet or superior strait. Inlet contracture occurs with a normal-sized infant if the anteroposterior is <10 cm or the transverse is <12 cm (or both). Clinically, inlet contracture is signaled by a floating vertex presentation at term or in labor, an inability to manually push the fetal head into the pelvis with gentle fundal pressure, the presenting part not well applied to the cervix in labor, an abnormal presentation (*e.g.*, breech, transverse lie), cord prolapse, poor progress in labor, uterine dystocia, excessive molding of the fetal head and caput succedaneum formation. Complications of inlet contracture include prolonged labor, prolonged rupture of the membranes, and pathologic retraction ring at the junction of the lower uterine segment and fundus

(Bandl's retraction ring—signifying impending uterine rupture). Usually cesarean is necessary for inlet contracture.

Compromise in the transverse diameter of the midpelvis (interspinous diameter) is currently the most common cause of pelvic dystocia. The degree of prominence, sharpness, and extent of encroachment of the ischial spine into the birth canal must be evaluated and the interspinous diameter of the midpelvis (normal is equal to or greater than 10.5 cm) has a lower limit of 9.5 cm for passage of an average-sized infant. Evaluation of the sacrosciatic notch is a useful adjunct to midpelvic measurement. It is essentially the length of the sacrosciatic ligament (from the ischial spine to the sacrum) and is normally greater than 3 cm. An additional useful evaluation of the midpelvis is afforded by sacral palpation to determine the contour, depth, and irregularities. This is usually noted by characterizing the curvature as *hollow* (deep or posterior), *average* (normally capacious), and *flat* (impinging on the space by ventral angulation, shallow) and any irregularity. Midpelvic contracture usually occurs as a result of an interspinous diameter of less than 9.5 cm and this may be suspected if convergent sidewalls and a narrow pelvic arch are present. With labor, a midpelvic contracture is suggested by prolonged second stage of labor, persistent occiput-posterior, deep transverse arrest, uterine dystocia, and excessive molding of the fetal head. Neglected midpelvic dystocia may result in uterine rupture or fistulae due to pressure necrosis. Cesarean section is the treatment of choice because with the compromised space, instrumented delivery may lead to fetal and/or maternal injuries.

Outlet dystocia without other pelvic abnormalities is rare; thus, a careful outlet evaluation assists in determining other problems of the bony pelvis. This is usually accomplished by determination of the biischial diameter, the posterior and anterior sagittal diameters, and the subpubic angle, and by evaluation of the mobility in the sacrococcygeal joint. The biischial diameter (bituberous, intertuberous) is the distance between the inner margins of the ischial tuberosities and constitutes the hypotenuse of the anterior pudendal triangle. The actual distance between the bony margins usually exceeds 11 cm; however, when measured through the soft tissues, a normal value is 8 or more cm. The posterior sagittal diameter of the outlet (normal is 8–9.5 cm) is determined directly with the rectal finger touching the sacrococcygeal joint and is the distance from the midpoint of the line between the ischial tuberosities to the external surface of the tip of the sacrum. Thoms' or Klein's rule states that when the sum of the biischial and the posterior sagittal exceeds 15 cm, an infant of normal size will usually pass through the outlet without difficulty. The anteroposterior diameter of the outlet (normal exceeds 11.9 cm) is the distance from the inferior border of the symphysis to the posterior aspect of the tip of the sacrum. The angle formed by the pubic arch (the angle of the rami at the pubis) is usually 110 to 120 degrees. In an android pelvis the angle is narrow (<90 degrees) and the biischial diameter is narrow. If the coccyx is grasped between the fingers of the examining hand, with the other hand placed in the cleft between the buttocks, the direction of the coccyx, its degree of movement at the sacrococcygeal articulation, and local tenderness may be determined. In summary, critical pelvic dimensions (for average-sized fetuses) include a diagonal conjugate greater than 12.5 cm, an obstetric conjugate (anteroposterior of the inlet) greater than 10 cm, a transverse of the midpelvis of greater than 9.5 cm, and a sum of the posterior sagittal and bituberous of more than 15 cm.

Based on these clinical observations, and in the extreme case x-ray pelvimetry, the pelvis may be classified into four major types (Caldwell-Moloy classification), although various combinations of types occur. The gynecoid pelvis is most favorable for vaginal delivery and occurs in over 50% of women. It is characterized by oval inlet (transverse diameter slightly greater than the anteroposterior diameter), straight sidewalls, nonprominent ischial spines, wide bispinous and bituberous diameters, a wide and deep curved sacrosciatic notch, a wide subpubic arch, and a concave sacrum. The android (malelike) pelvis is found in roughly one third of white and 15% of black women. The android inlet is wedge-shaped; the pelvic sidewalls are convergent; the ischial spines are prominent; the sacrosciatic notch is narrow, deep, and pointed; the subpubic arch is narrow; and the sacrum is inclined anteriorly in its lower one third. The android pelvis is likely to be associated with persistent occiput posterior position and deep transverse arrest dystocia. The anthropoid pelvis is found in approximately 85% of black women and one fifth of white women. It is marked by an oval inlet (but the anteroposterior diameter exceeds the transverse), the sacrosciatic notch is broad and shallow, the subpubic arch is narrowed, the pelvic sidewalls diverge, and the sacrum is inclined posteriorly. This type of pelvis is most likely to be associated with occiput posterior dystocia. The platypelloid pelvis is rare (less than

3% of all women) and is characterized by a very wide transverse diameter of the inlet, a curved and small sacrosciatic notch and a wide subpubic angle. Deep transverse arrest is common because the fetal head cannot enter the true pelvis.

The use of x-ray pelvimetry exposes the mother and fetus to 1 to 2 rad. Attempts to eliminate even that level of radiation has led to the restriction of x-ray pelvimetry to specific indications, including projected breech delivery, unusual bony pelvic configuration, malpresentation, unengaged vertex presentation at term in labor, failure to make progress in labor, and a history of difficult labor. Ultrasonic scanning may also assist in evaluation of fetal or soft tissues but cannot be used for bony measurement.

Pelvic Floor

The pelvic floor creates a resistance that must be overcome in the process of labor before birth can occur. It consists primarily of a strong pelvic diaphragm formed by the levator ani and coccygeus muscles with their fascia, along with a urogenital diaphragm that adds additional strength. The latter is comprised of perineal fasciae, the superficial muscles, and the transverse perinei muscles, both superficial and deep, which, together with the fasciae, provide significant support. The endopelvic fascia, which is a continuation of the transversalis fascia of the anterior abdominal wall, is reflected off the pelvic viscera where these organs pierce the pelvic floor. Envelopments of fibrous investments blend with the outer muscular coats of the organs along with other connective tissues to form the ligaments of support. These tubular connective tissue condensations incorporating muscular components give rise to definitive structures. The condensations of tissue on the lateral aspects of the isthmus of the uterus extending to the lateral pelvic wall provide the major support for the uterus and are called the *cardinal ligaments*. The condensations extending from the posterior aspect of the uterine isthmus to the sacrum are the *"uterosacral" ligaments* (lateral boundaries of the pouch of Douglas). Attenuation and lateral displacement of these ligaments predispose to the occurrence of a cul-de-sac herniation in the form of an enterocele. The condensations of fascia between the pubis and urethra give rise to a *pubourethral ligament,* which helps maintain urinary continence through its support to the sphincteric segment. The location of the endopelvic fascia, which forms tightly fitting collars about the several organs, determines its specific designation at the various sites. The fascia between the pubis and cervix is known as the pubocervical fascia; between the bladder and vagina as the vesicovaginal fascia; and between the rectum and the vagina as the rectovaginal fascia. The vesical, uterine, and rectal layers become continuous not only with the transversalis fascia from above but also the fascia of the pelvic diaphragm, the iliac fascia, and the obturator fascia.

The *broad ligaments* are two winglike folds of peritoneum that extend from the lateral margins of the uterus to the pelvic walls. The inner two thirds of the superior margins contain the fallopian tubes, while the lateral third forms the suspensory ligaments of the ovaries and transmits the ovarian vessels. Beneath the fallopian tube the broad ligament contains the parovarium. The parovarium is the remnant of the wolffian duct (Gartner's duct). The caudal portion, called paroophoron, is a vestigial group of mesonephric tubules, which may occasionally give rise to cysts of variable size (termed *hydatids of Morgagni*). Laterally the broad ligament is reflected upon the side of the pelvis. The inferior margin is continuous with the connective tissue of the pelvic floor and transmits the uterine vessels. The uterine end of the broad liagment is triangular, containing uterine vessels in the broad base, with a wide connective tissue attachment adjacent to the cervix called the parametrium. These tissues together with the paravaginal connective tissue provide major uterine support.

The *round ligaments* lie within the broad ligaments on either side and extend from just below the insertion of the tubes in the uterus to the inguinal canal, terminating in the labia majora after coursing through the inguinal canal.

Vagina

The vagina is a musculomembranous tube interposed between the bladder and the rectum and lying in the pelvic floor between the vulva and the uterus. The urethral portion is firmly united to the urethra and vesicovaginal septum; the vesical portion is loosely attached to the bladder. It is separated above and behind from the rectum by the cul-de-sac of Douglas. The upper end of the vagina forms a blind vault into which the cervix projects, with its opening pointing toward the sacrum. The vaginal wall consists of three layers: the mucous, the muscular, and the connective tissue layers. The mucosa is composed of stratified epithelium, of which the lowest layer is columnar. The submucosa is rich in blood vessels. The sphincter vaginae is a thin layer of voluntary muscle, but for practical purposes the levator ani muscle acts as the sphincter. In the adult the vagina measures 8 cm to 10 cm in length, although it is normally pliable and distensible in depth as well as bore. It forms a part of the birth canal at labor, represents the excretory duct of the uterus, and is the female organ of copulation.

Uterus

The uterus is a flattened, pear-shaped, hollow, muscular organ, partially covered by peritoneum and lined with mucous membrane. It consists of an upper triangular corpus and a lower cylindrical cervix. The fallopian tube comes off the cornua on either side of the corpus. The adult virgin organ measures 5.5 cm to 8 cm, 3.5 cm to 4 cm, and 2 cm to 2.5 cm in its greatest vertical, transverse and anteroposterior diameters, respectively, as compared with 9 cm to 9.5 cm, 5.5 cm to 6 cm and 3 cm to 3.5 cm in multiparous women. A normal multiparous uterus will not exceed 125 g, and the nulliparous uterus weighs even less.

CERVIX

The cervix is the portion that lies below the isthmus and the internal os. Its upper boundary is marked anteriorly by the lowest reflection of the peritoneum. Its intravaginal portion projects into the vaginal fornix and at its tip presents the external os. The cervix is composed of connective tissue containing muscle fibers, some elastic tissue, and many vessels. Its mucosa is composed of a single layer of high, narrow, columnar epithelium resting on a thin basement membrane. This epithelium is continued in the lining of the cervical glands, which are branching and racemose. The mucosa covering the vaginal portion of the cervix is directly continuous with that of the vagina and also consists of stratified epithelium.

UTERINE CORPUS

This is made up of three layers—serous, muscular, and mucous. The serous layer is formed by the adherent peritoneum. The peritoneum is nonadherent just above the bladder and laterally where it is deflected to the broad ligaments. Owing to the changes of menstruation, the endometrium varies greatly in thickness, measuring from 0.5 mm to 3 mm or 5 mm. It has no submucosa but is attached directly to the musculature. The surface epithelium is composed of a single layer of high, columnar, ciliated cells with a basement membrane and projects below the surface to form large numbers of small, tubular uterine glands. The cilia persist throughout the reproductive era and for some years thereafter, and the current is in the same direction as that of the tubes, namely, from the fimbriated end of the oviducts downward to the external os. The secretory activity of the endometrium is limited to nonciliated cells. The cells in the tubules have the same structure as the surface epithelium and extend down to the muscular layer. Between the glands is a loose stroma of stellate cells with many blood vessels and lymphatics and occasional lymphoid nodules.

The musculature of the uterus is made up of bundles of nonstriated muscle, united by connective tissue containing elastic fibers and richly perforated with blood vessels.

The *blood supply* of the uterus is derived from (1) the uterine artery, which arises from the hypogastric, enters the broad ligament, crosses ventral to the ureter, and divides into a cervical and a uterine branch; the last divides into fundal, tubal, and ovarian branches, and (2) the ovarian or internal spermatic artery (a branch of the aorta), which supplies the ovary and, after traversing the broad ligament, anastomoses with the ovarian branch of the uterine artery.

The veins correspond to the arteries and are very abundant. The blood from the ovary and the upper part of the broad ligament collects in the pampiniform plexus; the vessels from this plexus terminate in the ovarian vein. The right ovarian vein empties into the vena cava, while the left empties into the renal vein.

The *lymphatics* of the body of the uterus are distributed to the hypogastric and the lumbar glands; those from the cervix are distributed to the hypogastric glands.

Innervation of the uterus is derived principally from the sympathetic nervous system, but partly also from the cerebrospinal and parasympathetic systems. Both systems enter the plexus of Frankenhauser, which consists of ganglia of varying size on either side of the cervix just above the posterior fornix and in front of the rectum. The abundant nerve supply of the uterus appears to be regulatory rather than primary. The sympathetics cause muscular contraction and vasoconstriction, whereas the parasympathetics inhibit contraction and cause vasodilation. Pain from the uterus is carried by sensory fibers in 11th and 12th thoracic nerve roots, and that of the cervix and upper vagina is transmitted through the pelvic nerves to the second, third,

and fourth sacral nerves. Pain from the lower tract passes through the ilioinguinal and pudendal nerves.

Fallopian Tubes

Each fallopian tube consists of (1) a uterine portion (interstitial), (2) an isthmus, (3) an ampulla, and (4) an infundibulum. It varies in thickness from 2 mm to 3 mm at the isthmus to 5 mm to 8 mm at the ampulla. Except for the uterine portion, it is entirely enclosed in the peritoneum of the broad ligament. The funnel-shaped fimbriated extremity (infundibulum) opens freely into the abdominal cavity, the fimbria ovarica extending almost to the ovary. It is composed of an inner circular and an outer longitudinal layer and is lined with a single layer of high columnar epithelium resting upon a basement membrane. Cilia occur in patches. The mucosa is arranged in elaborate longitudinal folds resembling a Maltese cross or in complicated tree-like folds. Tubal mucosa undergo cyclic histologic changes similar to but less marked than those noted in the endometrium. Spontaneous contractions under the influence of hormones occur, and their greatest frequency and intensity are noted during ova transport at mid-cycle. The tubes are richly supplied with elastic tissue, blood vessels, and lymphatics.

Ovaries

Each ovary is attached to the broad ligament by the mesovarium and to the uterus by the ovarian ligament. The suspensory ligament of the ovary extends from its upper or tubal pole to the pelvic wall and is really a continuation of the broad ligament, through which the ovarian vessels and the nerves pass. Except for its hilus, the ovary lies freely in the abdominal cavity and is not covered by peritoneum. The size is variable, but usually during the childbearing period the ovary measures about 2.5 cm to 5.0 cm in length, 1.5 cm to 3.0 cm in breadth and 0.5 cm to 1.5 cm in thickness and weighs 4 g to 8 g. In later postmenopausal years the ovaries may not exceed 0.5 cm in diameter.

On cross section the ovary presents an external cortex and an internal medulla, the former containing the ova and the graafian follicles. The outermost portion of the cortex is dull and whitish and is designated tunica albuginea. The surface germinal cuboidal epithelium of Waldeyer forms the outermost layer. The medulla is composed of loose connective tissue continuous with that of the mesovarium. Both sympathetic and parasympathetic nerves supply the ovaries.

GRAAFIAN FOLLICLES

Before puberty the graafian follicles are found only in the deeper portions of the cortex. However, later they make their way to the surface, becoming thinner walled and obtaining a larger blood supply. Necrobiosis of the overlying tissues rather than pressure within the follicle gives rise to rupture gradually in an almost bloodless area called the stigma. The whole process of discharge of the ovum along with its zona pellucida and attached follicular cells probably takes only a few minutes. Normally, during each cycle, only one mature follicle makes its way to the surface and discharges its ovum, although this limiting mechanism is unknown.

From the outside inward, the mature graafian follicles consist of (1) a connective tissue covering (theca folliculi), (2) an epithelial lining (membrana granulosa), (3) the ovum, and (4) the liquor folliculi. Just before rupture the ovum separates from the follicular wall as fluid accumulates in the cumulus, and it floats freely in the liquor.

The *theca* is divided into a tunica externa of ordinary ovarian stroma and a tunica interna of yellow, granular theca lutein cells that play a part in the formation of the corpus luteum.

The *membrana granulosa* consists of a number of layers of small polygonal or cuboidal cells that at one point are massed to form the discus proligerus, in which the ovum is included.

The *follicular fluid* is partly the product of degenerated follicular epithelium and partly a transudate. The fluid is normally clear, albuminous liquor folliculi, which contains the specific internal secretion of the ovary—estrogen.

OVUM

As the ovum approaches maturity, it becomes the largest cell in the body (0.133–0.140 mm in diameter). Primary oocytes, resting in the prophase of their first meiotic division since approximately the fifth month of in utero development, undergo individual maturation; the process is completed shortly after the release of the egg at ovulation. Usually only one of a group of follicles continues to grow to produce a mature egg, which is extruded at ovulation. Others undergo atresia and develop into irregular hyaline bodies. There is a gradual decline from a mean of 439,000 oocytes in girls under 15 years of age to a mean of 34,000 in women over the age

of 36. It is *not* generally accepted that ova are continuously arising from the germinal epithelium throughout maturity.

It is important to recognize some of the essential structures within the mature ovum and in its surroundings. It has an outer enveloping corona radiata; a zona pellucida; a perivitelline space, which contains the first polar body shortly before ovulation; a small clear zone of protoplasm; a broad, finely granular zone of protoplasm; a central deutoplasmic zone; the nucleus with its germinal spot; and many spheroidal mitochondria. Shortly before ovulation the nucleus achieves a peripheral position and formation of polar bodies begins.

CORPUS LUTEUM

The corpus luteum is formed at the site of a ruptured graafian follicle. When the mature follicle ruptures, the ovum, the liquor folliculi, and part of the degenerated membrana granulosa escape, and the walls of the empty follicle collapse. However, in a short time the cavity becomes filled with blood, is rapidly penetrated by proliferating granulosa cells and forms a yellow corpus luteum. In the proliferative stages, strands of so-called K cells of Hertig migrate from the theca to penetrate the membrana granulosa as far as the central coagulum. The peripheral yellow ring enlarges until it almost entirely fills the follicle; this ultimately undergoes hyalinization, forming the corpus fibrosum. The mature corpus luteum measures 1 cm to 3 cm in diameter (prior to 23rd day of the cycle) and is characteristically bright yellow. The life cycle of the corpus luteum is characterized by stages of proliferation, vascularization, maturity, and retrogression; finally, if pregnancy has not occurred, it becomes a fibrosed structure known as a corpus albicans. The active life span of the corpus luteum of menstruation is about 8 days, and thus its secretory function begins to decline some 6 days prior to the next menstruation. In the event of pregnancy, the corpus luteum does not retrogress but becomes even larger, forming the corpus luteum of pregnancy. This structure and its steroid elaborations are necessary for implantation, but there seems to be no critical need for their existence beyond the earliest stages of pregnancy. The early trophoblast appears to secrete sufficient progesterone to sustain the conceptus. Degenerative changes and a diminution in secretion occur in the corpus luteum after the ninth day. Regressive changes take place up to menstruation when the central coagulum has been obliterated by connective tissue and blood pigment has been removed by leukocytes. Thus, spaces in the ovary left by the ruptured follicles are obliterated without the formation of scar tissue and progressive gonadal devitalization.

Menstrual Cycle

Menstruation is that part of the menstrual cycle of endometrial changes in which the endometrial lining of the uterus is sloughed off and expelled, together with a discharge of blood. Except during pregnancy and lactation, it normally occurs every 28 days from puberty to the menopause, lasting from 3 to 5 days, though the duration varies considerably. The term cannot be properly applied to anovulatory or dysfunctional bleeding, to the discharge of blood during pregnancy, or to that caused by the presence of a neoplasm or some other abnormality.

The menstrual cycle is ordinarily divided into three phases: (1) proliferative, from the 6th to the 14th days; (2) secretory (or progestational or luteal), from the 15th to the 28th days; and (3) menstrual, from the 1st to the 5th days. Although the post-ovulatory phase of the cycle is usually very close to 14 days, the follicular phase normally varies from 7 to 21 days. Changes in the activity of the endocrine glands and response in the uterus are continuous throughout the cycle, and considerable variations in pattern are normally observed. The postovulatory phases can be subdivided according to their histologic features since identifiable characteristics occur on an almost day-to-day basis. These changes have significance clinically since they permit ''dating'' the endometrium and assessment of sufficiency or insufficiency of progestational development.

Immediately following the menstruation the endometrium is very thin, but during the subsequent week or so under the influence of estrogen, it proliferates markedly. The cells on the surface become taller, while the glands that dip into the endometrium become longer and wider. As the result of these changes the thickness of the endometrium increases sixfold or eightfold. It is during this phase of menstrual cycle (from the 6th to the 14th days) that a graafian follicle each month is approaching its greatest development and is manufacturing increasing amounts of follicular fluid. The estrogenic hormone (*estradiol*) contained in this fluid causes reorganization, proliferation, and growth of the endometrium. It also causes growth of the uterine musculature and sensitizes the myometrium to oxytocic activity. Estrogen stimulates the growth of the spiral arterioles of the endome-

trium (thus improving blood flow) and induces rhythmic contractions of the fallopian tubes. The estrogenic hormone—in the form of estradiol—is secreted by the maturing follicle and, later, by the corpus luteum. During the preovulatory phase of the cycle, estradiol is produced in increasing quantity.

Following rupture of the graafian follicle (ovulation), between the 13th and the 16th days of the cycle, the cells that form the corpus luteum begin to secrete, in addition to estrogen, another important hormone, *progesterone*. This supplements the action of estrogen on the endometrium in such a way that the glands become very tortuous or spiral in appearance and greatly dilated. This change is due to the fact that they are swollen with a secretion containing large amounts of glycogen and mucin. Abundant glandular secretion results from the combined action of progesterone and estrogen. Meanwhile, the blood supply of the endometrium is increased, with the result that it becomes very vascular and succulent. Apparently, vascular patterns and physiologic mechanisms observed during the menstrual cycle constitute patterns of behavior and function observable in the myometrium and decidua during pregnancy and are responsible for many vascular and muscular actions and phenomena observed in the gravid state. Similarly, a steroid hormonal milieu underlies these manifestations. Under the influence of progesterone the cervical mucus becomes scanty, viscid, full of leukocytes, unable to form a fern pattern, and impermeable to spermatozoa.

Changes in the endometrium are directed at furnishing a bed for a fertilized ovum. Unless the ovum is fertilized, the corpus luteum is short-lived, and its activity regresses rapidly after about 8 days (or around the 23rd day of the cycle). This means withdrawal of estrogen and progesterone, the hormones responsible for building up and preparing the endometrium, and the endometrium undergoes a phase of premenstrual ischemia and involution associated finally with vasoconstriction of the coiled arterioles some 4 to 24 hours before the onset of menstrual bleeding. Collapse and desquamation of the superficial layers of the endometrium and both arterial and venous bleeding then occur as constricted vessels relax. Hemorrhage stops later when the coiled arterioles return to a state of vasoconstriction.

Just prior to puberty the cerebral centers and endocrine tissues reach a critical level of maturity. The central nervous system (CNS) has a profound effect on the endocrine system and messages are relayed to a specialized part, the hypothalamus, from visual, olfactory, and psychological areas. Decoded messages affect the neurohumoral process in the hypothalamus, which is an essential part of the secretion of releasing hormones or factors. For each of the trophic hormones elaborated by the pituitary gland, there is a hypothalamic-releasing hormone; inhibitory factors may also be secreted. Relative to gonadotropins, the hypothalamus secretes a decapeptide-releasing hormone known as leuteinizing hormone-releasing hormone (LHRH), or gonadotropic-releasing hormone (GRH). This hormone has the ability to stimulate the synthesis, as well as the release, of both follicle-stimulating hormone (FSH) and leuteinizing hormone (LH) from the pituitary gland. The portal vessels are particularly important in the transmission of the releasing hormones from the hypothalamus to the anterior pituitary. The region of the median eminence and preoptic area of the hypothalamus are the main centers for secretion of LHRH. The preoptic area is the center leading to the cyclic release of LH and FSH necessary for ovulation, whereas the tonic release of both gonadotropins is controlled by the center in the median eminence. The mechanism of neurosecretion in the hypothalamus involves two basic actions. The dominant mechanism under normal conditions involves certain catecholamines that stimulate the secretion of LHRH and prolactin-inhibiting factors (PIF). A second mechanism, controlled by a serotoninergic action, will inhibit the gonadotropin secretion and stimulate prolactin secretion. The nature of the latter control mechanism is not as well understood, but, at least in animals, there may be gonadotropin-inhibiting activities in the melatonin and serotonin secretions from the pineal gland.

The menstrual cycle is a function of a coordinated, intact hypothalamic-pituitary-ovarian axis. The estradiol signal in the recycling system operates at key moments and plays a critical role in both negative feedback and positive feedback relationships. Thus, the interplay between the ovarian follicle and the hypothalamus represents messages that lead to successful follicular development and triggering of ovulation. First, the negative feedback results in a critical initial rise in FSH during menses. A rapid rise in estradiol at midcycle triggers a surge of LH and ovulation through the positive feedback mechanism. Presumably, the nature of this LH response determines the life span of the corpus luteum; there will be inevitable degeneration unless conception occurs and human chorionic gonadotropin elaborated by the trophoblast emerges as a new luteotrophic stimulus. The latter hormone

should become operative at the eighth day after ovulation, which prevents regression. The fourth factor in the scenario is the endometrium, which should have been properly prepared to permit implantation and proper placentation.

If the ovum is fertilized, the first part of the cycle is like that of the normal menstrual cycle, but the collapse of the corpus luteum and the endometrium does not take place. The corpus luteum grows larger and continues its hormonic influence on the endometrium, which becomes the decidua of pregnancy. The integrity and the growth pattern of trophoblast are dependent upon a well-prepared uterus. Extensive ultracytochemical studies have been made of the human endometrial cycle that show that biochemical determinants of intracellular metabolic activity are required to support implantation and early nutrition of the conceptus. Among these are the well-timed appearances of glucose-6-phosphatase around the time of ovulation and early secretory phase and acid phosphatase in the lysosomes of glandular epithelium after the 21st day.

VERY EARLY GESTATION

Fertilization of the Ovum

During early embryonic life, the sex cords first break up into distinct clumps of cells, usually by age 6 weeks, and then develop into an organized pattern resulting in primary follicles (16th week), which incorporate germ cells soon to become recognizable as oogonia (7 million by the 20th week). Although most of these undergo atresia, a first meiotic division occurs in many by the time of birth, and at that point these cells, called primary oocytes, number about 1 million. They remain dormant in the prophase until puberty, although by that stage their number has been reduced to about a half million. Ultimately, ovulation consumes less than 500, and fertilization involves only a few.

The first maturation division *(meiotic division)* results in the formation of a large secondary oocyte and the minute first polar body. The polar body, which has scant cytoplasm, lies between the zona pellucida and the vitelline membrane of the secondary oocyte and is cast off while still in the ovary. Following this process and before the nucleus of the secondary oocyte returns to a resting stage, the second meiotic division begins, which results in the formation of a large mature oocyte and a second polar body. Ovulation occurs as the spindle begins to form in the secondary oocyte. In the second maturation division, the paired chromosomes separate so that half go into the polar body and half remain in the egg or ootid. In every species each individual cell normally has a characteristic number of chromosomes. The set number for the normal human being is 46, consisting of 2 each of 22 different autosomes in addition to the two sex chromosomes XX or XY. The constancy of this chromosome number is assured by the process of meiosis. Upon penetration of the vitelline membrane, male and female pronuclei, each with 23 chromosomes, unite to form the segmentation nucleus and restore the original 46 chromosomes. The primary sex ratio is established. Normally, fertilization of an ovum bearing the X chromosome by an X-bearing sperm results in a zygote with the XX constitution (female). A Y-bearing sperm fertilizing the same ovum would result in a male zygote with the XY constitution. The sex ratio of infants at birth favors the male (106 males to 100 females), and this numeric difference may be even greater at conception. The process of fertilization initiates the sequence of mitotic divisions resulting in cell cleavage and development of the zygote.

Only one of many millions of spermatozoa deposited actually penetrates the ovum, presumably by enzymatic action. Failing to meet a spermatozoon within 24 hours of ovulation, the ovum begins to degenerate. When fertilization does occur, the ovum continues to develop up to the stage of implantation and shedding of the zona pellucida.

The spermatozoa are carried into the uterine cavity—both by their own motility and by uterine contractions against the ciliary action of the uterus and the tubes. Fertilization usually occurs in the outer third of the tubes, the fertilized ovum normally being carried down the tubes to the uterus, not only by the ciliary current but also by peristalsis of the tubes. Proper synchronization between transport and endometrial preparation is important.

Sexual Differentiation. Genetic or chromosomal sex is determined at the moment of fertilization, but the gonads remain in an indifferent stage until about the 7th embryonic week. At that time, one set of differentiation is stimulated preferentially in response to gonadal development while the other set undergoes atrophy. The Y chromosome carries the testicular inductor in the human fetus. In the absence of the testicular inductor, the indifferent gonad develops as an ovary. Under androgenic influence (testosterone), there will be medullary dominance and midline fusion forming the scrotum and penile shaft; development within the wolffian system gives rise to the seminal vesicles, vas deferens, epididymis, and collecting system in the testicle itself. Without this androgenic influence, there will be a critical dominance that results in

preservation of the müllerian system. Apparently, there are also unidentified organizing substances, but the X chromosome does not appear to possess a counterpart gene opposite to the testis-inducing one in the Y chromosome. There must be two X chromosomes for the ovary to differentiate, since gonadal dysgenesis occurs if the second X is either missing or deformed. The germ cells of XO individuals (45 XO karyotype) reach the gonads in the normal manner, but are apparently lost through some unknown mechanism.

The consensus view about the derivation of the vagina is that the organ develops from the müllerian ducts in its upper four fifths and from the epithelium of the urogenital sinus in its lower fifth. The sinus epithelium forms a cord growing upward to displace, at least in part, the müllerian epithelium craniad and establishes the anlage of the future hollow tube. In the absence of a vaginal mass, the hymen is not formed. Incomplete fusion of the distal portions of the müllerian ducts results in various forms of partial or total duplication of the uterus, as well as septation of the vagina. The vagina is the last genital organ to be completed embryologically; masculinizing effects beginning relatively late may result in aberrations in its formation. Development of the external genital system and structures of the hind end are so closely related that isolated anomalies are rare.

The clinical implications of genetic faults and structural anomalies arising from embryogenic defects are discussed in the section on gynecology.

Implantation of the Ovum

This usually occurs on the upper part of the anterior or posterior wall of the uterus on about the 6th or 7th day after fertilization. The full decidual response of the endometrium is not elicited until the trophoblast has eroded the superficial uterine epithelium, presumably the result of histamine or histaminelike substances at the site of the blastocyst attachment. The early ovum is covered on all sides by shaggy chorionic villi, but very shortly those villi, which invade the decidua baasalias, enlarge and multiply rapidly. This portion of the trophoblast is known as the *chorion frondosum* (leafy chorion). On the other hand, the chorionic villi covering the remainder of the fetal envelope degenerate and almost dissappear, leaving only a slightly roughened membrane. This is called the *chorion laeve* (bald chorion). The majority of the villi are aborescent structures whose free endings do not reach the decidua. A certain proportion extend from the chorionic membrane to the underlying decidua, attaching the ovum to it; hence, they are designated as fastening villi. Where the invading trophoblast meets the decidua, there is a zone of fibrinoid degeneration called Nitabuch's layer. An inconstant deposition of fibrin, Rohr's stria, is found at the bottom of the intervillous space surrounding the fastening villi. After day 21 there is progressive proliferation of cellular trophoblast at the tips of the villi, and these columns anchor to the decidual plate to form the floor of the intervillous space. These anchoring villi give rise to proliferating "free" villi within the intervillous spaces, while capillary blood vessels multiply within them. The sprouting, free-floating, tertiary villi become the major surfaces for fetomaternal exchange.

Embedding of the ovum is the work of the trophoblast, which possesses the peculiar enzymatic property of being able to digest or liquefy the tissues with which it comes in contact. In this manner these cells not only burrow into the decidua and eat out a nest for the ovum but also digest the walls of the many small blood vessels that they encounter beneath the surface. Trophoblast invades some 40 to 60 spiral aterioles by the 6th week after conception. While the trophoblastic cells invade maternal endometrium and tap maternal blood vessels, the cytoplasmic vacuoles coalesce to form lacunae that rapidly become filled with maternal blood. The ovum finds itself deeply embedded in the decidua with lacunae of blood in its immediate environment. The fetal and the maternal blood systems, the former being developed by the 17th day, are separated only by the trophoblastic epithelium and a delicate layer of mesenchyme. Mitotic figures are noted in the cytotrophoblast, but they are absent in the syncytium. The rapid accumulation of nuclei in the syncytium is probably due to cellular proliferation in the cytotrophoblast followed by coalescence of daughter cells in the syncytium. The nourishment of the fetus is accomplished by the passage of foodstuffs from the maternal blood in the intervillous spaces through the walls of the chorionic villi to the fetal blood, and through the destruction and absorption of parts of the uterine decidua by the trophoblast, which is the parenchyma of the placenta. Additionally, progesterone, which stimulates blastocystic expansion, may serve as a mechanism for removing CO_2 by augmenting carbonic anhydrase activity.

Upward pressure from the pulsatile arteriolar spurts at the placental base exerts its force upon free-floating villi, creating a relatively hollow center within tentlike walls made up of closely packed secondary and tertiary villi (intervillous space). In effect, each fetal cotyledon is a terminal arterial glomus from which blood spurts and then filters slowly through the surrounding fetal villi into the intervillous space proper. By the 225th day the basal plate is pulled up between major cotyledons by anchoring villi to form septa, and there is continued growth and development of the definitive placenta. The chorionic frondosa contain some 200 primary and anchoring stem villi, although about 150 become functionless. Placental transfer occurs across the placental membrane by simple diffusion, by active transport mechanisms and by the passage of whole particles via fluid-filled vacuoles through a phagocytic syncytial process known as pinocytosis. A virtually continuous line of vesicles and vacuoles is present between the syncytial surface and the fetal capillaries.

Placenta

The placenta is the organ through which the embryonic mass is attached to the uterine mucosa and through which the embryo receives its nourishment. Collectively the ancillary organs of the developing conceptus consist of the placenta itself, the chorion, the amnion, and vestigial structures representing the allantois and yolk sac. In addition, there is the umbilical cord uniting the placenta with the fetal body. A number of anatomic arrangements or types of placenta are found in mammals to serve as the union between fetal and maternal tissues for purposes of physiologic exchange. When the chorion is vascularized by the allantois or its derivatives, as it is in humans, the placentation is referred to as the chorioallantoic type. More specifically, according to the Grosser classification, the human placenta is termed hemochorial, since the trophoblast is directly exposed to maternal blood. Other classifications of the human placenta refer to it as villous because of its villi; deciduate because of maternal decidua, which is shed along with the fetal placenta at birth; and discordal because of its circular shape. At term gestation there is considerable variation in placental size and weight; however, an average placenta is 15 cm to 20 cm in diameter and from 1.5 cm to 3 cm in thickness. It averages approximately one sixth the weight of the fetus and is generally approximately 500 g.

CHORION

The chorion arises from a single layer of ectodermal cells forming the wall of the blastodermic vesicle. The wall of the blastocyst, at first entirely smooth, develops polypoid projections known as *trophoblastic buds.* Initially these are quite solid, but later they are penetrated by a core of mesenchyme to form the early villi. Villi in primitive form are distinguishable as early as the 12th day of development, but it is not until the 14th day that maternal blood enters the intervillous space and the 17th day before both fetal and maternal blood vessels are functioning. Villous structures after *in situ* angiogenesis are termed tertiary. The embryo is connected with the connective tissue layer of the chorion by the abdominal pedicle, the forerunner of the umbilical cord, and in it the fetal blood vessels develop.

AMNION

This begins as a small sac covering the dorsal surface of the embryo but eventually enlarges and completely surrounds it, thus lining the interior of the chorion. The two membranes are slightly adherent but may be separated readily. The amniotic cavity is filled with amniotic fluid in which the embryo is suspended.

DECIDUA

The mucous membrane of the uterus that has undergone certain changes under the influence of the ovulation cycle to fit it for the implantation and the nutrition of the ovum, the decidua is usually divided into (1) the decidua vera that lines the main cavity of the uterus, (2) the decidua basalis beneath the ovum, and (3) the decidua capsularis that surrounds the ovum. However, at the 12th week of pregnancy the growing ovum entirely fills the uterine cavity, so that the capsularis and the vera are brought into intimate contact.

The decidua vera is composed of three layers: (1) a compact surface layer made up of large oval or polygonal cells with large lightly staining vesicular nuclei, (2) a spongy layer of dilated hyperplastic uterine glands, and (3) a zona basalis.

PHYSIOLOGIC CHANGES OF PREGNANCY

Respiratory System

Capillary dilatation throughout the respiratory tract leads to engorgement of the nasopharynx, larynx, trachea, and bronchi. Voice changes and difficulty breathing may ensue, along with symptomatic enhancement of respiratory infections. Chest x rays reveal increased vascular markings. With uterine enlargement the diaphragm is elevated (4 cm), the rib cage is displaced upward and the lower ribs flare, increasing lower thoracic diameter (2 cm) and circumference (up to 6 cm). The abdominal muscles have less tone and are less active in pregnancy, but elevation of the diaphragm does not impede its movements.

Relaxation of the musculature of the conducting airways results in an increase in dead space volume. Tidal volume increases 35% to 50% while total lung capacity is reduced by 4% to 5%. The functional residual capacity, residual volume, and expiratory reserve volume all decrease by about 20%. Larger tidal volume and smaller residual volume result in enhanced alveolar ventilation (~65%) during pregnancy. Expiratory capacity (5%–10% increase) reaches a maximum at 22 to 24 weeks of gestation.

The respiratory minute volume increases approximately 26%. There is a 50% increase in minute ventilation with a progressive increase in oxygen utilization up to 15% to 20% above nonpregnant levels. Alveolar CO_2 decreases, which lowers maternal CO_2 tension. Many of these alterations are thought to be due to the action of progesterone on the respiratory center, mediated through changes in the peripheral chemoreceptors in the carotid body. In sum, these maternal hyperventilatory alterations offer a protective environment to the fetus by decreasing carbon dioxide and enhancing oxygenation.

Cardiovascular System

The cardiac output increases approximately 40% (1.5 liters/minute) over the nonpregnant level, reaching a near maximum at 20 to 24 weeks of gestation and continuing until term. In early pregnancy the increase is primarily due to stroke volume (25%–30%), but the heart rate increases with lengthening gestation (to a total of 15 beats per minute). The pregnant uterus impinges on the inferior vena cava, materially influencing cardiac output with body positional changes. With diaphragmatic elevation, the heart is displaced upward and somewhat to the left, with rotation on its axis and lateral movement of the apex. Cardiac capacity increases by 70 ml to 80 ml and heart size by approximately 12%. With increased flow and anatomic changes, there are alterations in both electrocardiogram (EKG) and auscultatory findings. The EKG findings include a 15 to 20 degree shift to the left with reversible ST, T, and QA changes. The first heart sound may be split with increased loudness. A third sound may also be present. As many as 90% of pregnant women have a late systolic ejection murmur. Continuous murmurs along the left sternal border arise from the mammary (internal thoracic) artery.

Normally, systemic blood pressure begins and ends the pregnancy at approximately the same level. However, in midgestation there may be a small reduction in systolic pressure, and the diastolic pressure is generally reduced 5 to 10 mm. Significant venous pressure increases occur in the lower extremities with lengthening pregnancy. This is in part because of the uterine position on the inferior vena cava. With progressive occlusion of the vena cava, which decreases cardiac output, a fall in blood pressure may occur.

Peripheral resistance equals blood pressure divided by cardiac output. Since blood pressure either decreases or remains the same during pregnancy and cardiac output increases appreciably, peripheral resistance markedly declines during the midportion of pregnancy, returning to a higher level near the end of pregnancy. The increased cardiac output is directed primarily to the uterus (increased 500–800 ml/minute), kidneys (increased 400 ml/minute), and breast (increased approximately 200 ml/minute). There is also enhanced blood flow to the skin.

With labor, uterine contractions cause an increase in cardiac output, a slight decrease in heart rate, and approximately a 7% increase in stroke volume (lateral recumbent position). The pulse pressure increases with contractions, as well as the central venous pressure and cardiopulmonary blood volume.

Urinary System

During pregnancy, each kidney increases by 1.5 cm to 1.7 cm in length with concomitant weight increase, and the renal pelvis is dilated up to 60 ml (vs. 10 ml nonpregnant). The ureters are also dilated (right more than left). In all, 200 ml of residual urine may be present in the dilated collecting system.

The glomerular filtration rate (GFR) increases during pregnancy (~50%), and the renal plasma flow (RPF) increases by 25% to 50%. During rest, approximately 20% of cardiac output is delivered to the kidneys. Despite the increase in pregnancy GFR, the volume of urine passed each day is not increased, but an increase in creatinine clearance occurs (~50%). Glucosuria during pregnancy occurs in more than 50%, but proteinuria is unchanged. Bladder muscular tone decreases, with

capacity increasing up to 1,500 ml during pregnancy.

Hematologic System

Blood volume increases remarkably during pregnancy (45%–50%). Initially, this is nearly totally accomplished by enhanced plasma volume, but by term cellular volume is also increased by 15% to 33%. Because of the necessity for enhanced maternal red cell mass and fetal iron, an iron deficiency anemia may occur. The total leukocytes increase as high as 12,000/mcl in the last trimester and up to 16,000/mcl with labor. The clotting factors increase throughout pregnancy, particularly fibrinogen (50%) and Factors VII, VIII, IX, and X, with a marked increase at the beginning of the third trimester.

Gastrointestinal System

Generally, during pregnancy increased progesterone causes both reduced motility and decreased smooth muscle tone with particular effect on delayed gastric emptying. An additional notable effect is the uterine enlargement pushing the appendix superiorly and into the right flank as pregnancy progresses. This is particularly disadvantageous should appendicitis and rupture occur, in that the abscess cannot be walled off. Gallbladder emptying time is slowed and often incomplete. The resultant stasis may lead to stone formation. Functional alterations occur in the liver including doubling of the serum alkaline phosphatase activity, decrease in plasma albumin, and a slight increase in plasma globulins (notably α_2).

PRENATAL CARE

Prenatal care has a wider application than the words imply and may be defined as supervision and care of the pregnant and parturient woman that will enable her to pass through the dangers of pregnancy and labor with the least possible risk, to give birth to a living child, and to be discharged in such a condition that she will be able to nurse. Women who have demonstrated disproportionate obstetric problems should have the benefit of preconceptional workup and care and interpregnancy supervision, which includes responsible family planning. Every effort should be exerted to identify all risk factors and to program patient management on an individualized basis, as determined by the various adverse factors uncovered and estimates of the level of prenatal vulnerability. A general health screen is needed.

The emphasis in prenatal care differs somewhat in each of the trimesters. In the first, the diagnosis must be established, which may necessitate qualitative or quantitative tests for human gonadotropin in the urine or serum. A pelvic ultrasonic study may be necessary to establish the presence and location of the gestational sac, status of fetal development, number of fetuses, and the fetal age. The expected date of confinement must be established to judge the growth pattern. Uterine measurements are made serially beginning in the second trimester.

Proper antepartal care requires a preliminary medical and obstetric history and a complete physical examination, including blood pressure, weight, clinical measurement of the pelvis, urinalysis, urine culture, blood type, Rh determination, complete blood count, serologic test for syphilis, rubella titer, and culture for gonorrhea. When the Veneral Disease Research Laboratory (VDRL) test is positive (1%), especially with titers of 1 : 8 or less, it is important to follow up with a fluorescent treponemal antibody (FTA) serology. It is advisable to screen patients for a metabolic disorder by obtaining a blood sugar 1-hour post 50 g glucose load. In high-risk patients (drug abuse, human immunodeficiency virus [HIV] positive partner, bisexual partner) HIV screening is desirable. Detection of anti-Rh antibodies should be attempted in all Rh-negative patients; the zygosity of the husband should be evaluated. Antibody titers are checked bimonthly after the 20th week of gestation. Patients with group O blood should have the husband's blood group determined for possible ABO incompatibility in the fetus. A screen for bacteriuria is helpful and is mandatory if there is a history of urinary infection or abnormal urine sediment. A check for the presence of glucose and protein in the urine should be performed on each prenatal visit. If glucosuria is present, or if the blood sugar screening level is borderline or elevated, a glucose tolerance test is indicated. A routine chest roentgenogram (with proper pelvic shielding) is usually not rewarding as a screen procedure, but such evaluations are mandatory when chest symptoms are present. Vaginal and cervical smears are taken routinely as a screen for cancer. During epidemics the risk of clinical rubella infection increases from about 1 to 22 or more/1,000 pregnancies. A titer of 1 : 10 and above generally indicates nonsusceptibility. A lower titer calls for postpartal vaccination.

The patient should be instructed regarding diet, rest, exercise, bowel habits, bathing, clothing, smoking, substance abuse, alcohol, douching, breast care, coitus, recreation, and dental care. Education should begin about pregnancy, nutrition, nature of supervision and tests, safeguards, breast feeding, infant care, role and participation of father, and so forth, to explanation of risk factors and options for mode of delivery. Psychologic support and reinforcement must be provided in all patient encounters in order to make the experience meaningful and to optimize patient compliance in preventive measures (*e.g.*, smoking, drugs, alcohol, lack of rest, dietary indiscretions, abuse of medications), and so forth. The patient should also be cautioned tactfully about certain danger signals, which include vaginal bleeding, however slight; edema; persistent headaches; visual disturbances; pain; persistent vomiting; chills and fever; urinary discomfort; sudden escape of fluid from the vagina; and persistent constipation.

The normal patient is commonly seen at least once a month for the first 7 months, then semimonthly until the last month, when weekly visits are instituted. Patients with particular problems are usually seen more frequently.

Questions concerning immunization during pregnancy occur with sufficient frequency to merit discussion. Immunizing agents are of four types: live virus vaccines (whole or subunit), immune globulin preparations, toxoids, killed bacterial and viral vaccines. The live virus vaccines include poliomyelitis, measles, mumps, rubella, and yellow fever. Current recommendations for immunizations are summarized in Table 4-1.

The immune globulins include hepatitis A, hepatitis B, measles, tetanus, rabies, and varicella. Again, there is no known fetal risk from administration. Hepatitis A immune globulin is recommended for the gravida as soon as possible and within 2 weeks of exposure. Hepatitis B hyperimmune globulin is recommended primarily for infants born to hepatitis B surface antigen–positive mothers. Measles immune globulin may be used within 6 days of exposure for prophylaxis, but it is unclear whether it prevents the disease or merely conceals the symptomatology. Rabies hyperimmune globulin immunizing agent has no known risk to the fetus; is recommended during pregnancy for known exposure and is used with the rabies killed virus vaccine.

Tetanus hyperimmune globulin is also recommended for postexposure prophylaxis in conjunction with the tetanus toxoid. Neither agent has known risks for the fetus. Varicella hyperimmune globulin is not routinely indicated in healthy pregnant women exposed to varicella, but it has no

TABLE 4-1. Current Recommendations for Immunizations During Pregnancy

IMMUNIZATION	RECOMMENDATION
Cholera	Only to meet international travel requirements
Hepatitis A	Immunize gravida after exposure Newborns of mothers who are incubating or ill should receive one dose after birth
Hepatitis B	Newborn should receive hyperimmune globulin soon after delivery, followed by vaccination
Influenza	Evaluate gravida for immunization according to criteria recommended for general population
Measles	Live virus vaccine during pregnancy · contraindicated on theoretic grounds Pooled immune globulins for postexposure prophylaxis
Mumps	Theoretically contraindicated during pregnancy
Plague	Use only if there is substantial infection risk
Poliomyelitis	Not routinely recommended, but mandatory in epidemics or when traveling to epidemic areas
Rabies	Same as nonpregnant
Rubella	Contraindicated (although teratogenicity in follow-up of those inadvertently given the vaccine appears negligible)
Tetanus–diphtheria	Give toxoid if no primary series or no booster in 10 years Postexposure prophylaxis in unvaccinated tetanus immune globulin plus toxoid
Typhoid	Recommended if traveling to endemic area
Varicella	Varicella-zoster immune globulin for exposure Indicated for newborns whose mothers developed varicella within 4 days before or 2 days after delivery
Yellow fever	Immunize before travel to high-risk areas, but postpone travel if possible

known fetal risk from the immunizing substance. Tetanus–diphtheria has no confirmed risk to the fetus from the immunizing agent and is indicated during pregnancy if the gravida lacks a primary series, or has had no booster within the past 10 years.

Patients recognized as being at risk for toxemia should be supervised at intervals beyond the routine. At each visit the blood pressure should be taken and the urine examined carefully, especially for albumin. The patient should be weighed at each visit since sudden and excessive weight gain may occur as the first warning sign (before hypertension, edema, and albuminuria develop). Total weight gain in pregnancy for most women in the United States is about 27 pounds, although there is considerable variability. Weight gain is encouraged to be about 1 pound/week from the 16th gestational week to term. Salt is not generally restricted since its intake is not of value in either preventing or treating pregnancy-induced hypertension. Curtailment of weight gain must not impair the quality of the diet.

A minimum of 35 calories/kg/day is indicated during pregnancy. It is recommended that approximately 100 g of protein be consumed daily. Additional needs include the fat-soluble vitamins (vitamin A 5,000 IU; vitamin D 400 IU; vitamin E 15 IU), water-soluble vitamins (ascorbic acid 60 mg, folacin 800 mcg, niacin 14 to 18 mg, riboflavin 1.4 to 1.7 mg, thiamine 1.3 to 1.5 mg, vitamin B_6 4.1 to 4.5 mg, vitamin B_{12} 7 mg) and minerals (calcium 1,200 mg; phosphorus 1,200 mg; iodine 125 mcg; iron 36 mg; magnesium 450 mg; and zinc 20 mg). Lactating women require even more calories and greater amounts of vitamin A, niacin, riboflavin, iodine, and zinc. Moreover, the underweight or malnourished patient must be supported nutritionally to ensure an optimal weight gain.

The demands of metabolism, fetal growth, uterine growth, breasts, increased blood volume, lactation, and so forth, require that protein consumption be emphasized, along with adequate intakes of vitamins and minerals. It now seems clear that past emphasis on strict weight control and actual weight loss in pregnancy seems to be at least potentially hazardous and gives rise to low-birth-weight infants in the extreme. The fact that, at least in animals, the presence of undernutrition causes a reduction in the brain cell number calls for intensified effort to test the effects of nutritional states upon the human fetus. Some available epidemiologic evidence suggests that these same organic brain changes may occur in the human. Nutritional deficits may be either intrinsic or extrinsic. Each category may result in fetal growth retardation. Extrinsic causes such as placental vascular insufficiency give rise to asymmetric growth patterns in which the fetal brain is spared while other organs are undergrown. Intrinsic defects caused by maternal malnutrition may give rise to symmetrically retarded growth, including the brain. Both types of conditions obviously present problems in management, but the prognosis is different.

The growth pattern of the uterus should be noted at the time of each clinic visit, and any abnormality in shape, size, or tone should be noted. If there is any tendency for increased uterine tone more rest is advised, and coitus may have to be disallowed to reduce the uterotonic effect of orgasm and the prostaglandin action of the seminal fluid. The fetal heartbeat should be checked regularly after it appears. Supplemental iron therapy is indicated, since most women have marginal iron stores available that are insufficient to meet the increased demands of pregnancy. Calcium and vitamin supplements may be given as indicated. Fluoride administration may be desirable for women not drinking fluoridated water, to help reduce dental caries in the offspring. Since the high phosphorus content of milk may depress diffusible serum calcium and lead to muscular tetany, milk ingestion may be restricted and phosphorus-free calcium and vitamin D administered. In the third trimester blood counts are repeated and parenteral iron or other therapies are given as necessary to establish optimal hematologic and metabolic conditions for labor and delivery; a repeat 2-hour postprandial blood sugar is also advisable.

Attention is directed to any of the common complaints experienced during pregnancy. These include backache, varicosities, hemorrhoids, heartburn, pica, ptyalism, fatigue, somnolence, headache, leukorrhea, nausea and vomiting, and so forth. If mild in degree, of temporary duration and unattended by worrisome associated complaints, they are easily treated symptomatically, and the patient is reassured about their nature. Psychosomatic complaints during pregnancy and in the puerperium must be given careful attention, especially when there is a history of emotional problems. Specific programs of preparation for childbirth have become very popular; these emphasize preparatory education based on conditioned reflex in an effort to reduce the need for pain relief in labor and delivery or for manipulative procedures to achieve childbirth, (*e.g.*, Lamaze's methods).

About 2 weeks before term, accurate clinical pelvimetric measurements should be obtained, and the presentation and the size of the fetus should be determined by external and internal palpation; this may also reveal any abnormality of the generative tract. The degree of irritability of the uterus is noted. The presenting part is identified, and engagement is assessed. The cervical findings, including consistency, length, effacement, type of mucus, possibility of amniotic fluid leakage, and so forth, are evaluated. A recheck of hemoglobin is indicated in the last month of pregnancy. A more detailed evaluation is performed, if indicated.

Diagnosis of Pregnancy

The diagnostic criteria of pregnancy may be classified into (1) positive signs; (2) probable signs; and (3) presumptive signs, which naturally vary according to the state of pregnancy. Classically, the positive signs of pregnancy are (1) hearing and counting the fetal heartbeat; (2) perception of active fetal movements by the examiner; and (3) recognition of the fetal skeleton by x-ray examination. In light of ultrasonic and magnetic resonance imaging (MRI) technology the last criteria might best be restated: recognition of the fetus through the use of imaging technology. Probable signs of pregnancy include (1) positive pregnancy test; (2) outlining the fetus; (3) ballottement; (4) changes in shape, size, and contour of the uterus; (5) enlargement of the abdomen; (6) changes in the cervix; and (7) the detection of intermittent contractions of the uterus. Obviously, numbers 4 to 7 can be occasionally confused with uterine pathology, such as myomata. A variety of presumptive signs may also be noted: (1) cessation of menses, (2) changes in the breasts, (3) nausea and vomiting, (4) quickening, (5) Chadwick's sign, (6) pigmentation of skin and abdominal striae, (7) urinary frequency, and (8) fatigue. Obviously, these latter signs merely require that pregnancy be included in the differential diagnosis.

CALCULATION OF TERM

On the assumption that labor occurs 280 days from the beginning of the last menstrual period, the date of confinement (EDC) is estimated by adding 7 days to the date of the first day of the last menstrual period and subtracting 3 months (Naegele's rule). This is not totally accurate, but, other things being equal, usually it proves to be correct within a few days, despite the fact that patients with long cycles ovulate relatively later and pregnancy will terminate at a later date. In approximately 40% of cases, a deviation of 1 to 5 days before or after that date may be expected. In over 1%, labor is delayed 3 or more weeks after the calculated date.

DIAGNOSIS OF PRESENTATION

Presentation is determined by the four maneuvers suggested by Leopold:

1. Palpation of head or breech at fundus
2. Palpation of back and nodular extremities through abdominal wall
3. Palpation of head or breech between thumb and fingers to determine engagement and degree of flexion
4. Deep pressure toward the superior strait, showing the cephalic prominence on the same side as the small parts in vertex presentations;

on the same side as the back in face presentations

The examiner can appreciate the presentation from the data thus obtained.

Ascertainment of position from the fetal heart sounds is of disputed value. In obese patients ultrasound examination will be helpful in identifying the presenting part.

Laboratory Tests

Chorionic gonadotropin is produced shortly after implantation and is excreted in the urine. A commercially available test, based on inhibition of agglutination, employs polystyrene latex particles coated with a purified preparation of human chorionic gonadotropin (HCG) as the antigen and antiserum to HCG. When mixed with test urine on a slide and gently agitated, results are obtained in 2 minutes. Several commercial test kits are available containing latex particles or red cells that are agglutinated by HCG antibodies. Failure of agglutination after adding a woman's urine that contains HCG represents a positive test; it may be sensitive to small amounts, amounting to HCG levels of only 1,000 to 4,000 IU/liter. The tests become positive at 10 to 14 days after the first missed menstrual period. In normal pregnancy the diagnostic accuracy is 95%; in the absence of pregnancy, it is about 98.5% accurate.

Additionally, the availability of antisera to the β subunit makes it possible to detect HCG in the pregnant woman within a week of conception. A highly sensitive test of this type can be useful in the very early detection of pregnancy, in cases of suspected ectopic pregnancy, and in following women prior to and after therapy for trophoblastic tumors. The specific assay permits the measurement of minute amounts of HCG in the presence of LH. It should be emphasized that HCG titers below 5 mIU/ml may overlap with physiologic levels of LH with less sensitive tests. It is important to distinguish between the two hormones since the earliest rises denoting malignant disease will not be missed. With β-HCG radioimmunoassay (RIA) tests, the cross reaction is so minimal that for all practical purposes it is considered specific.

Ultimately, the definitive diagnosis of pregnancy is based on detection of the gestational sac, which can be accomplished very early through ultrasonic screening (particularly vaginal). It is regularly possible to detect a gestational sac within the uterus from about the sixth week after the last menstrual period. Real-time methods may pick up fetal heart pulsations between 8 and 10 weeks of gestation and limb movements at 10 to 12 weeks. Irregular and infrequent breathing motions can be observed at about 12 weeks. When Doppler techniques are used, it may be possible to detect a fetal heart beat between the 10th and 12th week after the last menstrual period.

TESTS OF FETAL MATURITY AND INTRAUTERINE STATUS

A number of screening tests are available for evaluation of fetal environment and *in utero* welfare. Estriol (urinary); human placental lactogen; and estrogen-creatinine ratios (urinary and plasma) are now being used infrequently. Currently the emphasis on determination of fetal well-being has shifted to biophysical monitoring including NST (nonstress test), CST (contraction stress test), and biophysical profile.

The least formal antepartum biometric testing is maternal assessment of fetal movement. One method is simply the daily notation of the time required for 10 movements to occur. If 10 movements have not occurred in 12 hours, or if it takes twice as long for 10 movements to occur as the week before, the count is abnormal and further testing is initiated.

An NST is frequently used as a primary means of fetal surveillance for the fetus at high risk. An NST utilizes external electronic fetal monitoring and is the observation of the fetal heart rate (FHR) changes occurring with fetal movements. The test is classified as reactive if at least 2 accelerations of the FHR are present (each of at least 15 beats per minute [BPM] above the baseline rate and lasting for at least 15 seconds) within a 20-minute period. A reactive NST with an otherwise normal tracing is a very solid indicator of fetal well-being. The compromised fetus will often show a prolonged nonreactive NST. Additionally, spontaneous decelerations (particularly if they exceed 40 BPM or are less than 90 BPM with a duration of longer than 60 seconds) are associated with a high incidence of fetal distress in labor (50%) and fetal demise (25%). Thus, this finding mandates careful evaluation and in many circumstances delivery. In questionable NST evaluations it is common to proceed to CST.

The CST utilizes uterine contractions to reduce placental blood flow mildly—the assumption being that a fetus with adequate reserve will tolerate transient reductions in placental perfusion, whereas the fetus with a decreased reserve will not tolerate the reduction and will demonstrate deceleration of FHR after the uterine contraction (late deceleration). A CST may be performed using either nipple stimulation or oxytocin infusion and requires 1 to 2 hours to complete. In situations where uterine stimulation may evoke risk (*e.g.*, predispositions to uterine rupture, premature delivery, or uterine bleeding), the relative risk/benefit of CST must be carefully weighed. Most authorities recommend taking into consideration not just decelerations of the fetal heart in relation to the contractions but also the presence or absence of FHR accelerations. Although the test has a low rate of false negativity, 25% to 50% of the fetuses with a so-called positive CST (late decelerations occurring with each of three contractions in a 10-minute period) tolerate labor.

The biophysical profile is a combination of an NST with ultrasonic assessments of fetal breathing movement, limb movement, trunk attitude and movement, and qualitative amniotic fluid volume. Each of these criteria are graded on the basis of 2 points for normal, or 0 to 1 point for abnormal, and a numeric value is assigned. The perinatal mortality rates with biophysical profiles of 8 to 10 are very low.

Amniotic fluid analyses have been very helpful in determining degrees of fetal hemolysis in isoimmunization problems (spectral OD at 450 mμ), in estimating fetal maturity (creatinine and disappearance of peak in spectral OD at 450 mμ), in determining fetal lung maturity by assessing phospholipids (lecithin/sphingomyelin [L/S] ratio and phosphotidyl glycerol) and in cytogenetic diagnosis by karyotyping fetal cells grown in culture media. Enzymatic studies capable of discovering *in utero* many inborn errors of metabolism can be made of amniotic fluid. Assessments of certain endocrine analyses, such as 17-ketosteroids, hold promise of detecting adrenogenital syndromes *in utero*. Chorionic villus sampling (CVS) is an alternative to amniocentesis for genetic or metabolic testing. CVS is commonly performed transcervically at 9 to 11 weeks' gestation (earlier than the usual amniocentesis) by inserting a sterile catheter into the uterine cavity under ultrasonic guidance. Chorionic villi are aspirated for analysis, and the results for many common problems may be available within a shorter time than taken for cell culture following amniocentesis. Most recently, it has been found that ultrasonically guided periumbilical blood (PUB) sampling of the fetus may be safely accomplished (complications generally less than 2%). This procedure is usually performed in the second or third trimester and is limited to a rather urgent need

for knowledge of chromosomal or metabolic abnormalities.

Fetal lung maturity may be assessed by determination of the L/S ratio. These phospholipids are secreted into the amniotic fluid by type II pulmonary alveolar epithelial cells. Typically until about the 35th gestational week these substances appear in approximately equal quantities. After that time, the secretion of lecithin rises abruptly while the sphingomyelin remains the same or gradually declines. Lipids in surfactant that is released by lamellar bodies into the amniotic fluid are represented by phospholipids (80%–90% by weight), of which lecithin is the major component (70%–80%). Phosphatidylglycerol may also be determined in amniotic fluid. Respiratory distress syndrome develops in less than 2% of newborns when the L/S ratio is greater than 2.0. In the range of 1.5 to 2.0, approximately 40% of infants will suffer this respiratory problem. It should be recognized that a rise in the L/S ratio is accelerated over that noted in normal pregnancy in association with a variety of clinical situations that cause fetal stress. The most important examples include placental insufficiency, hypertensive toxemia, and premature rupture of the membranes.

The routine use of ultrasound is recommended by some authorities. Serial studies are indicated when the past obstetric history is poor, the mother is older, bleeding has occurred, nutrition is poor (or alcohol, drug addiction, etc.), dates are uncertain, a serious maternal disease arises (*e.g.*, diabetes, hypertension, etc.), there is evidence of fetal compromise or defect, or evidence of placental problems. Serial ultrasonic measurements are useful to achieve accuracy in predicting the EDC as well as the additional dividends of detecting retardation of fetal growth, multiple gestations, malposition, and various anomalies. Generally, it can be assumed that 90% of fetuses with a biparietal diameter greater than 8.5 cm will weigh more than 2,500 g at birth. Ultrasonic diagnosis of intrauterine growth retardation has a clinical accuracy of about 75%. Errors caused by asymmetric growth are minimized by combining various measurements and comparing serial measurements.

FETAL HEART RATE MONITORING

The fetal heart rate offers two major advantages in assessment of fetal status: it is directly available and there are usually reliable changes in the fetal heart rate caused by fetal hypoxia and acidosis. However, the fetal heart rate, as would be the case in an adult, should be viewed as only one parameter and must be evaluated with all other available information to enhance accuracy. The fetal heart rate may be obtained by several methods: manual stethoscope, Doppler ultrasound, direct ultrasonic visualization (not practical for any length of time), phonocardiography (difficult to achieve), and direct electrocardiography. The method chosen is based on availability of equipment, the health care provider's comfort with the various techniques, and the patient's risk.

For detection of alterations, the heart rate is divided into the basal fetal heart rate (that which occurs without the alterations of stress) and periodic changes (heart rate response to various stresses). The fetal heart rate (FHR) in early gestation is approximately 20 beats per minute (BPM) higher than at term. The slowing occurs linearly throughout pregnancy. The baseline, or basal, fetal heart rate is the average rate prevailing apart from beat to beat variability and periodic changes; normal is 120 to 160 BPM. Tachycardia is a baseline FHR greater than 160 BPM lasting for more than 30 minutes and is further quantified as moderate (160–180 BPM) or severe (exceeding 180 BPM). Tachycardia may be the result of maternal fever, maternal hyperthyroidism, fetal infection, or fetal distress. Bradycardia is defined as a FHR of less than 120 BPM. Moderate bradycardia (100–119 BPM) may be associated with severe fetal distress, whereas severe bradycardia (FHR less than 100 BPM) is more likely either agonal or the result of a heart block.

In the mature fetal heart there is a beat-to-beat variation; that is, the time interval between heartbeats varies (short-term variability). Electronic fetal monitoring demonstrates this reassuring finding as small, rapid, rhythmic fluctuations with an amplitude of 5 to 15 BPM. Several conditions are associated with less beat-to-beat variation than normal, including the premature (but normal) fetus, the sleeping fetus, and medicated fetuses (e.g., alphaprodine, atropine, barbiturates, conduction anesthesia, diazepam, general anesthesia, meperidine, morphine, phenothiazines, and magnesium sulfate in large doses). Good FHR short-term variability in the absence of the above mitigating factors indicates adequate central nervous system oxygenation. If normal FHR variability is apparent 5 minutes before birth, irrespective of earlier periodic changes, a good Apgar rating is likely, assuming a mature fetus with no congenital anomalies. When significant unexplained FHR decreased beat-to-beat

variability occurs, therapy should be undertaken, including shifting the mother to a different position, administering maternal oxygen by mask, and maintaining normal blood pressure. With failure of these measures to improve beat-to-beat variability, fetal assessment by stimulation tests (e.g., motion, noise) or scalp blood sampling should be undertaken to further assess fetal well-being. Short-term variability also appears to have a rhythmic reproducible pattern, termed *long-term variability*. If present, long-term variability is a sign of well being but is altered by the same factors affecting short-term variability.

The periodic changes are acceleration or deceleration from the baseline FHR in response to fetal stimulation, movements, or uterine contractions. An acceleration occurs when the FHR increases more than 15 BPM for more than 15 seconds. Accelerations usually appear as smooth patterns on electronic fetal monitoring and are a good indication of fetal well-being. Accelerations may be triggered in the normal mature fetus by fetal body motion, acoustic stimulation, stimulation of the fetal scalp, and other stimuli.

Decelerations are periodic heart rate decreases from the baseline, usually in response to uterine contractions. When a spontaneous deceleration is noted on antepartum monitoring, it is an ominous finding. When viewed by electronic fetal monitoring, in relationship to uterine contractions, there are three deceleration patterns. The early deceleration patterns are uniform, occurring as mirror images of the uterine contractions, and usually repetitive. The onset of early decelerations occurs with the onset of the contraction, the nadir of the heart rate occurring with the apex of the contraction and the heart rate increasing back to baseline as the contraction ebbs. This deceleration is caused by compression of the fetal head and, as a result, is much more common with ruptured membranes. It usually requires no therapy and is viewed as a benign finding because long-term sequelae have not been associated with this pattern. However, early decelerations may indicate a problem if the patterns are severe, prolonged, persistent, or accompanied by thick meconium staining. Under those circumstances, therapy includes change of maternal position (lateral recumbent is best), ruling out umbilical cord compression (sterile vaginal examination), and, in some cases, administration of atropine to the mother (because it is caused by vagal stimulation, the fetus receives enough to block the response).

Late decelerations have the same uniform appearance as early decelerations, except for one difference; late deceleration's pattern occurs later than the contraction. That is, the onset of FHR deceleration occurs after the contraction onset, the nadir of FHR occurs after the apex of the contraction, and the FHR deceleration continues after the contraction has abated. Late deceleration is associated with uteroplacental insufficiency and is a consequence of hypoxia and metabolic abnormalities. *Thus, late deceleration is the most ominous fetal heart rate pattern.* In less severe cases the FHR may transiently exceed the baseline after the deceleration ends. With severely affected fetuses, the FHR takes longer to return to baseline from the deceleration and does not transiently accelerate. However, in some with severe compromise, the fetus will have a baseline tachycardia. Late decelerations merit therapy; this is usually to decrease uterine activity (*e.g.*, turn off oxytocin), correct maternal hypotension, hyperoxygenate, and expand maternal blood volume. Should these steps not be immediately effective, delivery must be undertaken.

Care in interpretation is necessary because significant changes during contractions may be subtle and the FHR may be within the normal range. This is exemplified by the postmature fetus, for often the findings of late decelerations are less obvious than at an earlier stage of gestation.

Variable decelerations are usually nonrepetitive, not uniform, vary widely in configuration, begin at any time in relation to the contraction, and often both onset and cessation are marked by precipitous changes in the FHR. Frequently, there is a transient acceleration before and/or after the deceleration. Variable decelerations are caused by umbilical cord compression and are classified as severe if they last more than 60 seconds or lead to a FHR of less than 90 BPM. If vaginal examination reveals no palpable cord, maternal positional changes do not resolve the pattern, and/or it is severe, then fetal scalp sampling may be necessary to determine the degree of fetal compromise. In the absence of fetal scalp sampling availability or with other compromising factors, immediate delivery may be prudent.

Combinations of FHR patterns also occur; the most common combined pattern is that of variable and late decelerations. This is a most ominous pattern and usually consists of variable decelerations with a late deceleration component appearing as fetal status deteriorates. Fetuses with this pattern are usually severely compromised and immedi-

TABLE 4-2. Mature Fetal Heart Rate Parameters

FEATURE	PARAMETERS	INTERPRETATION
Baseline Heart		
Rate	120–160 BPM	Normal
Tachycardia		
Moderate	161–180 BPM	Nonreassuring
Marked	>180 BPM	Abnormal
Bradycardia		
Moderate	100–119 BPM	Nonreassuring
Marked	<100 BPM	Abnormal
Short-term variability	5–15 BPM	Reassuring
Long-term variability	Present	Reassuring
Periodic Changes		
Accelerations	>15 BPM for >15 sec	Well being
Decelerations		
Early	10–40 BPM	Head compression
Late	5–60 BPM	Hypoxia/acidosis
Variable	10–60 BPM	Cord compression
Combinations		Nonreassuring

ate delivery should be considered if the simple steps outlined above for late decelerations do not cause the pattern to improve. Fetal heart rate parameters are summarized in Table 4-2.

PHYSIOLOGY AND CONDUCT OF LABOR

From the first trimester onward the uterus undergoes sporadic, nonrhythmic, painless contractions, the intensity of which is not great until near term, when they account for most cases of false labor. These are called Braxton Hicks contractions. The uterus also exhibits low-intensity contractions of great frequency and rhythmic pattern. Theories concerning the cause of the onset of labor include (1) progesterone deprivation, with release of the myometrial block and loss of potassium effect at the placental site, which causes hyperpolarization of the cellular membrane; (2) oxytocin theory—increasing sensitivity of the myometrium to oxytocin; (3) uterine stretch theory—any hollow viscus tends to contract and empty itself when distended to a certain point; (4) the fetal adrenal theory—by providing the placenta with C-19 precursors for estrogen metabolism may give rise to an endocrine milieu that favors the onset of labor; (5) the prostaglandin theory—in which certain of these hydroxylated 20-carbon fatty acids widely distributed in mammalian tissues are markedly elevated in both the amniotic fluid and the peripheral blood of spontaneously laboring women (eightfold increase over nonlaboring women). Smooth muscle contraction requires an elevated level of intracytoplasmic free calcium. An adenosine triphosphate (ATP) dependent system binds or releases calcium from the sarcoplasmic reticulum that surrounds the myofibril. Prostaglandins E_2 and $F_{2\alpha}$ inhibit the calcium binding in pregnancy and in nonpregnant women. The resultant rise in intracytoplasmic levels of calcium would promote myometrial contractility.

The character of labor involves intermittent contraction and relaxation phases, and as labor advances the interval between contractions decreases. At the acme of contractions intrauterine pressures may normally reach 50 mmHg or more. Proper uterine contraction requires the interaction of a contractile substance (actomyosin), a supply of energy (ATP), a stimulus to initiate contraction and a means of conducting the stimulus to contractile elements (distribution of ions in the membranes). Uterine action in labor, like that of the heart, is under intrinsic nervous control originating either in the muscle itself or in ganglia in the uterine wall; however, pacemaker activity is not nearly so defined in the uterus as in the heart, and there is no known bundle of His. Nevertheless, the dependence of normal labor on rhythmic, coordinated contractions suggests that the bioelectrical physiology is an important feature. Pacemaker activity tends to center in the area of the uterotubal junction, but excitation points and propagation of electrical impulses may wander or arise in any group of myometrial cells. There must be a so-called fundal dominance and downward gradient of force for progress to be made and cervical dilation to proceed normally.

In normal labor there is a latent phase of several hours' duration, during which the cervix effaces but dilates only slightly. An active phase ensues, with great acceleration in progress when the cervix dilates rapidly and progressively. A deceleration or slowing occurs just prior to full dilatation. Prolongation of any one of these three phases, resulting in protraction of labor, may connote a problem.

NORMAL LABOR AND DELIVERY

In labor, the irregular painless uterine contractions are replaced by regular uncomfortable ones that bring about cervical effacement and dilatation. Differentiation of pattern normally establishes an upper segment that is actively contractile, and a physiologic retraction ring separates this thick powerful area from the thin, more distensible, less active lower segment. Normally, before the onset of labor, the fetal head in most primigravidas has settled into the pelvic brim (often 2 or more weeks earlier). This process of fetal descent of the presenting part is referred to as *lightening* and is marked by an ability to "breathe easier" and by more frequent urination (decreased bladder capacity). There may be associated ineffectual uterine contractions (false labor pains), but the process of shortening of the cervical canal is usually begun (effacement of the cervix). With the beginning dilatation there may be discharge of the cervical plug along with the passage of a small amount of blood known as "bloody show." In multigravidas it is much more common for the cervix to efface less and to begin dilatation prior to labor.

Stages

Labor is divided into three stages. The first stage begins with the onset of uterine contractions and ends with complete cervical dilatation. The average first stage duration is 8 to 12 hours in a primigravida and 6 to 8 hours in a multipara. The second stage of labor extends from full cervical dilatation to birth of the baby and normally does not exceed 2.5 hours in the nullipara and 50 minutes in the multipara. Generally, labor's second stage is marked by more rapid descent of the fetal presenting part. The third stage of labor begins with the birth of the baby, ends with placental delivery, and generally does not exceed 30 minutes.

Assessment of labor's progress may be afforded by evaluation of cervical dilatation as a function of time. Thus, the first stage of labor may be subdivided into the earlier and longer *latent phase* (when cervical dilatation progresses slowly up to 3 cm in a nulligravida and 2 cm in a multipara), and the *active phase* (from the end of the latent phase to complete dilatation). The latent phase in a nullipara should not exceed 20.6 hours and in a multipara should not exceed 13.6 hours. Similarly, the active phase in a nullipara should not exceed 11.7 hours and in a multipara should not exceed 5.2 hours. During the interval from 4 cm to 9 cm dilatation (phase of maximum slope), the nullipara's cervix should be dilating more than 1.2 cm/hour. In the multipara the phase of maximum slope is from 3 cm to 9 cm, and cervical dilatation should proceed at more than 1.5 cm/hour.

Obviously, abnormalities of labor may occur. If the *latent phase is prolonged* (>20 hours in nulliparas, >14 hours in multiparas) the patient may have an unripe cervix, be in false labor, have a uterine dysfunction, have been oversedated or improperly anesthetized. In such circumstances it is uncommon for fetopelvic disproportion to be the problem, and rest, fluid replacement, and support will usually remedy the problem. In cases of uterine dysfunction, adequate labor contractions (usually by oxytocin augmentation) are curative. Similarly, the active phase may be prolonged (*i.e.*, <1.2 cm/hour in nulliparas, <1.5 cm/hour in multiparas); this is termed a ***primary dysfunctional labor***. In such cases the etiology is usually malposition, sedation, or excessive conduction anesthesia, although approximately 30% will be due to fetopelvic disproportion. Whereas the latter group is treated by cesarean section, the former is merely afforded supportive measures. Finally, cervical dilatation may progress normally to a certain point in the active phase when it simply ceases. This is termed a ***secondary arrest*** of dilatation and is associated with fetopelvic disproportion in approximately 45% of cases. The majority of these patients require cesarean for delivery, but in some a trial of oxytocin is valuable.

Prolonged second stages of labor must be carefully evaluated for uterine inertia, fetal malposition, or fetopelvic disproportion. Although uterine inertia is usually treated with oxytocics, the majority of patients with the two latter conditions may require cesarean section.

Mechanism

This is conditioned by the fact that the greatest diameter of the superior strait is oblique, that the midpelvis is larger and permits turning and that in the inferior strait the greatest diameter is the anteroposterior. It is apparent that some process of accommodation of suitable portions of the fetal head to the various planes is requisite to the satisfactory completion of childbirth. The positional changes of the presenting part constitute the mechanism of labor, and the cardinal movements are listed below:

1. Engagement
2. Descent
3. Flexion
4. Internal rotation
5. Extension
6. External rotation
7. Expulsion

(These seven steps occur in sequence.)

Anterior rotation of the occiput is caused by the twisting of the head upon the shoulders as the occiput is directed from an oblique diameter to the long diameter of the pelvic outlet (*i.e.*, the anteroposterior). The occiput turns forward 45 degrees in anterior positions, 90 degrees in transverse, and 135 degrees in posterior.

Restitution occurs following the birth of the head, which returns to its original position in relation to the shoulders.

External rotation is due to the anterior rotation of the shoulder girdle to bring the shoulders into the anteroposterior diameter of the outlet. The occiput rotates 45 degrees to the transverse position.

In about 10% of patients, the membranes rupture prior to the onset of labor. Delivery is ideally accomplished within 24, but certainly less than 48, hours thereafter if the fetus is mature in order to avoid chorioamnionitis. Usually there is no fear of prolapsed cord if the presentation is normal and the fetus is not hypoxic. Membrane rupture should be established by direct observation of fluid coming from the cervix, by demonstrating fetal epithelial cells in the vaginal fluid, vaginal fluid alkalinity, a tree-like crystallization of dried fluid, fat globules, or presence of lanugo hair on a smear. Occasionally, only the chorion will rupture while the amnion remains intact. However, collected fluid between the two layers may be lost in a manner similar to rupture of both membranes. This situation does not predispose to intra-amniotic infection.

While solid food is not allowed, oral fluids may be offered in early labor. The patient may ambulate until an analgesic is required. Later, a lateral recumbent position may relieve uterine pressure on the vena cava. Vaginal examinations may be made at variable intervals in context with supervision of the frequency, duration, and intensity of uterine contractions. FHR should be recorded every 15 minutes during the time of contraction, and for at least 1 hour afterwards. There should be no decelerations, the FHR should not be below 120 BPM and accelerations above 160 BPM should not occur.

Currently, there is enthusiasm for monitoring the fetal heart externally by phonocardiographic or Doppler auscultation through the abdominal wall or internally by electrodes attached to the presenting fetal part, although efficacy for low-risk cases is not proven. Tokodynametric external monitoring of the uterine contractions and monitoring by an internal intraamniotic transcervical catheter attached to an external transducer are also valuable methods of monitoring the labor. Certainly, all patients with high-risk pregnancy, suspected fetal distress, passage of meconium, premature labor, or *in utero* growth retardation, or whose fetal heart is abnormal by evaluation with the stethoscope, should have the benefit of these more objective assessments. Fetal hypoxia resulting in fetal acidosis can be detected by demonstrating an abnormally low pH in capillary blood obtained from the fetal scalp. Values below 7.20 are quite worrisome, particularly if the mother's blood gases are normal and there is an abnormal FHR pattern. Passage of thick meconium and risk of meconium aspiration syndrome are of further concern.

Bladder care is necessary to avoid distention, hypotonia, and infection. When labor is long, intravenous glucose and possibly electrolyte infusion may be required. If the membranes are intact, amniotomy may expedite a desultory labor and may be used selectively if the presenting part is well engaged. Obviously, appropriate analgesia properly timed and given in proper dosage, may help support the labor in addition to the critical emotional considerations. In the second stage of labor, the patient may be instructed to use her abdominal muscles to assist the uterine expulsive effort. Leg cramps from pressure of the fetal head on the pelvic nerves may be diminished by massage or changing the leg position.

The delivery should be managed in a controlled manner to prevent injury to the fetal head from sudden decompression with rapid expulsion and to avoid significant laceration of the maternal tissues. There is a gaping of the introitus with each contraction and the perineum may be put under great tension. At this time, there is considerable risk of a perineal laceration. A proper episiotomy may prevent this trauma in certain instances. A modified Ritgen maneuver is the proper and simplest procedure to follow.

The fetal neck should be checked for a loop of umbilical cord, since this may be observed in about a quarter of deliveries. The cord should be slipped over the fetal head, if possible, or cut between clamps if it is tight. An unrecognized shoulder dystocia is another potential problem in some cases, if aid is not given to the shoulders by depressing the fetal head gently downward and forward until the anterior shoulder appears beneath the pubis. Gentle assistance may be given to the posterior arm after the head is lifted gradually to bring the posterior shoulder over the perineum. This is another point when perineal lacerations are likely to occur. Should shoulder dystocia occur, it may be resolved by removing the patient's legs from the stirrups and flexing them on the abdomen (the McRoberts maneuver).

After delivery, lowering the infant below the introitus of the mother before cord pulsations cease results in a significant transfer of placental blood into the fetus (equivalent to about 50 mg of iron). The infant's head should be dependent to allow mucus to drain into the nasopharynx where it can be aspirated. The cord is clamped and cut and the infant is warmed, labeled appropriately, and given prophylaxis for gonorrheal ophthalmia neonatorum. Should meconium be present in the amniotic fluid, a combined obstetric and neonatal effort is necessary to determine if thorough suctioning below the laryngeal cords will be necessary to decrease the incidence of the meconium aspiration syndrome.

Delivery of Placenta

The third stage of labor is made up of two phases, namely, the phase of placental separation and the phase of placental expulsion. The sudden diminution in uterine size after delivery of the fetus is accompanied by a decrease in the area of the placental site. The placenta becomes thickened, buckles on itself, and becomes separated in the spongiosa layer of the decidua. In the majority of cases this takes place within a few minutes after the birth of the infant. Expulsion of the placenta may occur sideways into the vagina with the maternal surface appearing first at the vulva (Duncan mechanism) or, much more commonly, by inversion of the sac with the fetal surface of the placenta presenting at the vulva (Schultze's mechanism). These mechanisms apply only to the behavior of the placenta in the vagina, because the placenta is expelled from the uterus through the flabby lower segment in only one manner. Thus, separation of the placenta is due primarily to a disproportion between the static size of the placenta and the reduced size of the placental site, this disproportion being the natural result of the uterine contraction associated with the birth of the baby. The periphery of the placenta is the most adherent portion and, as a result, separation usually begins elsewhere, commonly with the formation of a hematoma in the decidual cleavage plane. Traction on the umbilical cord risks inverting the uterus. It is customary to administer 10 units of oxytocin intramuscularly immediately after delivery of the placenta. Manual removal of the placenta and exploration of the uterine cavity to assure that it is clean and intact is indicated for long retention, hemorrhage, and retained placental fragments or membranes. However, this practice should be avoided if possible in Rh-negative mothers, to minimize the risk of transfusing the maternal blood sinuses with antigenic Rh-positive fetal red blood cells.

When placental retention occurs, the possibility of placenta accreta should be considered. This condition is marked by the absence of the decidual layer that separates the placental villi and the myometrium. Placenta accreta is rare (1 in 2,000–7,000 deliveries) and is divided into three types: accreta vera (80% of cases) in which the villi are adherent to the superficial myometrium; placenta increta (15% of cases) in which the villi invade the myometrium; and, placenta percreta (5% of cases) in which the villi penetrate the full myometrial thickness. In addition to placental retention, placenta accreta is marked difficulty in placental separation and by hemorrhage. Although conservative therapy may be successful for the majority of cases, hysterectomy may be necessary for placenta percreta or increta and if hemorrhage is extensive.

Both fetal and maternal surfaces of the placenta should be examined carefully to ascertain that no placental remnants are missing (usually remaining in the uterus). Also gross placental abnormalities should be noted; for example, a succenturiate lobe (usually signaled by a major fetal surface vascular disruption at the placental margin) or a bipartite placenta. Insertion of the cord into the placenta is ascertained. If cord insertion is within 1 cm of the placental margin, it is termed a Battledore or marginal insertion but has little clinical significance. By contrast, in roughly 1% of cases the cord will not insert on the placenta but will insert on the membranes. This is called **velamentous cord insertion** and has two important clinical implications. First, 25% to 50% of infants born with a velamentous cord insertion will have developmental defects. Second, the unsupported vessels coursing through the membranes to the placental chorionic plate cause the very risky clinical condition **vasa previa**. The risk of vasa previa is that with labor a vessel will rupture and the fetus exsanguinate. This usually has few symptoms other than painless vaginal bleeding and perhaps fetal tachycardia. The Apt test or hemoglobin electrophoresis will allow differentiation between fetal and maternal blood.

Further inspection of the cord, starting with the cut surface first details if the cord has three vessels and is directed to ruling out other abnormalities: excessive length (greater than 100 cm), shortness (less than 30 cm), true knots, tumors, and discoloration (for example, with meconium). A two-vessel cord (absence of one umbilical artery) occurs in 0.85% of singletons, but in 6% of twins. About 14% of infants with this defect will die and over 50% of the deaths are associated with major structural anomalies. As time permits the placenta is weighed (normal is 400–600 g, approximately one sixth the weight of the newborn) and further inspected. It is normally 15 to 20 cm in diameter and 2 to 4 cm thick. The fetal membranes normally arise from the placenta at its margin, but in about 1% of cases the membranes emanate from a thick whitish ring central to the margin. This is termed a **circumvallate placenta** and is often associated with second trimester bleeding and abruptio placenta.

A special comment about "inversion" of the uterus is warranted on the basis of its preventability as well as the seriousness of this complication. Strong traction on the umbilical cord, together with vigorous downward pressure on the uterine fundus in instances when the placenta is firmly attached, may result in an inverted uterus, partial placental detachment, hemorrhage, hypovolemia with shock, or, occasionally, acute circulatory collapse. Pushing on the central area of the inverted uterus should be avoided. A smooth muscle–relaxing anesthesia (*e.g.,* halothane) should be employed. The uterus can usually be gradually replaced by digitally pressing upward against the junction of the inverted and uninverted position of the uterus. If the placenta is still attached, it should be manually separated but only after replacement and supportive measures consisting of oxytocin administration, blood replacement as needed, fundal massage, and observations for uterine atony. Only rarely is replacement by the abdominal approach necessary or is incision of the constriction ring in the neck of the inversion in the posterior midline required.

An interesting phenomenon of the immediate puerperium during its first hour is the occurrence of "postpartal chills," which occur in up to a fourth of patients, particularly those who have had an operative delivery under regional anesthesia. One hypothesis is that the chills represent a fetomaternal transfusion reaction, although the cause has not been established.

Episiotomy

Episiotomy is incision of the perineum prior to delivery of the baby. It serves several purposes. (1) It substitutes a straight, clean-cut surgical incision for the ragged, contused laceration that is otherwise likely to ensue; such an incision is easier to repair and heals better than a tear. (2) The direction of the episiotomy can be controlled, whereas a tear may extend in any direction, sometimes involving the anal sphincter and the rectum or the vascular periurethral tissues. (3) It spares the baby's head the necessity of serving as a battering ram against the perineal obstruction. (4) The operation shortens the duration of the second stage and spares the maternal soft parts and the pelvic visceral supports.

Episiotomy may be made in the midline of the perineum (median episiotomy), or it may be begun in the midline and directed obliquely away from the rectum (mediolateral episiotomy). The median episiotomy is more easily repaired, is attended by less bleeding and causes the patient less discomfort; however, median episiotomies are attended more frequently by extensions into the rectal sphincter and mucosa than the mediolateral episiotomies. The choice of the type of incision should be suited to the individual circumstances, although, the median type is usually preferred.

It is essential that any untoward event occurring during delivery or episiotomy be recognized in anticipation of immediate repair (*e.g.*, laceration of the anal sphincter or injury to the rectal wall). Otherwise, postpartal anal incontinence or development of a rectovaginal fistula may call for major gynecologic reparative efforts after a suitable waiting period in order to clear tissue necrosis, control infection, and provide time for the fistula tract(s) to epithelialize.

Care of the Lacerated Perineum

Perineal tears of the first degree implicate the mucous membranes of the fourchette and the skin and the subcutaneous tissue of the perineum; those of the second degree implicate the skin of the perineum, the constrictor vaginae, and the transversus perinei muscles, and sometimes the levator ani; those of the third degree implicate the sphincter ani muscle and, in addition, the anterior surface of the rectum. Involvement of the rectal mucosa is sometimes referred to as a fourth-degree perineal laceration.

In all cases, the immediate closure of perineal lacerations and episiotomies by suture is urgently indicated. If the vagina is lacerated, its edges should be brought together by deeply laid chromic catgut sutures. In complete tears the rectum and its mucosa should be united by buried catgut sutures and the sphincter ani firmly sutured by catgut. The operator must make certain that the lateral halves of the sphincter muscle, which usually are retracted laterally, are approximated in the midline.

Care should be taken to inspect the periurethral region, since longitudinal tears in this area can bleed profusely.

Finally, it has become customary to think in terms of a fourth stage of labor because bleeding and other problems may be of paramount impor-

tance after delivery of the placenta. Sometimes there is atony requiring oxytocins, manual massage, compression or evacuation of the uterus, blood transfusion, and attention to the prevention of sepsis. In other circumstances, careful attention to bladder atony and other considerations are paramount. It is important to institute perineal exercises in the postpartal period to help reestablish proper pubococcygeal muscle tone and urinary control.

"Natural Childbirth" and Family-Centered Birth Process

The knowledge of the hazards of heavy analgesia and anesthesia as previously outlined to both mother and newborn led to the classic concept of "natural childbirth" in the 1960s and the Lamaze method and other approaches in the 1970s. These approaches were intended to reduce the need for the pharmacologic control of pain during parturition and delivery. Since the mid-1970s, the approach to the birth process has been family-centered care. The emphasis in this modern approach is to incorporate the father as a participant in this family event with the infant at center stage and to stress parent–infant bonding from the time of delivery. This concept, which is embodied in the Leboyer approach, calls for immediate skin-to-skin contact between the mother and her infant as well as a warm-water bath for the infant while the entire family-centered experience is conducted in a darkened delivery room. These human factors are now being emphasized in a variety of settings in close proximity to more traditional facilities where the proper therapeutic measures can be instituted promptly should an unexpected complication arise. These practices are safe but contingent upon proper screening techniques to identify patients at risk who may need specialized or even high-technology care.

Postpartal Care of the Mother

In as much as hemorrhage is the major risk in the immediate postpartal interval, the uterus should be watched for at least an hour after delivery. If it is not firmly contracted, it should be massaged gently and continuously. If intravenous oxytocics fail to maintain sufficient uterine tone, and there is no maternal hypertension, ergonovine (Ergotrate) or methyergonovine (Methergine) may be administered intramuscularly to promote uterine tone, although prostaglandin suppositories are also a valid option.

The vulva should be washed with sterile water and soap and covered with a sterile pad held in place by a T bandage. Severe "afterpains" may be treated by oral narcotics and/or nonnarcotic analgesics. An ice bag applied to the perineum will be comforting and reduce the risk of hematoma. After it is ascertained that stabilization has occurred, the temperature and the pulse should be taken four times a day. The patient should be encouraged to urinate within 6 hours, but catheterization should be avoided unless absolutely necessary as it carries at least a 3% chance of being associated with subsequent pyelonephritis. Early ambulation is helpful in establishing normal urinary and bowel function. A mild cathartic or enema on the second or third day may be required. The patient should be instructed about proper toilet of the vulva. The diet should be well balanced, containing 2,500 to 3,000 calories. Under normal conditions salt and fluids need not be restricted.

Before and after each nursing, the nipples should be washed with sterile water and soap. Full milk production will be achieved in 10 to 14 days, but the quantity of available milk per feeding will vary with the mother's diet, emotional status, fluid intake, drug intake, and other factors. Encrusted nipples are most likely to become irritated or inflamed, and the application of lanolin cream after nursing assists in prevention of this sequence. If the nipples become cracked or painful, they should be treated with compound tincture of benzoin, lanolin, or penicillin ointment. The use of a sterile nipple shield is of some assistance. If mastitis develops, antistaphylococcal chemotherapy must be instituted promptly. Nursing from the infected side should be suspended and the breast expressed or pumped until the inflammation subsides. If fluctuation occurs, the abscess should be incised surgically, the incisions running from the areolar edge to the periphery to avoid cutting the ducts. If appropriate chemotherapy is administered at the first sign of mastitis, abscess formation almost always can be prevented.

Rh immunoglobulin should be administered to Rh-negative unsensitized mothers within 72 hours of delivery (standard 300-μg dose). Smaller doses (50-μg doses) may be adequately protective in first trimester postabortal women. The standard dose should be given antepartally after amniocentesis. A routine antepartal dose at approximately 28 weeks in addition to the one postpartally has lowered the incidence of sensitization from about 1.0% to 0.3%. Finally, the patient with suspected fetal to maternal hemorrhage should be investigated using a Kleihauer-Betke stain test of maternal blood to see if more than the standard dose is necessary.

The patient should have a blood count on the third postpartum day, and if her hematocrit was low or borderline before delivery or is subnormal after delivery, appropriate studies are performed to determine the type of anemia, usually iron deficiency, and appropriate therapy is employed. Determinations of serum iron and iron-binding capacity and, occasionally, study of the bone marrow may be required to establish the diagnosis.

Puerperal perineal pain, episiotomy, vaginal or perirectal pain, problem voiding with or without visible bleeding, fever, bladder, or rectal pressure, or subsequent anemia should raise the suspicion of *puerperal hematoma.* A mass is usually discernible if the hematoma is below the pelvic fascia. Rupture of a vessel above the pelvic fascia may create a proximal paravaginal tumor and spread into the broad ligament or retroperitoneally in any direction. There may be presentation above the inguinal ligament, or the hematoma may rupture into the peritoneal cavity. Painful and expanding hematomas of a moderate to large size must be incised and drained, and vessels sought out and ligated. Packing may be required, and blood replacement, as well as antibiotic coverage, is an essential aspect of management. Recently, circumferential pneumatic compression provided by means of an antigravity-type suit has been employed with success in the control of markedly expanding intrapelvic hematomas.

If the patient does not nurse her infant, the breasts should be bound and ice bags and analgesics employed as necessary. Estrogenic hormones can be used to suppress lactation. Currently, an ergot derivative (bromocriptine) is utilized for lactation suppression through its antiprolactin action. It may be associated with decreases in blood pressure, so it should not be administered until the vital signs have stabilized. After that the patient should be observed for side effects relating to its basic ergot capability (hypertension, headache are evidence of CNS toxicity). It is best administered with food and is generally administered twice daily for 14 to 21 days. Most normal women can be safely discharged from the hospital by the 2nd or 3rd postpartal day.

The puerperium is the period of 6 weeks following the termination of labor. Generally, during this time the generative tract returns to its normal condition, which includes involution of the uterus and placental site, as well as general adaptations involving the breasts, urinary tract, lower generative tract, abdominal wall, and peritoneum. In the absence of nursing, menses resume within 6 to 8 weeks, and, by 3 months, roughly 90% of women will have had the return of menstruation. It is not unusual for women to have a brownish discharge with even occasional spurts of blood in minimal quantities for several weeks, but usually there is lochia alba after 2 weeks. Complete involution and normal recovery should be assured by a 4- to 6-week postpartal checkup. In addition to the history and careful examination, the urine should be checked and a smear should be taken for cytologic study. Follow-up of any abnormal findings noted during pregnancy should be undertaken (*e.g.,* glucose tolerance test, CBC, cardiovascular renal studies). If present, cervicitis should be corrected.

Family planning is often discussed or implemented at the postpartal visit. The available methods include the rhythm method, spermicidal creams and foams, vaginal diaphragms, cervical caps, oral contraceptives, implantable progestins, and an intrauterine device (IUD). The choice of method must be suited to the individual case after appropriate evaluation and discussion with the patient. In general, orally ingested steroids surpass all other methods in efficacy. Other methods and techniques are now under extensive study. It must be kept in mind that regardless of method, responsible family planning and ''wanted'' pregnancies are indispensable prerequisites for achieving optimal perinatal results. A more detailed discussion of contraception is provided in the section on gynecology.

ANALGESIA AND ANESTHESIA FOR LABOR AND DELIVERY

Pain relief in labor may be of two main types: (1) *obstetric analgesia* and (2) *obstetric anesthesia.* Obstetric analgesia is the administration of certain drugs during the first and second stages for the purpose of lessening the suffering caused by the labor pains prior to the actual birth of the baby. Obstetric anesthesia is the administration of certain drugs at the time of delivery for the purpose of rendering the birth of the baby painless; it is employed chiefly in operative deliveries and is the same as surgical anesthesia. Certain drugs may be used both as anesthetic and analgesic agents, but in that event the dosage and the method of administration are quite different in the two types of pain relief.

The potential hazards of providing pain relief during labor and delivery for both the mother and the fetus call for skilled personnel, adequate safety standards and equipment in the delivery room, and resuscitation capabilities. In the mother the emergency complications may take the form of respiratory obstruction, aspiration of gastric contents, laryngospasm, hypotension, cardiac arrest, drug overdose, or sensitivity reactions. The potential of acute problems calls for a secure indwelling plastic catheter for intravenous fluids and drug administrations and availability of blood. The possibility of hypoxia and depression in the newborn requires that analgesics and anesthetics be chosen and administered properly, and that the minimum effective dose of drugs be offered on a timely basis with respect to the anticipated delivery.

Appropriate childbirth education should be available to all patients, and knowledge about pain relief, various methods, and value in good obstetric practice should be emphasized. During labor, appropriate analgesia can be provided systemically or by regional sensory blockade. The patient is relatively insensitive to pain but is awake and responsive and the effect upon the fetus should be minimal. The use of a narcotic (*e.g.,* meperidine) often administered in small intravenous doses with or without a tranquilizer is a popular approach once labor is well established, if the fetus is mature. Since all drugs cross the placenta readily, it is important to minimize fetal depression by choosing the proper drug, dosage, route of administration, and time of use based on peak concentrations. If despite these safeguards a baby is born with respiratory depression from the narcotic, this may be reversed using naloxone (Narcan). In the major regional blocks such as epidurals, care must be taken to avoid hypotension by maintaining left uterine displacement and preloading the vascular system with appropriate fluids. A continuous epidural block provides pain relief for both labor and delivery. The disadvantage of this procedure is the potential accidental puncture, risk of maternal hypertension, and resultant postspinal headache if an intrathecal injection is made.

For most spontaneous and low forceps vaginal deliveries, a pudendal block is a very safe, effective anesthetic if intravascular injections are avoided and maximum recommended doses are not exceeded. When a general anesthesia is required for specific indications, a nonparticulate antacid should be administered (by mouth) to the patient prior to starting the anesthesia. An endotracheal tube is inserted to maintain the airway against laryngospasm and aspiration of vomitus. A balanced form of general anesthesia utilizing thiopental for rapid induction, succinylcholine for muscle relaxation, and nitrous oxide for analgesia represents a suitable choice when administered properly because the fetus is usually minimally affected. Spinal anesthesia is likewise both popular and safe when proper techniques and safeguards are followed to avoid hypotension and excessively high levels. Generally, anesthesia limited to the saddle area will suffice for vaginal deliveries. The drug should not be administered intrathecally during a uterine contraction as a safeguard against high levels of anesthesia and systemic ill effects. Spinal anesthesia is usually not the preferred method if uterine relaxation is required. For that purpose, halothane produces rapid uterine relaxation. By the same token, postpartal hemorrhage from uterine atony becomes a risk with halothane administration. Unless general medical or obstetric conditions dictate more special handling, anesthesia for cesarean section can be achieved quite satisfactorily either by the balanced general technique described or by regional anesthesia in the form of a spinal or epidural block. Trained personnel in both anesthesia and the specialized care required in managing patients during the period of recovery should be constantly available.

The effects of hypoxia, narcosis, and trauma may be additive or synergistic insults for the newborn; in selecting proper methods of obstetric management, these several factors must be given consideration if the infant is to be spared severe birth damage. Maternal hypoxemia and hypercapnia may have immediate fetal effects resulting in both hypoxemia and acidosis combining the respiratory and metabolic types. The program of pain relief for the mother must be determined in concert with the maturity and status of the fetus as well as the proposed method of delivery and its prospects for provoking hypoxia or trauma.

Maternal deaths directly or indirectly related to anesthesia make up about 5% to 10% of the total number of deaths. Complications of obstetric anesthesia are generally regarded as the fifth most common cause of death, although in certain areas or in isolated studies they may rank higher. There is rather general agreement that aspiration of vomitus with inhalation anesthetics and unusually high anesthetic levels with spinals are the prime offenders. The problem of aspiration can be minimized if food is withheld at the initiation of uterine contractions, antacids are administered, and endotracheal tubes are used for any general anesthetic. The dosage employed in spinal and saddle block anesthesia should be less than that utilized for the nonpregnant patient of comparable size and weight. A test dose designed to rule out intrathecal effects is indicated before injecting a full anesthetic dose into the epidural canal. Other avoidable problems are administration of incompatible drugs, failure to administer proper fluid, electrolyte, and blood replacements, failure to maintain a proper airway, and failure to recognize serious medical diseases. Certain anesthetics such as halothane (Fluothane) produce marked uterine relaxation with the potential of subsequent postpartal hemorrhage and possibly maternal liver damage. In addition, fetal depression is a significant problem. Probably, such agents should be restricted to clinical situations requiring rapid uterine relaxation.

If an overdose of local anesthetic is injected accidentally into the subarachnoid space, "total spinal" anesthesia may result in death if prompt endotracheal intubation, artificial ventilation, and measures to support the blood pressure are not initiated. This serious complication ranks as a major cause of maternal deaths due to anesthesia, behind only aspiration of vomitus and cardiovascular collapse.

COMPLICATIONS OF PREGNANCY

Abortion

Spontaneous abortion is the termination of pregnancy before 20 completed weeks of gestation (fetal weight < 500 g) and probably occurs with an incidence of 15% to 40%. The interval may be divided with early abortion occurring before 12 weeks and late abortion at 12 to 20 weeks. Many other modifiers are utilized to describe the process. *Inevitable abortion* is when bleeding of intrauterine origin occurs with continuous and progressive dilatation of the cervix but without expulsion of the product of conception. *Incomplete abortion* is the expulsion of some but not all of the products of conception. *Complete abortion* is an expulsion of all of the products of conception. *Missed abortion* is when the embryo or fetus dies *in utero* before the 20th week of gestation, but the products of conception are retained *in utero* for 8 or more weeks.

Approximately 75% of spontaneous abortions will occur before 16 weeks and 62% before 12 weeks of gestation. The incidence of abortion is influenced by age of the couple, previous full-term normal pregnancy, previous spontaneous abortions, previous stillbirth, previous infant with malformations or known genetic defects, and known parental influences (*e.g.,* balanced translocation carrier, diabetes mellitus). Over 60% of first trimester spontaneous abortions have an abnormal karyotype. Other associations (listed in descending order of occurrence) include infection, anatomic defects, endocrine factors, immunologic factors, and maternal systemic diseases.

The symptomatology may vary from the simple slight bleeding and cramping with threatened abortion to pain, bleeding, cervical dilatation, and complete or incomplete expulsion of the products of conception. The differential diagnosis includes ectopic abortion, dysmenorrhea, unopposed estrogen stimulation of the endometrium, hydatidiform mole, pedunculated myomas, and cervical neoplasia. Treatment for threatened abortion is generally no more than bed rest (including complete pelvic rest). Inevitable, incomplete, and complete abortion may require intravenous fluids, oxytocics, and evacuation of the products of conception from the uterus. Missed abortion may require evacuation of the uterus by either medical or surgical means; the most commonly used method is prostaglandin E suppositories.

Hyperemesis Gravidarum

Hyperemesis gravidarum represents a pernicious exaggeration of the nausea and vomiting that many pregnant women experience. Normally the height of nausea and vomiting coincides with the maximum peak of HCG production in the first trimester and, perhaps on this same basis, one can associate troublesome symptoms with the relatively higher levels found in molar and multiple pregnancy. Refractory vomiting leads to starvation, weight loss, marked dehydration, low-grade fever, hypokalemic alkalosis, extreme electrolyte imbalance, and finally acidosis. Most ominous signs include fever, tachycardia, jaundice, delirium, and retinal hemorrhages. These grave cases are rare today, undoubtedly because of better emotional preparation and support of patients and because of appropriate family planning practices.

Among those with troublesome symptoms, the self-limiting nature of the problem together with simple measures, including reassurance, eliminating stressful commitments, adopting multiple small dry feedings, drinking only hot or very cold fluids between meals but often avoiding these altogether in the early morning, and use of an antiemetic drug, usually will be successful. Hospitalization is rarely necessary but may be useful for parenteral fluids and electrolyte adjustments as well as temporarily removing the patient from a stressful situation. Psychiatric consultation may uncover an underlying disorder and aid in overall therapy. Nausea and vomiting appearing after the first trimester merit

special investigation for an organic basis. The same is true of severe and refractory vomiting even in the first trimester. Possible underlying etiologic factors may include intestinal obstruction, gastrointestinal tumor or other disorders, hyperthyroidism, heavy metal poisoning, or other toxic states.

Hypertensive States of Pregnancy

Preeclampsia, eclampsia, chronic hypertension, chronic hypertension with superimposed preeclampsia, and transient hypertension are all included in the broad classification "hypertensive states of pregnancy." Preeclampsia is the presence of edema, hypertension, and proteinuria occurring primarily in nulliparas after the 20th week of gestation and has an increasing frequency near term. It occurs in approximately 8% of the general population and has the following predisposing associations: nullliparity, black race, maternal age less than 20 or over 35 years, multiple gestation, hydatidiform mole, low socioeconomic status, polyhydramnios, nonimmune fetal hydrops, diabetes, chronic hypertension, and underlying renal disease.

Preeclampsia is divided into mild and severe categories. *Mild preeclampsia* is marked by a blood pressure of 140/90 mmHg or a 30 mmHg systolic or 15 mmHg dystolic increase above previous levels. Other diagnostic criteria for preeclampsia include nondependent edema of the hands or face (dependent edema is considered a normal finding in pregnancy), weight gain in excess of 2 pounds per week, or a particularly sudden weight gain and proteinuria. Proteinuria is the last sign to develop in preeclampsia; indeed, nearly 30% of eclamptic patients do not have proteinuria. Edema is the least reliable sign. Indeed, nearly 40% of patients have no edema. The hemoglobin and hematocrit are elevated due to hemoconcentration, but severe cases may be marked by anemia due to hemolysis. Thrombocytopenia may be present. Fibrin-split products and decreased coagulation factors may be detected. Uric acid is usually elevated above 6 mg/ml. *Severe preeclampsia* is marked by the following: systolic blood pressure more than 160 mmHg or diastolic blood pressure of 110 mmHg or more (recorded on two occasions at least 6 hours apart with the patient at bed rest), proteinuria exceeding 5 g in a 24-hour period or 3 to 4+ on dipstick testing, less than 500 ml of urine in a 24-hour period, cerebral or visual disturbances, epigastric pain, pulmonary edema, or cyanosis.

Many pathophysiologic alterations occur during this extraordinary process; however, a central factor appears to be an alteration in the sodium–potassium pump at the cellular membrane resulting in intracellular retention of sodium and, thus, water. Plasma volume is reduced materially with preeclampsia. Whereas normal pregnant patients are resistent to the vasopressor effects of angiotensin II, women who develop preeclampsia lose their refractoriness many weeks prior to the onset of clinical symptomatology. In the kidney there is swelling in the glomerular capillary endothelium (glomeruloendotheliosis), which results in decreased glomerular perfusion and decreased GRF. In some patients red blood cell disruption may occur along with disseminated intravascular coagulation (DIC) and thrombocytopenia. In such cases elevated fibrin-split products are usually found. The acronym "HELLP" syndrome has been used to describe patients with *h*emolytic anemia, *e*levated *l*iver enzymes, and *l*ow *p*latelet count. These stigmata are found in approximately 10% of patients with severe preeclampsia.

The complications of preeclampsia include early delivery with resultant fetal complications due to prematurity, acute uteroplacental insufficiency resulting in stillbirth, or intrapartum fetal distress or a small-for-gestational-age fetus.

The treatment of mild preeclampsia is bed rest and delivery. Patients are usually hospitalized, although occasionally mild preeclamptics who can be relied upon to follow instructions may be treated as outpatients. A typical regimen consists of bed rest, daily urine dipstick measurements for proteinuria, and blood pressure monitoring every 4 hours. Patients must be aware that severe headaches, epigastric pain, or visual disturbances constitute grave warning signals and should be reported immediately. Other danger signals include increasing blood pressure or increasing proteinuria. Patients should be weighed daily, and 24-hour urine studies for creatinine clearance and total protein obtained twice weekly. Other important laboratory considerations include liver function studies, uric acid, electrolytes, and serum albumin. Coagulation factors (prothrombin time [PT] and partial thromboplastin time [PTT], fibrinogen, platelet count) must be obtained in patients with severe preeclampsia. Antihypertensive medicines are not generally used unless the diastolic blood pressure exceeds 100 mmHg and the gestational age is 28 weeks or less.

Serial ultrasonography (every 2 to 4 weeks) and weekly NST and CST are used to determine fetal status. Amniocentesis assists in determining fetal pulmonary maturity, and corticosteroids may be used to accelerate fetal lung maturity in patients with increasing disease and an immature pulmonary maturity. When preeclampsia is rapidly worsening, continuous fetal monitoring is advisable.

The overall goal of treatment of mild preeclampsia is to prolong the gestation to a point of fetal maturity for delivery. The goals of management of severe preeclampsia are to prevent eclampsia (convulsions), to control the maternal blood pressure, and to initiate delivery (definitive therapy). Some cases of mild preeclampsia and most cases of severe preeclampsia will be treated with magnesium sulfate. The exact mechanism by which it acts is unknown, but it decreases the amount of acetylcholine released at the myoneural junction, has a transient mild hypotensive effect, a transient mild decrease in uterine activity in labor, a tocolytic effect in premature labor, and potentiation of depolarizing muscle relaxants. The therapeutic level is 4.8 mg to 8.4 mg/ml. At a serum level of 10 mg/ml there is loss of deep tendon reflexes, and at 15 mg/ml there is respiratory paralysis. At higher levels, cardiac arrest occurs in asystole. Magnesium sulfate is usually given intravenously with a loading dose of 2 to 4 g followed by constant infusion of 1.5 g to 2.0 g/hour after it is ascertained that urinary output is within normal limits (as magnesium sulfate is primarily excreted by the kidney). Magnesium sulfate should be administered only with an infusion pump, and the patient must be checked every 4 hours to ascertain that deep tendon reflexes are present, respirations are at least 12/minute, and urine output has been at least 25 ml/hour. Should overdosage with magnesium sulfate occur, the antidote is 10 ml of 10% calcium chloride or calcium gluconate given rapidly intravenously.

The goal of antihypertensive therapy is to bring the diastolic blood pressure to 90 to 100 mmHg. The drug of choice is hydralazine (a direct arteriolar vasodilator), which causes a secondary baroreceptor-mediated sympathetic discharge. It results in tachycardia and increased cardiac output and is metabolized by the liver. The dose is 5 mg given intravenously every 15 to 20 minutes, and the onset of action is 15 minutes. The peak effect occurs within 30 to 60 minutes, and duration is 4 to 6 hours. In more than 95% of cases hydralazine will be effective in controlling blood pressure. In some cases it may be necessary to go to labetalol, sodium nitroprusside, diazoxide, or trimethaphan. Once the patient is stabilized, a decision is reached as to whether delivery may be effected by induction of labor or whether cesarean is necessary.

Eclampsia, which includes the signs and symptoms of severe preeclampsia plus the addition of seizures, occurs in 0.2% to 0.5% of all deliveries. Approximately 75% of eclamptic seizures occur before delivery. Approximately half of postpartum seizures will occur within the first 48 hours after delivery, but may occur as late as 6 weeks postpartum.

There may or may not be an aura preceding a seizure, and the seizures are of a tonic–clonic type. Apnea is notable during the seizure and immediately postseizure hyperventilation occurs. Fever is a very poor prognostic sign. Complications of a seizure include tongue biting, broken bones, head trauma, aspiration of gastric contents, and retinal detachments. Pulmonary edema may occur following the seizures.

The treatment for seizures is usually magnesium sulfate given in the loading dose noted above. If the seizure occurs longer than 20 minutes after the loading dose, an additional 2 to 4 g of magnesium sulfate are given intravenously. If a seizure occurs despite a therapeutic level, diazepam 5 to 10 mg may be given intravenously or amylbarbitol up to 250 mg intravenously. Once the seizure is controlled and the mother is stabilized, the process for delivery is initiated using the same general guidelines as for severe preeclampsia. Preeclampsia and eclampsia contribute materially to both maternal and perinatal morbidity and mortality. Maternal complications include cerebral hemorrhage, aspiration pneumonia, hypoxic encephalopathy, thromboembolism, hepatic rupture, renal failure, or anesthetic accident.

In patients with just preeclampsia the risk of recurrence is only 1 : 3, but if there is chronic hypertension mistaken for preeclampsia the risk of recurrence is 70%. There is only a 2% recurrence of eclampsia if the patient has had a previous hypertensive disorder not related to chronic hypertension.

Chronic hypertension complicating pregnancy varies according to the population. The average incidence is 1.5%. Of these patients, 80% have essential chronic hypertension, and 20% will have hypertension due to various renal diseases (*e.g.,* interstitial nephritis, acute and chronic glomerulonephritis, systemic lupus erythematosus, and diabetic glomerulonephritis). Only a few cases will be due to endocrine diseases (*e.g.,* Cushing's disease, primary hyperaldosteronism, thyrotoxicosis, pheochromocytoma) or coarctation of the aorta. Generally these patients are older (>30 years) obese,

multiparous, and have associated medical problems (*e.g.,* diabetes or renal disease). Black woman are at particular risk, as are women with a family history of hypertension. Typically, these patients have hypertension without other signs of preeclampsia, and the diagnosis is based on documented hypertension before conception, before 20 weeks of gestation, or persistence of hypertension longer than 6 weeks postpartum. Differentiating worsening hypertension from superimposed preeclampsia may be difficult.

The medical workup of these patients must include electrocardiography (left ventricular hypertrophy is found in 5% to 10%). Elevated serum creatinine, decreased creatinine clearance, and proteinuria are present in 5% to 10%. A chest x ray may reveal cardiomegaly.

Approximately one third of the patients with chronic hypertension in pregnancy will develop superimposed preeclampsia. These patients have an increased risk of abruptio placentae, DIC, acute tubular necrosis, or renal cortical necrosis. The fetus has a 20% to 30% risk of prematurity and a 10% to 15% incidence of intrauterine growth retardation.

It is agreed that antihypertensive therapy will benefit the patient whose diastolic blood pressure exceeds 110 mmHg. Treatment of mild chronic hypertension remains controversial. If treatment of mild hypertension is utilized, methyldopa (a central α-adrenergic agonist) is the only antihypertensive drug whose long-term safety for mother and fetus has been adequately assessed. More severe hypertension may require hydralazine, β-blockers, labetalol, or the calcium channel blockers.

In the mildly chronic hypertensive patient there is little true maternal risk and perinatal survival should be 90% to 95%. The primary complications are superimposed preeclampsia, abruptio placentae, prematurity, and intrauterine growth retardation. In the more severe hypertensive who has onset of superimposed preeclampsia before 28 weeks of gestation, the addition of renal insufficiency prior to pregnancy, hypertensive cardiovascular disease, or congestive cardiomyopathy provide a more guarded prognosis for both mother and fetus.

Abruptio Placentae

Placental abruption refers to obstetric bleeding from the premature separation of a normally implanted placenta prior to the 20th gestational week.

Prior to this the mechanism may be similar but the process is referred to as an abortion. Whereas abruptio placenta occurs in approximately 1/150 pregnancies, the severe form (which threatens maternal or perinatal survival) occurs in 1/500 pregnancies. Bleeding from this cause should be distinguished from placenta previa, uterine rupture, and nonobstetric causes of bleeding (such as infection, polyps, malignant lesions, etc.) and discharge of an endocervical mucous plug.

Although the etiology is unknown, placental abruption is found in association with maternal hypertension in about one half of cases. The predisposing factors may be vascular disease, pre-eclampsia, or chronic renal diseases. The previous occurrence of placental abruption is a risk factor. Others include smoking, a uterine tumor, a hyperirritable or overdistended uterus, or the sudden reduction of uterine volume as in delivery of one twin, or membrane rupture and escape of a large quantity of amniotic fluid (polyhydramnios). Other possible causes that have been cited include multiparity, trauma, malnutrition (including folic acid deficiency and low vitamin C levels), vena caval compression, and short cord.

When the abrupted portion of the placenta is centrally located while peripheral attachments remain intact, the bleeding is internal or "concealed." An extension of the hematoma to the placental edge where peripheral disruption occurs or an abruption arising at the periphery give rise to visible or "external" bleeding. In the most severe cases there may be extensive hemorrhagic infiltration beneath the serosa of the uterus, the tubes and the adjacent ligaments, and also between the uterine muscle bundles. The latter occurrence is known as the uteroplacental apoplexy of Couvelaire; the additional complication of uterine atony and further hemorrhage postpartally sometimes occurs.

The classic signs and symptoms of abruptio placentae are (1) vaginal bleeding (usually dark red); (2) intense abdominal or lower back pain; (3) a tetanically contracted uterus (usually expressed as "boardlike"); and (4) symptoms of shock. Less than one half of cases present so dramatically and, often, minor disruptions involving only one or two central cotyledons may go unrecognized until the placenta is inspected after its removal. Ultrasonic scan assists in establishing the diagnosis. With profuse vaginal bleeding maternal hemodynamic instability becomes the primary concern and more rigorous intervention (usually cesarean) is necessary.

There may be an apparent level of hypovolemic shock out of proportion to the observed blood loss, since there may be considerable concealed hemorrhage associated with uterine enlargement, dysrhythmic myometrial contractility, and severe pain. In the more severe grades of placental abruption associated with classic findings and shock, there may be DIC. Fibrin obstruction occurring in periglomerular arterioles, hypotension, lack of adequate renal perfusion, and perhaps arteriolar spasm from the release of myoglobin from damaged tissues may give rise to acute renal failure in severe abruptio cases.

A suspicion of placental abruption is an indication for blood to be drawn for a clot observation test and baseline coagulation studies. Defective clotting begins to occur when the concentration of plasma fibrinogen falls below 150 mg/100 ml. There is no role for expectant management once the diagnosis of a major placental abruption has been made.

The hematologic problem in the severe cases involves a consumption coagulopathy characterized by a depression in platelet count and decline in circulating levels of fibrinogen; Factors V, VIII, XIII; and, to a lesser extent, prothrombin. Rarely, there may be primary activation of the fibrinolytic system resulting in the lysis of fibrinogen by fibrinolysins before fibrin can be formed. This possibility accentuates the consumption coagulopathy and exacerbates the hemorrhage. The suspicion of this complication calls for the determination of fibrinogen-split products in the blood. If possible, fresh whole blood should be administered. If that therapy is not available, then packed red cells, fresh frozen plasma, and platelet packs are preferred. Success in eliminating the underlying problem (which usually means delivery) is evidenced by a decline in the concentration of fibrin-split products first and, subsequently, by a rise in plasma fibrinogen. It should be noted that subsequent postpartal hemorrhage, even involving uteri of the Couvelaire variety, seldom necessitates hysterectomy because the myometrium can be made to contract sufficiently to close off bleeding sites in most instances.

Even in the mild cases of placental abruption concern for the fetus will justify cesarean section as the preferred method of delivery. If labor has already commenced, the membranes may be artificially ruptured to hasten its progress, to ascertain if there is blood in the amniotic fluids, and so that appropriate fetal monitoring can be instituted. Placental abruption has a tendency to speed parturition. However, prompt delivery by cesarean section may be the best approach regardless of fetal status, if profuse bleeding, shock, and worrisome clinical signs are endangering the mother.

The prognosis for the mother varies with the severity of the placental abruption, but overall the maternal death rate in the United States is 1% or less. Among women surviving major shock, there may be postpartal necrosis with resultant destruction of the anterior lobe of the pituitary, which may be associated with a depression of gonadotropic, adrenal, and thyroid functions, as well as the development of cachexia (Sheehan's syndrome). The perinatal risks also vary with the degree and type of placental separation and the underlying maternal complications, hypertension, for example malnutrition. In addition to the risks of hypoxia associated with maternal shock and placental disruption, the complications of premature birth impose additional grave hazards. More than 50% of pregnancies with this complication result in infants weighing less than 2,500 g. Generally, the perinatal mortality rates are higher among black women than white women. Among those with partial placental separations, the rate is 15% to 30%. The risk is much lower when only a marginal sinus ruptures. Contrariwise, in the presence of total placental abruption, perinatal mortality rates are about 80%. Long-term morbidities among survivors are higher than like-weight individuals from other complications (*e.g.,* placenta previa). This is thought to be due to the additional risk of hypoxia from decreased placental transfer.

Placenta Previa

Placenta previa is encountered in about 1 in 200 deliveries. Placenta previa is defined as placental implantation in the lower uterine segment within the zone of cervical effacement and dilatation. About 20% will be total placenta previa where the placenta covers the entire cervix. The cause is not known, but the abnormality of placentation occurs more often in multiparas. It has been suggested that alterations in endometrial blood supply, variations in depth and nidational quality of endometrium, alterations in the uterine cavity size or contour, uterine scars, and receptivity of the endometrium may play a role. Obviously, surface area and distribution of placenta (multiple gestation, placenta membranacea, etc.) have an impact upon area of attachment and anatomic relations *in utero.* The types are designed on the basis of the relationship of

the placenta to the internal cervical os as follows: (1) complete, total, or central placenta previa (see above), (2) partial (the internal os is only partially covered by placenta), and (3) marginal (the edge of the placenta extends to the margin of the internal os).

The placental margin at or near the internal os is vulnerable, and a cleavage plane occurs in the decidua spongiosa. When separation occurs, particularly in response to increasing myometrial activity or cervical effacement, there may be external bleeding. The classic symptoms are recurrent episodes of bright red bleeding, usually painless, particularly in the earlier stages of pregnancy. With uterine contractions, bleeding may be accentuated and there may be discomfort. The latter clinical condition may be quite similar to a partially separated placenta implanted normally in the fundus. Generally, the initial episode of bleeding ceases spontaneously or continues as only minimal drainage. The blood loss is ordinarily not life-threatening to the mother unless an internal examination has been performed. However, recurrent episodes are the rule. In contrast with abruptio placenta, the bleeding is ordinarily entirely external and the degree of hypovolemia and anemia is proportional to observed blood loss. There should be no infiltrations of blood into the myometrium or other tissues and there is no tenderness or increase in the resting tone of the uterus.

Diagnosis. The most characteristic clinical presentation of painless, bright-red vaginal bleeding calls for the presumptive diagnosis. Since abnormal presentations are found in one quarter of the cases of placenta previa, the presence of a transverse lie or breech, particularly if the presenting part is high in the fundus, should provoke even more concern.

The definitive method of diagnosis is ultrasonic scan, maternal condition permitting. The technique is safe and carries an accuracy of more than 95%. However, as pregnancy advances, due to variable placental growth relationship to uterine expansion, the relationship of the placenta to the lower uterine segment may change.

Active Treatment. Definitive treatment (*i.e.,* delivery, usually by cesarean section) is indicated when labor ensues, when the amount of bleeding is hazardous to the life of the mother, or when the fetus is mature. Occasionally, late in pregnancy and with sufficient maternal blood loss to preclude a more leisurely evaluation, it will be necessary to go to a ''double-setup vaginal examination.'' This examination must be performed with some rigid safeguards since manipulations may disrupt more placenta and create life-threatening hemorrhage. Thus, these potential risks can be tolerated only if the fetus is clearly viable or if delivery is required to stop heavy blood loss. An examination of this type can be undertaken only under sterile circumstances in the presence of a double-setup capability, which means that the operating room has been adequately prepared for immediate vaginal or abdominal delivery. There should be provisions for infusions, blood transfusions, oxygen, anesthesia, instruments, nursing and neonatal personnel to proceed with active intervention if necessary.

Expectant management is indicated if it is necessary to postpone delivery until the fetus becomes mature. Preferably, the patient should remain at bed rest in the hospital under close observation with blood readily available. Sometimes, spontaneous heavy bleeding makes it necessary to abandon this conservative approach under emergency conditions. If a conservative plan of management is followed, it may be terminated electively when fetal maturity occurs as measured by ultrasound studies or amniotic fluid studies (L/S ratio, etc.).

Adequate blood replacement and treatment of shock are basic considerations in any management. All patients with total placenta previa should be delivered by cesarean section, and most who have even minor degrees of partial previa are better delivered by the abdominal route. The thinned out endometrium in the lower uterine segment predisposes not only to the possibility of previa but also to invasion of the myometrium by the trophoblast (*e.g.,* placenta accreta, increta, and percreta). Lower segment manipulations leading to partial placental disruption can lead to life-threatening hemorrhage.

Vaginal delivery may produce additional fetal hazards by compressing the placenta and creating partial obstruction of the fetal vessels or by enhancing placental separation. The additional hypoxia resulting from these vascular deficits may cause fetal compromise. The low-lying posteriorly implanted placenta may pose the additional risk of decreasing relative pelvic capacity to preclude pelvic entry of the presenting part.

Maternal risks involve primarily hemorrhage, shock, and puerperal infection, but the mortality rate in the United States is less than 0.25%. The perinatal risks are hypoxia, birth injury, and the consequences of premature birth, including respiratory distress syndrome and a slightly higher inci-

dence of developmental defects. The perinatal mortality rate is in the range of 15% to 20%.

Preterm or Premature Labor

Approximately 7% of deliveries in the United States are preterm (less than 37 weeks gestational age) and may or may not be small-for-dates. This is a very serious problem, for as a group the death rate of the low-birth-weight (LBW) neonate is 40-fold that of full-sized infants born at term, and both cerebral palsy (10-fold) and mental deficiency (5-fold) are increased in the LBW compared to the term neonate. Other sequelae of LBW include visual and hearing deficits, emotional disturbances, and social maladjustments. Preterm labor may be associated with many disorders or diseases; for example, smoking, substance abuse, previous preterm birth, incompetent cervix, uterine anomalies, multiple gestation, acute viral or bacterial infections, poor nutrition, and anemia. The clinical definition of premature labor involves four criteria: a gestation of more than 20 weeks but less than 36 weeks; regular, painful uterine contractions occurring at least twice every 10 minutes for at least 30 minutes; demonstrated cervical effacement or dilatation; and intact membranes. Other symptoms may include vaginal bleeding, increased vaginal discharge, and vaginal pressure.

When premature labor is being evaluated, it is necessary to ascertain that the membranes have not ruptured, that the fetus is truly premature, that fetal distress is not occurring, that cervical dilation has not exceeded 4 cm, and that there is not an abnormal fetal presentation (a frequent complication). The necessary laboratory studies include blood for CBC with differential, serum electrolytes, and glucose; urine for analysis and culture and sensitivity; and ultrasonography for fetal size, position, and placental location. Amniocentesis may be necessary in borderline cases for fetal maturity (L/S ratio, phosphatidylglycerol) as well as to check for amniotic fluid bacteria (7%–26% of premature labors have intrauterine infection).

To ascertain if contractions are occurring (see above), 30 to 60 minutes of electronic fetal monitoring are performed and it is ultrasonically confirmed that the gestational age is 20 weeks to less than 36 weeks. A history, physical examination, and tests (see above) are used to rule out any contraindication to sedation–hydration therapy. The period of observation details whether labor is present and whether the cervix has changed. Thus, cases may be categorized as follows: (1) no contractions, no cervical changes (no labor); (2) contractions, no cervical change (false or early labor); (3) no contractions, cervical change (incompetent cervix); and (4) contractions, cervical change (labor). Of all cases originally presenting with presumed premature labor 75% will not be in labor, will have an incompetent cervix, or will have contraindications to tocolysis. Of those with false labor, early labor, or labor, sedation–hydration therapy is begun, if there are no contraindications, with morphine sulfate 8 to 12 mg intramuscularly and 5% dextrose lactated Ringer's solution intravenously. At the end of the hour, which of the three treatment groups the patient will enter is based on cervical effacement and dilatation as well as uterine contractions.

If contractions continue and the cervix is progressively changing (only a small percentage of cases), one should proceed to first-line tocolytics, the goal of therapy being to arrest labor until the fetus is mature enough to achieve intact survival in the atmosphere. If there is no cervical change but uterine contractions continue, the patient may benefit from first-line tocolytics. This group is usually less than one half of patients, and even if suppression is currently successful, they still have a risk of subsequent labor and delivery. When uterine contractions cease and there is no cervical change, observation should continue for 6 to 12 hours. More than half of patients will be in this group and here, too, there is a continued risk of labor and delivery, but the majority of these patients may be monitored by an outpatient regimen. Prior to the use of tocolytic drugs several items are important: serial measurement of blood pressure and pulse rate, baseline ECG, and establishment of a fluid intake and output chart. The fetal heart rate is monitored electronically throughout tocolysis. The safest tocolytic is magnesium sulfate. It may be given in a bolus followed by continuous intravenous infusion. The vital signs, deep tendon reflexes, urinary output, and ECG are monitored closely (every 30–60 minutes). With careful monitoring, serious adverse effects of magnesium administration, for example, hypotension, sinoatrial or atrioventricular block, or cardiac arrest, are exceptional. However, each time a magnesium level is drawn (every 6 hours) a calcium level should also be obtained to ascertain that acute hypocalcemia has not occurred. The fetus should be minimally affected by this regimen. Intravenous Ritodrine, a more effective tocolytic than magnesium sulfate and FDA-approved for tocolysis, should be continued at effective dosage for at least 2 hours after cessation of contractions;

then it should be slowly reduced over 1 to 2 hours. A maintenance oral dose of Ritodrine may be used for weeks, if necessary. The adverse reactions of ritodrine are essentially those of all β-mimetic agents and are dose related. They include hyperglycemia, hypoinsulinemia, and hyperkalemia. Pulmonary edema may occur if ritodrine is given intravenously in saline solution, especially with excessive drug dosage or prolonged treatment, or when hyperhydration occurs. Unpleasant cardiovascular, gastrointestinal, or neurologic side effects must be expected but these are usually mild. Fetal tachycardia may occur with any β-adrenergic drug therapy. However, with proper selection of patients, correct dosage, and cautiously maintained tocolysis, there should be no harm to the infant.

Disproportionate Fetal Growth

Small-for-gestational-age (SGA) fetuses or neonates, sometimes referred to as having "intrauterine growth retardation," are less than the tenth percentile of weight, length, and head size for gestational age; while large-for-gestational-age (LGA) perinates are at or above the ninetieth percentile by the same criteria. Both SGA and LGA fetuses have altered body composition, altered distribution of organ weight, and altered body proportions. Both disproportionate growth perinates are at considerable risk for morbidity and mortality, although the risks are notably different.

Approximately 80% of SGA perinates are "asymmetrically" small, with relative sparing of brain, compared to other organs. The differential sparing is particularly prominent if deprivation occurs in the latter half of pregnancy. This form of SGA is caused by restricted growth potential and is usually caused by placental disorders (*e.g.*, infarction, previa, villitis, partial separation, malformations, twin-to-twin transfusion syndrome), coexisting maternal disease (*e.g.*, hypertensive states of pregnancy, anemia, renal diseases, malnutrition, pulmonary disease), or multiple pregnancy. The remainder of SGA perinates (~20%) are symmetrically small and are said to have decreased growth potential. The most common causes of decreased growth potential are constitutional (small maternal stature, female fetus, certain races), genetic disorders (*e.g.*, autosomal [trisomy 21, trisomy 18, trisomy 13], sex chromosomal [Turner's syndrome], neural tube defects [anencephaly], dysmorphic syndromes—usually autosomal recessive [Meckel's, Smith-Lemli-Opitz] congenital anomalies [Potter's syndrome]), congenital infections (*e.g.*, CMV, rubella, toxoplasmosis, malaria, listeriosis), substance abuse (opiates, cocaine, alcohol, tobacco), or drugs (warfarin, folic acid antagonists). Overall, the most common cause of SGA is decreased placental function as a result of placental abnormalities or the result of abnormal function of a normal placenta.

The pregnancy complicated by an SGA fetus may be marked by oligohydramnios, passage of meconium, enhanced pulmonary maturity for gestation, and ultrasonically detected fetal or placental abnormalities. It is crucial in any pregnancy at risk for SGA that baseline studies be established as early as possible. Critical points of diagnosis include accurate dating of the pregnancy, serial ultrasonography, genetic screening, maternal serum alpha-fetoprotein determinations, TORCH titers, specially indicated studies (*e.g.,* umbilical blood sampling), biometric testing, assessment for delivery and maternal studies as indicated by each circumstance. Stillbirth is not uncommon and delivery is hazardous for the SGA because of hypoxia and acidosis. Cesarean section should be used liberally for delivery. The overall perinatal mortality rate for SGA is 1.4- to 3-fold higher than that of average for gestational age (AGA) perinates. Neonatally the SGA is more prone to hypoxia, acidosis, meconium aspiration syndrome, hypoglycemia, hypocalcemia, polycythemia, hypothermia, congenital malformations, and sudden infant death syndrome (SIDS). The longer-term sequelae of SGA include lower IQ, learning and behavior disorders, and major neurologic handicaps.

The LGA fetus is generally associated with maternal diabetes, maternal obesity, postdatism, multiparity, previous LGA infants, and large maternal stature. Rarely, genetic or congenital disorders will be associated with the LGA perinate. Screening for LGA risk is performed by history and physical examination (25%–50% will be discovered), maternal glucose screening, and liberal use of serial ultrasonography. Attempts to control fetal size are most influenced by the appropriate use of insulin, for example, in gestational diabetics. At term the LGA baby generally exceeds 4,000 g and is very prone to birth trauma (6%–24%) such as shoulder dystocia and operative delivery. Indeed, shoulder dystocia, which occurs in 0.3% to 1% of AGA perinates, occurs with LGA at a frequency of 6% to 24%. Therefore, as the EDC approaches, labor induction should be considered. The incidence of cesarean for the LGA is 2- to 2.5-fold higher than for AGA. The maternal risk of LGA delivery is considerable and includes hemorrhage, operative delivery, and perineal damage. Neonatally the LGA is more prone to low Apgar scores, hypoglycemia, hypocalcemia, polycythemia, jaundice, birth injury, and feeding difficulties. Longer-term sequelae of LGA are obesity, Type II diabetes, and neurologic or behavior problems.

Prolonged Pregnancy (Postdates)

Prolonged pregnancy has continued for 294 or more days, or 14 days beyond the EDC, as calculated from the first day of the last menses, and occurs in about 5% of all pregnancies. Most commonly the cause is never determined, but prolonged pregnancy is predisposed in those who have had it before (twice as common), in fetal anencephaly (due to adrenal hypoplasia and altered hormonal production), and in certain families. Among postdate fetuses, 30% to 40% are dysmature; that is, they have or have had fetal distress from placental insufficiency. These fetuses are underweight with reduced subcutaneous fat, appear wrinkled with peeling skin, and are often meconium-stained. They are at increased perinatal risk, and oligohydramnios is frequently an associated finding. However, the majority of postterm infants appear to be normal or are macrosomic, continuing to grow slightly even after the EDC. Accordingly, it is essential to ascertain which fetuses are jeopardized and which are not.

Evaluation of the postterm pregnancy involves accurately dating the pregnancy (the EDC may not yet have been reached). Accurate dating is best performed prospectively (during the course of pregnancy), but quite often that is not the case. Thus, if three of the following four clinical criteria are met, the patient should not be considered postdates: less than 36 weeks have elapsed since a positive pregnancy test; less than 32 weeks have elapsed since Doppler recording of fetal heart (FHTs); less than 24 weeks have elapsed since observed fetal movements; and less than 22 weeks have elapsed since FHTs were noted by auscultation. Two satisfactory ultrasonographic fetal biparietal (or other) measurements, at least one month apart, can establish gestational age by ±1 week. The earlier in gestation the ultrasonic examinations were accomplished, the more accurate dating will be. The EDC cannot accurately be established or confirmed when the fetal biparietal diameter is greater than 9.5 cm by a single ultrasonography.

To affirm fetal well-being, fetal surveillance is essential after 294 days. Indeed, once the due date has passed and until week 42 it may be wise to implement all or part of the surveillance noted below (*e.g.*, weekly instead of biweekly determinations). Clinical parameters include full maternal evaluation, a biweekly recording of fundal height and abdominal girth (decreasing uterine contents signal oligohydramnios), maternal fetal motion counting, and visualization of the membranes (if possible) through the cervix to determine if meconium has been passed. Meconium is a nonspecific reaction to stress and should not be taken as a sign of fetal distress, but a warning signal that the fetus may be near the limits of placental reserve. Twice weekly biophysical profile testing (or minimally nonstress testing) is a useful evaluation of fetal well being. At least one definitive (level III) ultrasonography, specifically examining fetal size parameters, fetal organ systems, and the placenta (including grading), should be obtained. Contraction stress testing should be performed if any parameter above is questionable. Amniocentesis is rarely indicated, but may be useful in the patient who has totally unknown dates and presents without any prospective monitoring. Analysis of the amniotic fluid does not assist in determining the gestational age but can definitively describe fetal pulmonary maturity, even when a sample is contaminated by blood or meconium.

The safest time for delivery is 39 to 41 weeks. After week 41 there is steadily rising mortality (*e.g.*, stillborn, uteroplacental insufficiency), and potential morbidity. The mortality is 5% to 7% in infants delivered at or after 44 weeks, and by week 42 the risk is equal to that at less than 35 weeks. The ideal time for delivery is when the minimal risk of induction is surpassed by the ever increasing risks of postdates gestation and must be individualized. By this criteria, delivery at or shortly after 290 days' gestation is indicated, which is generally accomplished by induction of labor. If the cervix is not effaced, not dilated, not soft, is posterior and the presenting part is high (*i.e.*, a low Bishop score), it may be necessary to administer cervical prostaglandin E. Induction is most safely accomplished by rupture of the membranes, but if that cannot be accomplished, oxytocin may be administered. Upon rupture of the membranes, observation for meconium staining is important. The fetus should be constantly monitored during induction because the dysmature fetuses are prone to fetal distress and withstand labor poorly, particularly when oxytocin stimulation is used. There is a real risk of intrapartum asphyxia. Should fetal distress occur, maternal complications intervene, or the serial induction of labor fail, cesarean should be undertaken immediately.

Multiple Gestation

Multiple pregnancy, more than one embryo or fetus in a gestation, may be caused by division of a single fertilized ovum (identical, monovular, or monozygotic) or fertilization of separate ova by different spermatozoa (fraternal, or dizygotic). Monozygotic multiple gestations share the same genetic features but may have phenotypic variation of considerable degree, while dizygotic gestations bear only the resemblance of brothers or sisters and may or may not have similar enough genetic features to serve as organ donors for each other. Monozygotism is constant (~2.3–4/1,000 deliveries), but dizygotism has a number of predispositions, including a recessive autosomal trait via the female descendants, race (greatest incidence in blacks, intermediate in white, orientals having the fewest), cessation of oral contraception, artificial ovulation induction, greater maternal height or weight, increasing maternal age (peaks at 35–45), and white mothers of blood group O or A. The incidence of the father's being a twin has little influence on his offspring's potential to be multiple gestations. In a heterogenous population (such as the United States), approximately 30% of twins are monozygotic and nearly 70% are dizygotic. In heterogenous populations an estimate of the frequency of multiple gestation may be obtained by the knowledge that twinning occurs ~12/1,000 births (1 : 88). Subsequent incidences may be estimated by raising the ratio 1 : 88 to the exponential of the birth number minus 1. For example: triplets occur $1 : 88^{(3-1=2)} = 1 : 7,744$; quadruplets $1 : 88^3 = 1 : 681,472$; and so forth. Approximately 75% of twins are of the same sex, but in multiple births males predominate (45% compared to females' 30%).

Maternal morbidity and mortality is higher in multiple, compared to singleton, pregnancies. The conditions associated with this risk include enhanced anemia, more urinary tract infections, increased incidence of preeclampsia–eclampsia, greater predisposition to hydramnios, more frequent uterine inertia (from overdistention), and greatly increased chances of hemorrhage (before, during, and after delivery).

The perinatal mortality rate of twins is also three- to fourfold higher, and for each subsequent birth number much higher again, than for singletons. The two primary causes of this are prematurity and congenital anomalies. Considering both mono- and dizygotic fetuses, congenital abnormalities of all organ systems are as high as 18%, compared to the 3% to 5% of singletons. As the number of fetuses rises, their average size and length of gestation falls; on the average, twins are delivered at about 36 weeks, triplets at approximately 32 weeks, and quadruplets at less than 30 weeks. Intrauterine growth retardation (IUGR) is also more common in all multiple gestations, as opposed to singletons. Other general perinatal risks of multiple gestations include abnormal presentation and position, hydramnios, hypoxia because of cord prolapse (approximately 4%), placenta previa, premature separation of the placenta after the first twin, or operative manipulation. Collision, impaction, and interlocking of twins are additional but uncommon complications.

Compared to dizygotic fetuses, monozygotic multiple fetuses are even more likely to be jeopardized from general congenital abnormalities (a further threefold increase), incomplete separation, enhanced early loss of one or both fetuses (probably two thirds of all implanted multiple gestations end up with a single birth), enhanced IUGR and possibility of death in utero (the monochorionic placenta is likely less efficient than a fused dichorionic placenta), or a parasitic fetus without a heart (fetus acardiacus). Another unique monozygotic complication is the "twin-to-twin transfusion syndrome" in which the smaller cardiomegalic twin pumps its arterial blood into the lower pressure venous system of the larger, plethoric, and macrosomic twin. Cord problems are also enhanced in multiple gestation, including two vessel cords and velamentous cord insertion (7% incidence), and cord entanglement in a single monoamniotic sac (approximately 1% of all twins, but leads to about a 50% loss). The time of division is crucial to the outcome of monozygotic fetuses. Early separation, prior to the morula and trophoblastic differentiation (day 5), leads to separate or fused placentas, two chorions and two amnions. Division after trophoblastic differentiation but before amnion formation (5–10 days) is the pattern of two thirds of monozygotic twins and results in a single placenta, a common chorion, and two amnions. Later division (i.e., after amnion differentiation—days 10–14) leads to a single placenta, one chorion and one amnion. Division from day 8 to after day 14 results in conjoint ("Siamese") or incomplete twinning.

Early diagnosis of multiple gestation is desirable in order to provide the special care necessary for the mother as well as to prolong the gestation. The most precise method of diagnosis is ultrasonic imaging. Indeed, multiple pregnancy may be demonstrated by vaginal ultrasonography as early as the 8th week of gestation and should be routinely detected by other scanning methods by the 10th week. The clinical findings suggestive of multiple pregnancy include a uterus 4 cm or larger than expected for the length of pregnancy, uterine palpation of three or more large parts or multiple small parts, simultaneous auscultation or recording of two fetal hearts varying more than 8 BPM and asynchronous to the maternal heart, unexplained excessive maternal weight gain, hydramnios, eclampsia–preeclampsia, and subjective maternal increased fetal activity. The laboratory findings suggestive of multiple pregnancy include elevations of maternal HCG and/or alpha-fetoprotein, moderate reductions in hematocrit (as well as hemoglobin and red blood cell count), a blood volume increased over normal pregnancy values, and an increased incidence of glucose intolerance.

The differential diagnosis of multiple pregnancy includes single pregnancy, single pregnancy not compatible with gestation, hydramnios, hydatidiform mole, abdominal or pelvic tumors complicating singleton pregnancy, and complicated multiple gestation. Prevention of multiple pregnancy is possible by using barrier means of contraception for the first cycle off oral contraceptives and by more careful use of the ovulation induction agents. For example, clomiphene causes fewer multiple gestations, but dizygotic twins still occur in 5% to 10%. A new and somewhat controversial technique is that of "selective reduction" (i.e., selective termination) of some of the fetuses. This technique employs ultrasonic guided techniques for reducing the number of fetuses with the rationale that intact survival of a few is better than nonintact survival of many. The initial reports support usage in certain cases.

Maximizing nutrition and decreasing stress appear to assist in lengthening the gestation. Oral iron, high protein, high vitamin diet, and no weight gain limitation are all recommended in multiple gestations. Patients with multiple pregnancy are usually examined more often during pregnancy. Limiting physical activity may assist uterine blood flow. Although not always necessary, frequent rest periods after the 24th week have been suggested as a method of lengthening gestation. Blood counts are usually obtained more frequently. Repeated ultrasonic examinations screen for fetal defects, IUGR, proper growth, fetus-to-fetus transfusion syndrome, and fetal well being. These are usually obtained monthly from diagnosis until the 32nd week, when both the examinations and biophysical profile of each fetus may be useful on a weekly basis. Anticipate delivery blood loss (hemorrhage is increased fivefold over singletons) and seek donors acceptable to the patient in advance. Delivery of multiple pregnancies is best conducted in a unit with adequate assistance and neonatology. Both cervical cerclage and/or tocolytic agents have been used to delay preterm birth in selected cases. Beta-mimetic agents should be used with caution because of possible maternal pulmonary edema. Individual testing for pulmonary maturity studies may necessitate sampling each amniotic cavity.

During labor a number of special precautions are necessary. A large bore intravenous with lactated Ringer's solution should be started. Blood work should include CBC and type and cross match for a minimum of 2 units packed RBC or whole blood. The degree of aortocaval compression with subsequent hypotension may be profound; thus, it is prudent to keep the mother from lying on her back. Maternal oxygen therapy by mask (7 liters/minute) helps to guarantee proper maternal and fetal oxygenation. Each fetus is monitored electronically. Maternal analgesia and anesthesia is limited, with a preference for psychoprophylaxis or regional anesthesia.

Cesarean section is the preferred method of delivery for monoamniotic twins (10% delivery loss from cord entanglement), any birth number exceeding twins (*e.g.*, triplets), twins <2,500 g, or if the first twin is any presentation except vertex. Indeed, even twin gestations are at such risk that they should be delivered in a cesarean section room with full preparation (including maternal abdominal prep), equipment, and personnel in attendance for cesarean section. The presentation of both twins is ascertained by ultrasound to plan the delivery method. Continuous electronic monitoring is used for both fetuses. When Twin A is vertex and Twin B is vertex (slightly more than 40% of cases) both are usually delivered by vertex vaginal delivery. When the first fetus is delivered, clamp the cord promptly to prevent the second of monozygotic twins from partially exsanguinating through the first cord. A vaginal examination immediately after the first delivery is used to identify a possible prolapsed cord and to ascertain fetal position. If the second fetus is anything but vertex, external version is utilized to attempt conversion of the second twin to vertex. If the external version is successful, the membranes may be cautiously ruptured (to avoid cord prolapse) and labor will proceed to vaginal vertex delivery. However, if the external version is unsuccessful and the fetus is not a candidate for a vaginal breech delivery, cesarean should be performed immediately. When the external version is unsuccessful and the fetus is a candidate for a vaginal breech delivery (see Breech Presentation, below), that modality may be employed. When the first twin is nonvertex (approximately 20%), cesarean is used for delivery regardless of the second twin's position.

With all multiple gestations the three major preventable causes of morbidity are immaturity, trauma, and manipulative delivery (with associated asphyxia); thus, every effort is extended to prevent these problems. A second twin in distress and able to be delivered more quickly vaginally than abdominally may be an indication for the now rarely performed internal version; however, it is safer for the mother and baby if cesarean can be performed. For example, if the first twin has been delivered and the second suffers fetal distress (severe cord compression or premature separation of the placenta) and cannot be delivered easily or immediately, an emergency cesarean should be performed. Both neonates must be attended by a team experienced in neonatal management and resuscitation.

After delivery of the last fetus oxytocin 5–10 units IV slowly but promptly after delivery, followed by an infusion of dilute oxytocin will decrease the possibility of uterine inertia. It is also useful to elevate (out of the pelvis) and gently massage the uterus. Inspection, as well as dissection and sectioning for microscopy, of the placenta(s) and membranes, particularly the membranous "T" septum between the fetuses, may be immediately useful in determining zygosity. Monozygotic twins have a thin septum made up of two amnionic membranes with no intervening chorion or decidua. Dizygotic fetuses have a thick septum composed of two chorions, two amnions, and intervening decidua. In some circumstances it is necessary to resort to definitive genetic testing to determine mono- or dizygosity.

Coincidental Complications

Gravid women are naturally subject to all the diseases from which nonpregnant persons suffer. Most of these will not be aggravated by pregnancy, and the coincidental condition will not affect the normal course of gestation. The notable exceptions to this generalization are heart disease, diabetes mellitis, pyelonephritis, pneumonia, syphilis, and rubella. Current opinion suggests that pregnancy exerts no deleterious effect on tuberculosis, and that therapeutic abortion is rarely indicated. As a rule, tuberculosis of the mother does not affect the infant.

HEART DISEASE

Heart disease complicating pregnancy may be indicated by any of the following criteria: a diastolic, presystolic, or continuous heart murmer; cardiac enlargement; a loud, harsh systolic murmur (especially with an associated thrill); and severe arrhythmia. In determining the prognosis of cardiac patients, emphasis should be given to the functional classification, the age of the patient, signs or history of heart failure, atrial fibrillation, and complicating serious disease. Generally speaking, the prognosis is most serious in aortic or mitral stenosis, either alone or in association with insufficiency. Judging the severity of the heart condition by these several criteria, the unfavorable group of cases comprises about 20% of the total, yet these women with poor prognostic signs account for about 85% of the deaths attributable to heart disease.

Heart disease complicates pregnancy in about 1% of pregnant patients. The preponderance were rheumatic in etiology; however, in recent years, congenital cardiovascular lesions are being diagnosed more commonly and now the ratio of rheumatic to congenital disorders is <3 : 1. The success of cardiac surgery may decrease additional risks for patients who subsequently become pregnant (e.g., correction of patent ductus arteriosus, atrial septal defect, aortic stenosis, or simple coarctation of the aorta). In other circumstances surgical intervention may be more palliative, and pregnancy would impose prohibitive maternal risks (e.g., corrected pulmonary hypertension, partially repaired cyanotic lesions, Marfan's syndrome, complicated coarctation of the aorta).

Another consideration in the advisability or safety of pregnancy pertains to the ill effects upon the fetus of drugs used in treatment of cardiovascular diseases. The coumarins are teratogenic, and long-term heparin seems to increase premature births and perinatal deaths. Beta-adrenergic blocking agents given to patients with certain cardiac arrhythmias have the potential of initiating premature labor. Digitalis increases myometrial tone, and thiazide diuretics reduce plasma volume during pregnancy.

A further consideration is the risk in some types of heart disease of infection, particularly in those who have undergone valvuloplasty for rheumatic heart disease and those with prostheses, grafts, and residual defects postsurgery. Antibiotic prophylaxis in these cases is mandatory. Overall, congenital anomalies are noted in the newborns of mothers with significant heart disease about six times more often than the normal population.

The considerable physiologic burdens imposed upon the cardiovascular system during pregnancy have been previously reviewed. Most cardiac decompensations occur after the 7th month, and cardiac stress is accentuated even more during labor and delivery when the output increases to 60% to 80% over nonpregnant states. The early puerperium, in contrast to supine prelabor, may show a 15% to 20% drop in heart rate and a 5% to 15% reduction in blood volume.

In addition to the deaths that bear a relationship to the functional classification, especially classes III and IV of the New York Heart Association classification, certain cardiovascular complications, such as vascular accidents and bacterial endocarditis, may take an additional toll.

The principles of management are adequate rest, reduced emotional strain, prevention or correction of anemia, proper diet to avoid excess weight and fluid retention, avoidance of infection, recognition of early signs of heart failure, allowing labor to ensue spontaneously, meticulous care in labor, and allaying decompensation. The ideal delivery has the objective of avoiding great exertion on the part of the mother (minimize bearing-down efforts) while achieving a simple vaginal delivery (perhaps outlet forceps) under local or possibly carefully administered regional anesthetic. These patients are very vulnerable to trauma, shock, hemorrhage, and sepsis. Warning signs of early cardiac failure are decreased vital capacity, fatigue, orthopnea, resting tachypnea, rales at lung bases, and pulmonary congestion on a chest film. In the presence of heart failure, delivery by any known method carries with it a maternal mortality of more than 50%. Should frank heart failure develop, digitalis and bed rest in the hospital are required throughout the remainder of the pregnancy. During pregnancy, cardiac failure constitutes a grave hazard, since 15% or more of patients die. Valvotomy in pregnancy may be accomplished if necessary with relative safety for both mother and fetus. Recent reports dealing with large series of women undergoing pregnancy after placement of a prosthetic heart valve reveal a good perinatal outcome in about 72%; however, salvage is excellent (perhaps 95%) if oral anticoagulation therapy is not required. Uneventful pregnancies have been reported following insertion of a permanent pacemaker for complete heart block.

The early puerperium is a time of potential decompensation, collapse and death, since the cardiac output rises significantly and over a number of days fluid will be mobilizing. Bed rest and antibiotics are continued for 1 week postpartally.

The presence of heart disease must be identified at the onset of pregnancy to initiate appropriate therapy. Gestational disturbances making the diagnosis difficult include edema, fatigue, dyspnea, cardiac enlargement, left axis deviation, and occasional T-wave inversion on ECG, and apical or left sternal border systolic ejection-type murmurs.

Of special concern are those patients who have had cardiac failure previously, because repeated cardiac decompensation in pregnancy is very likely. Another grave category is represented by women with congenital cyanotic heart disease. Here, not only are the perinatal risks great but the maternal mortality rate is very high. In some instances, patients may be suitable surgical candidates even during pregnancy; however, in general, all women, particularly older women, classified as having class III and IV heart disease are extremely serious risks and should be considered for elective abortion prior to the eighth gestational week. Otherwise, hospitalization and bed rest through pregnancy is required, along with the closest supervision.

One of the most serious complications of cardiac disease in pregnancy is bacterial endocarditis, usually by *Streptococcus viridans*, enterococci, or *Staphylococcus aureus*. A combination prophylactic drug therapy has become popular (*e.g.*, penicillin, vancomycin, or ampicillin plus gentamycin, possibly alternatives of cephalothin, nafcillin, Keflin, or streptomycin). Such prophylaxis is indicated in any patient with a heart lesion, including mitral valve prolapse, although in the latter circumstances it is recommended only for delivery not during the entire course of pregnancy. In postsurgical patients, the prognosis depends upon any residual pulmonary hypertension or myocardial deterioration. Patients with repaired tetralogy of Fallot fare reasonably well in pregnancy if there is no pulmonary hypertension. Successful pregnancy has followed a cardiac bypass operation.

DIABETES MELLITUS

This is the most common and the most serious metabolic disease in pregnant women. The overall incidence of this maternal complication is <1%, although the incidence will be considerably higher in tertiary care centers (perhaps 2%–3%). Prior to the advent of insulin, about one half of diabetic patients were amenorrheic. When pregnancy did occur, maternal mortality was in the range of 25%.

Now, under optimal conditions, the maternal mortality is less than 0.5% with nearly all in the more severe groups. Diabetes' deleterious effect on pregnancy has several manifestations: an abortion rate twice the nondiabetic, a rate of congenital abnormality two- to threefold more than the nondiabetic, and perinatal death rate fivefold that of the nondiabetic. Other potential fetal sequelae include macrosomia, organomegaly, enhanced rates of respiratory distress syndrome, polycythemia, hyperbilirubinemia, hypocalcemia, hypomagnesemia, and neurologic instability. In the absence of adequate prenatal care, the perinatal mortality will be 40%, but it can be reduced to 3% to 5% under optimal conditions. Deaths increase towards term. In the presence of severe maternal vascular disease, the perinatal death rate may rise to as high as 50%.

Pregnancy is diabetegenic; that is, insulin demands are increased during the gestational state. This is due to a number of insulin antagonists, including chorionic somatomammotropin, which induces lipolysis, increases free fatty acids, and inhibits the cellular uptake of glucose and gluconeogenesis. In this biochemical process, glucose and protein are spared, presumably for fetal growth. As a consequence, there are increased maternal insulin requirements, especially after the first trimester. Estrogens also play a role by exerting a peripheral antagonism to maternal insulin, especially in the latter part of pregnancy. The placenta may contribute to the diabetic picture by producing insulinase. In normal pregnancy, plasma insulin levels are low in the fasting state but are elevated after a carbohydrate challenge.

First identification of the gravida at risk for diabetes is usually based on the medical history, physical findings, gynecologic background, past obstetric performance, and laboratory data. Obviously there are risk factors that make some individuals more vulnerable than others. A family history of diabetes in one close relative or two distant relatives should be taken into consideration. A gynecologic history of wound healing problems, resistance to infection, recurrent urinary tract infections, and refractory monilial vaginitis should be noteworthy. Obstetrically, a history of macrosoma, diabetes in a prior pregnancy, an unexplained fetal death, neonatal respiratory death, a child with anomalies, recurrent toxemia, gestational obesity, and polyhydramnios should be viewed with concern.

A screening procedure for diabetes is a routine procedure usually performed in early pregnancy and repeated in the third trimester. A common screen is accomplished by administering a 50-g glucose load to the gravida. A 1-hour blood sugar of more than 150 mg/100 ml has a high correlation with diabetes and requires further investigation. A 2-hour postprandial blood sugar level of 140 mg/100 ml is indicative of diabetes mellitus (or similar level 2 hours following ingestion of a solution containing 100 g of glucose). A sugar level in the 120 mg to 140 mg/100 ml range may suggest gestational diabetes. During pregnancy, postprandial glycosuria may be observed because the glomerular filtration rate is increased while there is no change in maximal tubular reabsorption, and the net effect is a decrease in the renal threshold for glucose. However, glycosuria with the pregnant woman in the fasting state may be a clue to abnormal glucose intolerance. A patient may have a normal fasting serum glucose and yet have an abnormal glucose tolerance test (GTT). A 3-hour oral GTT is indicated when the family or postobstetric (gynecologic) histories are suggestive or screening tests are positive, as well as in older obese patients, particularly if there is glycosuria. These screening and diagnostic procedures in an obstetric population at a medical center will uncover the 2% or 3% of women with overt diabetes who will require special attention. According to O'Sullivan's criteria, two of the four venous blood sugar levels should be elevated above the following baseline figures: fasting of 90 mg/100 ml; 1 hour = 165 mg/100 ml; 2 hours = 145 mg/100 ml; and 3 hours = 125 mg/100 ml. If plasma sugar is determined, the values are approximately 15% higher. If the fasting blood sugar is above 140 mg/100 ml, the diagnosis is established, and the GTT should not be performed because it could be dangerous. On the other hand, a negative study in early pregnancy in a high-risk or suspect patient calls for a repeat GTT after the 28th week of gestation.

Once the diagnosis is established, the disease should be classified because this will bear on the pregnancy outcome and prospects for perinatal survival. Class A, Priscilla White Classification, 1965, is associated with the best perinatal survival, above 95%. At the other end of the spectrum, patients with hypertension, proteinuria, and nephropathy have a survival rate of only 50% to 65%. Generally, perinatal mortality rates are less than 5% for all cases throughout the United States.

Among patients with gestational diabetes, approximately 25% to 30% will progress to chemical diabetes mellitus within 5 years. In pregnancy, there may be a rapid onset of diabetic symptoms even among previously undiagnosed patients. There is enhanced tendency for acidosis in preg-

nancy, and the presence of vomiting may create a confusing disturbance in the chemical balance. Maternal acidosis is the most ominous association with perinatal mortality. Other adverse factors are hyperglycemia, water imbalance, hypertensive disorders (up to 50%), excessively sized fetus (somatic and splanchnic growth), and hydramnios (10%). Monitoring the fetus should reveal several adverse findings with fetal jeopardy. Signs that are indicative of a deteriorating fetal status include deterioration of biophysical parameters of fetal well-being. The risk of fetal death rises substantially after the 36th week. Regardless of the initial classification according to White, Pedersen's poor prognostic signs in diabetic pregnancy include (1) pyelonephritis (premature labor), (2) ketoacidosis, (3) toxemia (25% incidence creating a 25% likelihood of fetal loss), and (4) "neglectors" who do not cooperate in the plan of clinical management. With respect to the classification, the complicated insulin-dependent diabetics who suffer the most guarded prognosis fall into classes D, E, F, and R (White's classification), for example, juvenile onset, proliferative retinitis, calcified vessels, coronary artery disease, nephropathy, and so forth, probably representing about 10% of the clinical diabetics.

The prime target in medical management is adequate blood sugar control prior to and throughout pregnancy. Preconceptual control (at least 3 months before pregnancy) decreases abortions and anomalies. Careful control throughout minimizes fetal macrosomia and newborn problems (potential for hypoxia, delayed pulmonary maturation, hypoglycemia, and hyperbilirubinemia). The daily amount of exercise should be maintained at a constant level. Diet must be rigidly controlled and insulin therapy precisely based on blood glucose levels. The daily calorie intake (30 to 35 calories/kg of body weight), which is achieved by consuming three meals and one to three snacks per day, is intended to permit a total weight gain of about 25 pounds, emphasizing a progressive linear gain of 350 g to 400 g/week after the first trimester. About 1.5 g protein/kg of body weight (higher for adolescents) is desirable, and about one half of the total calories should be provided by carbohydrate consumption, while avoiding concentrated sugars. A diet too low in calories will give rise to ketonuria. Ketoacidosis should be avoided meticulously by keeping fasting plasma glucose levels 100 mg ± 10 mg/100 and 2-hour postprandial levels below 120 mg/100 ml. Oral hypoglycemics are contraindicated in pregnancy due to their teratic potential. The insulin regimen is usually two injections daily of both NPH and regular insulin (2 : 1 ratio in the morning and 1 : 1 ratio in the evening) augmented in 20% increments to achieve better control as necessary.

Currently, even insulin-dependent diabetics are usually managed on an outpatient basis. Ideally, pregnancy assessment and control starts prior to gestation. It is only with impeccable control (as may be determined by normal hemoglobin A_{1C} measurements) that the diabetic sequelae in pregnancy can be avoided.

For an outpatient diabetic program to be successful, it requires careful initial assessment, a reliable patient, frequent blood sugar determinations by the patient, open communications, frequent outpatient visits, and a careful fetal-monitoring program. The initial assessment usually includes (in addition to the standard obstetric laboratory studies) a biochemical profile (SMA 6 and 12), electrolytes, creatinine clearance, urine culture, EKG, chest x ray, and in the more advanced classifications, retinal photography. Additionally, hemoglobin A_{1C} determinations afford an indication of integrated control in the weeks preceding the analysis. For the first few days the patient takes finger stick blood glucose measurements: fasting (before breakfast), preprandial at noon, at 2:00 P.M., and at 8:00 P.M.

After the initial control is established, these may be taken one a day in a rotating pattern so that in 4 days values are available for each of the times noted. Frequent communication and visits assure that the maternal-monitoring program is comprehensive and affords the opportunities to assess the fetus. A schedule of fetal assessment includes ultrasonic examination: early in gestation, at 20 to 24 weeks, and every 4 to 6 weeks after 26 weeks. Maternal assessment of fetal movements may be determined every day and NST employed weekly from 30 to 34 weeks, biweekly at 34 to 36 weeks, triweekly at 35 to 37 weeks, and more frequently (as indicated) after the 37th week. CSTs and biophysical profiles may assist if the NST is equivocal.

When appropriate (individualized for each patient), the fetal maturity is determined (usually by amniocentesis), and if the fetus is mature the labor is induced or cesarean section performed.

Definitive management of gestational (class A) diabetes is slightly controversial. However, at the present time it seems clear that only by the use of ADA diet and prophylactic insulin (25 U NPH in the morning) may macrosomia, operative delivery, and birth trauma be controlled. Women in the class A category who previously have experienced pregnancy-induced hypertension, overt diabetes in gestation or a fetal loss are best managed the same

as an overt diabetic. In these, antepartal fetal monitoring is also required. Delivery is achieved by or beyond the 38th week of gestation once euglycemia and fetal maturity are achieved. Labor may be induced as required. Hemoglobin A_{1C} levels, which are elevated in the presence of chronic hyperglycemia, can be used in series to roughly determine the quality of diabetic control. Preterm delivery before the 37th week by the vaginal route or cesarean section (if necessary) is dictated by bouts of acidosis, hypertension, worsening diabetic state, or fetal compromise. To avoid injury of these fragile infants, abdominal delivery is used liberally. Intensive neonatal evaluation and impeccable care are mandatory.

PATHOLOGY OF LABOR AND PUERPERIUM

Dystocia

Dystocia (difficult labor) may be defined as cessation of progress in parturition. The causes fall into three main groups:

1. Uterine forces that are not strong enough to overcome the natural resistance offered to the birth of the baby by the birth canal. Weakness of uterine action is called **uterine inertia** and is the most common cause of dystocia.
2. Faulty presentation or abnormal development of the fetus.
3. Abnormalities in the size or the character of the birth canal that form an obstacle to fetal descent.

Dysfunctional Labor

"**Hypocontractility**" in which uterine contractions occur less than twice per 10 minutes and average less than 25 mmHg, is the most common cause of **dysfunctional labor.** Progress in labor is arrested or retarded in terms of rate of cervical effacement and dilatation and descent and rotation of the presenting part. Abnormal cervical compliance (cervix remains firm and poorly effaced) has been implicated as the underlying cause in a small percentages of cases (approximately 3%). Patients with arrested labor must be evaluated for obstruction of the birth canal, fetal origin, placental origin, or, if in the second stage, poor patient effort, (which may be an effect of heavy analgesia). Dysfunctional labor may also present in the form of "**hypercontractility,**" which is manifested by more than five contractions in 10 minutes with or without elevated resting pressures (normal range of 8 to 12 mmHg). This abnormal uterine behavior may occur with placental abruption, and in some preeclamptic parturients.

Precipitate Labor

Fetal welfare is compromized when the intensity of uterine contractions is increased, intervals are shortened, and duration is increased. A combination of excessively forceful uterine contractions and minimal soft tissue resistance can give rise to precipitate labor, fetal anoxia and cerebral trauma, maternal lacerations, and postpartal hemorrhage caused by uterine atony. Early recognition of the problem, timely preparation for delivery under controlled conditions, and properly administered analgesia or anesthesia may minimize these risks.

Uterine Constriction Rings

In association with ineffectual uterine contractions, there may be annular, spastic muscular strictures that do not rise or change position as labor advances. Unlike the pathologic retraction ring of Bandle, they are not associated with obstructed labor and they cannot be palpated externally at the junction of the lower and upper uterine segments. The majority are palpable only on the uterine interior. Often, they arise from inappropriate manual or oxytocic stimulation. Relaxants including amyl nitrite, intravenous epinephrine, or deep anesthesia may eliminate the localized myometrial spasms, but more often abdominal delivery is required.

Intrapartal Infection

Normally, there appear to be natural defenses in the mother that are effective in preventing intrapartal infections. Obviously, host resistance in general is affected by the overall health status; the cervical mucous plug, intact membranes and perhaps antibacterial activity in the amniotic fluid are also important factors. These defense mechanisms are lost when the membranes rupture. Within 48 hours the great majority of patients will have positive amniotic fluid cultures. The longer the duration of membrane rupture prior to delivery the higher the incidence of "chorioamnionitis," and, in some cases, a rapid invasion of gram-negative bacilli will produce septic shock. Thus, an accurate diagnosis of ruptured membranes is crucial. Usually, by observation or inspection or utilizing the nitrazine paper test (positive results due to alkaline amniotic fluid), fern test (amniotic fluid allowed to dry shows ferning), and cytologic examination (presence of vernix caseosa cells) the diagnosis can be estab-

lished. Serial (usually daily) ultrasonic examinations for amniotic fluid index and biophysical profile are utilized to determine if chorioamnionitis has occurred.

Treatment is predicated on many variables; however, once chorioamnionitis develops, the fetus and the mother are at risk. Thus, it is recommended that regardless of gestational age the fetus with chorioamnionitis should be delivered. Often, there is a dilemma because immaturity of the fetus at the time of membrane rupture may mean the chances of extrauterine survival would not be great. This is of particular urgency in those of less than 27 weeks of gestation. With parental involvement the decision is often made for conservative therapy. In such cases this watchful waiting will offer the only chance of fetal survival but is all too frequently unsuccessful. In one recent series there were no survivors with rupture below 25 weeks. In those below 28 weeks there was a nearly 60% risk of chorioamnionitis, and 50% perinatal mortality, and only 30% of the survivors were neurologically normal at 6 months.

Unfortunately, prophylactic antibiotics do not protect the mother or the fetus. Tocolytic agents are generally contraindicated in the presence of ruptured membranes. A delay of some 18 to 24 hours after rupture of the membranes tends to provoke fetal lung maturity and lessen the likelihood of the respiratory distress syndrome. Within 48 hours of administering β-methasone therapy to the mother, even greater lung maturation can be achieved in the fetus. This seems particularly useful from 27 to 32 weeks of gestation. Thus, if there is no evidence of infection in the mother and the gestation is more than 26 weeks' and less than 34 weeks' duration, corticosteroid therapy and expectancy until pulmonary maturity might be an appropriate management. Bed rest is continued as long as there is active leakage. It is advisable to use external electronic fetal monitoring for some time after admission to evaluate the possibility of fetal tachycardia (distress) from occult cord prolapse. After an initial sterile speculum examination, no others are made. About 80% of these patients will go into labor spontaneously within 72 hours. Despite the risk of provoking a *Candida albicans* infection in the infant, antibiotic coverage during labor may reduce the likelihood of puerperal morbidity.

Once pulmonary maturity is assured, there is little to be gained by waiting. Thus, in an asymptomatic woman whose gestation is 35 weeks or more or with evidence of overt signs of infection at earlier stages, the presence of documented ruptured membranes may indicate induction of labor or, should this be contraindicated or unsuccessful, abdominal intervention. The appropriate cultures for mixed bacteria are taken initially after the diagnosis of membrane rupture is established. At any time amnionitis is detected (temperature above 99° F in the morning, white blood count above 12,000, fetal tachycardia above 160) delivery should be accomplished within 8 hours. Broad-spectrum antibiotics are given by infusion in labor.

Pelvic Contraction

The common types of pelvic contraction may be classified in four main groups: contraction of the inlet; contraction of the midpelvis; contraction of the outlet; and combinations of inlet, midpelvic, and outlet contraction. Inlet contraction is defined as diminution of the obstetric conjugate measurement (by roentgenogram) to 10.0 cm or less or diminution of the diagonal conjugate measurement (clinical) to 11.5 cm or less. When the interischial spinous diameter is 9.5 cm or less (by roentgenogram), there is transverse contraction of the midpelvis. In outlet contraction the angle formed by the pubic rami is narrow, and the ischial tuberosities are close together; thus, it resembles a male pelvis insofar as the outlet is concerned. Often it is called a funnel pelvis. It is customary to make a diagnosis of outlet contraction whenever the intertuberous distance is 8 cm or less by clinical measurement or 10 cm or less by roentgenographic measurement. The sum of the interischial tuberous diameter (TI) and the posterior sagittal diameter of the outlet (PSO) should be 15.0 cm or more by clinical measurement to be considered normal.

It should be noted that the size of the pelvis is only one important factor in determining whether or not a given fetus can be delivered through a given pelvis. Other factors involved in the eventual outcome include size of the fetus, moldability of the fetal head, fetal position and presentation, rigidity of the maternal soft parts, the uterine powers, and other clinical features. Clinical examination of the pelvis in context with an appreciation of these several factors as the mechanism and course of labor is observed provides adequate information to manage most patients successfully without resort to the use of x-ray pelvimetry, which has potential fetal hazards. A notable exception is the anticipated vaginal delivery of a breech presentation when x-ray pelvimetry may be mandatory. Ultrasound studies may assist in evaluating untoward problems involving the fetus. An oxytocin infusion in a carefully titrated administration is advisable only in patients in whom disproportion has been ruled out. If the infusion administered, a lack of progressive cervical dilation, or descent of the fetal head suggests an inadequate pelvis. A deceleration phase of more than 3 hours in primigravidas or 1 hour in multiparas is abnormal. A diagnosis of arrest of descent in the second stage is made by finding no progress over an hour's time.

Pelvic Dystocia

The treatment of dystocia due to abnormal pelves varies with the degree of contraction, the size of the infant and, in multiparas, the history of previous labors. Successful treatment depends on the ability to determine the extent of disproportion between the infant and the pelvis. However, in general, a normally developed full-term infant cannot be born spontaneously and alive when the true conjugate measures 10 cm or less. However, in modern obstetrics, fetal monitoring is instituted and the decision for intervening at an optimal time may be based more on the fetal status and clinical situation than any arbitrary set of pelvic measurements. Certainly, if the trial of labor is continued until there is a pathologic retraction ring of Bandle, indicative of an obstructed labor, the possibility of very serious fetal jeopardy already exists.

Dystocia due to abnormalities in the fetus include (1) excessive size, (2) fetal anomalies, (3) hydrocephalus, (4) multiple pregnancies, and (5) transverse lie. In "shoulder, oblique, or breech presentations," when placenta previa has been excluded, external cephalic version may be carefully attempted before or early in labor, provided that the patient's parity is not great, the fetal membranes are intact, and the presenting part is not markedly engaged. If this fails, then cesarean section is necessary except in the breech for vaginal delivery group. Any patient with a documented contracted pelvis should be subjected to cesarean section. The grave risk of uterine rupture with internal manipulations has made the procedure obsolete. Rarely, spontaneous evolution of a tranverse lie may occur—either by Douglas' or Denman's method—in which a small macerated fetus may be expelled spontaneously, or delivery may occur by a mechanism in which the fetus is doubled upon itself (*conduplicato corpore*).

Posterior Occipital Position

The majority of occiput posterior (OP) positions are delivered ultimately in the anterior position. However, at the onset of labor, posterior position of the occiput is a common finding. Persistent occiput posterior includes those cases that do not rotate anteriorly (only about 5%).

In the vast majority of OP positions, anterior rotation takes place spontaneously if patience is exercised. In a very small minority (and only after the cervix is fully dilated) one of the following procedures may be necessary: (1) manual rotation of the head to OA, followed by application of forceps; (2) forceps rotation to OA followed by reapplication of forceps (Scanzoni maneuver); and (3) delivery with forceps as a posterior. If the fetal head is considerably molded or the pelvis is anthropoid or android in type or shows midpelvic contraction, delivery by forceps as an occiput posterior may prove to be the least traumatic to the mother and the fetus, but each case must be considered and treated individually. However, since OP presentations enhance perinatal morbidity and mortality electronic fetal monitoring or fetal blood scalp sampling should be used to ascertain fetal well-being until these definitative therapies may be applied.

Breech Presentation

Breech presentations are classified as follows:

1. *Complete,* when the feet and the legs are flexed on the thighs, and the thighs are flexed on the abdomen, so that the buttocks and the feet present
2. *Incomplete,* when the foot or the knee, in any combination, presents through the cervix
3. *Frank,* when the legs are extended and lie against the abdomen and the chest, and the buttocks present

The diagnosis of breech presentation depends on palpating the hard ballotable head in the fundus with the irregular soft breech above the symphysis. Rectal or vaginal examination reveals the characteristic parts. The fetal heart sounds are heard through the back of the fetus at about the level of the umbilicus. The normal mechanism includes (1) engagement and (2) descent, ordinarily in one of the oblique diameters. Usually it is the anterior hip that first encounters the resistance of the pelvic floor, causing an internal rotation of 45 degrees that brings the anterior hip to the pubic arch. If the posterior hip descends first, internal rotation occurs through an arc of 135 degrees. Descent continues until the perineum is distended, when the posterior hip is

delivered over the anterior margin of the perineum by lateral flexion of the body, followed by the spontaneous delivery of the legs and the feet. As the shoulders reach the perineum they undergo internal rotation to the anteroposterior diameter. The flexed head enters the pelvis in one of the oblique diameters and then rotates so that the posterior neck engages under the symphysis. The head is born in a position of flexion, with the chin, the mouth, the nose, the forehead, the bregma and the occiput appearing in succession over the perineum.

The relatively high perinatal mortality (approximately 15%) of breech presentation is due mainly to the increased incidence of prematurity, fetal anomalies, complications of gestation and labor, the presentation itself being responsible for only about one third of the deaths, trauma and anoxia accounting for many of these. Prolapse of the umbilical cord is a particular hazard of the complete and incomplete varieties, the incidence being, respectively, about 12 and 22 times the usual incidence for vertex presentation (0.5%).

In the latter weeks of pregnancy, substitution of a vertex presentation may be attempted by external version. (See subsequent section devoted to this subject.)

Vaginal breech deliveries may be of three types:

1. A *spontaneous delivery* is one in which the entire infant is expelled by natural forces.
2. A *partial breech extraction* is one in which the infant is extruded as far as the umbilicus by natural forces, but the remainder of the body is extracted by the attendant. This method of delivery is the one of choice whenever feasible.
3. A *total breech extraction* is one in which the entire body of the infant is extracted by the attendant. This method should rarely be necessary.

Ideally, the breech should be allowed to advance spontaneously until the umbilicus has been born. The completion of labor is facilitated if the arms remain crossed on the chest and the head is sharply flexed. This is best obtained by avoiding traction and by moderate downward pressure on the fundus as soon as the breech begins to emerge through the vulva.

When delivery by traction is necessary, the traction on the legs and the body should be downward until an axilla becomes visible, when the body is flexed upward, delivering the posterior shoulder over the perineum. By depressing the body of the fetus the anterior shoulder is brought to emerge beneath the pubic arch. The head usually occupies an oblique diameter with the chin posteriorly and is best delivered by Mauriceau's maneuver. The index finger of one hand is introduced into the mouth of the child and applied over the superior maxilla, while the body rests upon the palm of the hand. Two fingers of the other hand are then hooked over the neck and, grasping the shoulders, make downward traction until the occiput appears over the symphysis. The body is now extended upward, and the mouth, the brow, the nose, and the occiput emerge successfully over the perineum. Piper forceps to the aftercoming head are favored by many obstetricians.

Current management is predicated upon the findings that vaginal delivery is risky and that, in general, perinatal mortality and morbidity can be improved by utilizing abdominal delivery more freely than in the past. The vulnerable groups include complete and incomplete (footling) breeches, among whom the incidence of prolapsed cord may be 10%, patients with premature labor or who have an *in utero* growth retardation problem (12%–14%) and primigravidas with average to large term-sized fetus. The trend now is to require specific indications and justification for vaginal delivery in breech presentations. The general contraindications to vaginal birth after previous cesarean are previous classical incision, macrosomic fetus, fetal malposition, and multiple pregnancy. Many authorities also indicate that the initial cause for the cesarean should be nonrecurrent, that there be no more than one previous cesarean, and that the postoperative course after the first was uncomplicated.

Generally, current criteria for vaginal delivery in the breech presentation include only frank breech presentation, a gestational age of 34 weeks or more, an estimated fetal weight of 2,000 g to 3,500 g, a flexed fetal head, an adequate maternal pelvis as determined by x-ray pelvimetry, and no maternal or fetal indications for cesarean section. Obviously, other circumstances may also be suitable, but are less ideal, for example, a previable fetus (<25 weeks of gestation), documented lethal congenital anomalies, and presentation so far in the delivery process that vaginal delivery is safer than attempting cesarean.

Recently, considerable attention has been directed to attempting to prevent the breech presentation in labor by performing external version in the third trimester. Although still mildly controversial, it now appears that even if tocolytics are necessary,

external version may be accomplished with relative safety and that there is risk–benefit justification on the basis of decreasing the incidence of breech presentations at term.

Face Presentation

Since face presentations result from extension of the fetal head, the characteristic sign is that the cephalic prominence is palpable on the same side as the back instead of on the small parts as in vertex presentation. The heart sounds are heard on the side of the small parts and are louder than usual.

Delivery occurs by (1) descent, as in vertex presentation, with internal rotation and flexion; (2) extension; and (3) external rotation.

If the pelvis is normal and the chin anterior, spontaneous delivery or an easy forceps delivery should be anticipated, no treatment being necessary. Internal rotation brings the chin under the symphysis, the head being delivered by flexion, with the nose, the eyes, the brow, the bregma, and the occiput appearing in succession over the anterior margin of the perineum. After the birth of the head the occiput sags backward and undergoes external rotation to the side toward which it was originally directed. The face must rotate, because delivery of a mature baby with the chin posterior is impossible. The initial position of the chin is posterior in about 30% of these cases.

Anterior rotation usually occurs spontaneously, though very late. When this is not the case (about one instance in ten), conversion into a vertex presentation may be attempted, provided that the face is not deeply engaged, the pelvis is normal, and the membranes are intact or recently ruptured. However, usually when the chin remains posterior, cesarean section is preferable. Finally, if the baby is dead, craniotomy may be necessary.

When a brow presentation is detected at the superior strait, it should be left alone until it promises to be persistent because the transient varieties will be born spontaneously as either a vertex or a face presentation. On the other hand, less than one half of the persistent cases—often attended by a true disproportion—can be expected to deliver uneventfully; thus, attempts at conversion or (usually) cesarean section are indicated on a basis similar to that outlined for face presentations.

Cesarean sections are advocated much more frequently in all cases of malposition and malpresentation of the fetus and when labor becomes abnormal or fetal distress develops.

Prolapse of the Cord

Cord prolapse is most common in conditions that interfere with engagement at the superior strait; hence, it is most common in transverse and foot presentations and less often found in frank breech. The overall incidence is 0.8% of deliveries. Variable deceleration noted in the fetal heart pattern identified through electronic fetal monitoring may help identify cord compression in occult prolapses. Persistent fetal tachycardia, noted on external electronic monitoring immediately or soon after spontaneous rupture of the membranes, may also signify the existence of an occult cord prolapse. The cord may sometimes be seen or, provided that the fetus is alive, may be palpated as a cord with distinct pulsations. Hypotension in the fetus for any reason may cause the cord to become limp and possibly prolapse. Perinatal mortality rates of 30% for all cases when the cord is visible can be anticipated, since many of these infants are premature.

If the cord prolapses after the cervix has become fully dilated, forceps are indicated only if the fetus can be delivered quickly and atraumatically. If the cervix is only partially dilated, the patient should be placed immediately in the knee-chest position, and by sterile vaginal manipulation an attempt made to replace the cord. The attempt is frequently unsuccessful, in which case the presenting part is pushed upward (to decrease pressure on the cord) and held there until cesarean can be performed. The chances for the child are poor without cesarean section, but this should not be attempted unless the fetal heart and the umbilical pulsations are strong after release of pressure from the cord. Oxygen should be administered to the mother. It is advisable to perform a sterile vaginal examination and to palpate for the cord when the diagnosis of abnormal presentation is first made. Close watch of the FHR is also imperative.

Rupture of the Uterus

Rupture of the uterus occurs once in approximately every 2,000 cases and is a grave accident, carrying a composite maternal mortality of about 10% to 15% and a perinatal mortality of about 50% to 75%. There are two main types, spontaneous and traumatic, and each of these, in turn, may be classified according to whether it occurs in pregnancy or in labor. Ruptures that occur spontaneously may further be categorized into three groups: (1) those with a previous cesarean section scar, (2) those with previous operative scars, and (3) those with an intact uterus. The distinction is important because the maternal mortality rate for ruptures of intact uteri is between 20% and 40%, while that associated with rupture of a cesarean section scar is less than 5%. It is customary to distinguish between "complete" and "incomplete" rupture, according to whether the laceration communicates with the abdominal cavity or is separated from it by peritoneal covering (subperitoneal hematoma).

Causes. Currently, spontaneous rupture of the uterus during labor is more common than traumatic rupture. In the past, nearly one half of the traumatic ruptures resulted from version and extraction. Other cases resulted from a Braxton Hicks version, difficult or unsuccessful forceps breech extraction, and the use of bags and bougies. The common antecedent factors in spontaneous rupture of the uterus are advanced maternal age and parity, contraction of the pelvis, a large fetus, and such obvious dystocial factors as abnormal presentation and impacted pelvic tumors. Excessive stretching of the lower uterine segment with the development of a pathologic retraction ring plays an important predisposing role. Pitocin stimulation of the uterus remains a significant factor in uterine rupture. Other predisposing factors in the spontaneous rupture of the intact uterus are congenital defects of the uterus, adenomyosis and a history of previous curettage, manual removal of the placenta and postabortive or postpartal sepsis. However, with the increasing incidence of cesarean section, *rupture of the scar has become the most common cause of uterine rupture*. The risk of uterine rupture following a previous cesarean section is about 2%. When the old scar merely disrupts and the myometrium is not freshly lacerated, the event is more properly referred to as a wound dehiscence than actual rupture, and the prognosis is much better. The overall incidence of uterine rupture is approximately the same following classic and low cervical operations; however, about one third of classic scars rupture in the later months of pregnancy and are apt to be complete and dramatic and to occur without warning, while the low cervical ruptures occur almost exclusively during labor and the signs and symptoms are insidious. A hematoma may develop within the broad ligament with few or no signs appearing until the patient begins to have pain and fever during the puerperium.

Symptoms. Rupture occurring in the later months of pregnancy usually causes sudden, sharp abdominal pains followed by collapse, but in some cases the immediate symptoms are mild. If rupture occurs at the time of labor, the patient usually complains at the height of a uterine contraction of a sharp shooting pain in the lower abdomen, followed by sudden relief. There may be external hemorrhage, cessation of uterine contractions, and sudden disappearance of the fetal heart beat. The lower uterine segment becomes more sensitive to pressure, the presenting part slips away from the inlet, and the firmly contracted uterus may be alongside the fetus. The symptoms of shock from hemorrhage are usually sudden and severe but may be delayed, especially if the rupture is in the lower uterine segment. Blood may appear in the urine.

If rupture occurs, immediate laparotomy is necessary. Hysterectomy is usually required, as is blood transfusion.

Postpartal Hemorrhage

Serious bleeding following the birth of the child is usually due to (1) uterine atony, (2) placental retention, (3) deep tears of the birth canal, or (4) a coagulation defect. In the latter category it is wise to consider von Willebrand's disease, which is the most common cause of coagulopathy in women. Nevertheless, the most common of all causes is uterine atony, which is responsible for over 90% of these cases. Among the other causes of postpartal hemorrhage, the most common are lacerations of the birth canal, operative delivery, deep anesthesia with agents that relax the uterus (e.g., halothane), and prolonged labor with maternal exhaustion. Postpartal hemorrhage should be anticipated and prepared for when any of these complications present or when there has been overstretching of the uterus, as in cases of an excessively large fetus, multiple gestation, hydramnios, or uterine tumors. Postpartal hemorrhage is defined as bleeding from the birth canal in excess of 500 ml during the first 24 hours after birth. Postpartal hemorrhage, as defined, is observed in about 10% of all deliveries.

In uterine atony there is a continuous flow, which may be very copious, and the uterus does not exhibit proper contraction. When due to retained placental tissue the blood may escape in gushes and frequently in large clots. If the bleeding commences immediately after delivery (third-stage bleeding), it may be due to tears or to partial separation of the placenta. If the hemorrhage (usually bright-red blood) continues after the uterus has been emptied and is well contracted, tears of the cervix, vagina, and perineum should be looked for and sutured at once. On the other hand, if the uterus does not

contract, the hemorrhage may be due to atony or the retention of a placental cotyledon, which will be suggested by careful examination of the fetal surface of the placenta and confirmed by careful uterine exploration. In the presence of marked bleeding before separation of the placenta has occurred, manual removal of the placenta should be carried out at once, certainly before appreciable blood loss has taken place. Also, if the placenta is retained for more than 30 minutes in the "absence" of bleeding, the placenta should be removed prophylactically. Recently there has been a trend toward even earlier manual removal if the placenta does not separate soon after delivery. On many services it is routine to explore the uterus after delivery of the placenta to assure complete evacuation as well as the intactness of the uterus. Certainly, it is advisable to explore the uterus if there is a question of incompleteness of placental removal, when bleeding continues after the placenta is expressed or following a difficult delivery when the uterine wall may have been injured.

Attempts to deliver the placenta by squeezing and kneading the uterus through the abdomen, as entailed in the original Credé procedure, are not only futile, but as a rule also traumatize the myometrium and often aggravate the difficulties. When the placenta has been removed and bleeding continues, 10 U oxytocin (Pitocin), given intravenously slowly and followed by a solution of 1,000 ml Ringer's lactate with 20 U oxytocin should control the bleeding. If this fails, and there is no preexisting maternal preeclampsia or hypertension, 0.2 mg ergonovine (Methergine) may be given intramuscularly. If bleeding persists despite bimanual compression and massage of the uterus, prostaglandin $F_{2\alpha}$ uterine injections or prostaglandin E suppositories will assist in uterine contraction and do not have the hypertensive effect of the ergot preparations. If symptoms of shock appear, the usual treatment of adequate blood replacement is indicated. Uterine packing has lost favor as a means of controlling hemorrhage, except as a temporary procedure in rare instances when hysterectomy is contemplated.

Delivery by Forceps

The most frequent indications for delivery by forceps are conditions in which it is desirable to spare the mother second-stage effort, in dysfunctional labor in the second stage, and in certain situations of fetal distress. Although to forestall prolonged pressure of the fetal head against a more or less rigid perineum and to spare the mother the strain of the last few minutes of the second stage, the use of so-called elective low forceps has become popular in recent years, particularly in primigravidas.

In general, it is considered good practice, in the absence of disproportion, to apply forceps if advance is not made after 1 hour if the head is on the perineum or is in a position for "low forceps," although each case must be individualized. It should be recognized that even in the second stage of labor, oxytocic stimulation, further delay or even abdominal intervention may be choices that are to be preferred to a difficult forceps delivery. The suggested time limits are appropriate points to evaluate the patient thoroughly but not necessarily to effect delivery in every case. The difficulty to be counteracted by the forceps operation and its inherent dangers to the mother and the fetus must be weighed against the hazards of allowing a protracted second stage with its significant fetal risks.

The following conditions must be fulfilled before forceps are applied:

1. The child must present correctly, either a vertex or mentum anterior.
2. The cervix must be fully dilated.
3. Membranes must be ruptured.
4. There must be no marked disproportion between the head and the pelvis.
5. The head must have descended to the level of the ischial spines or below.
6. The bladder must be emptied by catheterization.

The most important function of forceps is traction, although they are frequently employed to rotate the fetal head. Forceps operations are classified according to the level of the fetal head at the time that the blades are applied:

1. *Low forceps*—the application of forceps when the head is visible, the skull is on the perineal floor, and the sagittal suture is in the anteroposterior diameter of the pelvis.
2. *Mid forceps*—the application of forceps before the criteria of low forceps (as stated above) have been met but after engagement has taken place; that is, after the plane of the greatest cephalic diameter (biparietal) has passed the inlet. Every effort must be made to avoid this type of potentially hazardous vaginal delivery in the interests of perinatal welfare.
3. *High forceps*—the application of forceps before engagement has taken place. This variety

of forceps delivery has no place in modern obstetrics.

For general use the ordinary Simpson forceps are very servicable, but the particular forceps employed should be varied to suit the particular case. In certain midforceps extractions, axis traction is essential (Tarnier, Irving), and in certain cases of transverse arrest, the Kielland forceps have certain advantages. The Piper forceps generally are employed to deliver the aftercoming head in breech deliveries. In modern obstetrics, most clinical situations requiring major forceps operations are best handled by cesarean section. Occasionally, there may be an indication for the use of a vacuum extractor as a substitute for forceps when pelvic space is limited.

Version

Version consists of turning the baby in the uterus from an undesirable into a desirable position. There are three types of version: external, internal, and Braxton Hicks. According to whether the head or the breech is made the presenting part, the operation is spoken of as cephalic or podalic version, respectively. Today, cephalic version has been abandoned.

External version is an operation designed to change a breech or a transverse presentation into a vertex presentation by external manipulation of the fetus through the abdominal and the uterine walls. It is likely to be most successful when done about a month before full term. Recently, improved success rates have been reported using tocolytics. Both ultrasonic evaluation and NSTs have been advocated before and after the procedure. In rare circumstances, the placenta is partially separated, the uterine integrity is jeopardized, or the cord is entangled or knotted. The chance of success is greatest if the presenting part is unengaged and the membranes are intact. In the interest of reducing the relatively high incidence of cesarean sections, there has been some renewed interest in this procedure under carefully controlled circumstances. The rewards are high if successful.

Internal version is accomplished with cervical dilation complete. The whole hand of the operator is introduced high into the uterus and one or both feet are grasped and pulled downward in the direction of the birth canal. With his or her other hand (on the abdomen), the obstetrician may expedite the turning by pushing the head upward. However, the hazard of uterine rupture and the guarded fetal prognosis have led to the restriction of this procedure largely to delivery of a compromised second twin. The use of **Braxton Hicks, version**—compressing the lower uterine segment with the infant's buttocks in placenta previa or stretching the cervix with the infant's thigh so that labor may be initiated—has no place in modern therapy.

Cesarean Section

There are four main types of abdominal cesarean section: (1) classic, (2) low cervical, (3) extraperitoneal, and (4) cesarean hysterectomy. Low cervical is further subdivided into vertical and transverse and is the type favored generally, although other types are preferred in special circumstances.

Accepted indications for cesarean section include a serious disproportion between the size of the fetal head and the maternal pelvis or fetal malposition. In certain cases of contracted pelvis, the operation may be indicated if the trial of labor is unsatisfactory. A history of previous difficult labors is significant. Other important indications for cesarean section, in descending order of importance, are hemorrhagic complications (placenta previa, abruptio placentae), toxemias and intercurrent disease (especially diabetes), and fetal distress. There are other miscellaneous indications, such as certain cases of uterine inertia, pregnancy following major vaginal repairs, and carcinoma of the cervix. Generally, perinatal risks are weighed very high and when the welfare of the fetus or mother is potentially compromised by waiting, or if fetal monitoring shows the potential or actual distress in response to provoked or spontaneous myometrial activity, abdominal intervention may be desirable.

Except in the presence of an absolute pelvic indication, severe abruptio placentae or central placenta previa, cesarean section should not be performed when the child is dead or the mother is in poor condition. The maternal and the fetal morbidity and mortality are least if cesarean section is performed before the onset of labor; they increase progressively with the time the membranes have been ruptured and the duration of labor before the time of surgery. However, the modern chemotherapeutic agents have added a considerable margin of safety and flexibility to the use of cesarean section. Low cervical cesarean section, plus antibiotic therapy, has been used with good results in many infected cases. In these circumstances some clinicians employ an extraperitoneal technique.

The more liberal use of cesarean section in recent years (range of 25% to 30%) has unquestionably resulted in greater perinatal salvage; however, wider use of cesarean section should *not* be regarded as the ultimate solution for all antenatal problems. Surgical intervention undoubtedly introduces maternal risks (*e.g.*, anesthetic, hematologic, and infectious). Objective tests should be utilized in assessing fetal lung maturity when intervening. It should be borne in mind, also, that if this mode of delivery is to yield satisfactory results, it must be selected as a proper and timely technique of definitive management, not as a last resort after all others fail or after the fetus has sustained irreversible brain injury. Overall, there has been a recent trend toward reducing the rising trend for abdominal intervention.

Puerperal Infection

Puerperal infection, one of the three major causes of maternal death, is a postpartal wound infection of the parturient canal (usually of the endometrium) that may remain localized but often extends along lymphatic and vascular channels to produce systemic signs and symptoms. Puerperal infections are grouped under the general term **puerperal morbidity,** defined as a temperature of 100.4° F (38.0° C) occurring on two occasions, more than 6 hours apart, exclusive of the first 24 hours. In general, the most common cause of puerperal infection is the anaerobic *Streptococcus,* but the hemolytic *Streptococcus* is the most common cause of fulminating puerperal infection, as well as epidemics of the disease. Mixed infections are the rule, and other organisms include various staphylococci, *Escherichia coli,* gonococci, *Proteus vulgaris, Enterobacter, Peptostreptococcus, Bacteroides,* pneumococci, and clostridiae. *Clostridium perfringens* is an uncommon cause of puerperal infection, but has a dramatic course and high mortality. It is seen more commonly after criminal abortions than after deliveries near term. Gonorrheal puerperal endometritis, once considered the cause of 5% to 10% of all fevers occurring in the puerperium, is rarely seen today. The incidence of puerperal infection following vaginal delivery should not exceed 3%, although this figure may reach 25% or more in patients delivered by cesarean section.

The most important predisposing causes of puerperal infection are hemorrhage and trauma at the time of labor. Preexisting anemia, undernutrition, and other debilitated states make puerperal infection more likely. Retention of placental tissue is a common predisposing factor to infection.

The most common manifestation of puerperal infection is endometritis. Endometritis usually begins suddenly on the 3rd or the 4th day of the puerperium, with malaise, headache, chilliness or a chill and temperature of 103° F or more that remains elevated. The uterus may be enlarged and tender to pressure. The lochial discharge is variable, relating to the different organisms responsible for the infection.

If the infection is limited to the uterus, the patient slowly returns to normal. Rise in temperature indicates an extension, which may lead to abscess within the broad ligament, the posterior cul-de-sac or the anterior pelvis. The infection may extend through the uterine lymphatics to cause peritonitis, or pyemia may develop with typical spiking temperature or, rarely, septicemia with very rapid death. Thrombosis may arise in the pelvic veins and extend to the femoral, causing phlegmasia alba dolens (milk leg). Rarely, ovarian vein thrombosis may occur with its accompanying inflammation and give rise to protracted fever, pain, and disability. The most common organisms causing the septic type are streptococci and staphlococci. Other bacteria causing the condition are the colon bacillus, *Pseudomonas aeruginosa* and various anaerobes. Endotoxic shock following these latter infections carries a grave prognosis.

Prophylaxis. Most important are (1) maintenance of strict asepsis, (2) restriction of vaginal and rectal examinations, (3) omission of coitus and vaginal douches late in pregnancy, (4) prevention of anemia, (5) immediate repair of lacerations, (6) complete evacuation of placental tissue from the uterus at the time of delivery, (7) complete evacuation of placental tissue from the uterus at the time of deliveries, (8) supporting the patient's hydration, (9) proper bladder care, (10) proper postpartal perineal care, and (11) isolation of infected patients to protect others.

Since the advent of chemotherapy, adequate blood replacement, improved prenatal care, and modern techniques of management, fulminating cases of puerperal infection are rarely encountered.

Treatment. The type, intensity, and duration of specific therapy will depend upon the organism involved, drug sensitivities by *in vitro* tests, the extent of the infection and the presence of complicating clinical conditions (*e.g.,* septic shock, septicemia, thromboembolic disease). Appropriate cultures should be taken. The procedure of obtaining an intrauterine culture may, of itself, be beneficial because it promotes drainage. Oxytocins and, if necessary, ergot preparations may promote uterine

drainage. Collections of pus in the perineum, vagina or cul-de-sac will require adequate drainage. Transfusions are needed to correct significant anemia. In the more serious cases, monitoring fluid administrations, electrolyte replacement, urinary output, and fluid losses and invasive monitoring will be necessary if the patient is to be supported properly. Clinical suspicion of lower limb and pelvic thrombophlebitis will call for diagnostic tests, for example, Doppler ultrasonic flow detector or, occasionally, the more accurate but invasive method of ascending contrast phlebography. The presence of thrombophlebitis requires bed rest, use of anticoagulants, and antibiotics. Initially, heparin infusion is necessary, but oral warfarin may be begun in 36 to 72 hours, and the heparin discontinued. If there is femoral phlebitis accompanied by pain and fever, the involved extremity should be protected and alternating pressure devices utilized along with elevation until the acute process disappears. After that elastic support is needed (often for many months) to promote venous drainage.

When there is evidence of parametritis and pelvic cellulitis, it may be desirable to perform ultrasonic examinations to detect a cul-de-sac abscess because this must be drained to promote optimal recovery from the infection. Drainage or uterine debridement by curettage may be called for in endotoxic shock, which is treated according to the principles outlined for septic abortions. Otherwise, a curettage might be dangerous and generally it is best to avoid deep entry of disinfectant solutions or objects into the vagina. Manipulations should be avoided except for culture taking and checking on possible lacerations, hematomas, or collections of pus. Hematomas that are quite large, symptomatic, and continuing to expand should be incised and drained. There may be a combination of old blood and pus when the diagnosis is delayed a number of days. Occasionally, morbidity may be associated with a hematoma above the pelvic fascia, where the blood is paravaginal or spread into the broad ligament. Retroperitoneal extensions may give rise to an inguinal ligament presentation or to rupture into the peritoneal cavity. Any suspicion of hematoma in the form of unexplained pelvic pain, fever, tachycardia, hypotension, or anemia must be immediately investigated.

Puerperal infections may be delayed or refractory, characterized by persistent uterine red or purulent discharge (lochia). There may be continued bleeding with intermittent passage of old clots. There are usually pelvic complaints or backaches associated with subinvolution of the uterus and a low-grade endometritis. The underlying cause may be retained placental fragments or, occasionally, an infected leiomyoma of the uterus.

Endometritis does not always respond sensitively to antibiotics, particularly if cervical drainage is poor. While waiting for the antibiotic sensitivity report, a drug may be chosen on the basis of a Gram-stained smear of the cervical discharge. Recent hospital antibiotic sensitivity patterns can be taken into account in the selection of a drug, and it should be given in adequate doses intravenously. Mixed infections involving two or more organisms are common, and effective therapy may require a combination of drugs. Anaerobes frequently participate in mixed infections; their growth is promoted as secondary invaders into tissues that have become necrotic after initial infection by facultative pathogens. The appearance of anaerobic infections may be quite delayed after an apparent initial successful management. Details of management of pelvic inflammatory disease are discussed in the section on gynecology. The types of therapy in mixed pelvic infection (postpregnancy or not) are similar.

The majority of offending organisms are sensitive to ampicillin or to a combination of ampicillin and gentamycin given intravenously. Most of the anaerobes are susceptible to ampicillin, penicillin, and the cephalosporins. The presence of *Bacteroides fragilis* calls for the use of clindamycin or chloramphenicol. Massive doses of antibiotics (penicillin, ampicillin, or erythromycin) are used along with a hyperbaric oxygen chamber and subsequent surgical intervention in the presence of gas gangrene *(Clostridium perfringens)* infection. The possibility of *Neisseria gonorrhoeae* infections in the vaginal tract should be considered in screening patients for pathogens. The uncomplicated case is treated with oral probenecid (1.0 g) followed by intramuscular injections, at two sites, of aqueous procaine penicillin G (total of 4.8 million units).

THE NEWBORN

Fetal Circulation

The fetal circulation carries nutritive material from the placenta through the umbilical vein, whose smaller branch unites with the portal vein and empties into the liver, and whose larger branch, the ductus venosus, empties directly into the vena cava. On entering the right atrium, most of the blood passes through the open foramen ovale into the left atrium and thus to the systemic circulation, returning to the placenta by the umbilical (hypogastric) arteries. Blood from the head region delivered via the superior vena cava is low in oxygen and tends to pass in a direct stream into the right ventricle. Since the lungs do not function, the greater part of the blood in the right ventricle passes directly from the pulmonary artery into the aorta through the ductus arteriosus and is mixed with blood of higher oxygen content pumped from the left side of the heart.

Arterial blood passing from the placenta to the fetus is only about 65% saturated with oxygen. The maternal blood source in the intervillous space is mixed, thus reducing the effective saturation. The oxygen supply under normal conditions is adequate for the fetal needs, since a number of adaptive mechanisms are operative, such as an increase in fetal red cell count and hemoglobin, differences in fetal hemoglobin as compared with the adult type that result in a shift of the oxygen dissociation curve to the left, enabling an increased oxygen uptake at low gas tension, increased cardiac output several times that of the adult, and, finally, the mechanism allowing for anaerobic metabolism to help meet the fetal requirements. Therefore, the lactic acid content of fetal blood is only slightly greater than that of the mother. According to our present state of knowledge of the conditions under which anoxic survival is possible, the carbohydrate stores, particularly of the heart, may be of paramount importance. Oxygen tension in the fetal blood returning to the placenta may remain within the normal range for short periods despite considerable reductions in the oxygen level in the blood perfusing the uterus. In addition, the fetus has a number of autoregulatory, homeostatic mechanisms relating to placental blood flow, oxygen pressure gradients, and control of transport of various substances that are sensitive to external or internal environmental changes.

In a variety of clinical situations, however, there may be serious disruptions of these defense mechanisms, and the fetus may exhibit obvious signs of distress. Impairment of placental exchange can occur (1) in the maternal circulation, (2) in the placental membrane, (3) in the fetal circulation, or (4) in combination, with several of these insults operative. Anoxia arising from any one of these conditions represents the principal basic cause of perinatal death in 25% or more of cases.

The umbilical circulation ceases 5 to 15 minutes after birth, and blood from the right ventricle circulates through the lungs, causing mechanical closure of the foramen ovale. This is due to the increased volume of blood returning from the lungs as respirations are established and the diminished quantity of blood going to the inferior vena cava when the umbilical cord is ligated. The functionless umbilical vein becomes the ligamentum teres. The ductus venosus closes and forms the ligamentum venosum, and the obliterated umbilical arteries become the lateral umbilical ligaments. The ductus arteriosus closes as the lungs begin to function, becomes occluded, and forms the ligamentum arteriosum. A large volume of blood is pumped by the right ventricle into the previously collapsed pulmonary arteries, thus reducing pressure within the lumen. Thus, within several days after birth, the adult type of circulation, in which the venous and the arterial systems are separate, develops.

Care

Immediate care consists of clearing the nasopharynx, clamping and severing the umbilical cord, and placing the infant in a heated crib or resuscitator unit, where drying, further suction, oxygen administration, intubation, or other care is given as required. The cord is ligated or clamped some 2 cm from the abdomen. Chilling of the infant must be avoided. The infant is properly identified by beads or wrist band and footprints. It is important to perform a thorough examination as soon as possible with special emphasis on the respirations, heart rate, muscle tone, reflexes and color, as recorded on the 1- and 5-minute Apgar scores. Generally, infants with scores of 6 or above do not require any special treatment. Search should be made for a single umbilical artery because this is associated with anomalies in 15% to 20% of cases. The incidence in singletons is about 1% and up to 6% in twins.

The eyes of the newborn should be treated routinely with silver nitrate solution or antibiotic prophylaxis for gonorrhea.

Nursing may be started early in the postpartal period because of the stimulating effect even though only colostrum is present. The infant should nurse for 5 to 10 minutes at each breast during the hospital stay, usually at 3- to 4-hour intervals or on demand. The infant will usually lose about 5% to 8% of the birth weight in the first few days.

In some clinics, a "birthing room" or rooming-in policy has been adopted, whereby the infant is kept in a crib at the mother's beside rather than in the nursery. It stems from the modern trend to ambulate mothers early and to make all phases of childbearing as natural as possible. These natural practices are physiologic and promote a favorable "bonding" between the mother and her infant.

About one third of newborns will have mild icterus, usually between the 2nd and 5th days of life, probably caused by hepatic cell immaturity. The bilirubin is mostly unconjugated, and levels up to 9 mg to 10 mg/100 ml of serum are not uncommon. Icterus is usually more severe and prolonged among prematures. Breast feeding aggravates the problem. Care should be taken to exclude the possibility of hemolytic disease and other pathologic causes of jaundice.

Apnea Neonatorum

If the newborn has not begun to breathe within 2 minutes after birth, the condition usually is referred to as apnea neonatorum. In the milder cases the color of the infant is livid, and the muscle tone good—*asphyxia livida*. In the severe cases the child is pale and limp—*asphyxia pallida*.

Failure of the baby to breathe at birth is usually due to one of three main causes, or to some combination of them: (1) anoxia, (2) cerebral injury, and (3) narcosis.

The classic cardiopulmonary response of the fetus/newborn to asphyxia consists initially of increased respiratory effort (primary hyperpnea) followed by primary apnea. After about 1 minute, primary apnea is followed by gasping respirations at 8 to 10 per minute for several minutes, with respiratory efforts becoming gradually less frequent thereafter. Eventually secondary apnea ensues, and respiratory effort will not return until adequate resuscitation is performed. An infant in primary apnea will respond to simple stimulation by breathing; the infant in secondary apnea will not. Since one cannot know at birth whether an apneic infant is experiencing primary or secondary apnea, lack of response to brief stimulation indicates the need for immediate resuscitation procedures.

Treatment. The best treatment of apnea neonatorum is prevention (by combating anoxia and trauma) and anticipation (having trained personnel present to carry out whatever procedures are indicated by the condition of the newborn). It is important to keep in mind the following principles.

1. *Gentleness.* Rough treatment (vigorous spanking or shaking) is no more effective than gentle stimulation (*i.e.,* rubbing the back or feet while drying) and may harm the infant.

2. *Warmth.* A radiant heater over the infant is essential to maintain body temperature and avoid cold stress, which worsens acidosis and shock. The bed should be prewarmed in anticipation of the delivery.

3. *Drying.* Evaporative heat loss is rapid for the wet newborn. Warm blankets or soft towels should be used to dry the infant immediately after birth, then discarded to avoid having the infant lying on cold, wet blankets. This drying is sufficient stimulation to ascertain whether the infant is experiencing primary or secondary apnea.

4. *Posture.* A slight Trendelenburg position may favor gravity drainage of mucus.

5. *Establishment of an adequate airway.* The oropharynx and nasopharynx should be suctioned with bulb syringe and/or suction catheter to clear mucus, blood, and so forth. Routine suctioning of the gastric contents is not advisable unless specific indications are present (*e.g.,* polyhydramnios, thick meconium, bag and mask resuscitation) because of potential vagal response with bradycardia.

6. *Administration of oxygen.* The vast majority of apneic infants will respond to successful oxygen administration to the lungs. Bag and mask ventilation using 100% oxygen should be used initially unless there is an indication that the infant will need long-term ventilatory assistance by endotracheal tube (*e.g.,* small preterm infant) or that meconium must be removed from the trachea before assisted ventilation is started. The amount of pressure delivered to the lungs should be monitored to avoid overdistention and pulmonary air leak once adequacy of air exchange has been determined by auscultation, observation of chest movement, and infant response to resuscitation. Frequently in term infants, only a few breaths by bag and mask are required to initiate respiratory effort. Thereafter, oxygen should be blown by the nose until the infant is pink and good respiratory effort is maintained.

7. *Circulation.* If the infant is bradycardic (HR <60 or 60–80 BPM and not increasing) despite adequate respiratory resuscitation using 100% oxygen for 15 to 30 seconds, cardiopulmonary massage must be initiated at 120 BPM and continued until the heart rate is greater than 80 BPM.

8. *Drugs.* Naloxone (Narcan) 0.1 mg/kg per endotracheal tube or IV should rapidly re-

verse apnea due to narcosis. However, because of Naloxone's short duration of action repetition for recurrence of apnea may be necessary. The intramuscular or subcutaneous routes may be used but a delay in onset of 15 minutes is likely. Epinephrine (1 : 10,000) 0.1 to 0.3 ml/kg intravenously or by endotracheal tube is given if the heartbeat is absent. For persistent bradycardia (heart rate of less than 80 BPM despite 30 seconds of adequate ventilation and chest compressions), epinephrine (as above) is also administered. Sodium bicarbonate (4.2% solution), 2 mEq/kg administered slowly intravenously (over at least 2 minutes), may be given for documented or assumed metabolic acidosis only if adequate ventilation is established.

9. *Volume expanders.* Hypovolemia in the newborn is more frequent than previously recognized and may be the reason for neonatal depression. Signs of hypovolemia are pallor persisting after oxygenation, weak pulses with good heart rate, poor response to resuscitative efforts, or decreased blood pressure. The most common volume expanders are whole blood (usually not readily available), 5% albumin/saline, plasmanate, normal saline, or Ringer's lactate. Volume expanders are usually given in amounts of 10 ml/kg over 5 to 10 minutes and may be repeated if signs of hypovolemia persist.

10. *Postresuscitation.* After resuscitation, careful observation of the infant is advised and if the cause of depression is not apparent, further investigation should be conducted. The infant remaining in distress should be monitored and intensive care provided.

Hemolytic Disease (Erythroblastosis)

About 1% of all newborns have hemolytic disease. Although a host of factors in the blood are immunologically and genetically important, there are at least nine red cell factors representing significant genetically independent antigen systems. These "families" include ABO, Rh, MNS, Kell, Duffy, Kidd, P, Lewis, and Lutheran. There is a growing list of others, mostly rare, which are unclassified. Practically all blood factors are inherited as mendelian dominants.

With the discovery of three specific anti-Rh sera, a constellation of eight Rh types, which fall into two groups of four each, was distinguished; the distinction is related to the presence or absence of the antigen D (Rh$_o$).

About 85% of the population react positively with anti D (Rh$_o$) serum; roughly 15% have a negative reaction. For each of the Rh antigens there is an allelomorphic Hr antigen (Fisher-Race designation). Rh antigens dominate over other blood group antigens in the causation of erythroblastosis fetalis. They are inherited independently of all other blood group antigens.

Approximately 13% of all marriages in this country take place between an Rh-negative woman and an Rh-positive man. Isoimmunization occurs in about 7% of all Rh-negative gravidas, the great majority becoming sensitized by the fourth pregnancy. A homozygous Rh-positive male will give rise to all Rh-positive fetuses; there is a 50% chance of Rh-negativity in the offspring of heterozygous Rh-positive males (the former exceed the latter by about three to one). The likelihood of sensitization depends also upon the quantity of fetal red cells reaching the mother's circulation, the relative antigenicity of the Rh factor, variability of host responsiveness, and other factors. The various Rh factors, in diminishing degree of antigenicity, are D (Rh$_o$); c (rhl); E (rhll); c (hrl); e (hrll); and d (hr$_o$).

Extravasation of fetal cells into the maternal circulation is the antigenic stimulus; thus, isoimmunization may occur even in the first pregnancy (approximately 1.8% risk). The volume of fetal red cells transferred into the mother increases as pregnancy progresses and is much greater with a pathologic pregnancy (placental abruption, previa, toxemia, etc.); during labor, especially with obstetric intervention; and at the time of actual delivery, particularly if there has been a cesarean section or manual removal of the placenta. Sensitization may follow spontaneous or operative termination of early pregnancy. Survival time of fetal red cells in the circulation of adults has been found to be an estimated 80 days. A fetomaternal transfusion of more than 50 mm^3 has been found in at least one fifth of women at delivery. Apparently as little as 0.1 ml Rh-positive blood can produce sensitization.

The clinical degree of anemia, hyperbilirubinemia, and physical manifestations at birth is variable, and the prognosis varies accordingly. In the mildest form, the fetus is only anemic without other stigmata and the outlook is excellent. A more serious stage is designated *icterus gravis* in which there is jaundice, which deepens progressively. Hepatosplenomegaly is present. Many will survive with optimal exchange transfusion. The most serious stage is **hydrops fetalis,** which rarely responds even

to the most vigorous therapeutic regimen. In the more severe cases the placenta is also markedly edematous and boggy and exhibits large, grayish, friable cotyledons.

One of the postnatal phenomena of hemolytic disease is **kernicterus,** characterized by yellowish pigmentation of the basal nuclei, as well as other portions of the infant's brain. Approximately 6% of those who survive the first week of life develop signs of CNS damage, particularly premature infants and those in whom high levels of hyperbilirubinemia were evident over a protracted period. This risk can be minimized with prompt exchange transfusion repeated as often as necessary to keep the plasma bilirubin considerably below 20 mg/100 ml. Likewise, improved, more refined management has succeeded in reducing the overall perinatal mortality rate to 15% to 20% (even lower in intensive care nurseries).

Usually an indirect Coombs test is used to determine if a gravida is sensitized. Once it is sensitized, assessment of fetal involvement by amniocentesis is necessary. The amount of pigment in the amniotic fluid–spectral absorption curve, in which the optical density is plotted on semilog paper and the 450-nm peak is measured on a line drawn from the peak to an intersection with a tangent connecting the beginning and ending curves of the rise (Liley technique). The degrees of fetal involvement (mild, moderate, or severe) are represented by zones on the graph depicting the height of the peak of pigment in the amniotic fluid at different stages of fetal maturity.

By first documenting sensitization, noting the trend of the titers, and then performing serial examinations of the amniotic fluid, beginning as early as the 20th gestational week in patients with the poorest history and early prior fetal deaths, reasonably accurate estimates of the fetal condition can be obtained. Thus, management is based on objective tests as well as clinical notations regarding uterine growth and tone, presence or absence of hydramnios and evidence of maternal edema (mirror syndrome). Pelvic sonography will help in estimating fetal size, skeletal normality, and evidence of hydrops or hydramnios. Overall assessment, must take into account probable zygosity of the father, past obstetric history, antibody titer, spectrophotometric, and chemical analysis of the amniotic fluid for pigment, estimations of fetal maturity, and, of course, maternal complications affecting either fetal welfare or the timing of delivery.

When the history and clinical and laboratory findings indicate severe fetal involvement (in the absence of hydrops or significant hydramnios) by the 26th to 32nd week of gestation, thereby forecasting certain death of the fetus prior to the 33rd to 34th week, an intrauterine fetal transfusion should be performed and repeated at biweekly intervals until there is sufficient fetal maturity to yield a reasonable chance of survival, usually about the 36th week. Whereas this was performed in the past by intraperitoneal blood, it is currently often performed by ultrasonically guided direct fetal vascular transfusion. Amniotic fluid analyses are also important, when indicative of mild or no fetal involvement, in sparing the infant unnecessary premature delivery. Mildly affected fetuses occurring in sensitized mothers whose husbands are homozygous, even without a history of prior fetal erythroblastosis or perinatal loss, should be delivered a few weeks before term, usually in the 38th week. The choice of method of delivery in all cases, induction of labor or cesarean section, will depend upon the obstetric situation. However, it should be understood that these fetuses should not be subjected to any significant hypoxia or trauma since such insults increase their vulnerability to the deposition of bilirubin in the brain.

A small percentage of women who do not lack an Rh or an Hr antigen possessed by their husbands and show no evidence of immunization to these antigens have been reported as giving birth to infants suffering from hemolytic disease. Certain of these infants suffer from an ABO incompatibility, a situation in which the mother's blood contains anti-A or anti-B agglutinins incompatible with the fetal cells. Rh incompatibility and AB heterospecificity account for approximately 98% of all cases of hemolytic disease. The principles of management are identical in the two conditions, particularly with reference to the behavior of hemoglobin and bilirubin. For simple transfusion or exchange transfusion, group O Rh-negative blood is used.

The patient with multiple losses who has 80% or more chance of fetal death in any subsequent pregnancy, or one who has been subjected to intrauterine fetal transfusion, may desire tubal sterilization. A few may wish a pregnancy by an Rh-negative male donor.

One of the great advances in obstetrics, certainly in the management of Rh problems, has been the demonstration that high-potency, anti-D gamma globulin fraction administered to Rh-negative mothers antenatally at approximately 28 weeks' gestation and shortly after delivery (within 72 hours) has been successful in preventing the development of sensitizing antibodies. An effective commercial preparation is available for such purposes, to be administered to Rh-negative unsensitized mothers following the birth of each Rh-positive infant. A standard dose of 300 μg of Rh$_o$ (D) immune globulin has been prepared for routine use; this counteracts up to 15 ml of packed fetal Rh$_o$ (D) erythrocytes. If clinical circumstances make it likely that the fetomaternal hemorrhage exceeds that volume, or the concentration of fetal erythrocytes in maternal blood are excessive as demonstrated by the Kleihauer-Betke acid elution test, additional immune globulin may be required. The tragic prenatal losses, the tedious procedures of amniocenteses, and intrauterine fetal transfusion are very definitely being relegated to the past. The incidence of sensitization, however, has leveled off at about 1.0%. Thus, there will remain some mothers who require studies and possibly fetal transfusion.

Hyperbilirubinemia from Other Causes. It is important to recognize that hyperbilirubinemia of the newborn may arise from causes other than blood incompatibilities. All drugs administered to the mother should be evaluated for placental transmission, method of conjugation for excretion, hemolytic effect, ability to bind proteins, and effect on hepatocellular function. Ideally, the treatment for hyperbilirubinemia, caused by excessive dosage of vitamin K, sulfonamides, other drugs, hypoxia, disordered carbohydrate metabolism, or acidosis, is basically one of prevention.

Prematurity

From 7% to 10% of babies are born a month or more prior to the expected date of confinement. Among the lower socioeconomic groups, the incidence may reach 14% or more. Such infants usually weigh between 500 g and 2,500 g and are called premature. Their chance of survival is much less than that of mature infants and, as a consequence, premature infants account for more than half of all deaths in the first 30 days of life (neonatal period). Perinatal mortality rates vary between 15% and 20% overall, but the smaller the infant the poorer the prognosis. The clinical cause of premature birth is apparent in slightly less than 40% of cases. The conditions most frequently associated with the onset of premature labor are chronic hypertension, abruptio placentae, placenta previa, infection (usually urinary or genital), heart disease, toxemia, multiple gestation, and congenital abnormalities of the fetus and, formerly, syphilis. Premature rupture of the membranes is the triggering factor provoking premature labor or active intervention in 20% to 30% of the cases. Other known factors include incompatible blood groups, uterine pathology and anatomic defects, nutritional deficiency, endocrine dysfunction, and placental steroid defects. Prematurity is often repeated in a subsequent pregnancy.

The best clinical weapon against the ill effects of premature birth is prevention. Often, the underlying etiology is obscure and cannot be addressed. Many patients will be in advanced labor by the time they are first seen. Efforts to halt established labor are usually unsuccessful if the cervix is fully effaced and dilated more than 4 cm. The membranes are already ruptured in a substantial minority of cases and in others the maternal complication is an overriding clinical issue. In these circumstances, an arrest of labor might be highly undesirable.

Bed rest itself may be a preventive because myometrial irritability may be reduced. In circumstances involving uterine overdistention (e.g., multiple gestation, polyhydramnios, uterine tumor), bed rest may be an effective adjunct in delaying the onset of labor.

Synthetic β-adrenergic compounds (terbutaline) and sympathomimetic amines capable of stimulating uterine β-adrenergic receptors (ritodrine hydrochloride) are capable of inhibiting myometrial activity in 80% to 90% of patients. However, they have the disadvantage of producing both maternal and fetal tachycardia and hypotension in the mother. Indeed, therapy with the β-mimetics should not be undertaken without a thorough understanding of their pharmacologic potentials, a careful assessment of the patient's ability to tolerate their actions, and a hospital setting (facilities and personnel) able to adequately deal with their complications.

Recently, the inhibitory effects on uterine muscle contractility of magnesium sulfate have been recognized and utilized therapeutically in normotensive women experiencing threatening premature labor. The regimen is identical to that utilized in treating women with preeclampsia, and the same safeguards are required in terms of magnesium level control, urinary output, and periodic clinical assessments. Excessive serum levels can cause respiratory depression in the newborn, since magnesium traverses the placenta. Another popular development has been the expanding use of cervical cerclage as a means of enhancing competency of the cervix. The traditional indication was to constrict the dilating and effacing cervix at the earliest possible moment (before 3 cm dilation or 50% effacement) or as a preventive during the second trimester to correct a problem of repeated, painless, bloodless, late abor-

tions associated with bulging or prolapsing membranes. A synthetic tape (Shiredkar-Barter operation) or braided silk sutures (McDonald-Hofmeister procedure) may be used for this purpose. Lately indications have expanded (e.g., uterine anomaly).

Once premature labor is established, clinical management takes into account the particular vulnerabilities of the immature infant. Care must be exerted to avoid the all too synergistic insults of narcosis, hypoxia, and trauma. A generous episiotomy cut under a local or regional block might spare the fetal head and facilitate an easy spontaneous delivery. If there is a faulty labor, malpresentation, or reasons to believe that more operative manipulations than desired would be necessary in achieving a vaginal delivery, abdominal intervention should be considered. A more liberal use of cesarean section even in the delivery of very small infants has been made possible by the great advances achieved in recent years in increasing the chances of neonatal survival. In today's intensive care nurseries, live-born infants with birth weights of only 750 g to 1,000 g (25th–27th gestational week) have better than 50% chance of surviving.

In considering low-birth-weight infants, it is very important to distinguish between those whose weight is commensurate with the gestational age and those whose birth weight is low for the stage of gestation. The latter are referred to as *small-for-gestational-age* infants. By definition, their birth weight is below the 10th percentile for gestational age and they are said to have an *in utero* growth retardation. These make up about one third of all low-birth-weight infants. They may be genetically small or defective from a variety of insults (e.g., viral infections of the TORCH types) or they may have suffered *in utero* malnutrition. Uteroplacental vascular damage, preeclampsia, chronic infections (syphilis, rubella, etc.), chronic hypoxia (hemoglobinopathies), heavy smoking, chronic alcoholism, drug addiction, severe diabetes, and other maternal illnesses may underlie the fetal inanition and jeopardy. In some instances, there is a problem of postdatism beyond 42 gestational weeks. Serial ultrasonic studies are useful in detecting a trend of intrauterine growth retardation. Additionally, biophysical evaluation (e.g., NST, stress test, or biophysical profile) may detect those in jeopardy. Undergrown infants at birth are frequently hypoxic, hypoglycemic (two thirds), and polycythemic. Glucose infusion is ordinarily required.

Among immature (premature) infants, a respiratory distress syndrome (hyaline membrane disease) constitutes one of the gravest risks. This problem affects about 20% of prematurely born infants but only 1% to 2% of all live births. Premature infants do not produce adequate quantities of surfactant, which is a group of phospholipids elaborated by type II alveolar cells. Surfactant, is produced in large quantities after the 34th or 35th week of gestation. After birth these phospholipids are surface active and they reduce the alveolar wall surface tension, increase compliance, and promote partial alveolar distention with residual air, even at the end of expiration. Without these properties, alveoli tend to collapse (atelectasis) and eosinophilic hyalinelike membranes develop on the surface of the alveoli and in the terminal bronchioles, presumably due to capillary plasma–fibrin transudation. The submembranous epithelium becomes necrotic, vasoconstriction occurs, aeration is diminished and hypoxia (acidosis), and systemic hypotension develop. This chain of events can lead to death in 4 to 72 hours. Widespread availability of surfactant replacement therapy has substantially decreased mortality from hyaline membrane disease.

When meconium is present in the amniotic fluid, precautions are taken to decrease the incidence of the meconium aspiration syndrome. Although meconium aspiration may occur prior to delivery, the obstetrician generally suctions the baby's nose, mouth, and stomach immediately after delivery of the head to minimize further aspiration. Personnel capable of intubating and suctioning the trachea immediately after delivery should be present in the delivery room. The decision to intubate and suction is based on whether there is meconium below the level of the vocal cords. In this condition, there is mechanical obstruction, chemical irritation and inflammation, resulting in edema, hypoxia, atelectasis, and possibly pneumothorax.

Retinopathy of prematurity (ROP), originally termed retrolental fibroplasia, is a vasoproliferative disorder primarily affecting preterm infants of less than 1,500 g. Its prevalence is inversely proportional to birth weight, occurring in as many as 40% to 70% of survivors less than 1,000 g. Although there is an association with prolonged elevation of oxygen tension in the blood of preterm infants, that is no longer thought to be the sole cause. There are documented cases of ROP in infants experiencing only room air as well as a variance in incidence by location not only by area of the country, but even by hospitals in the same area.

The incidence of cerebral palsy and mental retardation is also increased among premature infants. The mortality rate is higher during the first 2 years of life, and even after that time there is a higher incidence of disorders considered to be associated with birth injury.

A special comment is required concerning the documented ill effects of alcohol ingestion during pregnancy. The chronic alcoholic patient will have malnutrition in varying degrees, particularly when ingestion of alcohol negates the desire for food and an adequate diet is ignored. Alcohol traverses the placenta readily, and newborns may suffer from withdrawal symptoms. In about one quarter of the cases, there will be extremely serious effects upon fetal growth and development *in utero,* depending upon the amount of daily consumption. There are no known levels of maternal alcohol levels below which embryotoxic and teratogenic effects are nonexistent. As little as 1 ounce of alcohol per week has been incriminated as a potential cause of abortion or as at least elevating the risks of early fetal loss. Major defects have been attributed to the daily intake of six bottles of beer. In the offspring of mothers comsuming alcohol, especially in the first trimester, significant fetal damage occurs in a dose-related fashion, for example 10% with two to four daily drinks; 20% with four to six drinks; and 30% to 40% over six drinks. A so-called fetal alcohol syndrome has been described, which is made up of several major defects, including growth retardation, microcephaly, and a variety of anomalies involving the face, palate, auricles, eyes, heart, genitourinary tract, skin joints, and external genitalia. The infants may fail to catch up following their *in utero* growth defect or fail to thrive neonatally. There may be persistent hyperactive behavior, poor coordination, and inadequate fine motor function independent of "withdrawal" symptoms.

A growing problem is the high incidence of drug abuse, particularly abuse of cocaine. Cocaine is relatively cheap and readily available. Studies have shown that as high as 10% to 15% of pregnant women are using this drug during pregnancy, regardless of race or socioeconomic status. Perinates of these pregnancies complicated by maternal cocaine use have an increased incidence of prematurity, intrauterine growth retardation, cerebral infarcts, necrotizing enterocolitis, congenital infections (especially sexually transmitted diseases), and sudden infant death syndrome. The neonates of such pregnancies may experience withdrawal symptoms and have long-term neurologic abnormalities.

Another potentially tragic condition affecting newborns is acquired immunodeficiency syndrome (AIDS), which can affect women and children (formerly thought to be limited to homosexual men). The disease may be acquired *in utero* or neonatally, occurring in the offspring of HIV-infected mothers. It has been reported in an infant transfused *in utero* for Rh incompatability. The transmitting virus has an epidemiology similar to hepatitis B infections. Asymptomatic carriers may transmit the disease through heterosexual contact. Additionally, HIV may be transmitted by breast feeding. Reduced immunologic defenses, drug abuse, and malnutrition increase susceptibility and expression of the disease. Affected children are at high risk of dying of opportunistic infections (*e.g., Candida, Salmonella*). These infants may show imbalances of mature T cells rather than the failed T-cell differentiation of a genetic cell-mediated immunity. No reliable specific therapy has emerged at this writing.

The concept of dysmaturity focuses on infants who are postmature, associated with an undergrown *in utero* compromised status. Dysmaturity can also characterize large-for-gestational-age infants. There may be excessive weight because of severe water retention or hydrops (*e.g.,* syphilis, erythroblastosis fetalis, maternal diabetes, or transposition of the aorta). A large-for-gestational-age infant can be compromised by complications usually associated with immatures (*e.g.,* increased prevalence of hyaline membrane disease among large infants born of diabetic mothers). Obviously, there are additional perinatal hazards of shoulder dystocia, birth trauma, operative obstetrics, hypoxia, and other problems.

The reader is referred to the section on pediatrics (neonatology) for more details about management of the newborn. The importance of early diagnosis in the newborn should be stressed (*e.g.,* structural status of the external genitals, anomalous development, patent orifices, possibility of a genetic fault, congenital adrenogenital syndrome, and neonatal thyroid dysfunction).

GYNECOLOGY

DISORDERS OF THE LOWER GENERATIVE TRACT

Leukorrhea

The proper environment for the vagina is maintained under the influence of estrogens and enough acidity to foster the growth of a normal bacterial flora. An acid pH of 3.5 to 4.0 is achieved in the presence of adequate lactobacilli (Döderlein's bacilli) and acidogenic corynebacteria. Endogenous estrogen causes proliferation of the stratified squamous epithelium of the vagina, which brings about a resistance to infection and trauma after puberty and during the premenopausal years. Normally, under estrogen stimulation, vaginal fluid contains a cellular debris resulting from a continuous process of desquamation. There may be an excess of mucus discharge in response to sexual excitement, increased estrogen stimulation, use of oral contraceptives, pregnancy, and pelvic congestion. There should be no real problem of soiling of underclothes or evidence of vulvovaginal irritation or offensive odor.

Menstrual fluid reduces the acidity of the vagina. Estrogen depletion, caused by castration or aging, produces mucosal atrophy, reduction in cellular glycogen content, and decreased acidity of the vaginal fluid.

The literal meaning of the term *leukorrhea* is a white discharge. In practical usage it is applied to a wide range of vulvovaginal exudates that vary in color, consistency, odor, and cause. The warm, moist condition of the vulva makes it vulnerable to irritation and infection when it is exposed to urinary and fecal soiling. Allergies, coitus, feminine hygiene practices, excessive douching, tight-fitting heat- and moisture-retaining pantyhose, abrasions (masturbation and other practices), and potential insults may predispose to symptomatic leukorrhea by changing the vaginal flora. The overall physical and emotional health, nutritional and metabolic state, and general level of activity will affect the vagina. There may be specific causes of leukorrhea that arise in the cervix, endometrium, and fallopian tubes, and these discharges may adversely affect the vaginal flora and decrease the pH. Mucopurulent fluids, arising from infected endocervical mucosa, are alkaline and will change the bacterial flora by altering the vaginal pH.

Vaginal infection is the most common cause of leukorrhea and represents the most common gynecologic complaint. Vulvar irritation resulting from contact with the vaginal discharge may give rise to the presenting complaint. There may be some pruritus, dyspareunia, and a sense of severe burning discomfort when the irritated areas on the vulva and perineum are exposed to urine. There may be mixed bacterial flora without predominant organisms, although one or more common pyogenic pathogens may be present in vaginal cultures. Nonspecific vulvovaginitis may be secondary to poor perineal hygiene, foreign bodies, mucosal atrophy, trauma, skin infections, or intestinal parasites or may arise in association with a systemic illness. *Escherichia coli, Proteus* sp., *Enterobacter aerogenes, Klebsiella pneumoniae,* and other organisms common to the intestinal tract may be found in vaginal cultures. Occasionally, pinworms migrate into the vagina from the anus and deposit ova, which may lead to vulvovaginitis because of contamination with *Escherichia coli* and other intestinal bacteria. Sexual molestation involving the female child almost always causes injury to the immature vagina, and such trauma may give rise to hematomas and infection. The thin vaginal mucosa prior to puberty is also susceptible to invasion by the gonococcus.

Many of the specific types of vulvovaginitis causing leukorrhea represent a wide variety of sexually transmitted infectious diseases. The offending organisms may be classified as bacteria, spirochetes, chlamydia, fungi, metazoans, mycoplasma, protozoans, and viruses. The specific diagnosis is required if the appropriate therapy is to be selected. The most common symptom of vulvar disease is pruritus. Some of the more specific common entities associated with leukorrhea are listed below.

TRICHOMONIASIS

Trichomonas vaginalis vaginitis is a sexually transmitted disease caused by a unicellular anaerobic protozoan flagellate that infests not only the vagina but also the lower urinary tract of both men and women. These organisms may occasionally be found in an asymptomatic female with normal vaginal acidity and bacterial flora. However, vulvovaginitis and urinary symptoms represent the typical clinical picture, and the *p*H of the vagina usually exceeds 5.0. The characteristic leukorrhea is frothy, greenish, profuse, and malodorous. However, the classic discharge may not be present in two thirds of the patients. The mucous membranes show generalized erythema and scattered small petechial hemorrhages ("strawberry cervix"). There may be vulvar edema and excoriations. The discharge may be blood-tinged, and the patient may complain of postcoital (cervical) bleeding. The diagnosis is made by demonstrating the motile flagellates in a saline wet-mount preparation. These protozoa are smaller than a mature epithelial cell but usually larger than polymorphonuclear leukocytes. In symptomatic women, it is possible to identify motile trichomonads in about 80% of cases. Nonmotile trichomonads may be seen in a Pap smear. Although several antitrichomonal suppositories are available, the preferred method is

the simultaneous treatment of both partners with metronidazole (Flagyl), in one 2 g dose (probably 95% cure rate). In resistant cases, and in the event of reinfections, oral therapy may be repeated at 250 mg metronidazole three to four times daily for 7 days. Drug resistance is rare, and reinfections are controllable using the same treatment plan. Since trichomonas infections and candidiasis often coexist, persistent symptoms may be caused by unrecognized monilial vaginitis. The couple should be warned about the possibility of intolerance to alcohol as an important side effect of metronidazole. This agent should be withheld during the first 20 weeks of pregnancy and during lactation. Indeed, the 2 g dose probably should not be used during pregnancy because of the higher blood levels achieved in the fetus.

CANDIDIASIS

Candida albicans vaginitis is a fungus infection arising from candidal organisms that may be normal inhabitants of both the vagina and the large bowel. There may be a disturbance of normal vaginal physiology that allows these ubiquitous organisms to overwhelm the normal bacterial flora. The *p*H may not be elevated. Large numbers of *Candida* may be introduced during coitus, or their growth may be promoted by metabolic disease (*e.g.,* diabetes mellitus), pregnancy or certain drugs (*e.g.,* antibiotics, corticosteroids, and oral contraceptives). The typical clinical picture is vulvar erythema, edema, maceration, and excoriation usually associated with the intense pruritus, as evidenced by scratch marks on the skin. The characteristic discharge is a thick, tenacious, often cheesy-white (curdy) "thrush patch" or plaque overlying a red mucosal base that may bleed when scraped. Burning may be intense in the acute stage, particularly following urination. Normally, there is no odor unless a secondary infection develops. The diagnosis is based upon the demonstration of filamentous forms (hyphae and pseudohyphae) of the *Candida albicans* organism in a wet slide preparation utilizing 10% to 20% potassium hydroxide. Blastospore forms can be identified on Gram stain. Sabouraud's or Nickerson's medium can be used to grow the organism. The sexual partner should always be examined, particularly in refractory or recurrent cases, and there should be no coitus without the protection of a condom. There are several effective anti-*Candida* preparations, including nystatin tablets (100,000 units), one or two vaginal inserts twice daily for 14 days; miconazole nitrate (Monistat), 2%

cream, one applicator full daily for 1 week; and a 0.25% to 1% aqueous solution of gentian violet. Repeated gentian violet applications risk chemical vulvitis. Imidazole agents miconazole, and clotrimazole are preferred therapies for recurrent cases. Nystatin–corticosteroid (Mycolog) cream can be used to eliminate vulvar pruritus and to treat the male partner.

GARDNERELLA VAGINALIS

This type of infection, formally referred to as *Haemophilis vaginalis* and, together with anaerobic bacteria, sometimes called "nonspecific vaginosis," has certain distinctive features. The vaginal mucosa appears normal, but adherent to it is a thin, homogenous, foul-smelling, yellow gray discharge. The typical odor is fishy and is accentuated by 10% potassium hydroxide. The vaginal *p*H is greater than 4.5. The fishy foul odor is caused by the anaerobes, which produce amines. The offending organism is a small gram-negative bacillus, which attaches itself to vaginal epithelial cells. In saline wet mount, "clue" cells are seen whereby epithelial cells show myriads of adherent bacteria around their borders, which become obscured and stippled. As many as 50% of the cells may show these distinctive markings. Lactobacilli and polymorphonuclear leukocytes are absent. There remains some confusion about this condition, since as many as 40% of asymptomatic women may be found to harbor these organisms. Whether or not these infections are sexually transmitted remains unsettled. Treatment consists of metronidazole, 250 mg twice daily for 7 days.

ATROPHIC VULVOVAGINITIS

In the absence of the stimulation of normal endogenous estrogen, the vaginal epithelium is quite thin and deficient in glycogen, and the bacterial flora becomes mixed in association with an abnormally high *p*H as the normal acidogenic flora is replaced. Multiplication of potentially pathogenic organisms, including many types of streptococci, coliform bacteria and others, is encouraged. There may be pruritus, external burning discomfort, dyspareunia, and often an associated urgency–frequency syndrome caused by atrophic urethritis. The discharge is highly variable in amount, color, and consistency, but it may be thick and purulent or serosanguineous. The *p*H of the vaginal fluid is usually in the range of 5.5 to 7.0. Vaginal cytology on wet-mount preparations on stained smears shows a predominance of intermediate or parabasal cells. The treatment consists of nightly applications of topical estrogenic creams for about 10 days and, for maintenance of the vaginal mucosa, periodic instillations twice weekly thereafter. A simple atrophic condition of the vulva must not be mistaken for a dystrophic lesion or perhaps an even more serious underlying condition, such as a malignancy, that has given rise to a bloody vaginal discharge. Estrogen orally or by local application is the therapy of choice for the atrophic vulvitis. Testosterone is a trophic agent for vulvar epithelium and may be effective. Two percent testosterone propionate in petrolatum applied three times daily is a common therapy.

VIRAL VULVOVAGINITIS

Human Papillomavirus (HPV). HPV has increased at an alarming rate for the past two decades and is now the second most common sexually transmitted disease (after chlamydia) as well as the most common viral sexually transmitted disease in the United States. In the overall incidence of sexually transmitted diseases, genital herpes is the third most common and gonorrhea the fourth. Well over a million new HPV infections are detected annually, and HPV occurs in 5% to 10% of young women and 1% to 2% of all women; however, a large proportion of HPV infections are asymptomatic, thus the true incidence of HPV is likely underestimated.

HPV is a small (7,800 base pairs) DNA, obligatory, intranuclear virus with a protein coat but no envelope. HPV has an infectivity rate (the transmission rate from a single exposure) of about 65%, but the correlation is often missed because it has such a long incubation period (6 weeks to 6 or 8 months). The usual mode of spread is by direct contact with viral entry through the skin, the mucosa, or a small abrasion. HPV may also be transmitted on inadequately sterilized specula or biopsy instruments. HPV infections can be either latent or productive. If HPV resides as a tightly coiled, circular DNA in an extrachromosomal nuclear location (episomal form) and only replicates once each cell cycle, it is classed as latent and is not histologically recognizable but may be detected by DNA probes. If large numbers of viral copies are produced as the cell terminally differentiates, it is productive (replicative). In symptomatic women, the diagnosis of HPV infection is usually by observation of typical clinical lesions on the external genitalia or mucosal surfaces of the internal genitalia. The typical finding of HPV infection on Pap smear or biopsy is a particular form of perinuclear halo called *koilocytosis.* Other cellular changes included an enhanced mitotic rate and nuclear polyploidy. More sophisticated laboratory methods of detection include probes for specific types of HPV DNA.

There are now more than 70 HPV types known, and the viral type determines clinical presentation, pathologic appearance, natural progression, and degree of malignant potential. The types most consistently associated with genital infections are 6, 11, 16, 18, 31, and 35. Generally type 6 or 11 cause condylomata acuminata (genital warts) and over 95% of external lesions are of low-malignancy potential. Internal lesions caused by types 6 and 11 usually demonstrate only mild dysplasia, while lesions caused by types 16, 18, 31, 33, 35, 38, 45, 51, 52, and 56 seldom cause external genital lesions but are associated with a high malignant potential when infecting mucosal surfaces (as well as *in vitro*). Overall, about 10% of HPV lesions progress to severe dysplasia and/or carcinoma of the cervix and over 95% of cervical cancers contain HPV DNA. Thus, while complex, the link between this infection and cervical dysplasia appears nearly incontrovertible.

Currently, therapeutic modalities for HPV infections includes podophyllin, trichloroacetic acid (TCA), bichloroacetic acid (BCA), cryotherapy, electrocautery, laser therapy, loop electrosurgical excision procedure (LEEP), and Podofilox (0.5%). Podophyllin, TCA, and BCA all require physician application, are most irritating, if not painful, and are rarely successful on a single application. Cryotherapy and electrocautery may be very useful in certain patients (*e.g.,* during pregnancy) but also usually require multiple treatments. Laser therapy, like surgical excision, is less commonly used today, while LEEP or Podofilox self-application by the patient are increasingly preferred.

Herpes Simplex Virus (HSV). Vulvar infections caused by HSV are sexually transmitted and represent the most common viral disease of the lower genital tract. The typical clinical picture is one of vulvar pain in association with vesiculation and skin maceration. The primary disability may be quite severe for 7 to 21 days before remission occurs; recurrences are common, although the symptoms may be less severe. There may be vaginal and cervical involvements without symptoms. When the infection is extensive, there may be excoriations and secondary bacterial infection. Lesions may also be seen on buttocks, thigh, and perianal areas. Fever may develop, and there may be enlarged inguinal lymph nodes. Burning may be present on voiding, or there may be urinary retention. If acute herpes genitalis occurs during late pregnancy, the potential for transmission of the virus to the infant during delivery is sufficiently serious to justify abdominal intervention, provided the membranes are intact or ruptured for less than 4 hours.

There is no specific clinical picture that can be considered diagnostic in all cases because lesions may be nonvesicular. Laboratory methods include the demonstration of giant cells or intranuclear inclusions in Pap and Tzanck smears, or HSV antigens in specimens by immunologic techniques. Virus isolation in tissue culture is the most sensitive diagnostic method, and the virus is identified by staining positive cultures using a direct fluorescent antibody technique. A serodiagnostic screening is useful only in detecting patients who have had primary infections in the past, but significant antibody cross reactivity exists between type 1 and type 2 Herpesvirus, and it may be impossible to differentiate between the two types. About 15% of these genital infections are caused by type 1 Herpesvirus hominis. Oral acyclovir, 200 mg every 4 hours for 5 days, has been found to shorten the duration of virus shedding, relieve symptoms, and reduce healing time. Laser vaporization of primary lesions is not helpful. Intravenous therapy with acyclovir may be used for extraordinary recurrent cases and for use in infants and immunosuppressed patients.

It is possible to confuse this type of vulvovaginitis with another self-limiting disease characterized by multiple gas-filled cystic structures involving the vagina and cervix. Vaginitis emphysematosa, which is the official designation, may be a manifestation of trichomoniasis; however, the lesions are often unattended by leukorrhea or irritation, and no treatment is usually required.

CHLAMYDIA TRACHOMATIS

Chlamydiae are obligate intracellular microorganisms that grow only within the host cell's cytoplasm, attach themselves to columnar (or transitional) epithelial cells, and usually invade tissues only superficially (except for L_1, L_2, and L_3 lymphogranuloma serotypes). Urogenital infections include nongonococcal urethritis and epididymitis in men and endocervical infections and pelvic inflammatory disease in women giving rise to Fitz-Hugh–Curtis syndrome (perihepatitis), infertility, pregnancy loss, and postpartal endometritis. Chlamydiae and genital mycoplasmas may coexist along with *N. gonorrhoeae.* Chlamydial infections usually have a longer incubation period. Cervical epithelial changes induced by oral contraceptives may favor the growth of chlamydiae. Mucopuralent cervical discharge may be the only symptom, and salpingitis may be present without adverse tenderness or lower abdominal pain. Speculation is that long-term infections may proceed silently and give rise to cervical dysplasia and tubal infertility. Serologic tests may demonstrate antibodies, and if there is a high level of specific IgM antibodies, a recent infection can be suspected. The most sensitive diagnostic method is to culture the organism on irradiated or idoxuridine-treated McCoy or HeLa cells. Cultures are best taken from the endocervical or endosalpingeal secretions. As less expensive and more easily applied fluorescent diagnostic screening has expanded, *Chlamydia* is now recognized by some experts as a common cause of acute pelvic inflammatory disease, alone and in mixed infections. Tetracycline (currently Declomycin) is the antibiotic of choice, although erythromycin or trimethoprim/sulfa may be effective. The male partner should be evaluated for urethritis and epididymitis.

Toxic Shock Syndrome

A potentially fatal illness related to menstruation and use of vaginal tampons, toxic shock syndrome has been attributed primarily to the toxins associated with an overgrowth of *Staphylococcus aureus*. The classic syndrome is characterized by the sudden onset of high fever, vomiting, watery diarrhea, sunburnlike rash, hyperemic mucous membranes, hypotension, lethargy, and confusion, usually occurring during menses. A death rate of 5% to 10% is attributed to this syndrome, and successful treatment will depend upon prompt recognition, volume repletion, administration of antistaphylococcal antibiotics (cephalosporins or penicillinase-resistant penicillins), and selected use of corticosteroids. In many, the syndrome will recur in a subsequent menstruation. All sizes and types of tampons and various vaginal foreign bodies have been implicated, and the syndrome has been observed in children, men, and nonmenstruating women. However, as a precaution, tampons should be changed frequently and not used overnight.

Benign Ulcerative Lesions of the Vulva

Granulomatous lesions of the vulva are often sexually transmitted and are infectious, although they may be cancerous either as a primary lesion or coexisting with the infectious underlying process. Granulation tissue is simply a reaction to the infection, and the superimposition of nonspecific inflammation is almost inevitable. A variety of investigative tests and procedures are required to establish the proper diagnosis and to initiate the proper therapeutic plan. The various diseases of clinical significance are outlined are below.

CHANCROID

This lesion is an irregularly shaped shallow vulvar ulceration with an incubation period of only about 3 or 5 days. An exudate aspirated from the buboes or pus obtained from the ulcer usually demonstrates *Haemophilus ducreyi*. Autoinoculation is common, and the vesiculopustular ulceration is usually very painful. When there are lesions about the external urethral meatus, the resultant scarring may lead to stenosis. The ulcers may multiply or be confluent and spread toward the thighs; usually there will be a thick foul discharge, draining buboes, and tender inguinal nodes. The *H. ducreyi* can usually be cultured on blood agar, and Gram stains of the material from open lesions or buboes with show gram-negative rods in strands. One can culture a biopsy specimen for the most accurate results. One or two weeks after an infection, Ducrey's intradermal skin test will become positive and will remain so for years. On culture there may be a mixed complex vaginal flora. These lesions usually heal quickly following ceftriaxone 250 mg IM, erythromycin 500 mg orally four times a day, or trimethoprim/sulfa therapy in usual doses for 7 to 10 days. Streptomycin may also be effective singly or combined with tetracyclines, but these drugs may mask the early signs of syphilis.

GRANULOMA INGUINALE

This ulcerative granulomatous disease involving the vulva, perineum, and inguinal regions is sexually transmitted. The causative organism is *Calymmatobacterium granulomatis*, and the incubation period is 8 to 12 weeks. Bacteria encapsulated in mononuclear leukocytes are known as Donovan bodies. Initially, there is a papule that ulcerates, and satellite ulcers may coalesce to produce a large lesion. Inguinal swelling and abscess (bubo) formation are common features, and ulcerative lesions may extend to involve the urethra and anal area. There may be vegetative lesions, ulcers, and introital cicatricial distortions leading to dyspareunia and pain on walking or sitting. The diagnosis is made on the basis of large mononuclear cells containing the Donovan bodies. Smear materials stained with Wright's, Giemsa's, or silver stain will demonstrate the cystic inclusions; in traditional hematoxylin and eosin preparations there will be small round or rod-shaped particles. The treatment of choice is tetracycline administered orally in doses of 500 mg four times daily for 2 to 3 weeks. In about 10% of the cases the disease will be recurrent.

LYMPHOGRANULOMA VENEREUM (LGV)

This infectious disease, caused by a chlamydia, is transmitted by coitus and is characterized by a chronic process often occurring in an anemic person in poor health. The organism is represented by the L_1, L_2, and L_3 serotypes of chlamydiae, and it has a biological aggressiveness capable of producing deep tissue invasion. These LGV serotypes attach to mononuclear cells and are disseminated to regional lymph nodes. The early clinical lesion is a painless erosion that proceeds to ulceration on the fourchette, urethral meatus, or medial surface of the labia. The ulcer itself may be irregular, shallow, poorly defined, and associated with lymphatic spread and finally a destructive phase which may lead to loss of urethra, vaginal narrowing and distortion, anorectal edema, ulceration and stricture, and systemic symptoms. The diagnosis is most reliably established by culturing the organism from tissues obtained at a suitable genital site. Serologic methods (micro IF or complement fixation) may suggest recent infection when there is an antibody change or a high level of specific IgM antibody. Other suggestive features include vulvar elephantiasis (esthiomene), hypoproteinemia, and reversal of the albumen–globulin ratio. The best treatment consists of doxycycline (100 mg twice a day for 21 days), although tetracycline, erythromycin, or sulfisoxazole may be an alternative. Various local and surgical therapies may be required because of abscesses and strictures.

VULVAR LESION OF SYPHILIS

Two thirds of the syphilitic lesions occur on the labia majora or minora, and many are quite small and lie within the labial folds. The infecting organism, known to be *Treponema pallidum,* gives rise to single or multiple primary lesions at the portal of entry about 21 days (range 10–90) after exposure. The characteristic features are a firm, painless ulcer with raised borders, lymphatic spread, inguinal adenitis, and discrete rubbery nodes. Treponemes

will pass through intact mucous membranes or abraded skin.

About 2 weeks to 6 months after disappearance of the primary lesion, a rash develops in the form of maculopapular, follicular, or pustular lesions. Secondary syphilis may produce generalized nontender lymphadenopathy associated with fever, weight loss, and malaise. Highly infectious, hypertrophied, wartlike lesions may appear on the vulva or perineum (condylomata lata). In about one third of these patients there will be superficial, painless mucosal lesions in the vagina or mouth (mucous patches).

There may be latent syphilis, which becomes noncommunicable and in 4 years or later produces destructive (tertiary) lesions in about one third of patients (fatal in one fourth and nonclinical in one fourth). The tertiary lesions are vascular and neurologic. A gravid female with latent syphilis may transmit the disease to her fetus.

Primary lesions may be found in areas of the perineum, nose, breast, and mouth and may be difficult to locate. Serologic tests for syphilis are usually nonreactive when the primary chancre first appears but become positive 1 to 4 weeks later. In primary syphilis, darkfield microscopic findings are positive, while serologic tests are positive in only about one quarter of the cases. VDRL is a nontreponemal, nonspecific reagin antibody. Up to 10% of false-positive serologic tests for syphilis may be caused by collagen diseases and viral, protozoal, or other spirochetal infections. The false-positive VDRL titers are usually 1 : 8 or less. Patients with a false-positive VDRL will have a negative treponemal antibody serology (FTA), since false-positive tests are rare.

The standard treatment for primary and secondary syphilis (or latent disease of less than 1 year's duration) is benzathine penicillin G, 2.4 million units intramuscularly (1.2 million units in each buttock); or aqueous procaine penicillin G, 600,000 units intramuscularly daily for 8 days. Treatment of a patient with a positive spinal fluid examination or latent syphilis of more than 1 year's duration would call for benzathine penicillin G, 2.4 million units intramuscularly once weekly for 3 successive weeks (7.2 million units total). Penicillin-allergic patients can be treated with tetracycline, 500 mg by mouth four times a day for 30 days, but the therapeutic failure rate may be higher with this regimen. If a reaction to therapy develops, usually within 24 hours (fever, tachycardia, myalgia, hypotension), it may be caused by massive spirochete destruction (Jarisch-Herxheimer reaction) and therapy must be stopped in the seriously affected patient. It is of great importance that the treated patient return within 6 months for a repeat VDRL to check adequacy of therapy. To confirm adequate therapy, the repeat VDRL titer should be negative or at least demonstrate a fourfold fall (*e.g.,* from 1 : 32 to 1 : 8). If the VDR titer has not fallen in this manner, the reason for therapeutic failure should be investigated, possibly including lumbar puncture to check for neurosyphilis.

VULVAR TUBERCULOSIS

The vulva may be infected by the excretion of tubercle bacilli from the genital tract, urine, stool, or infected sputum. Contact of the organism with damaged vulvar epithelium leads to ulceration. There may be a foul discharge and contact bleeding. Genitourinary tuberculosis in the sexual partner may rarely infect the female. Characteristic lesions include chronic ulcers with firm margins and irregular bases, granulation tissues at the fourchette, fistulous tract to the rectum, and inguinal adenopathy. Diagnosis is suspected when biopsy and histologic examination show the typical tuberculous granuloma, consisting of epithelioid cells, Langerhans' giant cells, and a collar of lymphocytes and plasma cells. Confirmation is achieved bacteriologically by smears, cultures, or animal inoculation. The standard treatment is multiple-drug therapy consisting of streptomycin and isoniazid according to standard therapeutic protocols.

OTHER LESIONS

Other benign ulcerative lesions of the vulva consist of sclerosing lipogranuloma, hidradenitis suppurativa, diphtheric vulvitis, noma (pudenti) vulvae, pyogenic granuloma, dexamethasone granuloma and, of course, superficial desquamations associated with various dermatoses, including acute monilial infections. In addition, there may be aphthous, small, yellowish, painful ulcers; shallow ulcers associated with the *Bacillus crassus* (Lipschütz ulcer); and Behcet's syndrome, which is a conglomerate of eye and mouth lesions along with painful small ulcers in the labia, vestibule, and vagina. Rarely, multiple draining sinus tracts appear in the labia of women with ulcerative colitis.

Lesions of the Vulva Involving Abnormal Pigmentation

The coloration of the vulva varies among individuals and racial groups; however, in general, the vulvar skin color depends not only on pigment (melanin or blood) but also on vascularity of the dermis and thickness of the overlying epidermis. A dystrophic lesion may take on different appearances in the course of its evolution or maturation. There may be erythema early and a distinct white appearance later on when there is decreased vascularity (sclerosis and atrophy) or hyperkeratosis (vasculature is obscured by the thickened epidermis). White lesions may be associated with loss or absence of melanin, either diffusely (vitiligo) or focally (leukoderma). Inflammation, congestion, vasodilation, and neovascularization may produce red lesions, particularly when there is superficial ulceration and the underlying vascular dermis becomes more apparent. Some specific vulvar lesions are typically velvety red (psoriasis and extramammary Paget's disease). Lesions that result in increased production or concentration of melanin or blood pigments will give rise to dark discolorations (bluish, purplish, brownish), for example, melanosis, melanoma, pigmented nevus.

VULVAR DYSTROPHIES

There is a spectrum of vulvar diseases that are associated with a variety of clinical terms, but these terms are being discarded in favor of a classification based on histologic features. When the vulvar epithelium is exposed to chronic irritations from long-standing infection, the clinical appearance in response to thickening and maceration may be localized or diffuse white raised lesions. These may extend to involve the perineum, perianal skin, and adjacent thighs. These conditions have been referred to as *"lichen simplex chronicus,"* or *neurodermatitis.* This type of dystrophy is designated as "hyperplastic" because the principle histologic features are benign epithelial changes consisting of thickening, acanthosis, hyperkeratosis, and inflammatory infiltration.

In contrast, there may be pronounced atrophy in association with a profound reduction in endogenous estrogen or in conjunction with a systemic skin condition known as *"lichen sclerosus et atrophicus."* Clinically, the vulvar skin becomes thin, inflamed, fragile, wrinkled, parchment thin, and contracted or stenotic. Histologically, the principle features are thin epithelium, homogenization, loss of rete, and dermal inflammatory infiltration. There may be a combination of the two ("mixed" type) types of dystrophies, and these lesions may be further subclassified according to the presence or absence of cellular atypism. A typical hypertrophic dystrophy is particularly worrisome as a premalignant lesion when there are abnormal maturational patterns and intraepithelial "pearl" formation. Intense pruritus may be associated with the several varieties of lesions, along with dyspareunia and dysuria if there is an associated atophic urethritis. Although symptomatic treatments encompassing topical applications of corticosteroid, testosterone, and antipruritic creams may be effective, preliminary biopsies taken at multiple sites suggested by toluidine staining are imperative to exclude areas of dysplasia and carcinoma *in situ* that may merge with frank cancer. Malignant lesions may be found coexisting with atrophic and hyperplastic dystrophic conditions. Concomitant monilial, parasitic, or bacterial vulvovaginitis should be treated.

VULVAR INTRAEPITHELIAL NEOPLASIA (VIN)

These focal or diffuse lesions, often found in association with atypical hypertrophic dystrophy or dysplastic lesions of the vulva, may be of the squamous- or of the transitional or intermediary-cell type. Either type may be at the periphery of an invasive lesion. Usually, the preinvasive lesion produces pruritus, burning, discomfort, dyspareunia, and sometimes dysuria. There may be considerable shrinkage of the introitus. One variant of the Bowenoid transformation is a lesion of definite intraepithelial malignancy that occurs only in the mucous membrane or at the mucocutaneous junction. This condition has been termed erythroplasia of Queyrat and has the capacity to terminate in frank squamous-cell carcinoma and metastatic spread if left untreated. These lesions in their several forms are best treated with a total vulvectomy with resection lines wide enough to provide at least a 1-cm clear margin.

VULVAR PAGET'S DISEASE

This uncommon vulvar disease derives its name from its histologic similarity to Paget's disease of the breast, although the two conditions are probably unrelated. In the breast there is an underlying primary mammary carcinoma, usually apocrine in type, which gives rise to an intraepidermal metastasis. In contrast, the vulvar lesion arises in the epithelium and it may be either unifocal or multicentric. The epidermis should contain clusters of cuboidal cells that show very pale cytoplasm containing mucopolysaccharides (Paget's cells). This intraepithelial cancer usually presents as a sharply demarcated, slightly elevated, somewhat indurated,

reddened lesion. There may be patchy excoriations and maceration and an appearance of eczema. These lesions may be found in the vulva of women during the reproductive years or in the elderly at any age. This occurs particularly in white patients and has a brick-red appearance. The associated symptoms of pruritus, burning, and tingling may have been present for many years before the nature of the condition was appreciated. If there is a malignant transformation, the progression will be downward from the epidermis along the several appendages or by lymphatic permeation, and there may be an underlying sweat gland carcinoma. The primary lesion may coexist with other histologic types. Total vulvectomy with adequate margins is adequate treatment unless the deep areas of the corium are involved and dictate an associated lymphadenectomy.

MELANOTIC LESIONS

The proportion of melanomas arising in the vulva is disproportionately high, and while these lesions are uncommon (1% to 3% of all malignant vulvar tumors), they tend to be highly aggressive. The labia minora is the most favored site. They may arise from pigmented nevi, which must be removed by excisional biopsies to diagnose or exclude melanoma. Similarly, melanosis may undergo malignant transformation after a number of years. The typical lesion is brownish, and the pigment is unequally distributed throughout ill-defined, irregular areas of spread. Treatment consists of adequate local excision. If malignant degeneration occurs, the surgical approach would be radical vulvectomy together with inguinal, femoral and, possibly, pelvic lymphadenectomy. In malignant melanoma, the overall prognosis for a 5-year survival is in the 35% to 40% range, but the prognostic variables depend on histologic picture, site of origin (worse with lesions near the vestibule), and size of lesion at the time of therapy.

BENIGN TUMORS OF THE VULVA

Condylomata Acuminata

See Human Papillomavirus *(HPV)*, p. 243.

Molluscum Contagiosum

This condition is a proliferative virus-induced skin disease with a predilection for the vulva. The lesions are usually multiple, benign tumors that vary in size from tiny growths up to about 1 cm. They are usually attached by a sessile base, although some are pedunculated. The tumors tend to be dome-shaped, and some may develop a central opening secondary to necrosis and infection. The epithelial cells degenerate because their cytoplasm succumbs to the formation of large inclusion "molluscum bodies" that contain the numerous elementary structures representing the virus. The disease is sexually transmitted, and autoinoculation is common. The lesions may be treated individually by freezing, desiccation, or curettage and cauterization of the base.

Hidradenoma

These rare, small benign tumors may be solid, but the typical lesions are cystic and they present chiefly on the labia majora of white women as sharply circumscribed, movable, partially translucent (partly dark), elevated masses, rarely larger than 1.5 cm. They will make their appearance only after puberty when the apocrine glands from which these tumors arise become functional. The tumors are firmly attached to the overlying skin, which becomes thinned out or necrotic from the pressure. A central opening, or so-called umbilication, may show a protrusion of papillomatous, red, granular tissue. There may be associated infection, bleeding, and pain. Histologically, the highly papillary adenomatous proliferations may be mistaken for adenocarcinoma, although the absence of anaplastic changes or stromal invasion should call attention to the benign nature of the tumor. These growths can be locally excised intact.

These cystic tumors may be grossly similar to others of epidermal or epidermal appendage origin, for example, epidermal cysts (arising from buried squamous epithelium), Fox-Fordyce disease (formation of microcysts from the retention of sweat in the apocrine gland ducts), sebaceous cysts, or syringomata which arise in the eccrine sweat gland structures. These conditions may give rise to intensive pruritus, and some may need to be locally excised. A benign cystic teratoma may be found in the vulva, and there may be no associated symptoms, or secondary infection is capable of evoking acute symptoms.

Bartholin's Duct Cyst

Obstruction of the Bartholin duct usually near its opening into the vestibule may give rise to cyst formation. A combination of congenital narrowing and inspissated mucus may be a much more common cause of obstruction than scarring secondary to primary bartholinitis from gonorrhea or other microbial organisms. Usually, the main duct is obstructed and the cyst is unilocular; however, multiloculations can occur if the deeper minor ducts or acini or the ductal system becomes occluded. Cysts enlarge in response to the secretions of sexual stimulation, and the mass may be tender and cause pain. The cyst may become infected, and abscess formation will give rise to marked inflammation of the overlying skin and severe vulvar pain. In addition to the gonococcus, *Escherichia coli, Aerobacter aerogenes,* various types of streptococci and other organisms have been isolated. Large symptomatic cysts usually having diameters of greater than the average of 1 cm to 4 cm or those associated with recurrent abscesses should be approached surgically. In most instances, simple marsupialization will suffice, and the original opening into the cyst wall will shrink to a small permanent tract for the escape of secretions. The appearance of a tumor mass in the region of the Bartholin gland after the menopause, or development of an enlarging firm tumor, even if the tissues are inflamed, should arouse suspicion of a neoplasm.

Benign Solid Vulvar Tumors

In addition to a number of benign solid epidermal and epidermal appendage tumors, one can encounter may neoplasms of mesodermal origin. These include tumors arising from smooth muscle in the round ligament (leiomyomas), proliferations of fibroblasts (fibromas), combinations of fat cells and connective tissue (lipoma), neural sheath (neurofibromas or granular cell myoblastoma), blood vessels (hemangiomata), capillary hemangioma, possibly pyogenic granuloma, and hypertrophied lymphatic channels (lymphangioma). Generally, large tumors or those causing symptoms can be excised. Excision of the granular cell myoblastoma may be the most troublesome because the margins of the tumor are indistinct and there is poor encapsulation. Wide excision will be necessary, and close subsequent follow-up to detect early recurrences in the area of the resection line. There may be a similar tumor in the lower respiratory tract which calls for evaluations of the chest as a routine. Cavernous hemangiomas are probably best treated expectantly unless there is ulceration, bleeding, or extension into the underlying muscle.

One may encounter primary and secondary vulvo-vaginal endometriosis presenting as dark-colored nodular lesions. The majority of lesions seem to occur in old scars from lacerations, episiotomies, or colpoperineorrhaphies, or from extensions of pelvic endometriosis, usually through the posterior vaginal fornix. The cervix may be involved as isolated lesions or as a part of a much wider disease process. Histologically, endometrial stroma and glands are demonstrable. Lesions may be fulgurated or locally excised and it may be best to suppress subsequent menstruation until the operative sites have healed.

Another benign solid tumor is the urethral caruncle, which is caused by ectropion of the posterior urethral wall secondary to postmenopausal mucosal atrophy or possibly by chronic irritation and infection of the meatus. The tumors may be pedunculated but they are generally sessile, and they rarely exceed 1 cm in diameter. The appearance may be red or fleshy and the tumor may be friable. Some lesions cause dysuria, pain, bleeding, dyspareunia, and tenderness. Histologically, they may be papillomatous, angiomatous, or granulomatous. Symptoms may be relieved with topical estrogen, or symptomatic larger tumors may be removed by local caustics, fulguration, or surgery.

INVASIVE MALIGNANCIES OF THE VULVA

Squamous-Cell Carcinoma

Squamous-cell carcinomas make up about 85% to 90% of vulvar malignancies and roughly 3% to 4% of all malignant tumors of the generative tract in women. These lesions occur in postmenopausal women (more than half being over age 60 years), usually after a long history of vulvar irritation, bleeding, venereal infections, discharges, granulomatous ulcerations, poor personal hygiene, or preexisting dysplasia (one third of the patients). There may be long physician and patient delays in appreciating the clinical significance of refractory pruritus and vulvar sores. About two thirds of the tumors arise in the labia majora and minora, but the lesion may spread to involve the whole vulva, perineum, and anal margin. The gross lesions may be exophytic or infiltrating, but the appearance does not seem to correlate either with the histologic grade of the tumors or presence of nodal metastases. The diagnosis is established by biopsy or excisional biopsy at a suitable local site.

The size of the local lesion at the time of therapy is a key prognostic variable. There will be lymph node involvement in more than half of the patients with local lesions over 3 cm in diameter. Midline lesions involving the clitoris, urethra, or rectum are most often associated with metastases extending directly into the obturator and other deep pelvic nodes. Otherwise, the primary route of spread is by way of the superficial and deep inguinal, deep femoral, and external iliac lymph nodes. Usually, if the Cloquet's node in the upper femoral canal is not involved, no higher glands will be involved. Contralateral spread may occur because there are rich intercommunicating lymphatics in the vulvar skin. In fact, the contralateral inguinal nodes may become involved first. The primary lesions may be localized, confluent, or multifocal, and the histologic appearance of the cancers may show a spectrum of types (grades I, II, and III) based on degree of differentiation, keratinization with distinct pearl formation and anaplasia. Stromal tissues with invasion may show a variable degree of inflammatory cell differentiation. The degree of dedifferentiation has prognostic significance in small lesions, but overall the gross size of the tumor at therapy is the more sensitive factor. Most authorities use the FIGO nomenclature for staging of vulvar carcinoma: Stage 0 is carcinoma *in situ;* Stage I is a tumor confined to the vulva of 2 cm or less in diameter and nodes not clinically suspicious of neoplasm; Stage II is a tumor confined to the vulva of more than 2 cm diameter with nodes not clinically suspicious of neoplasm; Stage III is a tumor of any size with adjacent spread to the urethra and any or all of the vagina, the perineum, the anus, and/or nodes clinically suspicious of neoplasm; and Stage IV is a tumor of any size infiltrating the bladder mucosa or the rectal mucosa (or both) including the upper part of the urethral mucosa, tumor fixed to the bone, fixed or ulcerated nodes in either or both groins, or other distant metastases. Young women tend to experience lesions on the fourchette most commonly, while in the elderly, midline lesions notably in the region of the clitoris are more common. Lesions that extend into the vagina are less favorable varieties, and when tumors involve the vulva bilaterally, nodular metastases are more frequent.

The optimal therapy is surgical, and the principle is to excise the lesion widely to encompass the entire tumor together with regional lymphatic tissues. The commonest type of treatment failure is a local recurrence resulting from inadequate removal of tissue and lack of a wide margin of cancer-free tissue on the specimen. The usual procedure is the en bloc radical vulvectomy and bilateral lymphadenectomy devised by Way, Bassett, and others.

Frozen section examination of the glands of Cloquet will determine the need to proceed to lymphadenectomy in the deep pelvis, in addition to the groin dissections involving both nodes and skin that are called for in the standard procedure. Radiation therapy and chemotherapy have limited place in the management of vulvar cancers, and seldom could a case be made for palliative surgery. Optimal treatment results in a 5-year survival rate of about 65%; however, if nodes are not involved, the expectation for survival rises to about 90%.

Basal-Cell Carcinoma

These slow-growing, locally infiltrating lesions are derived from primordial basal cells in the epidermis or hair follicles and account for about 2% to 3% of vulvar cancers. Their site of origin is normally in the skin of the labia majora, and they may be described as papillomatous, somewhat pigmented, or maculopapular eruptions. Since as many as one in five lesions give rise to a local recurrence, an adequate resection is the key to proper management. Distant metastases are not expected unless the tumor is of the basal/squamous-cell type. The latter are more aggressive and have sufficient potential for metastatic spread to justify radical surgical therapy.

Other Malignant Lesions

Other malignant vulvar lesions include melanoma (2% of vulvar cancers), cloacogenic carcinoma (arising from epithelial rests or remnants of the urogenital sinus or cloaca), mesonephric carcinoma (arising from the remnants of the wolffian or gartnerian ducts), sarcoma, hemangioendothelioma, lymphosarcoma, and various metastatic tumors (vaginal, cervical, endometrial, ovarian, trophoblastic, rectal, or urinary tract origins). Bronchogenic carcinomas, as well as other primary types, may spread to the vulva, and there can be leukemic infiltrations.

Carcinoma of Bartholin's gland deserves special attention because the diagnosis may be long delayed. The symptoms associated with carcinoma are the same as those noted in the much more common acute inflammatory conditions. Ultimately, there is degeneration of overlying tissues, and an irregular ulcer or sinus tract may be formed. Carcinomas arising from the duct of the gland are squamous cell in type and the histologic appearance is not different from the other epidermoid vulvar lesions. Tumors arising in the gland may be adenocarcinoma (most frequent variety), adenosquamous, or squamous in type. These tumors account for about 5% of vulvar cancers. The prognosis is generally poor, and the presence of malignant lesions of this type calls for radical vulvectomy, and partial vaginectomy as required, along with bilateral lymphadenectomy (inguinal, femoral, and deep pelvic).

CANCER OF THE VAGINA

Primary carcinomas of the vagina are largely epidermoid (roughly 75%), and the peak age of women with the disease is between age 60 and 70. Altogether, these lesions make up only 1% to 2% of gynecologic malignancies. An invasive tumor may be preceded by an *in situ* lesion for up to a decade or more. Early lesions high in the vaginal fornices may be inconspicuous, although cytology may be positive for malignant cells. The tumors may progress as ulcerative lesions, or they may become exophytic. There may be direct spread into the bladder or rectum, while proximal lesions tend to produce nodal metastases similar to those in the cervix (deep pelvis) and distal vaginal tumors spread like vulvar lesions into the lymphatic tissues of the groin. The likelihood of lymph spread and the prognosis are determined largely by the size of the primary lesion. Bleeding or foul discharge from ulceration are prominent early symptoms, and there is usually no associated pain. The treatment may be surgery or radiation therapy. The prognosis depends upon the stage of the disease when treated (70%–75% 5-year survival for Stage I, 25%–30% for Stage III).

Primary malignancies of the vagina may also take the form of adenocarcinomas, melanomas, and sarcomas. Young women, between the ages of 14 and 23, may have an increased incidence of clear-cell adenocarcinoma of the vagina associated with intrauterine exposure to diethylstilbesterol (DES) administered to the mother usually prior to the 17th gestational week. The prospect for this occurrence is fortunately quite low, probably 0.1 to 0.01 cases/1,000 exposed individuals. A benign vaginal condition associated with DES exposure, known as "adenosis," is much more common (60%). In addition, the squamous metaplasia that occurs in maturing lesions of adenosis has not been seen to develop into a squamous cancer. Thus, the current attitude toward the management of vaginal adenosis is conservative and quite optimistic.

Distant spread is rare and late in epidermoid vaginal cancers, while pulmonary and liver metastases with melanomas and sarcomas are more common, usually disseminating by the bloodstream. Embryonal rhabdomyosarcomas occur in young girls, and leiomyosarcomas and reticulum-cell sarcomas are seen in the adult female.

Secondary vaginal malignancies are common (more common than a primary vaginal carcinoma) and there may be extensions or metastatic spread from vulvar, cervical, endometrial, trophoblast, tubal, or ovarian cancer. A malignant lesion in the Bartholin gland, urethra, bladder, kidney, or rectum may extend into the vagina, but cancer from more distant sites is rare. Cases of adenocarcinoma have been reported to arise from mesonephric duct remnants, ectopic cervical glands, and vaginal endometriosis.

DISORDERS OF THE CERVIX

Cervicitis

Acute, subacute, and chronic forms of cervicitis probably represent the most common gynecologic disorders, and the cervix may participate in a variety of the infectious processes involving the vulva and vagina that have already been discussed. In addition to parasitic, bacterial, viral, and other pathologic agents, the underlying causes may be anal–vaginal contamination (poor hygiene), hypoestrogenic state, hypovitaminosis, pressure necrosis (pessaries), foreign bodies, obstetric lacerations or iatrogenic factors relating to perforations, and other injuries associated with instrumental procedures.

Symptoms may include purulent discharge, bleeding, irritation, dyspareunia, lower abdominal discomfort, secondary urethritis (if there is an associated vulvovaginitis), infertility (hostile environment for sperm, incompetency of the cervix, etc.), or even carcinoma, possibly related to granulomatous, HPV, or herpes simplex viral infections. The cervix may appear acutely inflamed with erythema and edema, or, in cases of chronic infection, it may have a denuded, red, granular (eroded) appearance at the mucosquamous junction. In longstanding infections, the cervix may be hypertrophied and elongated.

There may be positive laboratory studies for specific pathogens that call for a particular type of therapy. In addition to local or systemic antibiotic and other medical treatments, severe chronic cervicitis may rarely require surgical intervention in the form of electrocauterization (incision and coagulation), cryosurgery (tissue destruction by freezing), laser vaporization, endocervical curettage (after polypectomy), or conization. The preliminary diagnostic procedures must be adequate to exclude specific granulomatous infections before embarking upon these procedures (*e.g.*, tuberculosis, tertiary syphilis, granuloma inguinale) in addition to carcinoma. There may also be virulent pathogens residing in polyps, and a simple local excision may be associated with rapid spread to the internal genitalia. Adequate broad-spectrum antibiotics are required at the first suspicion of extension of local infection. Rarely, lymphogranuloma venereum, chancroid chlamydial infections, fungi, or parasites give rise to prominent cervical lesions that present as papillary tumefactions, fistulous tracts, or ulcerations.

Occasionally, mesonephric (wolffian) duct remnants lying deep in the stroma of the cervix will become cystic. Ectopic endometrium can also involve the cervix by implantation during surgery or possibly delivery or by direct extension of pelvic endometriosis through the cul-de-sac. A papilloma arising on the portio vaginalis should be excised and carefully examined histologically because a small percentage will be anaplastic. Cervical leiomyomata are capable of becoming highly symptomatic, particularly if they are large, and may give rise to dyspareunia, bladder or rectal complaints, ureteral obstruction or hematometra (pyometra) secondary to obstruction of the endocervical canal. Most cervical tumors of this type are associated with leiomyomas of the uterine fundus and can be treated surgically in context with the overall problem.

Cervical Intraepithelial Neoplasias (CIN) and Microinvasive Lesions

Cervical "dysplasia" (CIN) refers to a histologic condition in which there is cellular anaplasia, nuclear hyperchromatism, increased numbers of abnormal mitotic figures, and loss of polarity in the deeper layers, but only a part of the thickness of the squamous epithelium has been replaced by these abnormalities. These disturbances can be mild, CIN-1; moderate, CIN-2; or severe dysplasia to carcinoma *in situ*, CIN-3, depending upon the depth of the more superficial layers of cells still capable of maturation. In the severest form, only a few cell layers near the surface retain their normal status.

This falls short of total loss of maturation from the basement membrane to the surface that characterizes squamous-cell carcinoma *in situ*.

Although dysplastic lesions may regress, the more severe stages tend to progress more often and more rapidly than the minimal lesions. Exfoliated cells occurring in cervical–vaginal cytologic smears tend to show a degree of the same anaplasia, changes in the nuclear chromatin, as well as multinucleation and increased nuclear–cytoplasmic ratio. Usually, there is a fairly close correlation between the cytologic and histologic findings (better than 80%). However, management and diagnostic investigations as well as treatment, are predicated upon the fact that a "dysplastic" smear does not rule out an *in situ* carcinoma, and an *in situ* lesion noted on biopsy does not necessarily exclude an early stromal invasion. Although most early lesions of the cervix arise in the region of the squamo-columnar junction and are confined to the distal 2 cm of the endocervical canal, they can remain hidden from view. It appears that epithelial spread of intraepithelial neoplastic lesions is more commonly endocervical along the canal lining and into the glands. Thus, Stage 0 (*in situ* lesion), Ia (microinvasion up to 3 mm), and Ib occult clinical lesions may occur in grossly normal appearing cervices, or actually these several types may coexist. One definition of microinvasion (Stage Ia) is that the neoplastic epithelium invades the stroma in one or more places only to a depth of 3 mm or less below the basement membrane. Thus, there may be the full spectrum in one cervix between the normal and the clearly malignant and *in situ* carcinoma can be found at the periphery of an invasive lesion.

The incidence of squamous-cell carcinoma *in situ* of the cervix on initial population screening is probably about 7/1,000, while it is estimated that about 2% of women over age 40 will ultimately develop clinical cancer. The prevalence of cervical dysplasia is less than 4.0% in nonpregnant women, probably 1.5% to 3.5%. Cervical changes of the dysplastic type are much more common during pregnancy, but in the majority of patients the lesions regress postpartally. Although biological progressions from dysplasia to clinical cancer have been observed in a significant minority of cases, possibly one third, many lesions may remain static for many years. However, overall, the suggestion of progression is underscored by noting that the average age of a patient with clinical cervical cancer is about 45, while the peak incidence for *in situ* cancers is age 35, and dysplasias are usually noted in women from 25 to 35 years and perhaps even younger. Some grades of CIN (*i.e.*, moderate to severe dysplasia) seem to have an aneuploid chromosomal pattern and an abnormal nuclear DNA content similar to invasive lesions, which supports the view that these are truly precancerous lesions.

The epidemiologic variables related to causes and predisposing factors are not altogether clear; however, the most positive correlation exists between cancer and coitus at an early age involving multiple experiences with different partners. Cervical cancer is virtually unknown among nuns. Thus, cancer screening should begin when the female becomes sexually active or no later than age 18 years. Attention should be paid to matters of personal hygiene, since viral and chemical agents may be involved. An increased incidence of dysplasia has been noted in patients who smoke cigarettes. Undoubtedly, hereditary immunity and cultural practices (circumcision, etc.) are also operative because the incidence of cervical cancer is very low in Jewish women. Prior cancer in another organ, multiparity, low socioeconomic status, Herpesvirus type 2 infections, papillomavirus infections, and immunosuppressive therapy may be other factors.

A plan of management dictates that an abnormal cytologic examination in the presence of a normal-appearing cervix requires colposcopic examination and directed biopsies of any areas displaying atypism. In general, disturbing features on colposcopy calling for histologic evaluation include white epithelium, mosaicism, or the coarse punctate pattern of the surface capillaries, and, particularly, bizarre capillary configurations (possibly indicative of stromal invasion). The entire limits of the transformation zone and margins of the lesion or lesions must be clearly visible, or a diagnostic cone biopsy is mandatory. This occurs in 10% to 15% of premenopausal women and an even greater percentage of postmenopausal individuals. The same approach is indicated if there are significant discrepancies among the cytologic, colposcopic, and histologic findings. Selection of a specific treatment is made on an individual basis. If abnormal cytology is found in association with infection in the cervix or vagina, eradication of the infectious process and further cytologic studies are indicated.

Mild to moderate dysplastic cervical lesions may be treated with cryosurgery, provided there are no extensions into the endocervical canal and adequate follow-up is assured. Most recently loop electrosurgical excision procedures (LEEP) has been demonstrated to be a safe and atraumatic outpatient procedure to treat dyplasia by modified cervical conization. If a cone biopsy has been performed and all margins show only normal tissue, this should suffice as treatment, even for *in situ* carcinoma, if the patient is young and is desirous of childbearing. Other means of accomplishing the conization include laser vaporization or conization and cold knife conization. An extrafascial total abdominal hysterectomy would represent a definitive treatment for an *in situ* cancer or certain Stage Ia lesions. However, if there is microinvasion associated with deep cell nests, confluence of cell aggregates or lymph or vascular involvements, it is best to consider the lesion an occult Stage Ib (clinical type) and offer more radical treatment (see next section).

Cervical Malignancy

About 95% of cervical malignancies are epidermoid (roughly 87%) or the adenosquamous type (8%), while the remaining 5% present as adenocarcinomas, or very rarely as sarcomatous lesions. The usual histologic grading based on differentiation I to III is generally directly related to the biological potential. Undifferentiated tumors (grade III) tend to metastasize early. The adenocarcinomas are more difficult to classify in this manner. Most of these cancers arise from the glandular elements of the cervix, although some may be derived from the mesonephric (wolffian) duct remnants.

Epidermoid lesions may be infiltrative or exophytic, and ulceration associated with abnormal bleeding (acyclic) and odorous discharge may be primary manifestations. There may be irregular indurated edges with central friable necrotic tissues that may give rise to frank bleeding. Histologically, the squamous lesions may be of the small-cell type, large-cell keratinizing type, or the large-cell nonkeratinizing type. Extension into the vaginal fornices will usually occur in untreated cases, and, ultimately, there will be parametrial involvements (beginning with Stage IIb) and metastases to the deep pelvic nodes in a progressive manner. These may be spread anteriorly to invade the mucosa of the bladder or rectum (Stage IVa). Lateral spread may occur to the lateral pelvic wall (no cancer-free space, Stage IIIb), which may be associated with hydronephrosis or nonfunctioning kidney. The extent of vaginal involvement also influences the stage, since disease that does not encroach upon the lower one third is classified in Stage II, while lesions that do become Stage III.

The clinical staging I to IV determines the likelihood of nodal metastases. Squamous cell carcinoma confined to the cervix from a clinical view-point (Stage I) is associated with lymph node involvement in 15%; in those patients with parametrial extensions, this incidence rises to 30% to 40% for deep pelvic nodes and about 10% for paraaortic nodes. The nodes in Stages III and IV will be positive in 35% to 65%. This relatively high percentage of pelvic extensions even with Stages I and II demonstrates the fallibility of clinical staging techniques, for example, examination under anesthesia, cystoscopy, rectosigmoidoscopy, intravenous pyelogram, barium enema, chest roentgenogram, sonograms, lymphangiograms, and chemical profiles for renal and liver functions. Recently, various imaging techniques have improved the likelihood of discovering parenchymal disease and positive nodes; however, the inherent errors in these clinical evaluations have led some to sponsor pretherapy staging operative procedures to obtain tissue samples for histologic study of pelvic and paraaortic nodes and the parametria.

In patients with Stage Ib and IIa lesions (proximal vaginal but no parametrial disease), the 5-year survival rates for irradiation and surgery are essentially the same under optimal standards of care. Since the ovaries can be preserved (rare site of metastases), surgery has some advantages if the young woman is reasonably thin and a good operative risk. The proper procedure would be a radical hysterectomy and bilateral deep pelvic lymphadenectomy. An adequate resection of parametrial and paracervical tissues requires dissection and displacement of the ureters bilaterally. Lesser degrees of surgery are adequate only for Stage Ia disease, in which the changes for the nodal disease are negligible. Even the high-risk categories of microinvasion (occult Stage Ib) are probably best treated in a more radical manner, since nodal involvements may occur in 2% or more of the cases (possibly up to 15% as the lesion expands to an overt clinical lesion). The presence of pelvic infection (chronic salpingitis, diverticulitis, ulcerative colitis, parametritis, etc.) or presence of tumor (large uterine leiomyomata or ovarian pathology) would tend to contraindicate irradiation and favor the operative approach. The surgical approach has special appeal in all three trimesters of pregnancy, since the pregnancy will be eliminated along with early cancer (avoids additional potentially hazardous manipulations to evacuate the uterus either before or after radiation therapy). Extensive pelvic and intra-abdominal adhesions from prior surgery and disease states would likewise complicate radiation. The surgical approach may be used as a method of salvaging some patients with central pelvic recurrences following irradiation or surgery or those who may have been left with multiple fistula from slough after radiotherapy (even without residual disease). In these cases a pelvic exenteration is performed, which accomplishes removal of the bladder (with creation of urinary diversion), rectum (with sigmoid colostomy), vagina (residual cervix if present), remaining central parametrial and paravaginal tissues, lymph nodes (if appropriate), and even the vulvoperineal tissues as may be required. The direction and extent of tumor growth determines the nature of the operative procedure. There are major operative and postoperative complications in all cases of radical pelvic surgery. The mortality rate varies from about 1% or less up to 2.5% in the extended surgical approaches. An effort to preserve ureteral blood supply and prolonged catheterization of the urinary bladder should give rise to fistulas in only about 3% or less of patients. Vesicovaginal and rectovaginal fistulas should be even less common.

Except for the above considerations, radiation therapy is generally the best primary treatment for invasive cervical carcinoma, especially in Stages IIb to IV. In planning therapeutic management, a critical concern must be given to the dose of radiation given to the organs adjacent to the cervix and vagina. Although the latter structures can tolerate doses up to 24,000 rads, serious damage can be created in the major blood vessels of the pelvis and the bowel at about 7,000 to 9,000 rads and in the bladder and terminal ureter at about 10,000 rads or higher. The delicate balance between cancericidal dose levels and the possibility for injury to important uninvolved tissues becomes clear when it is realized that a dose necessary to kill cervical carcinoma is in the range of 6,000 to 7,000 rads administered over a period of 4 to 5 weeks. Furthermore, the tumor dose will fall off rapidly and a central safe source of radium delivered by intrauterine tandem and lateral forniceal colpostats may need more therapy at the lateral pelvic wall. A standard technique is to use radium locally to deliver about 8,000 rads to point A (2 cm lateral to the central canal of the cervix and 2 cm above the lateral fornix in the axis of the uterus) where the uterine artery crosses the ureter. Usually the dose needed is given in 144 hours broken into two sessions, 2 to 3 days each at a 2-week interval. The dosage may be reduced in older patients. In 1 month's time, a dose of 1,100 rads can be given to point B (same level as point A but 5 cm lateral to the central canal of the cervix), which corresponds roughly to the pelvic wall where the major deep lymph nodes are present along the

iliac vessels. External radiation generated by supervoltage equipment (^{60}Co, linear accelerator, betatron) can be delivered first (with or without central shielding of the pelvis) to be followed by one or two cesium applications, depending upon the stage of disease and individual circumstances. A panhandle extension of radiation could be given up to 4,000 rads if the lesion involves the paraortic region.

Generally, chemotherapeutic agents have not been effective in the treatment of cervical carcinoma. A variety of protocols have been used, but the results have been discouraging. Recently, cisplatinum has been used to treat squamous lesions, but the drug is nephrotoxic to a worrisome degree. Overall palliative care and emotional support are extremely important features in managing incurable cases. Unfortunately, among patients with recurrences, the majority (probably 75%) will have disease involving the lateral pelvic wall. Uremia resulting from bilateral ureteral obstruction is the most common cause of death. In selected cases, urinary diversion or palliative colostomy may be rewarding adjuncts in providing chronic care.

The 5-year survival rate for Stage I fall into the 85% to 90% range for most major centers, and there is about a 10% to 12% salvage in the Stage IV cases. The moderate stages evidence 5-year survival rates of about 65% for Stage II and 35% in Stage III, although some individual institutions achieve higher salvages. The presence of positive nodes greatly reduces the chances of survial at all stages including Stage I (drop of 40% or more).

Special comment about managing a patient with a bulky central lesion (barrel-shaped cervical carcinoma) is needed. The hypoxic deep stromal tumor cells are more resistant to ionizing irradiation and, since 5-year survivals in Stage I and II are reduced, follow-up extrafascial hysterectomy may be beneficial.

DISORDERS OF THE UTERINE CORPUS

Leiomyomata

Leiomyomata are the most common uterine tumors (20%–30% of all women over age 30, with blacks having the greatest incidence), and they develop from the immature mesenchymal cells or smooth muscle cells in the walls of myometrial arterioles. Occasionally, they arise in the cervix, round ligament, or broad ligament. The tumors contain connective tissues, but they are chiefly smooth muscle and are not derived from fibrous tissue sources. These tissues are estrogen dependent, and the fibromuscular elements may be highly susceptible to estrogen stimulation. All of them decrease in size dramatically postmenopausally. Growth hormone may provoke their development (under estrogenic stimulation) and the associated erythrocytosis. They range in size from seedling tumors to masses of enormous size that fill the abdominal cavity. They may be discrete, but usually are multiple, and each tumor tends to be demarcated from encompassing normal tissue and somewhat lighter in color. The varieties are submucous, intramural, subserous, separate from the uterus, and parasitic. The subserous varieties may lie within the broad ligament (intraligamentary) or come to rely on extrauterine blood supply from omental vessels. The pedicle under the latter circumstances may undergo atrophy and resorption, and the tumor becomes parasitic. Unrelated to the clinical situation there may be a variety of degenerative changes, *e.g.,* atrophic, cystic (liquefaction of marked hyalinization), calcific (precipitation of calcium carbonate and phosphate from circulatory obstruction), septic (subsequent to central necrosis), carneous (venous congestion, thrombosis, interstitial hemorrhage, aseptic degeneration, and infarction particularly during pregnancy), and myxomatous (fatty degeneration). Leiomyosarcoma occurs in less than 0.5% of patients with leiomyoma.

Symptoms will depend upon tumor size, nature of any degenerative changes, location, clinical state, and whether or not there is a pregnancy. Most women who have leiomyomata have small tumors and are asymptomatic. They require only observation and reassurance. Large tumors impacting on pelvic nerves may cause pressure and considerable pain radiating to the back and lower extremities. Abnormal uterine bleeding, usually in the form of hypermenorrhea or menometrorrhagia, is a common manifestation, and may result in anemia. Endometrial hyperplasia is present in about one third of the patients; thus, hysterectomy should not be performed without a prior endometrial sampling. Hysteroscopy is gaining in popularity as a means of diagnosing pathologic, anatomic, and anomalous conditions, as well as a means of treating some under direct vision (*e.g.,* excision, vaporization). A submucous tumor in particular may cause intermenstrual bleeding in addition to hypermenorrhea, and secondary dysmenorrhea may be a prominent complaint. With large tumors, there may rarely be polycythemia (erythrocytosis) of unknown etiology. Hysterectomy usually reverses the hemato-

logic problem. Endometritis or carneous septic degeneration may incite a systemic reaction with leukocytosis and increased sedimentation rate. Significant uterine enlargements and distortions may make it difficult or impossible to cancer screen or adequately curette the uterus or to control bleeding mechanically or hormonally. Acute torsions, infections, or infarction of a tumor may produce acute symptoms. The effects of pregnancy on the tumors and vice versa may be profound. The adverse effects on pregnancy may be early abortion, late abortion, abruptio placentae, placenta previa, premature birth, and degenerative changes leading to tenderness, pain, and a systemic reaction. In addition, there may be malpresentation, uterine inertia, dystocia, retained placenta, and sepsis. Women with significant leiomyomata should probably be offered family planning methods other than oral contraceptives, and postmenopausal women should be given supportive estrogens with great caution, since these hormones promote tumor growth.

Rarely, treatment consists of emergency surgical intervention in the event of acute torsion of a pedunculated tumor or intestinal obstruction in association with the ensuing inflammatory process. Other emergencies include infection and infarction. Supportive measures may require blood transfusions or iron therapies to correct anemias. Occasionally, a submucous leiomyoma provokes severe uterine contractions, which deliver the body of the tumor into the vagina while the elongated pedicle is still attached in the endometrial cavity. There is almost always infection present. It is best to excise the bulbous tumor near the cervix and delay hysterectomy if it is indicated until the infection is controlled.

For the most part, myomectomies are reserved for patients who wish to create or preserve a potential fertility. However, such procedures are likely to be associated with considerable blood loss. Intraoperative myometrial injections of pitressin or epinephrine 1 : 200,000 may be used to control bleeding. Additionally, the use of a Bonny clamp or tourniquet may assist in the effort to control bleeding. Postoperative sepsis, adhesions, tumor growth, or intestinal obstruction are potential sequelae of myomectomy, particularly when multiple large tumors have been excised. The rate of recurrence, even if all tumors are initially removed, is approximately 15%. Obviously, recurrent curettages for refractory bleeding in association with large intramural tumors are not effective means of controlling excess blood loss. Use of cyclic hormones is not rewarding, and radiation therapy to shrink down the tumor has very little place in overall management. Recently antigonadotropic hormones have been used in some symptomatic patients who are not good candidates for surgery and to shrink the tumor preoperatively to minimize blood loss.

The definitive treatment is abdominal hysterectomy. It should be recognized that tumors rising out of the pelvis (>12-week gestational size) deserve removal on the basis of their potential to cause symptoms, and a substantial minority will partially obstruct the ureter, leading to a silent hydroureter and hydronephrosis. Such damage calls for definite surgery even in asymptomatic women. The same is probably true when large tumors are present that rise above the pelvic brim (> 12-week gestational size), and confusion exists with respect to diagnosis (*e.g.*, solid ovarian tumor) or sudden growth has occurred.

Sarcoma

These mesenchymal tumors comprise less than 2% of uterine malignancies. It is customary to identify a homologous type that is derived from mesenchymal cells normally present in the uterus and a heterologous tumor that may contain cartilage, bone, striated muscle, and fat. There are also mixed tumors involving both homologous and heterologous sarcomas in addition to the mixed mesodermal (müllerian) tumors, which contain both sarcomatous and carcinomatous elements, but none of the teratomatous features.

Recently, it has been suggested that it may be best to discard the ambiguous terms *carcinosarcoma, sarcobotryoides,* and *cellular leiomyomas* and to restrict the classification to the more specific types known as *leiomyosarcoma, endometrial stromal sarcoma,* and *rhabdomyosarcoma.* Endolymphatic stromal myosis represents a low-grade variant of sarcoma. It grows around and within lymphatic vessels of the myometrium and is capable of extrauterine extension or local recurrence in 20% of the cases with compression of the ureters and bowel, if surgery is inadequate. If identification is impossible after appropriate diagnostic efforts, the tumor should be designated "unclassified." Another current attitude is the belief based on electron microscopic studies that leiomyosarcoma may be a distinct entity and that there is no malignant degeneration of a preexisting leiomyoma. The distinction between benign and malignant tumor is often difficult to make, although the number of mitoses per high-power microscopic field (HPF) is a helpful histologic criterion. Those with few mitoses per HPF are likely to be benign, while those with 10 or more mitoses per 10 HPFs are likely to be malignant and metastasize. So-called cellular leiomyomas are merely borderline or low-grade leiomyosarcomas.

Stromal endometrial tumors tend to bulge into the uterine cavity, produce necrosis and hemorrhage, and infiltrate the endometrium. Stromal myosis, which is the benign condition, occurs in the premenopause while the aggressive form known as stromal sarcoma is a postmenopausal occurrence. In most cases of sarcoma, the uterus is enlarged or there is a rapid enlargement within a preexisting uterine leiomyoma. Leukorrhea may be a presenting complaint, in contradistinction to abnormal uterine bleeding, and there may be pelvic discomfort. There may be progressive local extension. Epithelial components may be either squamous cell carcinoma or adenocarcinoma, or both, and heterologous elements include osteosarcoma with bone or osteoid formation, chondrosarcoma, or rhabdomyosarcoma. The poorest prognosis is associated with unencapsulated tumors, frequent mitotic figures per HPF, and cell types consisting of rhabdomyoblasts or osteoblasts. The grapelike, polypoid neoplasms noted in children (sarcoma botryoides) and the mixed müllerian tumors in adults are usually rhabdomyosarcomas. The metastatic lesions of sarcomas resemble adenocarcinoma in three quarters of the cases.

The prognosis is poor with hematogenous and lymphatic spread in most cases despite therapy. The standard treatment is total abdominal hysterectomy and bilateral salpingo–oophorectomy. In the case of mixed tumors with endometrial stromal lesions preoperative irradiation has been reported to be of value, but generally radiation therapy is not rewarding, especially with leiomyosarcoma. VAC chemotherapy, even though a very toxic combination, has been used in recurrent and progressive sarcoma. Some centers are using a combination which includes cis-platinum, doxorubicin (Adriamycin), and dacarbazine (DTIC) with some success. Rarely, endometrial stromal sarcoma will be responsive to large doses of medroxyprogesterone. Radical surgery is not indicated. The overall 5-year survival rate for uterine sarcoma is only 20% or less.

Endometrial Carcinoma

Traditionally, the ratio of the incidence of cancer of the body of the uterus to that of the cervix is 1 : 2 or 1 : 3. However, a sharp increase in the frequency of endometrial carcinoma during the decade of the

1970s and the more recent decline in cervical carcinoma has changed this relationship. Now endometrial carcinoma is the most common female pelvic malignancy. As a cause of gynecologic cancer death, it ranks third, and is preceded by carcinomas of the ovary and cervix. It is worrisome that the incidence in premenopausal, as well as older, women has increased, and it is estimated that about 3% of women in the adult reproductive age category will develop the endometrial lesion in their later years.

There appear to be precursors, predispositions, and various factors associated with the development of endometrial carcinoma. Heavy (obese), nulliparous women often suffering from diabetes mellitus and hypertension constitute a high-risk group. In some there will have been evidence of long-standing anovulation, delayed or so-called bloody climacterium, and changes in the endometrium indicative of adenomatous hyperplasia or carcinoma *in situ*. Chronic estrogen exposure from endogenous or exogenous sources may predispose malignant transformations in the endometrium in susceptible women or those with a familial predisposition. Presumably, estrone represents the most potential carcinogenic threat, and its major precursor is androstenedione, which is metabolized in peripheral fat in an augmented fashion among obese women and those with endometrial carcinoma. Presumably, chronic anovulation from any cause (polycystic ovary syndrome), estrogen-producing ovarian tumors, or prolonged estrogen intake represent risks even among relatively young women unless they are given progestin supplements. Granulosa–theca cell tumors of the ovary are associated with endometrial cancer in as many as 20% of the cases. In considering chronic estrogen usage, one cannot discount topical applications, because the hormone is absorbed rapidly into the bloodstream through the vaginal mucosa. The type of endometrium provoked by unopposed estrogen is also important because only about 5% or less of patients with cystic glandular hyperplasia will develop endometrial carcinoma, while a progression to malignancy in atypical adenomatous hyperplasia is a common occurrence (possibly 45%). The latter lesions often coexist, and in some cases no clear distinction can be made on histologic grounds.

The key clinical feature is abnormal uterine bleeding, particularly of the acyclic intermenstrual or postmenopausal types, although hypermenorrheic patterns and other forms of refractory dysfunctional uterine bleeding may have preceded the malignant endometrial transformation by a decade or more. At least one half of patients can be characterized by these presentations, both in terms of underlying etiology for the bleeding and predisposing menstrual disturbances. It is a wise policy to probe the endocervix (as in obtaining endocervical specimens for cytologic studies) in providing routine gynecologic care, particularly in women at risk for the development of adenocarcinoma. A cervical stenosis preventing the discharge of blood or pus (a vaginal discharge may also be a presenting complaint) can result in considerable delays in diagnosis. In these cases the initial symptoms of pain are associated with the development of a hematometra or pyometra.

Endometrial lesions may be focal or diffuse. The types are usually adenocarcinoma, adenoacanthoma (contain nests of benign squamous or metaplastic cells), or adenosquamous carcinoma, which contains both malignant glandular and squamous cells. Papillary serous adenocarcinoma could have early upper abdominal metastases. Adenocarcinoma often takes the form of a polyp, but the transformation of a "benign endometrial polyp" into an adenocarcinoma while its pedicle remains free of malignant change is a rare occurrence. Likewise, an epidermoid carcinoma arising from the endometrium in squamous cell rests, metaplasia, or cell patches within an atrophied uterus is extremely uncommon. Certain sarcomas may have their derivation in the endometrial stroma.

Most adenocarcinomas arising in the endometrium are fairly well differentiated; perhaps two thirds are graded I or II, and this histologic grade together with or without presence of malignant squamous cells, depth of the uterine cavity, depth of myometrial invasion and intraperitoneal cytology are the key prognostic variables. Spread of cancer can occur by surface growth into the cervical canal (Stage II) and into the myometrium (often associated with a uterine cavity depth of more than 8.0 cm, which distinguishes Stage Ia from Stage Ib and represents a worsening of the prognosis). With increasing myometrial infiltrations, lymphatic and vascular spread, as well as direct penetrations of tumor through the serosa, become major threats. When the outer one third of the myometrium is involved, there will be spread to the deep pelvic lymph nodes in about one half of the cases and to the paraaortic nodes in a significant minority. There may be a spread to the vagina (into the urethra, bladder, or rectum) and into the parametrial tissues. Tumors confined to the pelvis are Stage III unless the bladder, rectum, or rectal mucosa is directly infiltrated (Stage IV). Spread to the liver, bones, and lungs is not uncommon (also, Stage IV), which makes scans an important part of the metastatic survey.

Diagnostic procedures include exfoliative cytology or smears of endometrial cavity saline irrigation fluid (Gravlee Jet Washer), endometrial biopsy, or suction curettage. *In utero* inspection (hysteroscopy) is used in some institutions, but whether the procedure will encourage intraperitoneal spillage of tumor is being debated. Vaginal cytology as a screening diagnostic tool is less reliable in fundal than cervical cancers. The definitive diagnostic method is a differential curettage whereby tissues are obtained from the uterus in two specimens from scrapings first within the endocervical canal followed by a scraping of the endometrium. An adenocarcinoma may arise as a primary lesion at either site and the biological potential and the approach to management may be quite different. Also, when an endometrial cancer spreads to the endocervix (Stage II), the lymphatic metastases become quite similar to those of primary cervical carcinoma (internal, external, and common iliacs and obturators). Usually at the time of the fractional uterine curettage careful pelvic examination and inspection of the bladder (cytoscopy) and rectosigmoid colon (endoscopy) are done in an effort to "stage" the disease accurately. Proceeding to therapy on the basis of frozen section study of curetted tissues rather than awaiting reports on permanent sections can lead to clinical error. Sometimes, complications of the malignant disease will impose problems in following a standard management protocol. The metastatic survey may reveal large bowel obstruction (on barium enema), chest lesions (on pulmonary roentgenograms or laminograms), ureteral obstruction (on intravenous pyelogram), or the presenting problem may be salpingitis or pyometra. The latter calls for uterine drainage and appropriate antibiotics to clear the infection before the curettage is performed.

Definitive treatment should be an extrafascial hysterectomy, which incorporates a collar of proximal vagina, and bilateral salpingo–oophoretomy in all Stage I carcinomas of the endometrium. Patients with Grade II lesions should be considered for postoperative vaginal intracavitory radiation therapy with cesium. High-risk patients for recurrence (*i.e.*, Grade III lesions, deep myometrial invasion, positive nodes, and peritoneal washings) should receive external radiation to the pelvis of 5,000 rads over 5 to 6 weeks, including the vagina. If periaortic nodes are involved, a panhandle field should be used. Another acceptable alternative used by some

institutions in Grade III lesions is the use of cesium implant followed by surgery in 48 hours. Preoperative external radiation therapy of 4,000 rads followed by a single cesium implant of 3,300 mg/hour, followed by extrafascial total abdominal hysterectomy and bilateral salpingo–oophorectomy in 6 weeks is the treatment of choice. In the presence of Stage II disease, in some centers, a radical hysterectomy together with bilateral pelvic lymphadenectomy is used. Follow-up external irradiation to the paraaortic nodes can be administered. Occasionally, patients with Stage III or Stage IV disease are candidates for an exenterative surgical approach. More commonly, patients with widespread disease are best managed with chemotherapy. Long-acting progesterone administered intramuscularly may be effective in bringing about tumor regression and remission (perhaps in up to one half the patients with well-differentiated lesions involving the lungs). Various chemotherapeutic agents used to control metastatic disease have included 5-fluorouracil, Cytoxan, chlorambucil, melphalan, megase, or medroxyprogesterone (Depo-Provera) and others. However, the most promising single agent usually used in combination with some of the others is doxorubicin (Adriamycin), administered intravenously every 3 weeks contingent upon lack of toxicity (particularly myocardiopathy). Cis-platinum (nephrotoxic and neurotoxic), administered in combination, is a popular addition to the management protocol.

The overall 5-year survival rate varies with the stage. There should be roughly an 80% salvage when only the endometrium or superficial myometrium is involved. When the uterus is atrophic and only the endometrium is involved, *in situ* carcinoma, a "cure" can be expected in almost all cases even with surgery alone. When endocervical or extensive myometrial involvements occur, the 5-year survival drops to 50% or less, even with extensive therapeutic approaches; in the absence of extrauterine disease, little more than 15% to 20% of the patients will survive for that period of time.

Optimal gynecologic care for all women calls for the identification of those at special risk. Good medical supervision assumes that states of chronic anovulation will be recognized and remedied and that the administration of estrogen will be reserved for special indications and not abused. Proper practices of cancer screening should be pursued in context with continuing health surveillance. In the presence of endometrial hyperplasia, estrogen should be opposed by prescribing oral progesterone on a cyclic basis. Progesterone reduces estrogen receptors in the endometrium and depresses the receptor-mediated stimulation of these tissues. Even some of the atypical or very early cancerous lesions have been revised by this medical approach.

PELVIC INFECTIONS

General

Pelvic infections involving the internal genitalia, peritoneum, and adjacent structures are common occurrences in gynecologic practice, and their incidence is on the rise. These infections may be obstetric (postabortal, intrapartal, postoperative, postpartal), gynecologic (IUD related, postoperative, foreign body, catheter related, etc.), or pelvic extensions or inflammatory processes originating outside the genital tract (appendicitis, diverticulitis, urinary fistula, and so forth, or blood-borne condition). There can be local cellulitis, widespread peritonitis, abscess formation, pelvic thrombophlebitis, septicemia (septic emboli), thromboembolic phenomena, endotoxic shock, renal shutdown, and other formidable complications. Although the etiology is usually bacterial, pelvic infections may be viral, parasitic, fungal, or mixed.

Traditionally, so-called pelvic inflammatory disease was essentially synonymous with gonorrheal salpingo–oophoritis, and these infections were designated as initial attack or recurrent disease as well as acute, subacute, or chronic in type. It is now known that more than one half of these infections are mixed, and the various organisms involved include aerobic cocci, coliforms, and anaerobic bacteria. The latter tend to dominate (anaerobic progression) when the pelvic infection progresses to abscess formation. These organisms, which reside in the normal vagina and endocervix, including clostridia, bacteroides, anaerobic streptococci, and those indigenous to the gastrointestinal tract, tend to become virulent under these hypoxic environmental conditions. The eventual outcome in untreated cases may be a ligneous cellulitis, leakage or rupture of purulent contents into the peritoneal cavity, adherent tuboovarian inflammatory cyst, walled-off chronic abscess with recurrent flare-ups, distortions, adhesions, infertility, and a variety of incapacitating symptoms. Occasionally, abscesses obstruct the ureter, give rise to marked ileus or bowel obstruction, or extend to give rise to perinephric, subdiaphragmatic, or pleural gas collections.

A considerable amount of difficulty may be encountered in distinguishing gynecologic etiologies

from conditions arising in the gastrointestinal tract, appendix, gallbladder, pancreas, urinary tract, or elsewhere. Although anorexia, nausea, and vomiting may occur with acute salpingo–oophoritis, these symptoms are more characteristic of appendicitis. Change in bowel habits and especially presence of occult blood in the stool favor diverticulitis over salpingitis or appendicitis. The sudden onset of pain is more typical of ruptured viscus (tubal pregnancy) or torsion of an adnexal mass. Back or flank pain of a colicky type along with chills and fever suggests ureteral calculus (or urinary infection), particularly if there is radiation into the groin, microscopic hematuria, or pyuria. There may be backache with acute pelvic inflammation, but usually it is sacral and the pain radiates down one or both legs, and the patient may complain of an associated deep pressure. There may be marked abdominal tenderness, intermittent pain, and distention, but unlike intestinal obstruction, the bowel sounds tend to be hypotonic rather than hypertonic. Also, in acute salpingitis, the tenderness on motion of the cervix is likely to be exquisite. There may be fullness in the cul-de-sac associated with the cloudy fluid of a peritoneal inflammatory reaction or beginning pelvic abscess. An adnexal mass may be present, which may appear to be unilateral on palpation even though the contralateral tube is acutely inflamed.

Confusion with a degenerated leiomyoma or torsion of a subserous tumor can be a problem, especially if the mass is on a pedicle and there are no other uterine irregularities. The pelvic infection may even arise from the endometrium as in IUD-related sepsis, and an enlarged, boggy, tender uterus may arouse the suspicion of infected abortion or even of malignancy. Acute pelvic symptoms associated with marked tenderness in the absence of much temperature elevation or leukocytosis tend to favor other conditions, notably ruptured ectopic pregnancy. However, it is disconcerting that recurrent pelvic infections may not give rise to systemic responses, and there can be chronic abscesses in the pelvis without an elevated white blood count or sedimentation rate. Chlamydial pelvic infections may be relatively silent. Pelvic sonography may be very helpful in identifying structural disease in the tubes and ovaries. A β-HCG test will exclude pregnancy in questionable cases where ectopic gestation may be one of the diagnostic possibilities. Acute cholecystitis is likely to produce epigastric pain, colic, anorexia, nausea, vomiting, right upper quadrant tenderness, leukocytosis, and sometimes icterus (cholelithiasis). The presence of upper quadrant abdominal pain radiating into the back is suggestive of acute biliary colic.

It should be noted that gonorrheal perihepatitis represented by adhesions between the liver and surrounding structures can mimic acute cholecystitis almost exactly (*Fitz-Hugh–Curtis syndrome*). Generally, it is helpful to observe that, for the most part, gonorrheal infections involving the pelvis are usually associated with mild clinical pictures in sharp contrast with invasion of the pelvis by virulent mixed infection or sepsis in context with an acute surgical disorder. Nevertheless, these clinical clues notwithstanding, specific radiographs, ultrasonograms, culdocentesis, colpotomy, endoscopies, and other procedures and investigative methods, including exploratory operations, may be required before the diagnosis can be established in some cases, especially if there is no response to optimal antibiotic therapy.

In the event of a tubo-ovarian abscess that may follow an initial episode of acute salpingo–oophoritis, the gravest risk is leakage or sudden rupture. This seems to represent the greatest risk among older women. There may be the dramatic onset of tachycardia, tachypnea, oliguria, hypotension, disorientation, and sometimes hypothermia, indicative of septic shock. There will be four-quadrant abdominal pain, tenderness and rebound in association with a bulging cul-de-sac (pelvic abscess) and gross pus on culdocentesis. Without intensive monitoring, adequate support measures, and prompt surgical intervention, the mortality is very high.

Inflammatory masses in the pelvis that do not respond to medical therapy or decrease in size despite aggressive management may be leaking pus. Another possibility to be considered is pelvic tuberculosis, particularly if ascites has developed. There may be a history of chronic pelvic disease and infertility; eosinophilia in the peripheral blood would be suggestive. Menstrual disorders are common, often including amenorrhea, because tuberculous endometritis occurs in a very high percentage of cases with pelvic involvement. Detection of acid-fast bacteria in a Ziehl-Neelsen stain and positive cultures on Lowenstein-Jensen medium are diagnostic, and these evaluative methods can be applied to endometrial tissues, menstrual discharges, cul-de-sac fluid, or peritoneal biopsies. All serosal surfaces may show disseminated granulomatous disease. If the patient is mistakenly subjected to operative intervention before 12 to 18 months of appropriate medical therapy (combinations of isoniazid, aminosalicylic acid, streptomy-

cin, ethambutol, or others), suspicion of the disease should be aroused by certain distinguishing features. These may include unusually dense adhesions and lack of any clear planes of cleavage in the dissections. The tubes may be dilatated segmentally, but the ostia remain open. Fistula formations are highly suspicious findings.

There is the possibility that a septic abortion underlies a pelvic infection when there is a recent history of menstrual disturbance (especially missed menses), crampy pain, bleeding, foul vaginal discharge, or possible passage of tissue. A molar pregnancy may behave similarly. Occasionally, pelvic endometriosis associated with a chocolate cyst of the ovary and an inflammatory reaction causing fibrosis, contractures, serosal adhesions, and fixations may be mistaken for chronic pelvic infection and result in inappropriate therapies. The primary focus of endometritis and source of spread resulting in serious pelvic infection, including tubo-ovarian abscess, may be an infected polyp, submucous leiomyoma, or IUD. Sometimes, an IUD-related abscess is unilateral and restricted solely to the tube or ovary. Large pelvic abscesses, bilaterally as well as unilaterally, may progress to cause ureteral obstruction if proper drainage is not instituted through the cul-de-sac or extraperitoneally by the abdominal approach. Uterine perforation following biopsy, curettage, IUD insertion, and so forth may underlie serious pelvic infection. Pelvic infection (cuff abscess) may be a serious complication of hysterectomy and major vaginal operative procedures (intraoperative broad-spectrum intravenous antibiotics which may be continued several days postoperatively may be useful in reducing the likelihood of this occurrence). Critical sequelae in all these conditions are pelvic thrombophlebitis and septic emboli. A septic clinical course associated with high fever that does not respond to aggressive medical therapy suggests these complications. In particular, a marked persistent tachycardia may be a feature of pelvic thrombophlebitis, and the patient's clinical picture may not improve until heparin therapy is instituted. Pelvic veins become involved more often when anaerobic streptococci and bacteroides are the offending pathogenic organisms.

The principles of clinical management are based on the knowledge of likely causes of sepsis and the ability to assess the clinical picture properly, to provide proper coverage of the major bacteria involved in aerobic–anaerobic polymicrobial infection, to recognize associated complications (embolization, thrombophlebitis, foreign body, bowel injury, urinary leakage, etc.), and to intervene surgically when indicated (debridement, drainage of abscess, etc.). The four main categories of bacterial organisms requiring antibiotic coverage are (1) the gram-positive aerobes and anaerobes, (2) nonpenicillin-sensitive bacteroidaceae *(Bacteroides fragilis)*, (3) group D streptococci (enterococci), and (4) enterobacteriaceae. For life-threatening pelvic infections, triple therapy consisting of penicillin, clindamycin (or metronidazole), and gentamicin should provide proper coverage for these organisms. Ticarcillin disodium plus an aminoglycoside (tobramycin, etc.) is effective against *Pseudomonas* infections, as well as a broad spectrum of organisms. In about one third of the patients with gonorrheal salpingitis, there will be aerobic–anaerobic, polymicrobial organisms involved in the pelvic infection. Even patients with primary cases should be admitted to the hospital for intensive therapy with multiple antibiotics by infusion directed toward coverage of mixed infections, as previously outlined, for example, doxycycline, cefoxitin, and follow-up on medications, especially tetracyclines. In nonresponding or serious cases, even broader and intensified therapeutic coverage must be provided. Double-puncture diagnostic laparoscopy may permit an accurate diagnosis and make it possible to obtain cultures directly from the pelvis and tubal fimbriae, if initial management is unsuccessful or if there is a diagnostic confusion. Patients who fail to respond to medical management or develop a leaking abscess may require surgical intervention.

Generally, there is a favorable clinical outcome when acute salpingo–oophoritis is promptly and adequately treated in an appropriate manner. For some, however, there will be thickening and other tissue changes including hydrosalpinx or tubo-ovarian inflammatory cysts, which may give rise to acute or subacute flare-ups in addition to chronic pain, recurrent tenderness, deep-thrust dyspareunia, backache, rectal pain, menstrual disturbances, and general fatigue. Symptomatic heat, repeat courses of appropriate antibiotic therapy, analgesics, and careful follow-up will be adequate to control symptoms in some of these patients. Among those interested in childbearing, a form of tuboplasty may be indicated during a quiescent period under antibody coverage if there is tubal occlusion clearly demonstrated in the course of the infertility workup. If a large symptomatic adnexal mass persists, or if the patient remains symptomatic because of extensive chronic pelvic inflammatory disease, definitive pelvic extirpative surgery would be indicated, even among the relatively young. The most quiescent period possible must be selected for the

pelvic "operation," to avoid considerable postoperative morbidity.

Gonorrhea

Although documented cases of nonvenereal transmission of gonorrhea are on record, the disease is contracted almost entirely by coitus and the major site of primary infection in the female is the cervix. There is about an 80% to 90% risk of contracting the disease in the female following her exposure with an infected male, after an incubation period of probably about 2 weeks, although precise figures are unknown. Early symptoms may be quite subtle or absent, although some will present with a purulent urethral discharge, urinary frequency or dysuria, unilateral swelling of a Bartholin gland, or, possibly, sore throat or rectal discomfort if there has been pharyngeal or anal exposures. Most affected women will be asymptomatic carriers; however, it is probable that about 10% to 15% of untreated women will develop pelvic infection. Presumably, when spread to the tubes and ovaries does occur, it is subsequent to the development of an endometritis often in association with the first menstrual period after contracting the disease. This extension may occur silently or it may provoke acute pelvic symptoms and a systemic reaction.

Diagnosis of gonorrhea is presumptive when gram-negative diplococcal organisms are demonstrated on Gram stain, typical growth is seen on Thayer-Martin media, and there is a positive oxidase reaction. Selective media are highly effective diagnostic procedures, and sensitive serologic tests are available for detecting antibodies to *Neisseria gonorrhoeae* in special circumstances. A serologic test for syphilis should be obtained routinely, since the two venereal diseases may coexist. Also, chlamydiae, mycoplasmas, and mixed aerobic and anaerobic bacteria have been found coexisting with the gonococci, particularly in upper genital tract infections. *N. gonorrhoeae* can be cultured from peritoneal fluid obtained by culdocentesis in many patients with gonococci present in the endocervix (6%–61%). Direct cultures from the fimbriae may be taken through the laparoscope. By these more aggressive diagnostic methods, it is now apparent that the gonococci may be only one component of a mixed aerobic–anaerobic pelvic infection, perhaps in as many as two thirds of the patients. Gonococci tend to disappear from the cultures of women after several attacks of pelvic infection.

Treatment consists of ceftriaxone 250 mg IM. There are alternative management programs involving spectinomycin. This treatment is adequate only for uncomplicated infections. Since up to 45% of patients with gonorrhea also have a chlamydial infection, doxycycline 100 mg by mouth twice a day for 7 days, is given with ampicillin. Sexual partners are treated at once after examination and cultures. Patients with acute pelvic inflammatory disease should be hospitalized for intensive multiple antibiotic infusion therapy, for example, ampicillin, gentamicin, and clindamycin or other combinations involving cefoxitin, doxycycline, and so forth. Posthospitalization tetracycline, by mouth, is given to complete 2 weeks of total therapy.

ENDOMETRIOSIS, ADENOMYOSIS, AND DYSMENORRHEA

Endometriosis is a benign proliferative process consisting of functioning ectopic endometrium capable of invading and distorting normal tissues in the pelvis and elsewhere or occasionally spreading by lymphatics to the umbilicus and deep pelvic nodes or by hematogenous dissemination to the pleura and other sites. Pelvic pain, dysmenorrhea, dyspareunia, low backache, rectal discomfort, abnormal bleeding, and infertility represent the principal clinical features of endometriosis, although many patients remain asymptomatic despite extensive pelvic disease. There is little correlation between the severity of symptoms and the extent of pelvic involvement. The disease is common in women of all nationalities and can be found in teenagers as well as women in their 30s and 40s. The condition can only be diagnosed by direct visualization (usually laparoscopy), although it may be suspected from other imaging modalities.

It has been clearly documented that blood and detritus can flow retrograde through the fallopian tubes at the time of menses, and shed viable endometrium will sometimes implant on the visceral peritoneum or serosal surfaces of pelvic organs. Outlet genital tract obstructions (urogenital sinus aplasia with normal müllerian development) leads inevitably to pelvic endometriosis in neglected cases after the menarche. An inoculum of endometrium will implant more readily in some women than in others, but the length of exposure to such transplantations of viable tissues undoubtedly is a factor. This transplantation theory, proposed by Sampson in 1921, is made creditable by clear evidence of iatrogenically induced endometriosis at various operative sites following opening of the uterine cavity and contaminating the wounds with endometrial cells. In addition to the myometrium, there may be lesions in episiotomy wounds, abdominal incisions,

or in scar tissues arising from lacerations in the vagina or cervix.

However, not all sites of endometriosis can be explained on this basis. "Metaplasias of the coelomic epithelium," first proposed by Meyer and popularized by Novak, Meigs, and others, or a similar "müllerian cell rest theory" advanced by Russell have been put forward to explain ectopic foci of endometriosis at distant sites or in the retroperitoneal areas of the pelvis. A continuation of these processes may account for the various types of ectopic sites, and these may be spread by local propagation or through the lymph or vascular channels.

The ovary is the most common site of implantation, but other areas of involvement include the uterosacral ligaments and cul-de-sac peritoneum in the typical case. Other sites of predilection are the broad ligaments and posterior surface of the uterus, bladder peritoneum or that overlying the terminal ureters, and the serosa of the rectosigmoid colon. There is bleeding associated with functioning implants that gives rise to localized irritation, fibrosis, and adhesions. There may be pain of a crampy type associated with periodic intestinal distention, but also from the bleeding surrounding the deeply placed foci of endometriosis. The typical cul-de-sac lesions, including a fixed retroflexed uterus and adherent ovaries, give rise to dyspareunia, and when the rectovaginal septum is involved, painful defecation is a common complaint in addition to pain referred to the sacrum and coccyx. Serosal bowel lesions that create muscular involvements and contractures may be responsible for partial or total bowel obstruction. Rarely, the ureter will be obstructed by extrinsic strictures. Mucosal involvements are very uncommon. Rectal or bladder bleeding may arise from extreme submucosal inflammation and congestion without invasion of the lining. Uncommon, however, are ectocervical surface lesions or erosion through the vaginal mucosa overlying an extensively diseased cul-de-sac. There may be contact bleeding and bleeding at the time of menses at these sites.

Secondary dysmenorrhea is a classic presentation, but the cause is not clear. Although the mechanism of pain is known only under certain circumstances, dysmenorrhea may be caused by an increased local concentration of prostaglandin. Similarly, menstrual disturbances, usually taking the pattern of polymenorrhea (short cycles) and hypermenorrhea (excessive flow), are common even in the absence of extensive bilateral ovarian disease. There may be associated constant premenstrual, menstrual, and postmenstrual pain away from the midline in the region of the ovaries for periods up to one half the entire cycle, representing 2 weeks or more of incapacitating complaints. The ovary is usually adherent and very tender to palpation at these times surrounding the menstrual period. It may or may not feel cystic.

Sometimes, an endometrioma will rupture with very dramatic results characterized as an acute surgical abdominal emergency. For many, infertility will represent the most distressing problem. Among women who are infertile without apparent cause, laparoscopic investigation will reveal pelvic endometriosis often in association with perituboovarian adhesions in almost one third of the cases. In a few women the ovarian parenchyma will be destroyed by destructive endometriomas, or rarely the extent of tubal disease will obstruct the lumen; however, there is much more likely to be an egg "trapping" or "pickup" problem. The incidence of infertility tends to correspond to the extent of pelvic disease, but exceptions occur, since a few implants here and there on peritoneal surfaces without adhesions can be associated with infertility. Although there are several current hypotheses, including altered peritoneal fluid, altered concentrations of prostaglandin $F_{2\alpha}$, and possible immunologic factors, the mechanism(s) responsible have not been detailed.

Endometrial implants classically appear as dark bluish or brownish black cystic structures on the surface or embedded in tissues where there is a rather characteristic surrounding zone of fibrosis and contracture in the form of a "puckering." Histologic study of these lesions will show both endometrial glands and stroma, interstitial hemorrhage, fibrosis and inflammatory cells, including hemosiderin-laden macrophages, in the surrounding tissues. In long-standing cases or after the menopause these lesions may "burn out" and the glandular elements may disappear. In active disease, ectopic endometrium responds to cyclic ovarian steroid stimulation, although it may go out of phase and become hyperplastic. In stromal endometriosis, the glandular elements are absent even with active proliferation of the stroma. Rarely, an adenocarcinoma may develop in a focal area of ectopic endometrium, and few cases of sarcomatous degeneration have been reported. These entities are poorly understood.

In diagnosis, the occurrence of secondary dysmenorrhea in a nulligravidous woman in her 30s is endometriosis until proven otherwise. By the same token, asymptomatic endometriosis may come to light in the process of a routine pelvic examination, especially if there is a mass and tender nodules in the cul-de-sac. Pelvic and rectovaginal examination with a focus of attention on the cul-de-sac are imperative. Imaging studies assist only in confirming the presence of a pelvic mass; cystoscopy, intravenous pyelography, and rectosigmoidoscopy are helpful if damage to adjacent pelvic structures is suspected. Diagnostic laparoscopy can be used to take biopsies of suspicious lesions. An accurate diagnosis must be established before a therapeutic plan is instituted.

In managing a patient, the treatment plan will depend upon age of the patient, desire for childbearing, extent of pelvic disease, ovarian function, type of tubal involvement, general medical status, and emotional status. The range of clinical problems will vary enormously. On the one hand, there will be the 15-year-old female with extensive endometriosis and distal vaginal agenesis coexisting with normal gonads and müllerian duct differentiation. On the other hand, there will be the highly symptomatic woman in her 40s who has no interest whatever in childbearing but wishes to be rid of pain. Thus, it is necessary to integrate the stage of the process (which will assist in determining possible treatment) with the patient's reproductive desires and symptomatology. While there are several classifications available for review, the basic considerations revolve around patients who will or will not be expected to respond to conservative management, consisting of observation, administration of analgesics and endocrine therapy, in terms of both comfort and desire for childbearing. Currently, it is recommended that endometriosis in the pelvis be classified according to extent as suggested by the American Fertility Society. A score system has been devised to be used after diagnostic laparoscopy or laparotomy to assign the severity of the process in accordance with the size of the lesion or conglomerate lesions, the type and location of the disease process (e.g., adhesions, ovarian cysts, fixation, obliteration of cul-de-sac) and the organ(s) involved. The extent of disease is designated as mild (1–5 points), moderate (6–15 points), severe (16–30 points), or extensive (31–54 points), based on these considerations. The second major consideration involves those individuals who fall into a more advanced group, characterized by advanced disease, larger lesions, usually more symptoms, and the need for more aggressive, often surgical, therapies if there is to be a realistic chance for childbearing. There seems to be a direct relationship between the extent of disease according to the classification and the success of therapy for fertility.

In the palliation group, there are no endometrial implants as large as 5 mm in diameter and there are no avascular adhesions, scarred fimbriae, adherent bowel, uterine fixation, or involvements of the bladder, appendix, lymph nodes, surgical wounds, vagina, or umbilicus. Only in these cases of mild and moderate degrees of disease should hormonal suppression be attempted, and even in these only temporary remission should be anticipated. Basically, modern approaches to pharmacologic control of endometriosis have settled on several modalities:

1. Estrogen–progestogen (Ovral, Demulen, Norlestrin, etc.), consisting of combination-type oral contraceptive agents that contain the least amount of estrogen necessary to suppress ovulation and the amount of progestogen needed to induce a pseudodecidual reaction, necrosis, and resorption in the ectopic endometrium

2. Treatment with continuous low-dose oral androgens, which remain subvirilizing while they suppress growth of ectopic implants without preventing ovulatory menses

3. Danazol, which has similar properties to other 19-nontestosterone derivatives and inhibits all the enzymes responsible for steroidogenesis and prevents the LH surge for ovulation. The dosage is 800 mg given in two divided doses, for periods of 4 to 6 months. Sixty percent of patients or more have a resolution of disease. Pregnancy rates vary between 46% and 72% and recurrent disease occurs in about 20%.

4. Depo-Provera, 150 mg intramuscularly every 3 weeks, especially with distant lesions.

5. A popular current therapeutic approach consists of antiprostaglandin agents used to counteract myometrial hypertonicity (dysmenorrhea) and to oppose the antifertility effect of prostaglandins on tubal mobility, corpus luteum, and egg release or transport.

6. Gonadotropin-releasing hormone (GnRH) agonists cause profound hypoestrogenemia by down-regulation of pituitary GnRH receptors. Although quite effective, the low estrogen levels and side effects (hot flushes, vaginal dryness) limit usage to relatively short intervals.

If restoration of childbearing potential and relief of symptoms represent the primary therapeutic goals, surgical treatment promises a considerable chance of success, especially if dense adhesions or large chocolate cysts are present. Certain fulgurations or laser vaporization of implants and lysis of adhesions in the adnexa can be accomplished through the laparoscope, but occasionally conservative operations through a conventional laparatomy generally will be required. The objectives are to lyse adhesions involving the uterus, tubes, ovaries, and cul-de-sac, and any bands between the bowel or bladder and internal genitalia. All ectopic endometrial implants are excised, fulgurated, or vaporized. A meticulous reperitonealization is attempted, and the uterine fundus is suspended to mobilize the adnexal structures in an effort to prevent their adhering to the cul-de-sac peritoneum. If there is severe dysmenorrhea in association with minimal cul-de-sac disease, a presacral neurectomy may be effective in reducing pain. The conservative procedures are successful in restoring fertility in up to 80% of carefully selected cases, but success rates in the 40% to 80% range are acceptable, depending upon extent of disease. One disadvantage to this surgical approach is the high likelihood of persistent or recurrent disease that makes a second operation necessary (25% or more of cases).

Extensive involvements of bladder or bowel may require surgical resection of lesions from these important organs. Occasionally, endometriosis is so extensive even in a young woman that the risk of failure of the various conservative operative approaches would be prohibitive. Definitive surgery consisting of total abdominal hysterectomy and bilateral salpingo–oophorectomy is best for women with advanced disease or those who are highly symptomatic and have completed their family. Even in young women, this type of curative surgery may be required if there are refractory symptoms or evidence that lesions are obstructing the ureter or adversely affecting other important organs. One of the iatrogenic causes of symptomatic failure is the overly zealous treatment of menopausal symptoms with estrogen after definitive surgery, which keeps certain residual implants alive. Also, there may be tags of functional ovary left, and these pieces of tissue may produce enough estrogen to keep the ectopic endometrial implants alive. In these rare cases, the unfortunate necessity for a second attempt at ovarian extirpation may be needed, if hormonal suppression and conservative measures cannot control symptoms.

Adenomyosis consists of ectopic endometrial islands within the myometrial layer of the uterus that appear as discrete localized lesions (adenomyomas) without distinct capsules or more commonly as diffuse involvement extending into the muscle to variable degrees. The islands may or may not connect with the basal endometrium. There is usually hypertrophy and hyperplasia around the islands of ectopic endometrium, and this thickening causes a globular enlargement of the uterine fundus. Although this condition has been referred to as "endometriosis interna," it is probably misleading to link adenomyosis and "endometriosis externa" as if they were similar in origin or in patterns of symptoms. The etiology of adenomyosis is not known, but it appears to arise primarily in parous women over age 30, and usually becomes symptomatic in the fifth decade (about 70% of the cases). It is a relatively common condition (20% or more of hysterectomy specimens). The ectopic endometrium in the myometrium is similar to the basalis layer, and the tissue probably does not bleed during menstruation; only about 15% to 20% of patients will respond to progesterone therapy. Adenomyomas commonly coexist with uterine leiomyomas (more than one half the cases) and less often are associated with pelvic endometriosis. The characteristic symptoms are hypermenorrhea and dysmenorrhea. There may be a sense of pelvic pressure in association with an enlarged, softened, tender uterus. Chronic anemia from excess menstrual flow occurs in some patients. Attempts to regulate the menses hormonally are generally unsuccessful. Uterine curettage or hysterectomy is required to rule out other causes (submucous leiomyoma, endometrial polyp, adenocarcinoma, etc.), but cannot be expected to resolve the problem of hypermenorrhea. Hysterectomy establishes the diagnosis and represents the most satisfactory method of treatment.

Pelvic congestion syndrome, described by Taylor and often referred to as Taylor's syndrome, tends to arise in patients of the hysterical personality type and is associated with a variety of symptoms mimicking adenomyosis and other organic conditions arising in the uterus and pelvis. As in adenomyosis, the uterus may be symmetrically enlarged, softened, and tender and the associated symptoms may be menstrual disturbances, pelvic pressure, and dysmenorrhea. The presence of marked congestion, including a somewhat patulous cyanotic cervix along with marked tenderness and pain on palpation of the boggy uterus and supporting structures, represents the classic features. There may be associated tissue edema and muscle spasms giving rise to lower abdominal pain, low backache, cramps, and dyspareunia on a cyclic, intermittent, or nearly continuous basis. Usually, the uterus is retroverted, and the pelvic veins are engorged and tortuous. The veins within the broad ligaments may take on the appearance of a container of worms. These patients who suffer from a major functional overlay do not respond to symptomatic therapies very well, and the problem is not basically one to be approached surgically without considerable thought.

Premenstrual syndrome (PMS) is attracting much more attention today because of its prevalence and associated discomfort, which interferes with work and pleasure for affected women in the premenstrual phase of the cycle when steroid levels are falling from their luteal peak levels. The increased secretion of aldosterone premenstrually may give rise in susceptible women to edema, weight gain, abdominal bloating, and breast congestion. Hyperresponses of the sympathetic nervous system may provoke depression, mood swings, insomnia, irritability, and somewhat impaired ability to reason. Their personality types seem to be distinct from those complaining primarily of dysmenorrhea. Headache is a prominent symptom. Hyperprolactinemia has been considered in the etiology of this syndrome, but this factor is unsettled. The patient's whole life situation is evaluated and discussed. Symptomatic treatment consists of salt restriction and diuretics, lithium carbonate to control the emotional instability, vitamin B_6, methyltestosterone for 5 days to curb severe headaches or, perhaps, cyclic progesterone.

Painful menstruation is the most common gynecological complaint and a leading cause of disability that causes absenteeism from school and the loss of many millions of working hours annually. There may be an organic basis (secondary dysmenorrhea), or incapacitating cramps may be idiopathic and not related to any identifiable gynecologic disorder *(primary dysmenorrhea)*. Patients suffering severe menstrual cramps of the primary type tend to have a significant psychologic overlay, including recurring fear. Establishing rapport with the patient and gaining her confidence with simple psychotherapeutic methods represents an essential part of the management by creating faith in the therapeutic approaches. In addition to possible emotional factors, physiologic disturbances in the form of strong, uncoordinated uterine contractions have been demonstrated in some patients. There is a likely connection between elevated uterine tone and higher levels of prostaglandin production by the endometrium. Levels are higher after ovulation during the secretory phase and highest during the menses. Prostaglandin levels are lower in the proliferative stage and lowest in atrophic endometrium and after oral contraceptive therapy. The latter approach constitutes a rational therapeutic approach and cyclic medications administered for 6 months will be successful in 90% of cases. The use of prostaglandin inhibitors (indomethacin, maproxen, etc.) given 24 to 48 hours in advance of the anticipated onset of discomfort may be effective for the same reason. This type of therapy is a logical alternative to oral steroids when side effects arise and analgesics or hypnotics are poorly tolerated. Anticholinergic medications (isoxsuprine) given to relax the smooth muscle of the uterus may also be successful therapies. Rarely, refractory cases may require surgical attention. The sympathetic and parasympathetic autonomic nerve supply for the uterus is concentrated in the presacral nerve, uterosacral ligaments, and nerve endings and ganglia in the region of the internal cervical os. Thus, the surgical approaches have been to produce pressure necrosis of the sensory nerve endings in the endocervix (insertion of a stem pessary), transection of the uterosacral ligaments either vaginally or abdominally, or presacral neurectomy. Complete relief of pain can be expected in about one half of these difficult cases.

GESTATIONAL PATHOLOGY

Tumors of the Trophoblast

Hydatidiform mole (molar pregnancy) is a disorder characterized by villous grapelike vesicular enlargements capable of filling the uterus and enlarging it to the size of a 6- to 7-month gestation. There may be genetic factors associated with its occurrence since the incidence may be high in some areas (Taiwan, 1 : 82 pregnancies), relatively uncommon in some (United States, 1 : 1,500–2,000 pregnancies) and intermediate in others (Mexico, 1 : 200 pregnancies). It is thought to be caused by loss of maternal genetic material (into the polar bodies) so that the entire genetic component in the developing fertilized eggs is of paternal origin. Excessive trophoblast proliferation occurs and the syncytiotrophoblast, which is the source of chorionic gonadotropin, will produce higher titers than in normal pregnancy, and this finding is diagnostic of the disease. The investment with syncytium is complete, and the cytotrophoblast becomes quite prominent and will persist even after the 4th to 5th month if the mole is not evacuated. There is a tendency for these molar pregnancies to develop in females at either end of the reproductive era, either under age 20 or above age 40. The malignant potential of these tumors varies with the race. In the Orient, as many as 15% of hydatidiform moles behave as malignant, while in the United States, only about 1% to 4% become choriocarcinomas. A classification based on pathologic findings is unrewarding because the histologic pattern does not reflect the biological potential of the tissues. In about 15% of the tumors, the histologic features will be those of a benign hydatidiform mole, but the trophoblast will be aggressive in its ability to erode into the surrounding tissues (invasive mole).

A strongly positive pregnancy test, even in high dilutions, is suggestive of mole or multiple pregnancy. The HCG titer may exceed one million IU/24 hours at a peak time of 60 to 70 days, when the normal pregnancy range is approximately 400,000 IU. The titer may remain persistently high or may even rise up to 120 days and beyond, when normally there is a gradual fall to much lower levels. In molar pregnancy, there is a type of thyroid-stimulating hormone (TSH) activity usually without clinical evidence of thyrotoxicosis associated with elevated thyroxine (T_4) levels.

Clinical signs and symptoms associated with molar pregnancy consist of excessive nausea and vomiting (roughly one third of cases); uterus larger than one should expect by dates (about one half); uterine bleeding or dark-red or brownish vaginal discharge, usually by the 18th week (90% or more); pain of uterine origin from overdistention (one third of the cases); preeclampsia associated with hypertension, edema, and proteinuria (more than one third of retained moles); absent fetal heart tones, quickening, or palpable fetal parts after the 5th month; and extrusion of vesicles. On examination there may be an unusual fullness, softness, and thinning of the lower uterine segment; in the ovaries bilateral theca-lutein cysts may be caused by the excessive HCG stimulation (one half the cases). Dramatic symptoms attend the serious complications of hemorrhage, intrauterine infection with the potential of septicemia, and the rare occurrence of spontaneous rupture of the uterus.

The most satisfactory diagnostic method is the ultrasound scan, which shows a "snowstorm pattern" of echoes or a mottling effect in the uterine cavity coupled with absence of a fetus. Amniography is hazardous, but injection of Hypaque will show a "honeycomb pattern" and no fetal parts.

The great majority of patients require no treatment other than evacuation of the molar tissue, since routine follow-up care will show a rapid fall of the HCG until the highly sensitive radioimmunoassay of the serum beta subunit of HCG is negative (roughly 80% of cases). The risk of recurrent mole in a subsequent pregnancy is less than 2.0%.

Certain diagnostic evaluations are required to rule out metastases in anticipation of determining the type of management. In addition to HCG titers, roentgenograms of the chest (tomograms as necessary); intravenous pyelogram; liver, spleen, brain scans; electroencephalogram and, possibly, computerized tomography (CT) scans and arteriograms would represent an appropriate workup.

In the absence of labor, uterine evacuation by suction curettage followed by sharp curettage under the protection of oxytocin infusion is the proper approach for most patients. Attempts to rely upon prostaglandins to stimulate labor have not been rewarding. Hysterotomy, which was the traditional means of evacuating large uteri, is rarely necessary today. When the molar pregnancy occurs in the older age group or there is no interest in further childbearing, women who are good operative risks may be treated by total abdominal hysterectomy. The HCG regression time is roughly cut in half over that of cases handled by curettage and there is a lowered incidence of residual disease.

Histologically, the typical tumor shows advanced hyperplasia or anaplasia of the trophoblast, edema of the stroma (hydropic degeneration), absence of fetal capillaries, and no evidence of an embryo, cord, or amniotic membrane.

In the partial or "incomplete" mole, only a fraction of the chorion is involved and pregnancy may continue, although premature birth, severe intrauterine growth retardation, and symptomatology of a molar gestation are notable. Such cases are usually found to be triploidy on chromosomal analysis; thus, it is unfortunate that the misnomer "mole" has been applied to this condition. In binovular twins it is possible for a normal fetus and placenta to coexist with a molar gestation.

Careful posttherapy surveillance consists of weekly HCG titers (β-subunit) until three consecutive normal values are obtained. Pelvic examinations, including careful inspection of the vagina, should be conducted biweekly. Periodic chest roentgenograms are mandatory because metastatic spread involves the lungs most commonly (60%). Metastases to the vagina are next most common (40%). All other sites are involved in less than 20% of cases, but the more important organs include brain, liver, and kidney. It is extremely important to eliminate pregnancy and the confusion it would cause by administering oral contraceptives for at least 1 year.

Utilizing the β-subunit method of determining the HCG regression time, one does not expect the hormone to disappear until about 90 days following mole evacuation by suction curettage. However, after hysterectomy with the mole *in situ*, that time period is reduced to less than 60 days. One would expect the HCG to fall progressively during that period after a rather precipitous initial fall. This pattern is more important than the actual regression time up to about 3 months. A plateau, or rising titer, serves as a basis for treatment. This occurs only in about 20% of the cases. More than one normal test must be insisted upon because a negative report one week may be followed by a positive titer the next. Demonstration of a metastatic lesion at any time would of course indicate malignant trophoblast disease and call for primary therapy or change of drug.

Methotrexate is the standard drug used singly, but actinomycin D is equally effective and perhaps somewhat less toxic. The interval between courses is usually about 2 weeks as dictated by toxicity, particularly bone marrow suppression, although a variety of allergic and gastrointestinal complaints may arise. Generally, prior to each course of chemotherapy, a complete blood count and platelet count are performed. Treatment is permissible when the hemoglobin is over 10 g/100 ml, white count over 3,000/mm^3, and platelet count over 100,000/mm^3. The serum glutamic-oxaloacetic transaminase (SGOT), BUN, and serum creatinine should not be rising. If response is not apparent or if toxicity arises to one drug, the other should be tried. It is customary to give one therapeutic course after the HCG titers have been normal for 3 weeks. Hysterectomy might be necessary when the uterine wall is perforated by an invasive mole or the patient is refractory to chemotherapy. Remission can be anticipated in nearly all patients with nonmetastatic disease.

The highest-risk patients include those with advanced duration of disease before therapy (<4 months), brain or liver metastases, failed prior chemotherapy, exceptionally high titers of HCG if there is no apparent association with pregnancy (possible teratomatous origin) or those in whom the disease follows a nonmolar pregnancy (60% of cases). In these patients, as well as those who are nonresponsive to single-agent chemotherapy, multiple drugs must be given (methotrexate, actinomycin D and cyclophosphamide, or others) as well as irradiation of the brain metastases. Even in these high-risk categories, a favorable response can be achieved in about 75%. The myometrium itself is a site of metastatic disease in about 10% of patients, and its persistence in the absence of other lesions calls for hysterectomy. Usually surgical treatment is reserved for complications. Choriocarcinoma, which once was universally fatal, can now be controlled or even cured after appropriate therapy (greater than 85%), although toxic effects of the medications may be troublesome.

Ectopic Gestation

Ectopic gestation is a conceptus that implants itself at a site other than the usual one on the endometrium of the uterine fundus. Any of these ectopic implantation sites are ill-suited for proper nourishment and development of the conceptus. Thus, for the most part, the outcome is almost invariably one of loss of pregnancy and potentially represents a very grave risk for the mother. This complication of gestation accounts for 7% to 10% of all maternal deaths and represents one of the important causes of deaths relating to hemorrhage. Thus, it may be a factor in up to 12% or more of maternal deaths.

The reported incidence of ectopic pregnancy ranges from 1 : 80 to 1 : 200 live births; however, the precise incidence is not known because early conceptuses may die and be absorbed without arousing clinical attention. Tubal pregnancy is by far the commonest type of ectopic gestation, usually represented by an implantation site in the ampullary segment. Much less commonly, the conceptus implants in the interstitial isthmic or infundibular portions. A variant of the interstitial ectopic gestation is represented by implantation of the conceptus at the uterine end of the tube, which incorporates within the growing mass a significant proportion of myometrium. This so-called cornual pregnancy is rare, but it is significant because rupture tends to occur late in the second trimester and may be attended by dramatic hemorrhage. Similar consequences may occur when pregnancy occurs in a rudimentary uterine horn. Other rare types of ectopic gestation consist of cervical pregnancy, abdominal pregnancy (primary peritoneal implantation or secondary implantation following tubal rupture), and ovarian pregnancy. Ectopic pregnancy may also coexist with a normal intrauterine pregnancy or a pregnancy in the contralateral tube (heterotopic pregnancy).

The outcome of tubal pregnancy may be rupture resulting in free intraperitoneal or contained retroperitoneal (broad ligament) hemorrhage. There is erosion of capillaries or more major blood vessels in the course of trophoblastic penetration of the tubal wall, leading to rupture of the viscus. The entire conceptus, including the chorionic villi, may be found in the clot surrounding the tube rather than in its lumen. Other sequelae include completed tubal abortion, which may go unrecognized; partial extrusion of the conceptus through the ostium (incomplete tubal abortion); or, perhaps, even repeated hemorrhages around a dead conceptus, leading to a so-called tubal blood or carneous mole. If the conceptus survives tubal rupture or incomplete tubal abortion leaving the chorion and usually the amnion attached to the wall of the tube, the placenta may become entirely extratubal and attach itself to surrounding intra-abdominal structures as it grows (secondary abdominal pregnancy), or the placenta may be attached to bowel and omentum in addition the broad ligament, bladder, and internal genitalia. Under these circumstances, there may be ovarian attachments, but this does not represent an ovarian pregnancy. Primary ectopic gestations occurring in the ovary must conform to the classic diagnostic criteria of Spiegelberg. The fetal sac must occupy a portion of the ovary, and the ovary with its sac can be demonstrated in histologic section while the entire fallopian tube is intact and normal on the affected side. The gonad with its gestational sac must be connected to the uterus by the ovarian ligament. Grossly, these early conceptuses may resemble a corpus luteal hematoma.

A common cause of ectopic gestation is tubal abnormalities, causing structural or functional impairment. Characteristically there may be intrinsic damage resulting from prior salpingitis (gonococcal, chlamydial, mixed bacterial, tuberculous, etc.), or extrinsic distortions arising from peritubal adhesions (postabortal sepsis, ruptured appendix, endometriosis, etc.). Occasionally, extrinsic uterine or adnexal masses may kink the tube or there may be congenital anomalies that interfere with transport of the ovum and tubal function (accessory tubal ostia, diverticulae, etc.). Failed tubal ligations, tuboplasty operations, microsurgical tubal reversals following a previous sterilization procedure, and prior tubal pregnancy represent circumstances that place patients at high risk for ectopic gestations, for example, range of 5% to 12%, depending upon the condition, up to an incidence perhaps as high as 50% when a Silastic ring fails.

In a large number of ectopic gestations no mechanical or structural etiology can be established. In some, endocrine disorders may be causative, for example, delayed ovulation, corpus luteal defects with altered estrogen-progesterone activity, action of prostaglandins, catecholamines, and so forth, presumably interfering with tubal and cilial motility. Ovulation induction, failed progestin-only contraception, and pregnancies following the "morning-after pill" have all been associated with a disproportionately high rate of ectopic gestation.

Additionally, pregnancy occurring with IUD use has a disproportionate (4%–9%) ectopic risk.

All these potential etiologies have given rise to a threefold increase in the incidence of ectopic gestation, now accounting for about 1% of all conceptions. The disturbing realities involve not only the risk of maternal mortality but also dismal consequences for further childbearing, for example, only about one half of these women will achieve a term pregnancy, and any subsequent gestation has about a 10% chance of recurrent extrauterine gestation.

A satisfactory outcome, if achievable, is contingent upon early diagnosis predicated upon awareness and an alertness to pursue investigative measures before the classic signs and symptoms of tubal rupture occur. The first symptoms may be those of early pregnancy. There may be a missed menstrual period, or the last one may have been short or light (occasionally normal and not delayed, however). Early death of the trophoblast and steroid hormone decline will give rise to a decidual breakdown and intermittent vaginal spotting (sometimes heavy). In some cases, a decidual cast will be passed. In the great majority of cases, there will be no remaining decidua at the time of significant clinical symptoms.

Classic symptoms include abdominal pain, which may be diffuse and relatively mild until tubal rupture causes sharp exacerbation. At this time, there may be abdominal distention, muscular spasm, guarding, rebound tenderness, cul-de-sac fullness, and signs of hemorrhage shock. The patient will feel faint, and she may have shoulder pain or pain on inspiration as blood accumulates between the liver and diaphragm. Occasionally, there is bluish discoloration of periumbilical skin (Cullen's sign). The pelvic examination may provoke such pain and tenderness that a definitive mass cannot be identified (probably one half or less of the cases). A bulging cul-de-sac, can usually be appreciated by rectovaginal examination. In these circumstances, culdocentesis will yield unclotted blood in a high percentage of cases, and this procedure is usually diagnostic, especially if the hematocrit value is greater than 15%. Clots free in the cul-de-sac have undergone fibrinolysis. Usually, the patient will have a hematocrit of less than 30% while the white blood cell count is usually below 10,000/mm^3. If the patient is febrile, fever is usually low grade. With adequate blood replacement it is best to proceed immediately with laparoscopy. Further delays to pursue other investigations or vigorous pelvic examinations while being unprepared to intervene can lead to disastrous results.

In the stable patient in whom the diagnosis is in doubt or an unruptured tubal pregnancy is suspected, a less urgent management plan is justified to employ appropriate diagnostic procedures. A positive test for HCG (particularly the β-subunit) confirms the presence of a pregnancy but gives no indication of the site of nidation. The test may be negative in chronic ectopic gestations, which may present with signs of superimposed infection. An ultrasound of the pelvis is helpful in identifying adnexal masses, including some tubal pregnancies, but in early cases its greatest value lies in excluding the presence of an intrauterine gestation. The combination of a positive β-subunit HCG and absence of intrauterine pregnancy provides strong evidence in support of a tubal gestation. A follow-up examination under anesthesia together with a diagnostic laparoscopy if needed will be confirmatory of ectopic gestation or identify other possibilities. These latter steps are important because β-HCG levels may overlap normal values and increase serially comparable to that of an intrauterine pregnancy. Also, artifacts are seen on the pelvic sonogram which may simulate very closely a gestational sac. Very rarely, a heterotopic pregnancy may lead to even greater confusion. One of the diagnostic problems is corpus luteal cyst or hematoma (possibly ruptured) along with an intrauterine pregnancy. In the absence of pregnancy, a corpus luteal cyst rupture or hematoma may present in the same fashion as a ruptured ectopic gestation (e.g., amenorrhea, spotting, abdominal pain, unilateral tender pelvic mass).

The best management is early diagnosis and prompt surgical treatment. In cases with more extensive tubal damage, the standard treatment in a ruptured tubal pregnancy is salpingectomy with cornual resection followed by reperitonealization over the resection line usually utilizing the adjacent round ligament and broad ligament for this purpose. The ipsilateral ovary is not sacrificed. A ruptured interstitial pregnancy involving extensive damage to the cornu may require hysterectomy. Salpingostomy or expression of a tubal mole or incomplete abortion may be justified in women desirous of childbearing. Indeed, with proper training and instrumentation linear salpingostomy may be performed through a laparoscope. Later, a tuboplasty may be performed as needed, although the risk of a recurrent ectopic gestation will be substantial. Although still experimental, some centers are reporting success using locally injected or systemic methotrexate to treat nonemergent ectopic gestations.

DISORDERS OF THE FALLOPIAN TUBE

Fallopian Tube Malignancy

Malignancies of the oviducts (fallopian tubes) are overwhelmingly metastatic from other organs (about 90%), but primary lesions may occur, usually as adenocarcinomas (95% of the cases), even though they represent the rarest malignancies of women's genitalia. The predisposed woman is a nulligravida who is usually postmenopausal with a history of chronic salpingitis. The presence of an elongated, slightly tender mass in the adnexa, usually unilateral, less than 10 cm in diameter, and associated with lower abdominal discomfort from tubal distention and colicky pain followed by a profuse watery, serosanguineous or yellowish discharge and reduction in the size of the mass (hydrops tubae profluens) is highly suggestive of a primary malignant tumor of the oviduct. The tube is usually distended by a papillary adenomatous malignant lesion, which spreads by protruding through the fimbriated os and the lymphatic channels rather than invading through the myosalpinx. Ascites is not common, and abdominal enlargement and intestinal obstruction occur late. Postmenopausal bleeding is a common occurrence, and tubal cancer should be suspected when endometrial curettings are benign and examination of the pelvis reveals a fusiform or sausage-shaped mass. Vaginal cytology, ultrasonography, CT scan, magnetic resonance imaging (MRI) scan, and laparoscopy may lend credibility to the diagnosis of this rare pelvic condition. Characteristically, the diagnosis is delayed and not made preoperatively. A small malignant tumor found incidentally at the time of surgery for another condition might have a favorable prognosis. Otherwise, the outlook is grave despite total hysterectomy and bilateral salpingo–oophorectomy. Follow-up pelvic irradiation is recommended, but the 5-year salvage rate of less than 15% indicates the limited value of this modality or following a chemotherapeutic plan. The newer agents used in combination in a manner similar to protocols for endometrial adenocarcinoma may be more effective than past therapeutic regimens (*e.g.*, Adriamycin, cis-platinum, Cytoxan).

Other Conditions of the Oviducts and Paraovarium

Rarely, there will be unilateral or bilateral absence of the fallopian tubes, unilateral duplication with a single cornual entrance, multiple open tubular structures with independent fimbriae, atresias, unconnected tubes, absent fimbriae and other anomalies. Infertility is common, and tuboplastic efforts are usually not very successful. Related anomalies elsewhere in the müllerian duct (uterus) and urinary tract occur frequently.

Occasionally, there may be "ectopic ovarian accessory tissues" in the broad ligament near the cornu of the uterus or the normal ovary. They usually present as nodules of less than 1.0 cm in diameter, and they are predisposed to neoplastic transformation. Ovarian tissues may be found retroperitoneally near the kidney and in the groin in a hernia sac. Supernumerary ovaries should be removed when they are encountered.

Cysts may develop in the mesosalpinx from paramesonephric structures and come to lie between the tube and hilus of the ovary. Many of these are blind accessory lumens of the tube. The blind outer wolffian duct may become cystic and pedunculated (hydatid cyst of Morgagni). Rarely, they may produce acute symptoms by becoming necrotic or infected or by causing torsion of the tube and ovary. Benign, thin-walled, parovarian cysts may be single or multiple and occasionally may become large enough to produce pressure symptoms or acute distress if infarction becomes a complication associated with torsion. The ureter may be displaced or buried in the posterior wall of the cyst, making surgical removal of the intraligamentary (retroperitoneal) mass a tedious exercise. Often, surgery is undertaken in the mistaken belief that an ovarian neoplasm is present. A diagnostic laparoscopy may be helpful in distinguishing the two conditions prior to definitive surgery. Symptomatic cysts should be removed, but the majority are small, nonpalpable, and not associated with pelvic complaints.

DISORDERS OF THE OVARY

Benign tumors of the ovary may be cystic or solid. The cystic ones may be nonneoplastic (follicle, lutein, germinal inclusion, and endometrial cysts) or neoplastic (cystadenoma, pseudomucinous or serous, and benign cystic teratoma or dermoid). The solid ones are papilloma, fibroadenoma, fibroma, fibromyoma, angioma, lymphangioma, mesothelioma, chondroma, and osteoma. Other solid tumors, probably benign, are Brenner tumors, adrenal tumors, and hilus cell tumors.

Malignant tumors of the ovary may also be solid or cystic. The cystic varieties are pseudomucinous and serous papillary cystadenocarcinomas and epidermoid carcinoma arising in dermoid cysts. Primary solid carcinomas of the ovary take the form of adenocarcinoma, papillary, medullary, scirrhous, alveolar, plexiform, carcinoma simplex, mesonephroma, and chorioepithelioma. A special group of embryonic or dysontogenetic tumors includes granulosa cell carcinoma, thecoma, luteoma, arrhenoblastoma, and dysgerminoma. Other special malignant tumors are teratoma, sarcoma, and melanoma. Metastatic carcinomas may be of the following types: adenocarcinoma, Krukenberg tumor from the gastrointestinal tract, epidermoid carcinoma, and hypernephroma.

Ovarian Cysts

Formation of cysts following atresia of a follicle is physiologic. Occasionally, one or more cysts may enlarge at the expense of the others, forming a thin-walled mass up to about 5 cm in size and filled with a clear transudate. Hemorrhage into the cavity of a cystic, atretic follicle is common (follicle hematoma). Follicle cysts are the most frequent ovarian cysts, but they are the least important clinically, although they may cause temporary menstrual irregularities and alterations of flow. Occasionally, rupture may cause acute pain or even peritoneal irritation.

Lutein cysts may take the form of granulosa lutein cysts (corpus luteum cysts) and theca-lutein cysts (frequently associated with hydatidiform moles). The corpus albicans cyst is a variant or sequel of the corpus luteum cyst. Hematomas may develop in any of these structures. Corpus luteum hematomas, frequently associated with delayed menstruation, pain, and palpable mass, are not infrequently confused with tubal pregnancy. Occasionally, their rupture gives rise to considerable hemoperitoneum and acute abdominal symptoms, requiring emergent operative intervention.

Neoplastic cysts: The **pseudomucinous cystadenomas** are usually unilateral and grow very slowly, though they reach enormous dimensions. The histogenesis is thought to be from teratomatous elements within the ovary. They are multilocular and are lined with high cylindric epithelium that may be discolored by hemorrhage. They rarely become malignant or adhere to the intestines, being essentially benign and operable. Only about 10% of these tumors are papillary. If the cyst content is spilled on the peritoneum, it sometimes forms implantation metastases that cause adhesions by their continued gelatinous secretion (pseudomyxoma peritonei).

About 5% of these tumors undergo malignant degeneration. The treatment is surgical removal of the tumor unilaterally (if the tumor is unilateral, free, nonpapillary, and intact), or by total abdominal hysterectomy together with bilateral salpingo–oophorectomy in older women, or if there is a question of extension or bilateral involvement.

Serous cystadenomas, on the other hand, usually appear unilocular, though the larger ones are lobulated and multilocular. They arise from the germinal epithelium on the surface of the ovary. Many take the form of innocuous simple serous cysts without the more complex histologic features of the true serous cystadenoma. The latter may be lined with a low cylindric epithelium with papillary processes in both the inner lining of the cyst and the outer surface. The epithelium may show many of the characteristics of tubal epithelium. Psammoma bodies may be scattered throughout the stroma. They are filled with a clear, yellowish, serous fluid. Characteristically, these tumors grow in both ovaries, though not always simultaneously, and often spread between the leaves of the broad ligament. Those of the nonpapillomatous type usually are benign, but the papillary tumors have a tendency to malignant degeneration, as well as to form implantation papillomas on the peritoneum with prodigious ascites. When implants are present or there are papillary growths, a hysterectomy and bilateral salpingo–oophorectomy should be done; otherwise, a unilateral operation may suffice in young women, provided that the contralateral ovary is normal.

Dermoid cysts, or *benign teratomas,* are also common tumors, especially among young women with neoplastic cystic tumors. Only about 1% develop a malignant lesion arising in the squamous epithelium. The tumor is smooth-coated and pearl gray and shows, on cut section, a semifluid sebaceous material; hair, teeth, bone, and cartilage may be seen. Dermoid cysts are bilateral in nearly one fourth of the cases. There is a predominance of ectodermal elements, though mesodermal elements usually are also found, and occasionally even well-differentiated entodermal structures. Occasionally, thyroid tissue is present in the tumor in sufficient quantity to obscure or even exclude the presence of other elements. This tumor, the so-called struma ovarii, is usually a benign cystic variant, but in 5% to 10% malignant cases are found. These tumors may be missed in the course of a pelvic examination, as they may ride high up on their long pedicle. When suspected, diagnostic laparoscopy or pelvic sonography may be definitive in characterizing the nature of the cyst.

Teratomas may also be malignant, the fetal elements being of undifferentiated type, usually representing all three germ layers, whereas the simple dermoid cyst has only two (ectoderm and mesoderm). The teratoma is basically a solid tumor, although it may have cystic elements, while the dermoid is the reverse. Solid teratomas constitute the very small percentage of ovarian teratomas that are not cystic, probably over 1% or 2%. An extremely rare variant is the teratocarcinoma. Dermoid cysts are expanding lesions and destroy ovarian tissue by continued pressure. The cysts may be asymptomatic or, because of the long ovarian pedicle, may undergo torsion with acute symptoms or may undergo septic degeneration. Treatment is surgical, making every effort to leave intact all functioning ovarian tissue. The contralateral ovary should be inspected and transilluminated to exclude the possibility of leaving behind a small dermoid that could easily be enucleated. The malignant varieties are treated by total extirpation of the internal pelvic organs, but the prognosis is generally poor. The tumors do not ordinarily respond to irradiation or cytotoxic drugs.

Torsion is one of the most important complications of ovarian tumors; it occurs in 10% to 20% of all cases. The growth of an ovarian tumor causes it to rise out of the true pelvis, so that it may fall forward and rotate 90 degrees. Unequal growth in the cyst walls, trauma, intestinal peristalsis, or pregnancy may increase the degree of torsion. Generally, torsion of 180 degrees produces symptoms, though the cyst may twist on its pedicle two or three or even five or six times. The torsion first causes venous blocking, the arterial circulation producing a rapid increase in size, and results in hemorrhage into the lumen and areas of infarction; the damaged surface soon becomes adherent to the intestine and the omentum. If the torsion is acute, the symptoms are like those of acute peritonitis, with rigid, extremely sensitive abdomen and signs of shock. If there is no infection, the attack sometimes abates, but it generally recurs. Adhesions to the intestine may result in intestinal perforation, with peritonitis. If the tumor suppurates, it may rupture into the abdominal cavity. Uterine bleeding is common. If the patient seeks medical attention promptly, and the appropriate surgery is performed, the patient usually has an uneventful recovery; otherwise, suppuration, rupture, and general peritonitis may ensue with dire results. At the time of surgery it is important to avoid undue manipulation and untwisting the pedicle to minimize the risk of embolization.

Ovarian Carcinoma

This disease ranks next to uterine cancer in relative frequency insofar as the various forms of women's reproductive organs are concerned. The cancer may be primary or secondary to a lesion in other organs. It may be solid or cystic, the latter being more common (serous cystadenocarcinoma is the most common lesion). The great majority arise in previously benign cystadenomas. Cancerous lesions are bilateral in about half of the cases. It is estimated that about 15% of all ovarian tumors are malignant. The pathologic types have been outlined previously. From a histologic viewpoint the epithelial tumors are classifiable as serous, mucinous, endometrioid (similar to adenocarcinoma of the endometrium) mesonephroid lesions of the ovary (clear-cell carcinoma), and tumors that cannot be assigned to one of the above categories. Ovarian carcinoma spreads frequently to the tubes and the uterus and onto the pelvic peritoneum. The lumbar lymphatic glands are frequently involved, and metastases occur by bloodstream to such distant organs as the lungs and the brain. Symptoms appear late and are of insidious onset. The presence of a mass or ascites may be the first indication of disease. Menstrual dysfunction and pelvic pressure or pain may occur but are often absent. Ascites is relatively common. Weakness, anemia, weight loss, and gastrointestinal symptoms appear late.

The embryonic group of ovarian carcinomas may present special genital symptoms according to the type and the age and onset. The most common of this group is the feminizing mesenchymoma or estrogen-producing tumor (granulosa cell, thecoma, or luteoma). The granulosa-cell carcinoma is the most common variety, and it may arise at any time in life. Premenarcheal girls experience premature sex development and uterine bleeding and hypertrophy of the uterus and the endometrium. In older women the hyperplasia may develop atypical features or carcinoma of the endometrium. The counterpart of this tumor is the masculinizing ovarian neoplasm, arrhenoblastoma. There is a progressive defeminization and then masculinization of the patient. It should be mentioned that steroidogenesis may be disordered, and the hormonal effects may not coincide with the pattern suggested by the histologic picture of the tumor. Rarely, adrenal tumors of the ovary, hilus cell tumors, and gynandroblastomas are responsible for masculinizing symptoms. As a rule, the secondary sex changes gradually reverse after the tumor is removed. Another rare embryonic tumor, the dysgerminoma, is sexually indifferent, although it frequently arises in patients with pseudohermaphroditic defects. About one fourth of these embryonic tumors exhibit evidence of clinical malignancy. A conservative unilateral operation appears to be justified in young women in whom future pregnancies are important. However, some dysgerminomas are highly malignant and any suspicion of clinical malignancy (or positive evidence by frozen section) warrants a complete operation.

Prior to treatment, a malignant ovarian tumor must be staged and a systematic preoperative workup, including diagnostic procedures and a metastatic survey, must be completed. In Stage I growth is limited to the ovaries, as follows: Substage Ia, one ovary involved without ascites; Ib, both ovaries involved without ascites; and Ic, one or both ovaries involved and presence of ascitic fluid containing malignant cells. In Stage II there has been pelvic extension of the tumor: IIa, to internal pelvic organs only, or IIb, to other pelvic tissues. In Stage III there is widespread intraperitoneal abdominal metastases, and in Stage IV there is distant spread outside the peritoneal cavity.

The treatment and the prognosis for ovarian cancer will depend on the type of tumor, its histologic grade and degree of malignancy, the stage, presence of metastasis, and the age and general condition of the patient. The primary treatment is surgery, supplemented in selected cases by a follow-up course of cobalt irradiation or chemotherapeutic agents or both. Recurrent ascites can frequently be controlled palliatively by cobalt irradiation and peritoneal cytotoxic drugs. Colloidal gold used for this purpose has limited value. Intra-abdominal injections are followed by changes in the portion of the patient to permit maximum diffusion and time contact with the cytotoxic agent. If the capsule of the ovary is intact, cobalt radiation treatment is of little value. Even when the cancer has extended throughout the pelvis or to distant organs, it is advisable, whenever feasible, to excise the great bulk of the primary tumor and omentum because the procedure may result in good palliation or even temporary regression of implants at distant sites. Satisfactory palliation may also be achieved in certain patients with chemotherapeutic agents such as the alkylating agents. Cobalt irradiation may have a limited role that is useful in selected cases.

Surgical treatment for ovarian carcinoma Stage I is a satisfactory approach, but the 5-year survival is only about 65% (range 50%–80%). Adding external irradiation does not result in any substantial improvement in that figure. These early cases often have para-aortic node metastasis (approximately one case in five). Therefore, pelvic irradiation alone would not be expected to improve salvage. The use of radioactive gold or chromic phosphate should probably be restricted to protective therapies in Stage I disease when there is no gross intraabdominal spread, but the malignant tumor has ruptured or peritoneal washings are positive. The significantly improved salvage rates (90%–95%) seem to validate the value of this type of supportive therapy. Irradiation therapy in patients with spread to pelvic organs (Stage II) seems to improve survival (30%–70%), but the problem of para-aortic and subdiaphragmatic spread restricts the value of this modality since the liver and kidneys can tolerate only doses usually not considered to be cancericidal (about 2,500 rads). For the most part, all of these modalities have given way today to various chemotherapeutic protocols, which are better suited to the biological behavior of the disease.

Unfortunately, ovarian malignancies are usually nonresectable when they are first recognized. They disseminate early and the extent of spread calls for reliance upon surgery to "debulk" the tumor to the smallest volume possible prior to appropriate chemotherapy. This is referred to as *cytoreduction.* Chemotherapy is most effective when all gross tumor appears in nodules and lesions in sizes of less than 2.0 cm. In contrast with the endometrium (under 9%) and the cervix (about 12%–13%), there are distant lesions in ovarian carcinoma at the time of diagnosis in about two thirds of the cases. Single-agent therapy with melphalan or chlorambucil will offer a favorable tumor response in 12 to 18 months in two thirds or more of the cases (except in poorly differentiated tumors). Cyclophosphamide and thiotepa have been effective as well in perhaps 50% to 60% of the cases. Nonresponsive patients can be offered combination chemotherapy consisting of actinomycin D, 5-fluorouracil, and cyclophosphamide, given in daily regimens for 5 days repeated every 4 weeks unless toxic effects justify delay or discontinuation. The possibility of cardiomyopathy leading to heart failure calls for a limit on the total dosage of doxorubicin (approximately 550 mg/M^2 body surface). Hexamethylmelamine, Adriamycin, and cis-platinum, often used in combination with other chemotherapeutic agents, are enjoying current popularity, particularly the latter two, as a second line of defense in recurrent cases. The tendency now is to be more aggressive even in selecting the initial plan of therapy.

Nearly all patients today receive surgical therapy to reduce the bulk of tumor to the smallest volume possible so that the maximum effectiveness of adjuvant chemotherapy can be realized. After about 12 courses of chemotherapy the patient can be evaluated for discontinuation of the drug or for possible modification if residual disease is present. Accordingly, a "second look" exploratory laparotomy may be useful to inspect, palpate, and biopsy suspicious lesions or nodes in the pelvis and abdomen.

The management of advanced ovarian malignancy is very complicated. Drug toxicity may give rise to serious hematologic, cardiac, nephric, or gastrointestinal damage causing significant modification of drug regimens, long delays between administrations, or early discontinuation of therapy. Electrolyte, fluid, blood, magnesium replacements may be required repeatedly in some cases. Bowel obstruction is a particular problem, and the risk of fistula formation may call for a palliative bypass procedure to accomplish an ileotransverse colon side-to-side anastomosis. Occasionally, diverting ileostomy or colostomy, nasogastric and enteric decompression, fluid administration, paracenteses, thoracoenteses, hyperalimentation, and pain control may present complex management problems in addition to the requirement to provide the necessary emotional support.

The 5-year survival rate for all cases of ovarian cancer probably does not exceed 25% to 30%. For this reason, the emphasis should be on a high index of suspicion, early diagnosis, and prompt surgical intervention. Persistent masses of more than 5 cm to 6 cm in size in the region of the ovary, particularly if there are solid components, should arouse the suspicion of malignancy until proved to be benign. Inspection of the pelvis through the laparoscope is helpful in establishing the diagnosis. Pelvic ultrasound and other imaging modalities (CAT scan, MRI) to study the pelvis and abdomen are important diagnostic methods. In addition, cul-de-sac aspiration and cell block studies, as well as a careful examination under anesthesia, may be required. All women over 30 years of age should have periodic pelvic examinations every 12 months and, at the same time, should have a cytologic examination of the vaginal posterior forniceal pool. It should be borne in mind that an easily palpable ovary in a postmenopausal woman when the gonad is normally atrophic may represent enlargement by an early neoplasm. A cystic or solid adnexal mass in a female beyond the reproductive years is a call for alarm, as is a solid tumor at any age.

REMOTE EFFECTS OF THE INJURIES OF CHILDBIRTH AND GYNECOLOGIC THERAPY

Although insufficiency of the pelvic floor may arise from pelvic and vaginal surgery or on a congenital basis, the great majority of such defects result from the injuries of childbirth. These defects are accentuated in the postmenopausal era when poor estrogen support of the tissues gives rise to pelvic insufficiency of muscles and fascia. The specific defects may be classified on an anatomic basis as follows:

I. Injuries to the levator sling (disruption of endopelvic fascial layer in the rectovaginal septum)
   A. Rectocele (most common, bearing-down sensation, constipation)—requires manual expression of fecal material in rectal pouch
   B. Enterocele–herniation of peritoneum between uterosacral ligaments through the pouch of Douglas into the rectovaginal septum
II. Injuries to the anterior vaginal wall (vesicovaginal septum is stretched or torn)
   A. "Urethrocele"—stress urinary incontinence and disappearance of the posterior angle between the posterior surface of the urethra and the bladder base. In reality this condition is better defined as a urethral detachment from the normal lower posterior pubic location caused by incompetency of the pubourethral ligament resulting in a subpubic rather than retropubic location of the proximal sphincteric urethra.
   B. Cystocele—protrusion of bladder downward into the vaginal canal; stasis and infection of urine, pressure symptoms (residual urine)
III. Injuries involving uterine support (injury or stretching of the cardinal ligaments)
   A. Descensus or prolapse of the uterus—pressure, decubitus ulcer of cervix with bleeding
      1. First degree. The cervix lies between the level of the ischial spines and the vaginal introitus.
      2. Second degree. The cervix protrudes through the introitus while the corpus remains in the vagina.
      3. Third degree. The cervix and the body of the uterus have passed through the introitus, and the vaginal canal is inverted.
      4. When the entire uterus protrudes beyond the vaginal introitus, it is referred to as *procidentia,* which sometimes is referred to as a fourth-degree descensus.

B. Retrodisplacement of the uterus—possible backache, dyspareunia, rectal complaints, especially if fixed and enlarged
   1. Retroflexion. The body of the uterus lies posteriorly while the cervix retains its usual position in the vagina; the body is flexed posteriorly in the region of the isthmus.
   2. Retroverted. The fundus rotates posteriorly and the cervix anteriorly, maintaining a normal axis.
   3. Retrocession. The entire uterus has sagged backward into the posterior pelvis.
IV. Genital fistulas (trauma of operations, pressure necrosis in prolonged labor, trauma in childbirth, or extension of malignant disease)
   A. Urinary tract fistulas—vesicovaginal, vesicocervical, or vesicouterine
      1. Vesicovaginal. This is the most common type of fistula. They most often follow hysterectomy or extension of cancer from the cervix and elsewhere. Injuries of childbirth are no longer a common cause. It frequently follows therapeutic radiation.
      2. Ureterovaginal. This has become more frequent in recent years because of increased use of major pelvic surgery, particularly hysterectomy.
   B. Rectovaginal fistulas—rectal injury in childbirth, extension of cervical cancer, radiation necrosis
V. Injuries to the cervix uteri (lacerations, eversion, ectopion, erosion, chronic cervicitis, chronic discharge per vaginum; possible antecedent for cervical malignant disease)
VI. Injuries to pelvic joints
   A. Separation of the symphysis pubis—pain on locomotion
   B. Dislocation of the coccyx—soreness and tenderness

The concept of the role of the levator muscles and the importance of providing a smaller aperture with an adequate obturator form the basis of modern vaginal surgery. The pelvic diaphragm is formed by the fan-shaped levator ani muscles blending together in the midline to surround and support the three openings in the pelvic floor. Fibroareolar connective tissue providing both ligamentous and fascial supports passes beneath the bladder and forms a sheath around the vagina and rectum. Components of this supporting endopelvic fascia include pubo-vesicocervical, paravaginal, and perirectal sheaths, as well as condensations incorporating the cardinal and uterosacral ligaments. It should be borne in mind that a great number of multiparous women have some degree of relaxation of the pelvic floor; however, only a small percentage are symptomatic and require special gynecologic attention. Moreover, presenting symptoms must not be attributed to an obvious anatomic defect until other conditions have been excluded. For example, urinary incontinence, even in the presence of an obvious urethrocele, may be due to intrinsic or extrinsic bladder or pelvic conditions or even to a neurologic or emotional disturbance. Thus, a careful workup is often required, usually including cystoscopic, cystographic, cystometric, urodynamic studies, complete urinalysis and cultures or, occasionally, upper urinary tract studies.

In patients with stress incontinence, the vesical neck assumes the most dependent portion of the bladder and becomes the point of maximal impact transmitted from the dome to the base. This can be evaluated with a stress voiding cystourethrogram; with the patient standing and straining, the posterior urethrovesical angle may be increased beyond the usual 95 to 105 degrees. In the standing position the downward angulation of the proximal urethera in relation to the vertical is also increased beyond the usual 30 degrees or less if the defect is advanced (angle of inclination). Thus, the proximal urethra is usually wide in diameter, funnel in shape, and poorly contractile. When the posterior urethral angle is increased, the anatomic defect on x ray has been referred to as type I in contrast to type II, which is characterized by both an increased posterior urethrovesical angle and an angle of inclination. It should be understood, however, that these measurements and designations in and of themselves are not as important as assessment of the functional anatomy and may represent progressive relaxation, not two conditions, which will be discussed later. When scarring is likewise present, there may be an additional loss of mobility, motility, and elasticity and loss of sphincteric action since the elevated intraurethral tone relative to the bladder is diminished. In the presence of bladder infection, there is an increase in detrusor irritability, and urge incontinence develops as well as stress incontinence.

It should be borne in mind that urgency and urge incontinence are symptomatic hallmarks of urinary tract infection, and associated factors are obstruction, neurologic disease, congenital malformations, tumors, polyps, and drug therapy. Posturinary dribbling suggests expression of urine from a urethral diverticulum, although this symptom may also be a sign of urethral stricture. Weakness of detrusor action, or obstruction of the outflow of the urethra, or combinations of the two may be responsible for urinary retention and overdistention of the bladder, so-called overflow incontinence, which may be caused by a variety of abnormalities. Neurogenous chronic overdistention and retention must never be overlooked as classic causes of incontinence. Diabetic neuronitis is becoming a frequent and important cause of difficulty. Thus, it is apparent that in no other disorder of the genitourinary tract are the medical history and general, as well as pelvic, examination more important.

There is no single therapeutic approach to the management of patients with pelvic floor insufficiency. Some will respond to reassurance and perineal exercises. The use of a pessary for such conditions as retrodisplacement of the uterus, urinary incontinence, and uterine prolapse is palliative rather than a definitive plan of management except, perhaps, in elderly women who are not candidates for surgery. Most of the specific anatomic defects occur in combination, so that the surgeon usually has more than a single objective in reconstructing the pelvic floor. Moreover, the proper selection of surgical management in cases of pelvic insufficiency will depend on the age and the general condition of the patient, the desirability of preserving menstruation and childbearing function, the degree of descensus uteri, the condition of the uterus (including the cervix), the presence and the degree of cystocele and urethrocele, the presence and the degree of rectocele or enterocele, previous vaginal surgery and, above all, the presence and the duration of distressing symptoms. The symptoms do not always parallel the degree of pelvic relaxation.

Urinary loss that is potentially amenable to a successful reparative surgical effort must have strictly an anatomic basis. Urine is lost only in relation to stress or positional changes. Normal bladder function is present after involuntary losses. The patient is comfortable with voiding; there is no dribbling or bed wetting; the problem is gravitational, not associated with urgency and frequency. Most of all, the condition is a social problem about which the patient is concerned.

Checking the patient in the lithotomy and erect positions gives a fairly accurate comparison of the degree of severity of urinary incontinence. Elevation of the urethrovesical junction to a high retropubic position is a maneuver common to most of the tests devised to inhibit the loss of urine after water instillation, that is, the Bonney test, two fingers; the Marchetti test, two Allis forceps applied to the vesical neck region of the vaginal mucosa in an area previously anesthetized; and the Read test, two rubber-covered clamps applied to the same region. It should

be understood that these tests performed traditionally as a routine in workup are not always reliable and must not be the determining factor in selecting a type of management.

Determination of bladder capacity, caloric and tactile sensations, residual urine, cystometry, and direct observation of the anatomy and the functional relationships through urethrocystoscopy are essential preoperative investigations. Additionally, sophisticated tests are now available for cystometric examination. Important among these evaluations are the exteroceptive sensation tests demonstrating an intactness of touch and temperature perceptions as well as a rapid and sphincter response to a pinprick of the bulbocavernosus muscle, which indicates a proper functioning pudendal nerve parasympathetic motor pathway. Another evaluative technique is based on the fact that neurogenic bladders have a normal smooth muscle stretch reflex in response to instillation of 100 ml of water at a flow rate of 60 ml/minute (rise of 5–18 cm of water). However, when urecholine is administered in small doses (2.5 mg, subcutaneously), bladder hypersensitivity at the neuromuscular junction and ganglionic synapse results in pressure responses of 15 cm of water or more over control values. If there is a neurologic defect in all types of major disorders (e.g., cortico-regulatory tract, sensory limb of the lower reflex arc, motor limb of the segmental reflex arc), or any combination of the three, absence of sensation in the saddle area is noted in all neurogenic bladders except the uninhibited type (CNS damage). The neurogenic bladder may be the only sign of a neurologic deficit. Lesions above the micturitional reflex center at the sacral cord level of S_2, S_3, and S_4 give rise to uninhibited neurogenic bladder (higher centers, multiple sclerosis, tumor, etc.), or reflex neurogenic bladder (upper motor neuron cord lesion associated with high cervical disease or syringomyelia). Lesions occurring below the micturitional reflex center may be motor paralytic (anterior horn cells; multiple sclerosis or Guillain-Barré syndrome); sensory neurogenic bladder (tabes dorsalis or diabetes mellitus); or autonomous neurogenic bladder (disk, tumor, meningomyelocele, trauma, etc.). Reflex neurogenic bladder and uninhibited neurogenic bladder have small bladder capacity and uninhibited contractions, whereas sacral lesions lead to a flaccid bladder and overflow incontinence.

Electromyography of the periurethral tissues shows that urinary continence is associated with surface continuity of the urinary tract, proper pressure gradient between the urethra and bladder favoring the former, and normal detrusor muscle activity. Motor unit firing increases progressively until bladder capacity is reached. When the normal patient either thinks of urination or actually performs the act, the motor impulses to the urogenital diaphragm abruptly stop. Normally, no uninhibited voiding contractions are noted in the bladder during filling in the cystometric evaluations or at capacity when the patient is in discomfort. There is no abnormal detrusor hyperactivity or involuntary contraction in response to coughing, heel bouncing, or percussing the bladder as it is filled. When these reactions are present, the bladder is usually unstable (dyssynergic) and the patient experiences a false type of stress urinary incontinence in which losses occur in response to detrusor contractions coming on after a slight delay following the stimulus (coughing, sneezing, laughing, changing positions, running, and walking). Once the urinary stream is provoked in relation to urgency and frequency, there may be an urgency incontinence that is not controllable by will. Classically, organically based stress urinary incontinence is associated with a measure of control in which the urinary stream can be stopped in the process of voiding. The patient with the unstable bladder loses urine in large volumes, in contrast with small instantaneous leakages in immediate response to intra-abdominal pressures in anatomically based problems. The unstable bladder is quiescent at night, but women losing urine on a gravitational basis will also not experience enuresis except possibly in changing positions in bed rather abruptly.

Carbon dioxide urethroscopy is quite important in assessing the sphincteric urethral segment, particularly in recurrent incontinent cases. Opening pressures of the sphincteric urethra may be low (25–50 cm of water). Closures of the segment may be sluggish, asymmetric, and incomplete in the presence of marked periurethral scarring. These cases usually represent problems of loss of sphincteric urethra, which may give rise to considerable urinary incontinence, despite a retropubic anatomic position. Often, these patients will require a combined transvaginal and retropubic operative approach to break up the adhesive bands and to mobilize the vesical neck. It is important to individualize the workup and to select potential operative candidates very carefully.

It is estimated that about 10% of patients with urinary incontinence have an unstable bladder; in about one half of these, there will be an anatomic defect in addition. A bolus of urine sitting in a funneled dependent proximal urethra will often trigger detrusor hyperirritability and give rise to an urgency-frequency-urgency incontinence syndrome. These few patients represent exceptions to the rule that anatomically based urinary incontinence of the true stress type have a normal voiding pattern. Another exception is the patient who has a cystocele, urinary retention, and infection in addition to a dependent vesical neck. Here, too, urgency, frequency, and even dysuria may be overriding symptoms.

Every effort should be exerted to make the initial surgical procedure the definitive one, for the likelihood of success is never again as good. It is unacceptable to insist on a single operative approach and try to make every patient adapt to a stereotyped problem of management. The traditional failure rate of 15% to 20% with the initial operation emphasizes this lack of individualization of symptomatic cases. An even more distressing figure has been the recurrence rate of 50% after 5 years.

Plicating the pubovesicocervical fascia and the internal vesical sphincter (Kelly or Kennedy operation) has represented the traditional approach for most cases of urinary stress incontinence, a policy now needing revision as will be outlined later. If there is also relaxation of the vaginal and rectal walls, the procedure may be combined as an anterior and posterior colporrhaphy. Likewise, the cervix may be amputated, and the cardinal ligaments plicated onto the anterior stump if the cervix is elongated (Manchester operation); however, this approach does not enjoy much favor in this country. When there is a significant degree of uterine prolapse, it is usually better to perform a vaginal hysterectomy. The Spalding-Richardson composite operation in which the cervical isthmus is spared and used in the reconstruction to gain better pelvic support is rarely used today. In certain elderly women, it is possible to do a simple colpocleisis (Le Fort operation) to correct uterine prolapse.

When the patient's principal difficulty is descensus of the vesical neck and stress urinary incontinence, a retropubic urethral suspension (Marshall-Marchetti-Krantz operation) may be the preferred approach. When the periurethral tissues (pubourethral ligaments) are sutured into the Cooper's ligament (Burch technique) there is a potential danger of overangulation of the urethrovesical angle and possibility of enterocele formation. The traditional Marshall-Marchetti-Krantz procedure calls for the suspensory sutures to be placed in the pubic periosteum. These sutures have a low but real risk of causing symptomatic periostitis. The retropubic approach is particularly advantageous when the abdomen needs to be entered for some benign pelvic condition. Patients with a dependent vesical neck with considerable funneling may need plication retropubically before the ventral suspension is performed. Primary cases with true stress urinary incontinence, particularly those with funneling, dependent vesical neck and straightened PUV angle, are best handled by the retropubic approach. If other endopelvic fascial defects are present (e.g., cystocele, uterine descensus, enterocele, rectocele), the approach may of necessity be both vaginal and abdominal.

When a previous repair has failed, one may use a fascial sling to provide a suspensory support to the urethra, thereby producing the necessary acute angulation of the urethra at the vesical neck (Goebell-Stoeckel operation and its Aldridge and Studdiford modifications). After complete mobilization of the urethra and paraurethral tissues, monofilament, nonabsorbable sutures can be placed by a special instrument to suspend the urethrovesical junction retropubically by exposing the spaces of Retzius transvaginally (revised Pereyra procedure). The short, heavy-boned, obese woman or one whose condition is complicated by chronic coughing or sneezing may be handled best by a combined incontinence operation performed as the primary procedure. Likewise, the combined approach may be the procedure of choice in recurrent cases which necessitate tedious dissections to mobilize a scarred fixed sphincteric urethra and vesical neck. This operation combines an anterior colporrhaphy with a suprapubic ventral urethrovesical suspension after complete mobilization of the urethrovesical segment. In addition, after all periurethral adhesions are lysed, the urethral fascia is pleated from above as well as below to eliminate funneling in the proximal portion and to lengthen the organ. Also, if the bladder descends appreciably below the lowest margin of the symphysis during the effort of straining (more than 4 cm), or if there is considerable scarring and fixation of periurethral tissues, the retropubic ventral suspension operation must be substituted for or combined with an anterior colporrhaphy if a high success rate is to be anticipated. To be successful, the urethra must be of normal tonicity, it must be well supported and yet be free to move and contract normally, and the proximal urethra must be located in front of the main target point in the transmission of the force in intra-abdominal pressure from the dome to the base of the bladder, where pressures as high as 75 mmHg or more may occur during times of abrupt stress.

Posthysterectomy prolapse of the vagina can be caused by an inadequate suspension of the vault to the cardinal ligaments or by overlooking an enterocele. Often the prolapsed vagina has an associated cystocele and enterocele sac in the descended part. An extensive vaginal reparative procedure is required to relieve distressing symptoms. The current procedure of choice is sacrospinous ligament vaginal fixation, but a vaginal sacropexy may be another alternative.

In the last analysis, the best treatment is prophylaxis by providing good antepartal care (adequate nutrition), good intrapartal care (conservative obstetrics, prophylactic forceps, and episiotomy), and good postpartal care (bladder care, prompt treatment of lacerations, infections, and so forth, and perineal exercises). Perineal exercises may be of value either as an effective means of correcting mild stress incontinence in patients with slight anatomic defects or as preoperative or postoperative supportive measures in surgical cases and after childbirth.

Urinary Tract Injuries

Urinary tract obstructions, fistulization, and extravasations involving the urethra, bladder, or ureter may be serious complications of gynecologic disease, childbirth, and therapeutic intervention. There may be extensions of destructive granulomatous or cancerous lesions, irradiation damage, or direct tissue injuries sustained in the course of instrumentations and various operative procedures performed on genital tract organs in the immediate vicinity of urinary structures. Strangulations and tissue necrosis with slough following misplaced ligatures, acute angulations, and crushing injuries produce fistulas and extravasation of urine with tracts communicating between affected organs and structures. The direction of urine drainage may be external, intraperitoneal, or retroperitoneal, depending upon the nature and site of injury. The various types of fistulae are designated on the basis of the affected organs between which are communicating tracts, for example, urethrovaginal, vesicovaginal, or ureterovaginal, occurring singly or in combination. Usually, gynecologic surgery involving hysterectomy is the etiologic factor in most fistulas found in the terminal ureters or bladder. Resection of a suburethral diverticulum, anterior colporrhaphy, and certain urologic procedures are more likely to give rise to urethrovaginal fistulas. The ureters may be damaged in the course of eradicating pelvic disease associated with massive adhesions (pelvic inflammatory disease or endometriosis), when the ureter is displaced (broad ligament cyst or leiomyoma), or by devascularizing it in the course of stripping it out of its bed in the process of pelvic lymphadenectomy and radical hysterectomy for malignant disease. Extensive bladder adhesions following prior low cervical cesarean sections can make mobilization for a repeat cesarean birth or hysterectomy a risky undertaking. Postpartal urinary fistulas arise from prolonged labor resulting in ischemic necrosis from extreme continued pressure of the presenting part or, possibly, from a traumatic instrumentation. In modern obstetrics these causes are rare (less than 0.1% of deliveries), although bladder injury in the course of repeat cesarean births remains a potential problem. Rarely, in the course of various pelvic operations there may be multiple injuries involving the bowel (uretero- or vesicoenteric or rectal fistula), uterus (uretero- or vesicouterine or cervical fistula), and free abdominal cavity (uretero- or vesicoperitoneal fistula).

The site or sites of damage, extent of injury, and the subsequent pattern of urinary drainage will determine the nature of symptoms and signs, therapeutic approach, and prognosis. The timing of the problem is also affected by the etiology, since unrecognized structural defects produced at operation may give rise to urinary leakage through the vagina, wound, or abdominal drain site almost immediately. Intraperitoneal leakage may produce acute peritonitis and ileus. Severe colicky flank pain referred into the groin, costovertebral angle flank tenderness, and fever suggest ureteral injury with obstruction. When urinary leakage is delayed until 10 to 28 days postoperatively, progressive ischemic necrosis and tissue slough secondary to ligature or crushing injury are a likely possibility.

Proper management must be based on an appropriate urologic investigation to determine the extent, nature, and cause of the urinary injury. A bladder instillation of methylene blue coupled with intravenous phenosulfonphthalein (PSP) administration is a useful method of distinguishing between a vesicovaginal fistula (blue drainage) and a ureterovaginal fistula (red drainage). A three vaginal sponge test is used to check on these dye leakages. Excretory urography, cystourethroscopy, retrograde pyelography when a ureteral catheter can be passed, and CT or MRI scans as necessary are important diagnostic methods. The possibility of multiple injuries must be considered, which may call for uterine, bowel, and other studies. Prompt diagnosis is required to prevent an array of potentially lethal complications, including obstructive

uropathy, hydronephrosis, perirenal or psoas abscess, peritonitis, thrombophlebitis, anuria, and uremia.

Emergency treatment may consist of measures to combat shock, blood loss, and dehydration and to relieve acute urinary obstruction by an appropriate drainage method (catheter, gallbladder; "J" or "T" tube in the ureter; nephrostomy, etc.). A vesicoperitoneal fistula with a deteriorating clinical situation necessitates an immediate laparotomy to stop the intra-abdominal leakage or developing urinoma and abscess formation. Otherwise, fistula repairs should be delayed until all the necrotic and inflamed tissues have resolved to create a clean epithelialized tract. This waiting period may require 4 to 6 months, although some time may be conserved by administering cortisone to accelerate the healing process. Surgical principles include proper exposure; complete excision of the fistula tract(s); mobilization of the tissues; accurate closure without tension on the suture line; avoiding trauma, hematoma, and infection; and proper urinary drainage postoperatively until healing has occurred.

The great majority of the posthysterectomy vesicovaginal fistulas can be successfully closed transvaginally by partial colpocleisis (Latzko procedure). Multiple tracts and fistulas close to the uretheral orifice will usually require a transvesical approach. Severe scarring, poor blood supply, and large defects may require using adjacent muscle tissues with their independent blood supply in the repair when the potential for healing is in doubt. A concomitant ureteral injury would require a combined abdominal–vaginal approach. Severely damaged or severed terminal ureters are best treated by excising the diseased segment and reimplanting the healthy proximal end into the bladder (ureteroneocystostomy). A splinting catheter can be used for 10 to 14 days.

The best treatment obviously is one of prevention. In the better medical centers in the United States, the incidence of urinary tract injuries on gynecologic services should be less than 1.0% following major gynecologic surgery. Modern technics to protect or augment ureteral blood supply in the course of radical hysterectomy and to suspend the ureter have reduced fistulization from about 10% to 15% down to less than 4% in a number of studies. There should be no hesitancy to isolate or catheterize the ureters as a preliminary to difficult pelvic dissections, to inject dye into the bladder during or after the procedure before the abdomen is closed, or even to open the bladder to identify its margins in the "frozen" pelvis. If prevention of tissue injury is not possible, the best reparative results are at the time of damage in context with the initial operation. Subsequently, the decisive postoperative variable in success of repair is timing because no effort by any technique will be successful in diseased tissues. Rarely, small fistulas will heal in time and some will respond to local therapies. However, for the most part, the approach is surgical with anticipated successful results in the 90% range for the initial effort.

Rectovaginal Fistulas

Rectovaginal fistulas may develop from obstetric trauma, injury in the course of gynecologic procedures (posterior colporrhaphy, etc.), proctologic surgery, destructive diseases (malignancies), irradiation damage, trauma (straddle injuries, etc.), instrumentations, and others (Crohn's disease, etc.). Successful repairs depend upon adequate blood supply, a proper waiting period to improve tissue integrity after fistulization, preventing fecal contamination of suture line and infection (possible preliminary fecal diversion as required, antibiotic coverage, etc.), mobilization of tissues, excision of fistula tract(s), and closure without tension. Preliminary bowel preparation and cathartic cleansing as well as antibiotic bowel prep may be desirable. In low fistulas, the rectal suture line can be protected by a turned-down Warren flap of upper vaginal mucosa or by pulling down a mobilized segment of anterior rectal wall (Noble-Mengert technique). The Bricker vascular colonic pedicle flap technique may be required, or low colonic anastomosis must be performed with irradiation damage.

GYNECOLOGIC ENDOCRINOPATHIES

Disorders of Menstruation

Irregular or excessive bleeding from the uterus is one of the most common symptoms that the gynecologist is called upon to treat. Abnormal bleeding may manifest itself by profuse, prolonged or too frequent periodic flow or by bleeding between periods. Menstrual disorders may be classified as follows:

I. Disorders of incidence of menstruation
   A. Polymenorrhea—intervals are short
   B. Oligomenorrhea—intervals are lengthened
   C. Amenorrhea
      1. Primary—patient has never menstruated, and the diagnosis is not made before age 16
      2. Secondary—cessation of menses for 3 months or longer
      3. Physiologic—before puberty (or age 16), during pregnancy or lactation, after menopause
      4. Cryptomenorrhea—mechanical obstruction of the egress of uterine flow
      5. Uterine origin—good ovarian function, but uterus does not respond
      6. Functional—disturbance of the hypothalamic-pituitary ovarian axis

II. Disorders in amount of menstrual flow
   A. Hypomenorrhea—scanty menstrual flow
   B. Hypermenorrhea—profuse or prolonged flow (menorrhagia); also, there may be a disturbance in the functioning of the corpus luteum with irregular shedding of the endometrium and prolonged flow.

III. Periodic intermenstrual bleeding—ovulatory bleeding (midcycle)

IV. Premenstrual spotting—luteal phase (defect caused by impaired function of the corpus luteum)

V. Anovulatory uterine bleeding
   A. Anovulation—this is the most important single cause of abnormal bleeding in the absence of demonstrable pelvic lesions. Anovulatory periods are common at the time of puberty and during the climacterium, although they may occur from a variety of causes at any time during menstrual life. The atypical character of the uterine mucosa may be brought about by the prolonged action of moderate amounts of unopposed estrogen over a long time, or it may result from relatively short periods of hyperestrinism.
   B. Hyperplasia of the endometrium (cystic, cystic and adenomatous, adenomatous, typical or atypical)—in menopausal or postmenopausal women, atypical lesions may be noted that frequently predispose to or coexist with adenocarcinoma.

VI. Arrhythmic uterine bleeding (metrorrhagia)—there may be continuous bleeding (starting at the time of the expected menses), acyclic interval hemorrhage, intermenstrual spotting, bleeding after amenorrhea, or atypical irregular hemorrhage. This bleeding may be due to a variety of local and systemic conditions, but in older women cancer must be excluded. This type of abnormal bleeding occurs in more than one fourth of all nonpregnant women of childbearing age who seek treatment for bleeding disorder. Breakthrough irregular bleeding is one of the frequent side effects of oral contraceptives, particularly those with the lowest estrogen content. It is estimated that about 40% of patients over 40 years of age have some uterine or pelvic pathology that may contribute to the symptom of abnormal uterine bleeding. The common causes of arrhythmic bleeding are carcinoma of the cervix, submucous leiomyoma, endometrial hyperplasia, cervicitis, cervical or endometrial polyps, endometrial cancer, systemic diseases, and a small, miscellaneous groups of unknown etiology. Thus, a thorough uterine curettage is imperative in these cases to exclude cancer as a diagnostic consideration.

Since most abnormal bleeding is due to either organic causes or complications of pregnancy, these possibilities must be excluded. Many other cases are ascribable to psychogenic causes or no definite cause can be detected. Thus, it is a serious error to assume immediately that the cause is a disturbance of ovarian endocrine mechanisms without subjecting the patient to careful study. Moreover, an obvious ovarian dysfunction may be due to a primary defect or to some pathologic lesion, or it may be secondary to malfunction of other endocrine glands, notably the pituitary, the thyroid, and the adrenals. A systemic illness may present itself initially in association with dysfunctional uterine bleeding as the prominent symptom.

Menstruation Regulation and Dysfunction

The ovary is fully capable of an adult response before puberty, but these normal functions do not occur until there is a diminished sensitivity to the hypothalamic centers to a negative inhibitory feedback of gonadal steroids. When this sensitivity is gradually lost after about age 8, the gonadotropin secretion increases, promoting estrogen production as the follicular units mature.

The usual sequence of events are breast development (thelarche), pubarche (sexual hair growth), peak height velocity, and menarche, which occurs between the ages of 10.5 and 15.5 years (mean of 12.6 years in the United States). Puberty is considered "precocious" if signs of secondary sexual development appear before age 8 or menstruation (or estrogen-withdrawal bleeding) occurs before age 9 (normal range 9.1–17.7 years). When this early sexual development proceeds along the normal maturational progression, the precocity is "isosexual" (about 90%). Precocious puberty is "constitu-

tional" when it is without identifiable cause. The actual age of pubertal development and onset of menses is controlled by genetic factors, socioeconomic conditions, nutrition, and general health.

Reduction in FSH, LH, and estrogen levels to prepubertal values is noted in anorexia nervosa, and amenorrhea may be an early symptom. A decreased fat-lean ratio or vigorous athletic activity may delay the menarche and give rise to primary amenorrhea. There will, therefore, be variation in the time and sequence of these events. In addition, there may be precocious pseudopuberty in a small number of cases caused by hormones arising from sources other than the normal gonads, for example, hypothyroid disorder, adrenal adenoma, ovarian estrogen-producing tumor, choriocarcinoma (gonadotropin-producing lesions), or cerebral neoplasm, trauma, or infection.

Of special interest is the McCune-Albright syndrome, presumably caused by a congenital defect in the posterior hypothalamus; it results in loss of normal inhibition of gonadotropin production and release. The result is true precocious puberty found in association with café au lait spots and polyostotic fibrous dysplasia (cysts) of bone, which produce fractures following minimal trauma. True precocious puberty may also be found with diffuse encephalopathy and idiopathic epilepsy (Sturge-Weber syndrome). Certain tumors of the cortex may destroy the area (near the visual and olfactory centers) responsible for inhibiting the posterior hypothalamus in the prepubertal individual. Lesions in the posterior region of the tuber cinereum or near the mammillary bodies, may produce precocious puberty (e.g., hamartoma, ganglioneuromas). Neurofibromatosis (von Recklinghausen's disease) is associated with café au lait spots and precocious puberty. In some cases, pineal tumors in children give rise to premature development. The same is true of juvenile hypothyroidism. In addition to elevated TSH, there may be elevated gonadotropins (precocious puberty and polycystic ovaries) as well as elevated prolactin (galactorrhea). These changes are reversed when proper thyroid replacement therapy is instituted.

In the true form of puberty arising from estrogens elaborated by the ovaries, there is a sequence of progressive events characterized not only by formation and maintenance of secondary sexual characteristics but also by biological events representing certain tissue changes in response to endogenous estrogen (e.g., cervical mucus, vaginal cornification, and proliferative endometrium). During the early months after the menarche, uterine bleeding episodes are likely to be heavy and irregular since they represent anovulatory cycles. Finally, the definitive developmental response occurs; it is represented by the appearance of a positive feedback estrogenic mechanism on the hypothalamus. At this level of maturity in the hypothalamic-pituitary-gonadal axis, true menstrual function occurs by the creation of a midcycle LH surge and ovulation, which ends the so-called period of "adolescent sterility" and disordered bleeding pattern. Elaboration of progesterone resulting from ovulation and development of the corpus luteum has the effect of growth limitation on the endometrium. The corpus luteum has a normal life span of about 12 to 14 days, and during that time the structure secretes both estrogens and progesterone. In the absence of pregnancy, these hormones decline as the corpus luteum degenerates and menses follows as a consequence of universal, orderly, and progressive events occurring in the endometrium. In response to rhythmic waves of vasoconstriction of increasing duration, there is widespread ischemia, disintegration, and slough of the endometrium.

This recycling mechanism associated with normal menstrual physiology is dependent, therefore, upon the ability of gonadal steroids to evoke in the hypothalamus a negative feedback to promote gonadotropin (FSH/LH) secretion and a positive feedback to release GnRH to create the subsequent cyclic LH plus FSH peaks necessary for ovulation. The tonic GnRH center lies in the median eminence of the hypothalamus and the cyclic positive feedback hypothalamic center is located in the preoptic area. The ovaries must be responsive to the gonadotropins, and in turn the steroids elaborated must be able to affect the proper cyclic changes in the endometrium associated with preparation for egg implantation. Thus, any defect or disturbance of function arising in the hypothalamus, pituitary, ovaries, uterus, or extragonadal hormonal disorders involving the thyroid or adrenal glands may lead to abnormal menses. The disordered pattern may vary from frequent heavy periods (polymenorrhea with hypermenorrhea) to infrequent light periods or absence of menses (oligomenorrhea with hypomenorrhea, or amenorrhea). These dysfunctions often associated with chronic anovulation are more prevalent at either end of the reproductive era, although they do occur at various times during adult menstrual life. Fortunately, most patients with precocious puberty remain anovulatory for long periods, although pregnancies have occurred in the "true" type at very early ages, for example, one term delivery by cesarean section in a child at age 5.

In addition to the factors previously noted, a number of nonspecific causes may be found that include significant swings in weight, anemia, emotional stress, and all the ill effects of certain drugs sometimes found in association with galactorrhea (tranquilizers, antidepressants, methyldopa, reserpine, and others).

In the face of a mature hypothalamic-pituitary-ovarian axis, chronic anovulation is often found in association with two major types of pathophysiologic disturbances, regardless of the specific underlying defect. On the one hand, the estradiol signal to the hypothalamus may be inadequate to evoke the LH surge through a positive feedback mechanism. On the other hand, estrogen levels may not fall sufficiently to achieve the proper FSH response for ovarian follicular stimulation. In context with these defects, postpubertal girls may remain anovulatory because of lack of a mature mechanism achieving ovulation through the positive feedback, and, in the premenopausal woman, the disturbance may have its genesis in the lack of ovarian follicles to secrete sufficient estrogen to provoke an LH surge. Impaired metabolism and clearance of estradiol (hepatic disease, hypothyroidism, etc.) may not permit the proper nadir in steroid levels to occur. There may be extragonadal peripheral conversion of C-19 precursors, such as androstenedione, which are capable of producing both estrone and testosterone. Obesity associated with a considerable amount of androstenedione conversion in adipose tissue or stress resulting in increased adrenal contribution of estrogenic precursor can sustain the blood level of estrogen at a time when decline is necessary for recycling and negative feedback on the FSH.

A state of chronic anovulation results in a tonic rather than a cyclic condition in which the constantly slightly elevated levels of estrogen bring about static, somewhat elevated LH and lowered FSH. The follicular apparatus in the ovary is stimulated continuously but not sufficiently to achieve the proper growth and maturation. Multiple follicle cysts at various stages of development and dense stromal tissues derived from atretic follicles tend to perpetuate the problem of chronic anovulation by producing androstenedione, which is continuously converted into estrone in the peripheral tissues. The resultant perpetuation of follicles in all stages of development and atresia, dense functional stroma and the grossly thickened tunica albuginea represent the features of the classic polycystic ovaries. The pathophysiologic features found in association with the chronic anovulation may be various patterns of abnormal menses ranging from irregular heavy periods in more than one quarter and oligo-amenorrhea in more than one half of these patients. These patients are usually obese and more than two thirds have some degree of hirsutism, although only one third or less will be virilized. These basic problems of anovulatory dysfunction in association with abnormal bleeding, infertility, and possibly hirsutism may arise from a variety of causes including gonadal as well as extragonadal, but the common denominator is a steady state of asynchronous gonadotropin and estrogen production. This problem is quite different from hypergonadotropic hypogonadism (ovarian failure) or hypogonadotropic hypogonadism (central failure). Markedly high or significantly low serum gonadotropin levels and clinical or genetic stigmata characterize these latter conditions. For example, gonadal dysgenesis gives rise to high serum gonadotropin levels because of lack of follicular tissue on a genetic basis.

Chronic anovulation causes breakthrough bleeding from a faulty endometrium. Usually the endometrium is overgrown and the glandularity and vascularity outstrip the stromal support matrix. The fragile tissues break down in a random fashion and healing can only be temporary because the orderly physiologic process of rhythmical vasoconstriction and stasis does not occur. The bleeding may be acyclic, highly irregular, and very heavy at times. There may be periods of amenorrhea followed by profuse bleeding and possibly cramps. In younger women, these disturbances arouse the suspicion of incomplete abortion, endometrial polyp, or, less commonly, submucous myoma. Chronic anovulation gives rise to endometrial hyperplasia and to adenocarcinoma even at an early age in the susceptible person who is subjected to long-term unopposed estrogen stimulation. Adequate study of endometrial tissues is mandatory to exclude malignancy in such women above the age of 35.

Another pattern of menstrual disturbance associated with intermittent light bleeding of variable duration results from an unfavorably high ratio of progesterone to estrogen (progestin therapy or low-dose estrogen therapy as in prolonged use of oral contraceptives). The lack of a proper tissue base for endometrial growth, structural support, stability, and healing calls for estrogens to promote hemostasis. Usually, hormonal therapy is so effective in correcting all types of dysfunctional bleeding that a failed response in 24 hours should arouse the suspicion of an underlying cause (*e.g.,* polyp, placental fragments, blood dyscrasia, tumor, malignancy). Administration of estrogens in high doses should be considered as temporary therapy to be used only in the initial control of profuse bleeding. Long-term management depends on the underlying cause. A critical issue in determining the approach pertains to the amount of endometrium present. In cases of long-standing bleeding there may be little endometrium and responses to progesterone or even progestin–estrogen combinations may not be effective in these exhausted tissues without proper preliminary estrogenic support. Similarly, a thorough curettage of the uterus will not solve the problem since it does nothing to correct the underlying pathophysiology unless there is organic disease. Moreover, one may produce synechiae (fibrous adhesions) in the uterus that could cause secondary amenorrhea (Asherman's syndrome).

Among the most important aspects of management is the patient's history. It is best to judge the normality or abnormality of the menstrual pattern based on the patient's own past menstrual history. The presence or absence of molimenal symptoms may be an indication of ovulation or its disappearance. An attempt is made to discern any clinical stigmata or genetic cause that would be associated with abnormal menses. Check for evidence of malnutrition, psychologic stress, systemic illness, gynecologic disease, or endocrinopathy. Sometimes, the symptoms are subtle and the menstrual disorder may be the first or possibly only manifestation of a serious medical problem. Investigation of the diet and documentation of shifts in weight are necessary. A check for galactorrhea is required, and a careful pelvic examination should exclude organic pathology of the internal genitalia or complications of pregnancy. Routine laboratory studies should exclude anemia, blood dyscrasia, liver impairment, metabolic disorders, and renal dysfunction. Thyroid tests are often obtained, as are adrenal studies if there is hirsutism. If there is galactorrhea or infertility, serum prolactin levels and radiographic evaluation of the sella turcica with polytomography or CT scan should be obtained to rule out the presence of a pituitary adenoma.

Luteal phase defects with premenstrual spotting in association with a deficient corpus luteum may require thyroid and adrenal studies (acquired adrenogenital syndrome). After complete assessment, including plasma testosterone, luteinizing hormone, prolactin levels and, possibly, morning and evening cortisol determinations, patients with hirsutism may be suppressed in the hope of establishing a satisfactory treatment. A dexamethasone suppression test is helpful in assessing the suitability of corticosteroid therapy. Depending on these results, it may be possible to reduce the growth rate of the hair. Elevated plasma testosterone levels may be suppressed with estrogen-progesterone–containing compounds (oral contraceptives). Antiandrogens that prevent androgens from expressing their activity on target sites hold promise for the future.

Many women with hirsutism have increased testosterone production rates, elevated free testosterone levels, and increased testosterone metabolic rates. About 30% of hirsute women have increased androgen production from both the ovary and the adrenal; in some, hypothyroidism is present and when that problem is corrected, an associated adrenal or ovarian disorder associated with anovulation is corrected. When dehydroepiandrosterone and its sulfated compound are prominent secretory products, adrenal tumors or congenital adrenal hyperplasia are possible. With extremely high testosterone levels in the serum (above 500 ng/100 ml) and when androgen levels are fixed or unresponsive to suppression or stimulation testing, there is a significant probability of adrenal adenomas or carcinomas. Further studies are required. The same is true of hirsutism or when signs and symptoms of Cushing's syndrome are present with an abnormally elevated plasma cortisol after attempted suppression with dexamethasone, or failure to suppress elevated plasma testosterone with progestin therapy (ovarian tumor is a possibility). In the latter cases, a laparoscopy or pelvic sonogram might be helpful. Virilizing ovarian tumors include arrhenoblastomas, testicular tubular adenoma (Sertoli cells), hilar cell tumors (Leydig cells), gonadoblastoma, and combinations.

When the bleeding is heavy and the hemoglobin falls below 10 mg/100 ml and requires replacement of blood volume, hospitalization may be required to achieve initial hemostasis. Depending on the circumstances, high-dose estrogen therapy utilizing conjugated estrogens in 25-mg increments administered intravenously every 6 hours will usually cause heavy bleeding to subside within 12 hours. Oral high-dose progestin–estrogen combination pills can also be used in less dramatic problem cases for periods of 1 week. Failure of cessation or abatement of heavy blood flow calls for uterine curettage, even in the teenager, to rule out the possibility of organic uterine disease. In older women this procedure should precede hormone therapy in most cases to rule out malignancy as a prerequisite in the management. Underlying factors are studied and treated as necessary while cyclic hormone therapy is continued through three to six cycles. Establishing or reestablishing ovulatory menses is a goal only in the young and in those who are desirous of childbearing. Oral medroxyprogesterone administered in 10-mg doses on a cyclic basis on days 15 or 20 to day 25 of the cycle will prevent hyperplasia in refractory anovulatory cases.

Patients with isosexual precocious puberty who present no specific etiology susceptible to a direct therapeutic approach are not easily managed. Use of a synthetic progestin (Depo-Provera) or a steroid with apparent antigonadotropic action suppresses the pituitary, but there is no decrease in bone maturation. The use of synthetic GnRH analogues, which are capable of desensitizing the child's pituitary gland to her own hypothalamic GnRH, has been successfully used for treatment of isosexual precocious puberty including slowing of bone maturation.

When there has been no sexual development by the age of 14 or an absence of menarche by age 16, puberty is delayed and there must be a search for possible genetic faults or a hypothalamic-pituitary-ovarian axis disorder. Patients with gonadal dysgenesis showing short stature and a single missing X chromosome have a Turner's phenotype, for example, webbed neck, shield chest, widely spaced nipples, cubitus valgus, sexual infantilism, short fourth metacarpal, low nuchal hairline, pigmented nevi, lymphedema, hypoplasia of nails, coarctation of the aorta or ventricular septal defect, craniofacial and cognitive defects, and so forth. Overall, mosaicism is more common than single cell lines. There may also be ovarian failure in chromosomally competent females (46, XX gonadal dysgenesis), some of whom seem to suffer from a single-gene autosomal recessive inheritance observed in multiple sibships.

The appropriateness of height and bone age and the use of Bayley-Pinnean or Tanner tables to predict future adult height are proper evaluative methods. If there is short stature, there must be a check for the usual causes: malnutrition, chronic infectious disease, gonadal dysgenesis, and panhypopituitarism. There may be a familial history of growth tardiness with eventual normal stature. The average growth in height after the menarche is about 2.5 inches. In some individuals exhibiting menstrual dysfunction, there may be disturbances in sexual behavior, social adjustment, marital relations, and family status, which may require psychiatric assistance.

Overall, about two thirds of patients exhibiting dysfunctional uterine bleeding are either pubertal or premenopausal; about 30% of the cases occur during the childbearing years. The problem occurs in approximately 15% of females and accounts for a great majority of the justifications for uterine curettages, in addition to many endometrial ablations or hysterectomies. However, the latter must not be a means of eliminating refractory bleeding in the absence of pathology unless conservative medical measures have been exhausted. The potential problems of dysfunctional uterine bleeding can be both immediate (shock), remote (consequences of operative procedures, shock, or blood transfusion) and potentially dangerous over time (carcinogenesis of long-term unopposed estrogens either endogenous or offered exogenously on a chronic basis). The overall goals in specific therapies include (1) control of the present bleeding episode, (2) establishment of normal cyclic bleeding pattern in the future, (3) reestablishment of ovulatory cycles in the young if desirous of childbearing, and (4) establishment of cyclic progestational endometrium in those women not currently desiring fertility. Polycystic ovaries may require ovulation induction therapy for childbearing. Regularization of the bleeding pattern with polycystic ovaries is usually achieved with oral contraceptives when pregnancy is not an immediate goal.

In patients with amenorrhea, if bleeding can be induced by the injection of 50 mg or 100 mg of progesterone, one may generally assume that the amenorrhea is not due to any serious derangement of the pituitary, the ovary, or the uterus. However, if bleeding does not occur, the cause may be any one of the three. In this instance, if bleeding occurs after estrogen withdrawal (following 21 days of therapy), cause is due either to ovarian or to pituitary dysfunction, provided that the thyroid and the adrenal glands are normal. If bleeding does not occur, the factor is nonresponsiveness of the endometrium and can be demonstrated by hysteroscopy, hysterosalpingogram, and endometrial biopsy (tuberculosis or synechiae). Endometrial synechiae (Asherman's syndrome) represent adhesions and scarring within the uterine cavity usually following curettage for incomplete abortion or postpartal hemorrhage. Serum gonadotropins will usually distinguish the ovarian and the pituitary factors; a high titer indicates deficient ovarian function (agenesis, dysgenesis or hypofunction), while absence of or a low titer indicates pituitary or hypothalamic hypofunction. These assumptions are based on the fact that all other endocrine, systemic, and local factors have been proved to be normal by previous workup. For example, when amenorrhea is merely one manifestation of a problem of defeminization or masculinization, the problem is much more complex. The basic problem may be pituitary (basophilic adenoma, Cushing's syndrome), adrenal (cortical hyperplasia, adenoma, or carcinoma), or ovarian (arrhenoblastoma, adrenal tumor of the ovary, gynandroblastoma, hilus cell tumor, or the Stein-Leventhal syndrome). Obviously a much more extensive workup is required, including an adrenocorticotropic hormone (ACTH) or adrenal suppression test and others.

In the study of patients with primary amenorrhea, it is now possible to clarify better the various conditions characterized by low serum gonadotropins and to establish the reversibility or irreversibility of the hypogonadotropic state. The response of the pituitary FSH-LH hormones to an infusion of GnRF distinguishes between primary hypothalamic and pituitary disorders. Ovarian competence can be evaluated by a challenging administration of human menopausal gonadotropin (HMG). One irreversible form of hypogonadotropism distinguishable by these special studies is characterized by primary amenorrhea, sexual infantilism, normal cytogenetic status, anosmia, and inability to synthesize gonadotropins, presumably because of a defect in the hypothalamus (Kallmann's syndrome).

INFERTILITY

Approximately 10% to 15% of married couples of childbearing age in the United States have difficulty in achieving a pregnancy. This percentage may be increasing, since late marriages are more commonplace and now one half of the population is age 31 or over. Infertility is defined as failure to conceive after 1 year of regular coitus without contraception, in contrast with sterility, which is total inability to conceive. About 80% of normal couples are capable of achieving pregnancy within 1 year; however, after another 6 months that percentage will rise only to about 85% to 90%.

Thus, it is generally advisable to investigate couples for infertility after 1 year of unprotected coitus if childbearing is their interest. A workup can be conducted sooner if clinical stigmata or symptoms raise other therapeutic objectives. Fecundability, which denotes the probability of conception, is maximal at about age 24 in both the male and the female. Among infertile couples, modern investigative capabilities make it possible to identify one or more potential causes in about 90% of the cases. Appropriate therapy incorporating current modalities, both medical and surgical, will succeed in achieving pregnancy for only about one half of these. Infertility can be attributed to a male factor either as the definitive cause or one of the contributing causes in about 40% of cases. Both partners possess antifertility factors in almost one third of the couples. A significant minority of patients will conceive without therapy at some time during the workup (perhaps 35%), perhaps because of alleviation of anxiety and other emotional problems. By the same token, the tedious workup, including various tests and procedures to obtain specimens and requirements for the couple to perform on schedule, may remove the favorable effects of spontaneity in lovemaking or even result in impotence in the man. It may be possible to evaluate the true motivation of the partners under these circumstances and to sort out the various fears, guilt, ambivalences, and misinformation. Proper counseling and attention paid to these psychologic aspects by attempting to establish and maintain a proper relationship between the husband and wife are central issues in the overall management plan. It is essential for the husband to be present at the initial interview and after he and his wife are studied separately and as a couple, he must be a party to the management planning sessions. In addition to emotionally based issues, prognostic variables affecting therapeutic success are age, frequency, and technique of coital exposure, duration of infertility, number and type of antifertility factors, past reproductive performance in secondary infertility, quality of care, and patient compliance.

The cornerstone of the infertility work-up initially is a careful history and thorough physical examination of both partners. Although the investigative process should follow an orderly pattern, focusing first on the potential of a male factor, these basic evaluations may give immediate insights into potential etiologies and focus on certain targets in formulating a management plan for either partner. Routine laboratory screening may direct attention to problems affecting the workup, therapy, and prognosis (*e.g.*, anemia, diabetes, cervical neoplasia, urinary or prostatic infection, gonorrhea, and other conditions). More specialized tests, including those for specific endocrine disorders, need to be performed when clinically indicated. A check for subclinical hypothyroidism, which is a common endocrine-related antifertility factor, may be part of the routine investigation (measurement of serum TSH).

A management program of basic studies includes the following evaluative tests and procedures:

1. Evaluation of semen (usually two or more specimens): Determine the number, motility, and morphology of the spermatozoa. Sperm counts below 10 to 20 million/ml, total sperm counts below 25 million per ejaculate, and normal motile sperm of less than 12.5 million per ejaculate are frequent findings in infertile men. In addition, there may be enzymatic and certain chemical derangements, including serum fructose, which is normally produced in the seminal vesicles. If it is not found in the semen, there may be a congenital absence of the duct system. Presence of autoagglutinating antibodies in the semen may give rise to clumping of the spermatozoa, while poor motility may be an indication of autoimmobilizing antibodies. The latter defect is a more serious prognostic factor. Abnormal sperm morphology with tapering forms predominating and greatly reduced sperm motility may be associated with varicocele. Detection and correction of this condition as a cause of oligospermia and asthenospermia represent a major advance in male infertility. High ligation of the internal spermatic vein may be followed by improved counts and sperm motility and resultant fertilization capability in 40% or more within the first year.

2. Postcoital test: This test is performed on about the 12th to 14th day of the menstrual cycle, which is the time of peak spontaneous cervical mucous flow. Normally, there is a clear watery mucous with tenaciousness or stretchability (spinnbarkeit) in response to an estrogen level peak that promotes sperm penetration. A proper test reflects on sperm production and transport, coital technique, quality of the sperm and their motility, and the cervical transport. The worrisome features include thick, opaque, nontenacious mucous (inadequate estrogen stimulation or defective cervical glands), presence of pus (cervicovaginal or seminal-urinary infection), absence of sperm (azoospermia, failure of male transport mechanisms, or faulty coital technique), and poor sperm motility (asthenospermia, faulty mucous representing a physical barrier to penetration, or immunologic incompatibilities). Absence of sperm is seen in retrograde ejaculation (check urine for spermatozoa).

3. Tests of tubal patency: Tubal patency is usually determined by hysterosalpingogram or dye instillation and determination of peritoneal spillage under direct laparoscopic view. In the latter, it is frequently combined with hysteroscopic visualization of the uterine cavity. The hysterosalpingogram has the advantage of demonstrating both tubal patency and uterotubal morphology (distortions by diseases, tu-

mors or anomalous development). Unfortunately, misinterpretations may occur in a significant minority of cases. Antifertility factors involving congenital defects (septum), pathologic entities (submucous myoma), endometrial adhesions, infectious processes (tuberculous endometritis), placental polyp, foreign body (unsuspected IUD), and other conditions may be disclosed in these investigations. Sometimes after a hysterosalpingogram, filmy adhesions about the tubes will become disrupted and normal mobility is restored.

4. Test for ovulation: The standard methods to test for ovulation include the basal body temperature (thermogenic effect of progestin produces a biphasic curve), serum concentrations of progesterone during the midluteal phase of the cycle (expensive), and the endometrial biopsy taken on day 21 to 23 of the cycle (date the endometrium for appropriate secretory changes indicative of ovulation and progestational development). In the event of anovulation, adequate tissue studies of the endometrium will be required to check for hyperplasia and for evidence of malignancy in the older female. A uterine curettage may be needed. Chronic anovulation calls for weight (diet) assessment and evaluation of potential emotional factors. Amenorrhea calls for determination of gonadotropins and prolactin serum levels as well as cytogenetic (chromosomal) studies as indicated (see section on gynecologic endocrinopathies for further detail). The presence of hirsutism and virilism in particular would justify a more sophisticated workup (see the previous section). A unilateral ovarian enlargement likewise necessitates steps to rule out a functioning neoplasm. The response of an elevated 17-ketosteroid excretion level to dexamethasone suppression is helpful in distinguishing relevant entities. Suppression to a value consistent with normal ovarian function (2 mg/24 hr) is consistent with adrenal hyperplasia, while lesser depressions (to 5–11 mg/24 hr) are more compatible with persistent anovulation. An increased urinary pregnanetriol level suggests 21- or 11-hydroxylase deficiency (acquired adrenogenital syndrome), particularly when 17-OH progesterone levels are elevated. Very high levels of 17-ketosteroid excretion (greater than 30 mg/24 hr), or of serum testosterone or androstenedione, suggest tumor in either the ovary or adrenal, and these levels would not suppress appreciably. An elevated dehydroepiandrosterone or its sulfated compound (DHEA-S) is likewise suggestive evidence of adrenal tumor.

Polycystic ovaries may be associated with hypothyroidism (which should be checked for routinely, including tests for thyroid antibodies) but, also, in about 20% of these cases, there is hyperprolactinemia. These elevated levels may interfere with LH release, or may possibly disrupt steroidogenesis at the gonadal tissue level; however, there seems to be little correlation between prolactin values and those of the androgens and estradiol-17α. Fear or anxiety and a host of drugs, including phenothiazine derivatives and oral contraceptives, sexual practices (suckling), and a variety of lesions involving the hypothalamus, thyroid, adrenal, or pituitary glands may be at fault. Polytomograms, CT scan, or MRI of the sella turcica may detect some microadenomas of the pituitary, and these evaluations should be a standard part of the workup, particularly when galactorrhea is demonstrable. Bromocriptine is a synthetic ergot alkaloid that is a specific inhibitor of the release of prolactin, as well as TSH, capable of reducing elevated prolactin levels, suppressing galactorrhea, and inducing ovulation. It is a dopamine receptor against which it is believed to stimulate the release of prolactin-inhibiting factor from the hypothalamus, which then regulates the synthesis and release of prolactin from the anterior pituitary. The drug is used to induce ovulation in hyperprolactinemic patients with or without the galactorrhea–amenorrhea syndromes, once a pituitary adenoma has been excluded. Luteal phase defects due to this cause will also respond to this treatment.

5. Diagnostic laparoscopy: Inspection of the pelvis via the laparoscope adds a considerable dimension to the quality of the infertility workup. Detection of tubal and peroneal adhesions that immobilize but do not obstruct can best be accomplished by endoscopy. The actual dynamics of the tubes subjected to transuterine dye injections can be appreciated, and the precise location and extent of adhesions or blockage can be determined in most instances. Often these subtle changes are not apparent on physical examination, and there may be no history suggestive of prior pelvic disease. Adhesions associated with minimal endometriosis may be characterized in this way in many

instances. Similarly, pelvic infection arising from an IUD, after abortion, or following appendicitis or peritonitis of pneumococcal or fungal etiology may result in "silent" adhesions. Chlamydial pelvic infections may lead to adnexal damage without evidencing an acutely symptomatic episode.

Following these five major diagnostic approaches to infertility, the cause or causes of not conceiving are identifiable in 80% to 90% of cases. In some, pregnancy will occur during the course of the workup, perhaps even before a particular problem has been identified. However, in others, no cause will be found on these basic investigations. A few more etiologic antifertility factors will be unearthed by very specialized tests. Among these cases of so-called infertility of unknown etiology or "normal infertile couple," cultures for particular organisms (*T. mycoplasma*, tubercle bacilli, fungi, etc.), refined assessments for immunologic incompatibilities and chromosomal studies for pertinent genetic defects may pay dividends in some clinical situations. Sometimes, the multifactorial nature of the problem is not recognized until a more in-depth study of the couple is made. This same type of restudy is required if treatment is given to correct a particular problem such as anovulation fails after an adequate trial. A small percentage of patients with 45 XO complements may have spontaneous menses, normal height, and breast development. Those with a mosaic pattern of XX and XO gonadal dysgenesis with normal stature and appearance constitute an even greater likelihood of escaping detection. In about 5% to 10% of couples with repetitive abortions, either the wife or the husband will have balanced translocation. Antenatal diagnosis for chromosomal disorders can be offered. About 5% to 10% of fetal deaths involve an abnormal chromosomal complement, although that figure might be higher if macerated fetuses could be studied appropriately. Only about 1% of liveborn infants have these defects.

In the workup the more simple conditions with the best clinical prospects in the husband and the wife must not be overlooked through lack of an organized approach or preoccupation with the exotic. For example, plastic procedures on the penis, surgical correction of ductal obstruction, creation of artificial spermatoceles, and administrations of clomiphine, HMG, HCG, testosterone, and other approaches will yield some favorable results in selected cases. However, far better success can be achieved by eliminating faulty coital practices, de-

tecting and treating hypothyroidism, eradicating a genital infection, and discovering and ligating a varicocele. Remedying adverse heat effects on the testicles; advising on rest, exercise, consumption of alcohol, tobacco, caffeine, and drugs of various types; and offering emotional support may likewise contribute to the likelihood of success. These same principles pertain to the female partner. When sperm-agglutinating or sperm-immobilizing antibiotics are present, an attempt can be made to reduce the antibiotic titer in the woman by use of a condom by the male partner for 6 to 12 months. The effectiveness of this type of treatment is not established.

Hormonal therapies may be effective modalities in correcting anovulation, corpus luteum insufficiency, thyroid dysfunctions, adrenogenital syndrome, adrenal hyperplasia, gonadotropin deficiency, poor cervical mucus, and galactorrhea (hyperprolactinemia). A "hostile" cervical mucus with poor spinnbarkeit and atypical ferning can be improved by administering estrogen from day 7 through day 15 of the cycle. A luteal phase defect may be improved by the use of postovulatory cyclic progesterone, or with ovulation induction, if no specific etiology has been established calling for a more targeted remedy. In patients with mild adrenal cortical hyperplasia, a trial of dexamethasone will often represent the best hormonal treatment. A documented hypothyroidism might take first priority of attention because its correction often reestablishes ovulation despite apparent multiglandular defects. The mainstay in the induction of ovulation in the absence of thyroid deficiency, in adrenal disorder in the absence of thyroid deficiency or in adrenal disorder or hyperprolactinemia (galactorrhea) is the use of clomiphene citrate. Candidates for this therapy must be estrogen sufficient, and the hypothalamic-pituitary-ovarian axis and uterine integrity must be intact. If large polycystic ovaries (Stein-Leventhal type) are present, they may be hypersensitive to this therapy and the drug must be administered with care to avoid significant ovarian enlargement, abdominal distention, pain, nausea, vomiting, and many other side effects. When used in 5-day courses (usually days 5 to 10 of each cycle) and gradually increased in dosage at 50-mg increments beginning at 50 mg and stopping at a maximum of 200 mg, induction of ovulation can be expected in about 70% to 80% of properly selected patients. That figure can be increased to about 90% if refractory cases are offered (HCG) to mimic an LH surge given as a single intramuscular dose (5,000–10,000 IU) on about the 6th day following the completed course of clomiphene citrate. Follicular maturation can be judged by estrogen levels and by ultrasound studies of the gonads. Under very special circumstances, a more complicated and potentially dangerous hormonal regimen of HMG and HCG may be required, but the risks of a hyperstimulation syndrome can be life-threatening and are prohibitive except in the hands of the expert. In addition, multiple ovulation may result.

The discouraging feature is that while 90% of women may ovulate, only about 50% or less will conceive. Patients require reevaluation when they do not respond. Under clomiphene therapy, they may become somewhat hypoestrogenic, as evidenced by poor cervical mucus, which may require exogenous augmentation. Patients with low gonadotropins or hyperprolactinemia may not respond well to clomiphene. Surgical intervention is restricted largely to patients who are refractory to hormonal therapies provided the ovaries are not low normal or small in size. Progestogens (medroxyprogesterone acetate or dydrogesterone), GnRH, or antigonadotropin (danazol) may be administered in an effort to restore fertility in women with pelvic endometriosis. Conservative surgical procedures in patients with endometriosis may be more successful in restoring fertility than these hormonal approaches in selected cases. Restoration of childbearing potential occurs in 40% to 80% of cases, depending upon the individual circumstances, but one drawback is the risk of a second operation if there is progression of the disease. Laser and microsurgical techniques are providing better chances for success than in the past.

There are surgical approaches to female infertility problems that can be directed to a number of problems relating to the uterus, for example, hysteroplastic procedures (uterine unification and resection of septum), myomectomy, and cervical cerclage for incomplete cervix. Uterine synechiae can be treated by surgical debridement under hysteroscopy, insertion of an IUD, and estrogen therapy. Tubal infertility, characterized by blockage or immobility, results from scarring secondary to infection or inflammatory responses to pathologic conditions and peritoneal irritants (blood, etc.). There may be pelvic infections arising from or associated with uterine causes, and in many of these the outlook is poor for restoring reproductive function, for example, tuberculous endometritis and endosalpingitis, IUD-related pelvic abscess, fungus infections of the pelvis, septic degeneration in submucus myomas, and perforated uterus with abscess formation or pyometra. Generally, infections of the tubes are less amenable to surgical correction than adhesions affecting the tube extrinsically.

A number of plastic procedures are now applicable to the problem of tubal infertility, and, recently, advances in microsurgical techniques have upgraded the chances of success even in cases requiring partial resections and reanastomosis. Salpingolysis, requiring only division of peritubo-ovarian adhesions, carries the best results (50%–80% success rate). Fimbriolysis, salpingoplasty with or without a fimbrial prosthesis, and salpingostomy for fimbrial occlusion offer reasonably good chances for success. However, midsegment reconstructions and uterotubal implantations are other feasible techniques in selected cases, but salvage is generally in the 20% to 40% range. Tubal "reversal" (reversing a tubal sterilization) can be attempted, with the prospects for better results in ligations achieved by ligature and resection of small segment than by electrocautery, which may have inflicted extensive tubal damage. A short residual tubal segment portends poorly for success, and inadvertently operating on a patient with residual salpingitis will doom any plastic attempt to failure.

If there is a male developmental anomaly preventing intromission or normal ejaculation, artificial insemination may be attempted utilizing husband's sperm where possible (AIH), or donor (AID). When the husband has a very large semen volume, a split-ejaculate insemination may be used to exploit the fact that the first portion contains 75% of all sperm.

One of the most exciting advances is the development of an extracorporeal (in vitro) fertilization capability whereby ova are harvested prior to the time of ovulation by various techniques, fertilized in special culture media, and implanted into the uterine cavity transcervically. The technological advances afforded by this technique are utilized for other procedures, including gamete intrafallopian tube transfer (GIFT).

ABNORMAL SEXUAL DEVELOPMENT

Dysfunctional gynecologic presentations are frequently associated with developmental sexual abnormalities that must be considered if a wide range of disorders of the female is to be managed safely and effectively. In practice, the question of chromosome abnormalities, intersex and congenital anomalies of the female genital tract must be suspected in a host of abnormal presentations involving abnormal generative tract and reproductive functions.

These considerations have been mentioned in other sections under discussions of menstrual dysfunctions, amenorrhea, ambiguous external genitalia, disturbed puberty, infertility, reproductive wastage, and several types of carcinogenesis. Abnormalities are generally identified with a frequency inversely related to the age of individuals. A relatively high incidence of chromosomal anomalies is found in early spontaneous abortuses (roughly 40%). Defective developments in the ovary or testis may create morphologic and functional disturbances manifested at any time during the embryonic (up to the 56th day), perinatal, or pubertal periods of life. Particular maldevelopments may involve the gonads, müllerian ducts, genital tubercle, and urogenital sinus.

The Y chromosome appears to carry the testicular inductor in the human. An antigen promotes germ cell migration from the yolk sac to the genital ridges, as well as maturation, aggregation, and tubular differentiation. Genetic or chromosomal sex is determined at the moment of fertilization, but the gonads remain in an indifferent stage until about the 7th embryonic week. At that time, histodifferentiation in the female requires a little longer. The male set is stimulated preferentially while the female set undergoes atrophy if the testis-inducing Y chromosome is present. Testosterone favors mesonephric duct development (wolffian ducts) while elaboration of müllerian inhibiting factor by the fetal testes brings about regression of the paramesonephric duct system. The X chromosome does not possess a counterpart gene to the Y chromosome. There must be two X chromosomes for the ovary to differentiate, since gonadal dysgenesis occurs if the second X is either missing or defective. Thus, if the testicular inductors are absent, female differentiation will occur. The ovary is not essential for this type of development. Originally, germ cells of the 45 XO karyotype contain the same number of germ cells as the normal 46 XX type, but at some point, by unknown mechanisms, chromosomal sex material is lost. When the inductor is present, the testis is developed in its definitive form by the 10th to 11th week of intrauterine life. Hilar structures and the great proliferation of Leydig cells (distinctive interstitial cells) reach a peak at about 19 weeks. Seminiferous tubules without lumina are apparent, and their growth results in coiling and crowding prior to the lumina formation and the appearance of spermatogonia and Sertoli's cells. In gonads destined to be ovaries, one of the distinguishing features at about the 7-week stage is the presence of masses of oogonia. Ultimately, deeper ones become surrounded by somatic (granulosa) cells of the primitive follicles. These structures are very prominent by the 17th gestational week.

The uterus and vagina slowly arise as distinctly identifiable structures during the 4th and 5th months of fetal life. The uterus, including the cervix and upper two thirds of the vagina, are müllerian duct derived. The lower one third of the vagina is derived from a cord of epithelium that arises from the urogenital sinus and grows upward to displace at least in part the müllerian epithelium cephalad and establishes the anlage of the future hollow tube. Canalization proceeds from the caudal region in the cephalad direction and the fornices develop clefts to complete the definitive vaginal form. When sinus proliferation does not take place or grows to a certain point and atrophies, vaginal agenesis or transverse septae may occur. In the absence of a vaginal mass, the hymen is not formed. In some cases, there is normal müllerian duct developed resulting in a functional uterus, cervix, and proximal vagina above the distal atresia, which becomes a serious problem at the menarche (hematometra, endometriosis, etc.). Incomplete fusion of the distal portions of the müllerian ducts results in various forms of partial or total duplication of the uterus and proximal vagina. In addition to septation of the upper vagina and incomplete fusion of the sinovaginal bulbs (arrests in development occurring between the 8th and 12th week of fetal life), there may be transverse bars, adenosis, and various anatomic and histologic abnormalities occurring at the vault. The vagina is the last genital organ to be completed embryologically, and masculinizing effects occurring relatively late may adversely affect its development.

DES exposure *in utero* in the first trimester creates morphologic and anomalous changes in both the cervix and the vagina in a majority of young females, and very rarely there will be clear cell adenocarcinomatous development. There may be cervical and vaginal structural defects in the female as well as abnormal morphologic genital defects in the male as a result of DES exposure, and there may be attendant problems relating to reproductive success. Some nonneoplastic changes include vaginal adenosis, cervical ectropion, vaginal and cervical ridges, and morphologic changes in the cervix (cock's comb, collar, rim, etc.), fallopian tubes, and uterine corpus. Male offspring have been observed to have testicular, epididymal, and semen alterations, as well as upper genital tract abnormalities, but no neoplastic lesions have been reported. In exposed females, the peak incidence for clear-cell adenocarcinoma is age 19, with a risk of this development up to age 24 of 0.01% to 0.1%. The range in age has been 7 to 28, at this writing. Adenosis does not progress to a malignant condition and dysplastic and metaplastic lesions in the cervix are not progressive to *in situ* squamous cancer, and there is a tendency for maturation over time. Nonneoplastic alterations of one type or another particularly among offspring exposed in the first trimester occur in a majority of the study cases (variously reported in the range of 40% up to 90% in some reports). Transverse vaginal septae and bands of tissue in the upper segment may give rise to dyspareunia, while various deformities of the cervix may predispose to its incompetency in pregnancy. Cervical ectropin (erosion and eversion) and morphologic defects and vaginal adenosis and structural anomalies have been reported in a majority (up to 60%–90% in some reports) of DES-exposed offspring during the age period 14 to 24.

Anomalies are multiple in roughly one in four defective fetuses, and maldevelopments in the generative system are often coincident with those of the urinary organs. Development of the external organs of the genital system is so intimately interrelated that isolated anomalies are rare. In addition to sympodia, which represents an absence of the entire hind end of the body, other defects include agenesis of the perineum and phallus, exstrophy of the cloaca or of the bladder, imperforate anus, rectoperineal or rectovaginal fistulas, rectal agenesis, posterior displacement of the urogenital sinus, duplication of the external genitalia, and other anorectal and perineal anomalies.

Anomalies of the external genitalia in association with a 46 XX karyotype are usually associated with female pseudohermaphroditism. The classic underlying condition is congenital hyperplasia of the adrenal gland, but other causes may be female fetuses subjected *in utero* to maternal progestin or androgen therapy, or possibly, to an androgen-secreting gonadal tumor. Despite the illusion of the urethra opening into the vagina or the vagina into the urethra, these structures are intact and open separately into a common passage consisting of a persistent urogenital sinus. The vaginal and urethral openings present well within the common passageway, and there is one external opening located at the base of the phallus. The labia are fused and the clitoris is enlarged in male phallus. The uterus and tubes are not affected. This problem is easily corrected surgically by resecting the urogenital membrane, providing access to the vaginal introitus and

exposing the external urethral meatus. A cliteroplasty accompanies the procedure. Children should have simple surgical correction before the age of set sexual identity (about age 2). Androgenization from any cause during the first 8 to 12 weeks of *in utero* life can give rise to these ambiguous external genitalia in the normal genetic female fetus, for example, iatrogenic source (progestins administered to the mother), maternal androgen sources, and so forth. However, the most common problem in congenital virilizing adrenal hyperplasia is fetal-21-hydroxylase deficiency. The physical appearance of these female infants is one of male external genitalia with cryptorchidism. When there is 11-β-hydroxylase deficiency, not only will there be masculization of the genitalia but also hypervolemia and hypertension as life-threatening conditions in undiagnosed cases. Lack of the enzyme 5-α-reductase, which prevents the conversion of testosterone to the biologically active dihydrotestosterone, may produce in the genetic male fetus ambiguous genitalia resembling that of the female.

The complete form of testicular feminization is associated with no androgen response. Underdeveloped testicles that are cryptorchid in type contain immature germ and Sertoli cells but no evidence of spermatogenesis. Normal male values of serum testosterone are present, but there is an "androgen insensitivity" because enzyme defects interfere with testosterone-binding protein and tissue responses. The tissues do respond to estrogens produced in the testes and to that converted from androstenedione. There is a problem of sex assignment because usually there is normal external female development and these patients naturally are reared in that sex. In the case of partial response to androgens, there may be ambiguous genitalia. However, there is no müllerian development, and in these circumstances, the vagina is short and ends in a blind pouch. These genetic males are phenotypic females with normal secondary sex characteristics except for sparse genital and axillary hair. The breast development is female in type, but there may be discrepancies in size between the two and small nipples with pale areolae. Inguinal hernias are present in more than one half of the patients, and often the gonads are found in the inguinal canal. The gonads have a malignant potential, justifying castration after puberty and estrogen hormone replacement. The clinical situation is confused by a number of incompletely masculinized male pseudohermaphrodites. The presence of a normal vagina, uterus, and tubes differentiates the Swyer syndrome. In the Reifenstein syndrome, there is a phallic enlargement at birth, along with a severe perineal hypospadias. After puberty, hypogonadism occurs with gynecomastia. The pseudovaginal periscrotal hypospadias condition is associated at birth with a normal steroid condition that rules out adrenal disorders.

Anorchia is similar to the Swyer syndrome, except that the affected individuals lack internal genitalia and a vagina. Patients with the uterine hernia syndrome are individuals who appear to be normally male, but a well-developed uterus and tubes may be found in an inguinal hernia sac.

It is apparent that confusion in the gender role with its attendant emotional stress is a common problem among children with contradictory sex structures. Reinforcement of the gender role in the selected sex of rearing, including the erotic component, which is independent of the gonadal and chromosomal sex, is essential in programming management. From a surgical viewpoint, the assignment of sex may depend upon the morphology of the phallus and whether or not a penis adequate for successful coitus can be constructed. The technical factors are all important. Construction of a satisfactory artificial cavity for coitus is the simplest operative undertaking (McIndoe procedure with creation of rectovesical artificial space and split-thickness skin graft over a mold). Construction of an artificial penis with both erectile and erotic capacities has not been achieved to this same level of success.

In assessing the newborn, it is of interest to note that the number of cells with nuclear sex chromatin in normal female neonates will be falsely low in the first 2 days of life. 17-Ketosteroid and pregnanetriol excretion levels may be needed to distinguish between congenital adrenal hyperplasia (associated with elevated levels and other types of hermaphroditism). By the same token, labial adhesions may resemble labioscrotal fusion. The preferred treatment is simple application of estrogen cream to the adhesions. If some type of operative separation is performed, the results will be painful inflammation and recurrence of adhesions. Occasionally, hypertrophy of the labia resulting in a distorted gross appearance is associated with excessive masturbation and deep-seated psychologic disturbances.

In male hermaphroditism, laparotomy may be required for both diagnosis and therapy. Disadvantageous sex structures should be removed. When these individuals are reared as females, testes should always be removed at puberty, regardless of hormone production, because a variety of tumors,

including malignant ones, may develop in these abnormal gonads.

True hermaphrodites possessing both testicular and ovarian gonad tissues have immaturely developed structures of both sexes, although at puberty female functions usually become paramount. Surgical revisions as necessary may be required to establish function usually favoring the female capacities.

FAMILY PLANNING

In global terms, there may be socioeconomic indications for birth control to cope with increasing population, excess pollution, and an inevitable decline in natural resources and quality of life. The world's population has more than doubled since the end of World War II, from 2.4 to 4.8 billion. Contraception may be mandatory on medical grounds to safeguard a particular individual whose life would be put in jeopardy by a pregnancy. Contraception may be used to prevent a harmful genetic trait or a condition that gives rise to a hopelessly deformed offspring. Effective contraception has been sponsored to reduce adolescent and out-of-wedlock pregnancy and unwanted pregnancies among married couples, and in an effort to avoid the disastrous consequences of illegal abortion. The quality of married life and the ability to realize goals for the family may be predicated upon the ability to control the reproductive process. Traditionally, the folk and conventional practices of family planning have not been successful. These have included coitus interruptus, rhythm method, prolongation of lactation, and postcoital douches of various types. The barrier contraceptives consisting of the condom and diaphragm are much more reliable contraceptive methods, and they are of course medically safe, but mechanical and technical problems reduce their effectiveness. Nonetheless, the failure rate overall is low (two to three pregnancies per 100 women per year of exposure) with the vaginal method (cervical diaphragm), if prescribed and used properly, and probably this record can be improved by using spermicidal preparations for lubrication. A polyurethane foam barrier sponge permeated with a spermicide has enjoyed popularity, but the failure rate is high, perhaps 12% to 15%. The failure rates of vaginal spermicidal preparations, most containing nonoxynol-9, are only slightly higher than that of the condom and diaphragm. Cervical caps and vaginal rings have not enjoyed much recent approval. Other currently popular methods consist of oral contraceptives, repeated injections of progestational steroids, implantable progestagens, IUDs (both medicated and nonmedicated), surgical sterilization of the female transabdominally by laparotomy or laparoscopy, and male sterilization. In addition, there may be induced abortions by suction or surgical curettage, intra-amniotic instillation of an oxytocic agent (midtrimester), use of abortifacients (prostaglandin F_2, $F_{2\alpha}$, and E_2), or, rarely, hysterectomy. Laminaria (endocervical stent) may be used to "ripen" the cervix and partially dilate the canal to expedite labor and uterine evacuation. Suction curettage within 2 weeks after a missed menstrual period may be instituted under the designation of "menstrual regulation" to prevent unwanted pregnancies before the fact of gestation is established.

Oral Contraceptives

Oral contraceptives used to inhibit ovulation contain a combination of synthetic estrogen, usually in the form of ethinyl estradiol or mestranol, and progestin, usually norethindrone, dl-norgestrel, norethynodrel or ethynodiol diacetate. Under this therapy there is no rise of FSH or follicle growth in the first half of the menstrual cycle, and at midcycle there is no LH surge or ovulation. The course is a 21-day hormonal regimen whereby one pill is taken daily during days 5 to 25 of the cycle and the patient bleeds by withdrawal 3 to 5 days later to commence the new cycle. The on-and-off intervals, which must be remembered, can be avoided by using hormonally inert pills for the last 7 days. Newer compounds combine progestogen and estrogen in different contents in the two or three phases of the cycle (biphasic or triphasic), to mimic the physiological steroidal changes whereby estrogen dominates in the first half and progesterone in the second.

Except for sterilization, oral contraceptives are the most effective method for preventing pregnancy (less than 0.1 pregnancy/100 woman-years). The efficacy is based on the prevention of the release of gonadotropin-releasing hormone (GnRH) from the hypothalamus, and, probably, after a period of time, the synthesis and release of gonadotropins becomes refractory to the normal amount of GnRH stimulation. However, these steroids provoke a variety of systemic effects, the 1-year continuation rate is probably only about 70%, and included among the side effects are alterations in hepatic function tests, hematologic and coagulation tests, thyroid evaluations, glucose tolerance tests (15%–40%), serum folate values, metyrapone test, and others. Side effects may be gastrointestinal symptoms, breast discomfort, fluid retention and weight gain, megaloblastic anemia (diminished absorption of folate polyglutamates), pyridoxine deficiency, depression (sometimes reversible with vitamin B_6) and, rarely, chloasma (2%–5% of cases). The potential effects of pill usage are the slightly increased risks of thromboembolic disease, thrombotic stroke, and myocardial infarction (primarily among smokers). The likelihood of these serious complications is minimal but more common among women with hypertension, advancing age, type II hyperlipoproteinemia, obesity, previous toxemia of pregnancy, diabetes mellitus, varicose veins, chronic disease, and immobilization. There appears to be an increased risk of postsurgery thromboembolic complications, gallbladder disease, and benign hepatomas. Some patients will become hypertensive for the first time while taking oral contraceptives, presumably because of alteration of the renin–angiotensin mechanism. There may be a steepening of the corneal curvature (lowered tolerance to contact lenses), allergic reactions, augmented vaginal (cervical) secretions, and other conditions. Recent studies seem to indicate that formulations containing the smallest content of estrogen (0.03 or 0.035 mg) are associated with the lowest number of deaths overall as well as from vascular complications. Recently, the positive effects of oral contraceptives have been given more publicity, for example, fewer fibroadenomas, less fibrocystic disease, and lowered incidence of ovarian cysts, endometrial cancer, and tubal infections. Presumably, in the latter, changes occurring in the cervical mucus offer protection against bacterial invasion. There is some evidence suggesting that oral contraceptives protect against the occurrence of rheumatoid arthritis. Absolute contraindications would be thromboembolic, cerebral, or coronary artery disease, suspected carcinoma of the breast, known or suspected estrogen-dependent neoplasia, undiagnosed abnormal genital bleeding, or known or suspected pregnancy. Visual loss, severe headache, icterus or pruritus, cholelithiasis, development of hypertension, and significant breakthrough bleeding are causes for alarm. Normally, fertility following pill usage is not a worrisome feature, since 95% of the patients who are destined to ovulate will do so by the third cycle.

The "mini-pill," or nonstop progestin (norgestrel, 0.35 mg daily), is an effective oral contraceptive despite the fact that a high percentage of the menstrual cycles are ovulatory. The chief advantage of this approach is elimination of estrogen, its side effects, and the problems inherent in ovulatory withdrawal bleeding. Overall, the pregnancy rate ranges between 2 and 7/100 woman-years, and, whereas the precise mechanism of action is unknown, out-of-phase endometrial activity and hostile cervical mucus have been suggested as antifertility factors.

Diethylstilbestrol, ethinyl estradiol, conjugated equine estrogens, or other estrogenic substances given alone and progestins administered alone or in combination with estrogens have been used as postcoital, or "morning-after," pills with varying degrees of success. The effectiveness of a high dose of estrogen is based on its ability to suppress ovulation when ingested 2 to 6 days in advance of the event, or by accelerating transport of the fertilized ovum through the tube to reach the endometrium before it is properly prepared for implantation. Currently, it is believed that even after early fertilization, a high level of estrogen disrupts the process of embryogenesis. The failure rate ranges up to nearly 2.5% in some reports, and there may be significant side effects of estrogen use in these high doses. Recently, ethinyl estradiol, and DL-norgestrel in substantial doses have been used in combination to achieve a very low failure rate. Contraceptive effectiveness is also very high when hormone injections are given to prevent ovulation by suppressing the pituitary and eliminating the midcycle surges of luteinizing hormone. For this purpose, a popular choice is medroxyprogesterone acetate (Depo-Provera) administered intramuscularly in 150-mg doses every 90 days.

Intrauterine Contraceptive Devices

Insertion of IUDs to prevent conception is safe, effective, and inexpensive. Long-term protection is afforded without any attentiveness on the part of the patient that medications require. However, because of high costs of defending litigation against the IUDs, their availability is currently limited. The traditional intrauterine contraceptive devices were nonmedicated, but more recently the device was used as a vehicle for an active agent capable of enhancing local effects on the uterus. Copper is widely used for this purpose, and this metal, as well as zinc, evokes a profound leukocytic infiltration in the uterus that renders the endometrial environment unsuitable for implantation of the blastocyst. Progesterone-containing IUDs are also available.

The basic mode of action of IUDs remains unknown. IUDs do not prevent bacterial invasion, and salpingitis or pelvic abscess can occur in wearers. Devices with complex multifilament tails have been said to be potentially the most dangerous because bacteria can ascend from the vagina between individual fibers through a "wicking" action. For this reason, such devices have been replaced with those with monofilament tails. Recent studies tend to show that the greatest risk of infection occurs shortly after the time of insertion. At the earliest sign of infection, the IUD should be removed. For those without symptoms, the risk of long-term use seems to be less than that of periodic removal and replacement. The women most vulnerable to infection are nulligravidas of low socioeconomic status. There is also the added risk of ectopic pregnancy among long-term users, compared with pregnancies occurring in the uterine cavity.

One of the most serious complications associated with the insertion of an IUD is perforation of the cervix or uterine fundus. The significant side effects are cramping pain, uterine bleeding, early infection (first few weeks after insertion), or expulsion. If pregnancy occurs with the IUD *in situ,* the risk of spontaneous abortion is roughly 50%. Similarly, there is an increased risk of septic abortion, ectopic pregnancy (3%–9%), and preterm delivery (four times increased incidence). Overall morbidity resulting in hospitalization of IUD wearers is about 5/1,000 woman-years of use, which is five times the rate of pill users. If pregnancy occurs, with an IUD in place and the IUD cannot be removed by simple traction on the tail, an abortion should be offered to the patient because of the extraordinary incidence of extremely serious sepsis, usually in the second trimester. If the device can be removed, the chance of sepsis from this site is minimal and there is a greater chance of pregnancy continuation than if the device is left *in situ.* Sometimes, the device will be expelled spontaneously, and in this case the chances of abortion are greatly reduced, as they would be in therapeutic removal. Overall, the pregnancy rate for IUDs per 100 woman-years is in the range of 2.7 (0.4–5.8) and the 1-year-continuation rate is about 70% (50%–90%).

Sterilization

Surgical sterilization is a definitive, still very popular method of contraception that is legal in all states in the United States. Tubal closure represents the most consistently effective permanent method of controlling childbearing. Transabdominal operative techniques, including conventional laparotomy procedures or minilaparotomy, can be performed in the immediate puerperium or in an interim period at any phase of the menstrual cycle. The sterilization can also be performed concomitantly with an induced abortion. The classic techniques of tubal occlusion include the various types of tubal transection, ligation, and retroperitonealization of stumps (e.g., Pomery, Madlener, and Irving techniques). More recently, sterilization via the laparoscope on an ambulatory basis has become very popular, and by means of that endoscopic transabdominal approach it is possible to fulgurate (coagulate) the tubes with or without division or excision and to clip or band them. The latter methods have the theoretical advantage of more successful reversibility. In each one of the operative techniques, accidental pregnancy is likely to be tubal. Current methods of tubal sterilization are very safe, for example, fewer than 4 deaths/100,000 procedures per year in the United States. Overall, the pregnancy rate per 100 woman-years is in the 0.04 to 0.08 range, which is a slight improvement over the antifertility effectiveness of the combined type of oral contraceptives. Partial vasectomy is the most effective male contraceptic technique.

Abortion

In some countries, voluntary abortion has become the principal method of controlling the size of the family. In the United States, there is one legal abortion for every three live births. About 10% of the teenage population become pregnant each year, and a significant number of abortions occur in the very young who are not prepared for childbirth and child rearing. The duration of pregnancy at the time of anticipated interruption determines the preferred method. Termination of pregnancy at the 12th gestational week or less is most efficiently achieved by suction curettage with negative pressures ranging to about 30 cm to 50 cm H_2O. Maternal mortality rates are exceedingly low (2/100,000 patients or less), and the morbidity associated with infection, bleeding, and perforation of the uterus should be 5% or less. Midtrimester abortions can be accomplished by instilling 200 ml of 20% saline solution into the uterine cavity (80%–90% success rate within 48 hours), but side effects, complications, and emotional stress factors are very common. The use of oxytocin for induction of labor is unreliable, and the latent period and interval to abortion can be quite long. Prostaglandin therapy may be highly efficient in inducing labor, and vaginal suppositories are now the accepted method of abortion when there is fetal demise. Hysterotomy or hysterectomy should be considered only in the context of the presence of coexisting pelvic disease. Overall, complications associated with midtrimester abortions (approaching 20% after intra-amniotic instillations) are so prevalent that the primary emphasis in family planning must be upon contraceptive methods or early interruption if accidental pregnancy occurs.

CLIMACTERIUM, MENOPAUSE, AND POSTMENOPAUSAL SYNDROME

The term *menopause* refers simply to the permanent cessation of menstruation. The physiologic termination of menses, which results from a progressive decline in ovarian function over a period of years, usually occurs by age 52 in the United States. The atresia of germ cells, which has now depleted functional follicular units, has far exceeded those used up in ovulation, which account for only 450 or less, but the process is not understood. Occasionally, premature ovarian failure occurs, which results in premature menopause without discernible causes (approximately 1 menstruating woman in 20). Rarely, debilitating systemic illnesses, psychiatric disability, pelvic irradiation, and ovarian ischemia from pelvic surgery may cause early gonadal insufficiency. An abrupt bilateral oophorectomy may produce more severe acute symptoms than the more gradual physiologic process. There may be significant pathophysiologic changes resulting in autonomic nervous system instability, vasomotor changes, emotional upsets, and certain objective changes characterized by involution of the reproductive tract, urinary system, mammary ducts, and body hair, as well as increased bone resorption. At this stage of life, there is a slight increase in the development of hyperthyroidism and maturity-onset diabetes mellitus.

Preceding the actual menopause there may be polymenorrhea, hypermenorrhea, prolonged menstrual flow, and perhaps metrorrhagia suggestive of uterine malignancy after a chronic period of anovulation. Symptoms may be emotional instability, atrophic urethrocystitis (urgency, frequency, dysuria, urgency incontinence, pyuria, occasional hematuria, and possible meatal pouting and caruncle formation), and atrophic vulvovaginitis and cervicitis. There may be diurnal hot flashes (flushes) and night sweats. The skin may lose its elasticity and turgor, breast size may regress, bone resorption (symptomatic osteoporosis) occurs in about one quarter of postmenopausal women, and there may be symptoms and signs of atherosclerosis (more severe in women who were castrated before age 40). More than 50 symptoms have been attributed to the changes of the postmenopausal state, although a cause-and-effect relationship is doubtful for most.

Laboratory data tend to support the level of estrogenic deprivation. The vaginal cytologic smear may show a lowering of the cornification counts, although this measure is crude and it is now clear that many postmenopausal women derive significant plasma levels of estrogen from extragonadal sources. The most significant postmenopausal endocrine alteration is the great increase in the secretion of pituitary gonadotropins involving both FSH and LH production (FSH increased threefold over the increase in LH). Although sporadic gasps of menstrual function may occur before the final episode, the endometrium should be atrophic and clearly benign. Roentgenograms of the lungs, bones, and blood vessels show only the changes ordinarily associated with the normal aging process.

A variety of clinical conditions may mimic all of the signs and symptoms noted, which calls for appropriate evaluation of signs and symptoms as well as potential laboratory studies to sort out the proper diagnosis from among a host of masquerading diseases. Nothing can be done to stall a physiologic menopause, although there is discretion in creating an artificial termination of menses in context with pathologic entities of the internal genitalia. Probably, the potential consequences of artificial menopause can be justified in women who must be subjected to hysterectomy at age 40 or over. At that stage of life, the elective removal of ovaries to prevent ovarian cancer, which will be a risk of increasing proportions throughout life is probably justified.

Although vulnerable women cannot be identified with precision, there is the likelihood that endometrial cancer can be triggered by prolonged estrogen therapy. Mitigating influences may be low doses, cyclic administrations, opposing the estrogen with progesterone therapies in each cycle, and emotional support to reduce the need for support. The experience of withdrawal blood loss after progesterone therapy suggests that there is adequate estrogen stimulation to the uterus. On the other hand, progestins may relieve vasomotor symptoms in a patient whose uterus is not primed with estrogen to the level of provoking withdrawal bleeding when these hormones are administered. Catecholamines may be involved in central thermoregulatory func-tion, and the therapy probably should be more specific than simple estrogen replacement, although the objectives in management seem to be rather broad. Progestational therapies, while relieving some symptoms, will not replace entirely the estrogen deprivation in the minority who may not have endogenous sources in adequate amounts from extragonadal sources. The majority of patients will not need exogenous steroid therapy, but in those who do, estrogen therapy in modest doses for prescribed periods can be given without a documented increased risk of hypertension, atherosclerosis or heart, renal, and cerebral disease.

One of the potentially serious complications of the postmenopausal state is the "silent" disease of advancing osteoporosis, which first may be heralded by collapsed spinal vertebrae or hip fracture from a minor injury. Estrogen promotes and participates in the uptake of calcium into bone. However, the supplementation of estrogens postmenopausally is only one factor in minimizing bone loss (estimated loss of bone mass 1%–1.5%/year). The diet of calcium-rich products needs to be augmented, for example, milk, cheese, and yogurt. Proper exercise is also important, since inactivity promotes bone loss even in young women. Bone formation requires vitamin D and phosphorus as well as calcium and estrogens. Thus, proper mineral and vitamin intake needs to be encouraged. Calcitonin secreted by the thyroid controls bone resorption while parathyroid hormones and corticosteroids promote calcium loss. Unless there are specific contraindications, low-dose subuterine priming doses of estrogen may be given cyclically under careful monitoring, probably along with 5 to 10 days of progesterone on a cyclic 1- or 2-month basis to counteract the acknowledged risks, for example, strokes, vascular clots, endometrial cancer, or bleeding. Irregular bleeding requires directed endometrial sampling to exclude malignancy.

QUESTIONS IN OBSTETRICS AND GYNECOLOGY

What are the principal objectives of obstetric care?

What is the definition of maternal death?

What are the principal causes of maternal mortality?

What has been the trend in maternal mortality rates in the United States over the last 5 decades?

What factors are responsible for these trends?

What are the direct causes of maternal death? Indirect causes?

What are the principal causes of perinatal mortality and morbidity?

What are the recent trends in perinatal mortality in the United States?

What is the proportion of fetal deaths among perinatal deaths? What factors influence the risk of a fetal death?

Describe the true pelvis.

How is the true obstetric conjugate estimated?

Classify pelves according to type and describe the morphologic features of each.

Draw a sagittal section through the female pelvis, showing the vagina and the uterus and their relationship to the bladder and rectum.

Describe the relationship of the peritoneum to the uterus.

What is the main support structure for the uterus?

Describe the uterine ligaments.

What is the uterine blood supply?

Describe the fallopian tubes grossly and histologically.

Diagram a graafian follicle, indicating its principal parts.

Discuss the relation of the corpus luteum to the graafian follicle.

Describe the life cycle of the corpus luteum.

Describe the menstrual cycle and discuss the physiology of its production.

What is the relation of the hypothalamic-pituitary-ovarian axis to menstruation?

Where is the ovum fertilized?

Describe the retrogressive changes in the corpus luteum if pregnancy does not ensue.

What is meant by maturation of the ovum?

Describe some of the essential structures within the mature ovum and in its surroundings.

Describe the process of implantation.

What are the phases of the menstrual cycle?

Discuss the endocrine support of normal menses.

What are the vascular phenomena involved in the menstrual cycle?

What are some of the key histologic characteristics of the endometrium in the menstrual cycle?

Describe the nuclear events in oogenesis and spermatogenesis.

What is the characteristic chromosomal pattern of cells in the human?

Describe the process of implantation.

What is the chorion? Amnion? Decidua? Trophoblast? What are Langerhans' cells? Syncytial cells?

How is the embryo nourished before implantation? After implantation?

How does one classify the human placenta?

What triggers the endometrial decidual response after conception?

Discuss the maturation of the placenta from a vascular and functional viewpoint.

Describe the hemodynamics and metabolic exchange capabilities within the intervillous space.

What are the transport mechanisms within the placenta?

Outline proper prenatal care.

Give the positive signs, the probable signs, and the presumptive signs of pregnancy.

What are the common laboratory tests that are employed to establish the diagnosis of pregnancy? What is the hormonal basis for these tests? Which one is highly sensitive and specific?

Discuss diet in pregnancy and effect of maternal nutrition upon fetal growth and development

Discuss the current laboratory capabilities for estimating fetal status, welfare, and maturity; indications?

What is a stress test? A nonstress test?

Describe the diagnosis of fetal presentation.

What are the stages of normal labor? What is the so-called fourth stage?

Describe the mechanism of normal labor.

How is placenta normally delivered?

Describe episiotomy. What is the purpose of this procedure?

Describe the care of the lacerated perineum.

What are the principal techniques used in obstetric analgesia and anesthesia?

Discuss the purpose of systemic analgesia. Outline a plan of management.

What factors influence the choice of technique?

Describe the postpartal care of the mother.

Discuss common methods of family planning.

Define abortion; premature birth.

Define habitual abortion.

What constitutes good preventive medicine in obstetrics as it applies to the problem of repeated abortion?

What are the principal causes of spontaneous abortion?

Give the prophylaxis of abortion; give the signs, the symptoms, and the treatment of threatened abortion.

What clinical factors are known to influence the outcome in patients who are threatening to abort? What are the hazards of missed abortion?

What is the role of amniocentesis? Of pelvic sonography?

Classify the toxemias of pregnancy. What are the early warning signs? Discuss the etiology.

Discuss the principles of management of preeclampsia; of eclampsia.

What are the special problems of chronic hypertensive vascular disease complicating pregnancy?

Discuss the significant factors that determine the prognosis for patients with heart disease during pregnancy. Outline the principles of management.

How does pregnancy influence the clinical course of diabetes? What are the principal obstetric problems of the diabetic patient?

What are the principal causes of antepartum hemorrhage? How are they treated?

What are the clinical signs and symptoms of severe abruptio placentae? What factors determine fetal prognosis? What are the principal hazards to the mother? Outline a plan of management in cases of abruptio placentae.

Which factors favor the occurrence of placenta previa? Describe three types. How is it diagnosed and treated?

Discuss the diagnosis of extrauterine pregnancy. Specify types. Give the diagnosis and the treatment.

What are the major types of dystocia? Classify the types of uterine inertia. Discuss its management.

What are the current biophysical intrapartal fetal monitoring capabilities? What are the indications for their use?

Outline the various worrisome fetal heart rate patterns that reflect fetal insult or jeopardy. What are the underlying causes?

Which factors must be considered in determining whether or not a given fetus will negotiate a given pelvis?

Define the common types of pelvic contraction.

What are the special problems of a shoulder presentation? Outline a plan of management.

Give the diagnosis and the delivery of ROP.

Discuss the diagnosis, the mechanism, and the delivery of breech presentation. What are the principal fetal hazards? When should one perform a total breech extraction?

What is the current role of cesarean birth?

How is face presentation diagnosed and delivered? Discuss the clinical outcome of brow presentations.

Give the treatment for prolapse of the cord.

Give the etiology, the diagnosis, and the treatment of rupture of the uterus. What are the important predisposing factors in spontaneous uterine rupture? When should one contemplate a vaginal delivery in a patient who has had a previous cesarean section?

What are the principal causes of postpartum hemorrhage? How is it treated? What are the indications for manual removal of the placenta?

What are the indications for the application of forceps? Which conditions must be fulfilled before forceps are applied? How are forceps operations classified?

What is the clinical attitude toward external version? Internal version?

What are the indications for cesarean section? Contraindications? Types? When is a cesarean section indicated primarily for fetal indications?

What operative methods are available for female sterilization?

Into which main groups do puerperal infections fall? Discuss the prophylaxis and the treatment of puerperal infection. Define puerperal morbidity.

What are the common organisms involved? What are some of the late sequelae of puerperal infection?

Describe the fetal circulation. What are the maternal–fetal oxygen relationships? What are the compensatory mechanisms of the fetus to help meet its oxygen needs? Describe the changes in the infant's circulation after birth.

Describe the care of the newborn.

What are the causes of apnea neonatorum? What are its signs and treatment? What constitutes good prophylaxis?

Discuss the special problems of prematurity. What are the principal causes of premature labor? What are the principal hazards to the infant?

How is premature labor best managed? What drugs are most effective in forestalling or arresting premature labor?

What are the clinical forms of hemolytic disease of the newborn? Discuss each type. What are the pathologic findings? Outline the objective of management of isoimmunized women. Upon what evaluation is the timing for induction of labor based?

Discuss the immunologic basis for this disease. What is the significance of antibody determinations? Discuss the significance of kernicterus.

How does one estimate the severity of the fetal hemolytic process? What therapeutic capabilities are available? What method of prophylaxis is currently available? What is the basis for the approach?

Discuss ABO incompatibility.

What are the special characteristics of gonococcal infections? What are the principal types of acute lower tract infections? Outline the symptoms, the diagnosis, and the treatment.

Discuss the clinical varieties, the diagnosis, and the treatment of acute upper tract gonorrheal infections.

What are the principal types of salpingitis? Discuss the differential diagnosis.

What are the pathologic varieties of chronic upper tract infections? Discuss the role of surgery in the management of such cases.

What are the immediate hazards of acute pelvic inflammation? Subsequent remote hazards?

How do gonococcal and streptococcal pelvic infections differ? Mixed infections?

Discuss the common tuberculous lesions of the pelvis. Outline the clinical symptomatology and the diagnosis. Give the appropriate plan of management.

Classify and discuss the etiology of the ulcerative lesions of the vulva.

What are the vulvar dystrophies? What are their significance?

Describe the common varieties of vaginitis, the predisposing clinical factors, the characteristic physical findings, the diagnostic procedures, and the treatment.

What are the principal benign tumors of the vulva?

Describe the urethral caruncle. What are the histologic types?

What are the clinical characteristics of squamous-cell cancer of the vulva?

Give the etiology, the symptoms, the types, the diagnosis, and the treatment of uterine myomas. How do they influence pregnancy? Discuss the histogenesis of uterine sarcoma.

What are the diagnosis and the treatment of cervical polyps? Discuss the differential diagnosis.

Discuss the importance of detection of cancer in the cervix. Outline technique of detection and of diagnosis. What are the principal attributes of cytologic method? When is colposcopy indicated?

What risk does *in utero* exposure to maternal diethylstilbestrol impose upon young adult women?

Discuss carcinoma *in situ,* its histologic features, significance, and treatment.

When should the cervix be conized?

Describe the gross appearance of clinical cancers of the cervix. What are the principal symptoms?

What are the histologic types of cancer of the cervix? How does the lesion spread?

List and define the clinical stages of cancer of the cervix. What constitutes an adequate workup for these patients?

What are the objectives of radiation therapy? Describe the methods of achieving these objectives. What is a cancer-lethal dose at point B, and why is this an important consideration?

Outline the role of surgery in the management of cancer of the cervix. What is considered to be an acceptable 5-year survival rate for the various clinical stages?

What palliative measures are available in uterine cancer management? Cervix? Endometrium?

What are the expectations of chemotherapy in these lesions?

What clinical conditions are associated with a higher incidence of cancer of the endometrium?

Describe the histologic and the clinical types of adenocarcinoma. What are the common symptoms? What diagnostic procedures are indicated? How does the fundal cancer spread? Discuss management and prognosis.

What agents are useful for endometrial cancer?

Define and discuss the significance of endometriosis. Discuss the etiology and the predisposing factors. What are the common sites of involvement? Discuss the characteristic symptoms and the physical findings. Discuss the differential diagnosis. What is the fundamental fact upon which treatment is based? Outline a plan of management for these cases. What is adenomyosis, its symptoms, and management?

How are infertile patients with pelvic endometriosis treated?

What is the derivation of hydatidiform moles? Describe the histologic characteristics. Discuss the clinical and the diagnostic features. Discuss the role of hormone studies. What is the differential diagnosis? What is the risk of malignant degeneration? How helpful is pelvic sonography? At what stage of pregnancy?

What are the special hazards of chorioadenoma destruens? What are the clinical and the pathologic features of choriocarcinoma?

Classify ovarian tumors according to type. What are the functional cysts of the ovary?

Discuss the benign neoplastic cysts of the ovary, their derivation, histologic features, and clinical significance.

What are common complications arising in the benign ovarian cystic teratomas?

How does one stage the disease in malignant ovarian tumor?

What are the outstanding clinical characteristics of malignant ovarian tumors? What are the most common types? Discuss treatment and prognosis.

Classify the embryonic group of ovarian carcinoma, the clinical features according to type and the age of patient, and the malignant potentialities.

What clinical and histologic variables influence outcome in the treatment of ovarian cancer? What is the role of chemotherapy? What are the most effective agents?

Classify the remote injuries of childbirth according to anatomic defects. What is the most common genital tract fistula?

Define the retrodisplacements of the uterus. Define the various degrees of uterine prolapse.

What are the causes of genital tract fistulas?

What general principle forms the basis of modern vaginal surgery?

Discuss the usual clinical and laboratory workup of patients who chief complaint is urinary incontinence. What is the differential diagnosis? What are the modern testing capabilities? What are the clinical features of an unstable bladder?

The proper selection of surgical management of pelvic insufficiency is dependent on what factors?

What is the principle objective in restoring normal urethral and vesical neck anatomy? What are the surgical approaches?

Discuss the principal prophylactic measures that tend to maintain pelvic sufficiency.

Classify according to type the common disorders of menstruation. Give a definition of each specific type.

What is the most important single cause of abnormal bleeding in the absence of demonstrable pelvic lesions? Discuss the etiology of this condition, its histologic features, and its significance according to the age of the patient.

What are the common causes of acyclic bleeding and the relative frequency of such bleeding? Discuss the diagnostic workup and the significance of this condition.

Discuss the differential diagnosis and workup of patients with abnormal uterine bleeding due to anovulation. What are the principal goals in management? Outline the principles of hormone therapy in these patients. What are the hazards of chronic anovulation?

What are the causes of amenorrhea? Workup? What is the significance of galactorrhea? What special evaluative methods are used? How does one check on the various hypothalamic-pituitary-ovarian axis defects?

Discuss the differential diagnosis in female patients with defeminizing or masculinizing signs and symptoms. What workup is recommended to distinguish the conditions?

Discuss the principal clinical features, the etiology, the diagnostic workup, and the treatment of patients with polycystic ovaries. Describe the pathologic findings in the ovaries. What are the clinical results of surgical management? The results of hormone management? What endocrinopathies may underly the polycystic ovarian condition?

Define the term *infertility*. What are the incidence and the significance of this problem? What are the important causative factors in the male? In the female? Discuss a systematic program of investigations for these patients. Outline the general and the specific principles of management. What results can be expected?

How does one establish the presence of a tubal factor responsible for infertility?

Discuss abnormal sexual development by cause. What treatments are appropriate for abnormal sexual development?

What is the chromosomal defect in gonadal dysgenesis? How can an affected fetus be determined in utero?

What are the most effective methods of contraception? Indications for each? Side effects, hazards, contraindications? Level of effectiveness?

Multiple-Choice Questions

Indicate the best response. Answers are at the end of this chapter.

1. When should a female patient have her first complete pelvic examination?
   (a) As a newborn
   (b) As a child
   (c) When she begins to have sexual experiences regardless of age
   (d) At the time of menarche
   (e) At age 16
2. Puberty is the attainment of reproductive powers and may not be completed in all respects until about age 16 in females. Which is the last of the sophisticated developments in this progression of changes?
   (a) Menarche
   (b) Pubarche
   (c) Growth spurt
   (d) Hypothalamic cyclic center (positive feedback estrogen mechanism)
   (e) Thelarche
3. Which one of the following potential causes of maternal death is always classified as a "direct maternal death"?
   (a) Heart disease
   (b) Infection
   (c) Embolization (thrombotic)
   (d) Hemorrhage
   (e) Toxemias (preeclampsia)
4. Puerperal infections are generally caused by which type of organisms?
   (a) Beta-hemolytic streptococci
   (b) *Staphylococcus aureus*
   (c) Anaerobic organisms
   (d) *Bacteroides fragilis*
   (e) Clostridia

5. A fetal death occurring between the 20th and 28th gestational week when the birth weight is between 500 g and 999 g is classified as:
   (a) Intermediate fetal death
   (b) Abortion
   (c) Late fetal death
   (d) Immature fetal death
   (e) Perinatal death

6. Which of the following is a positive sign of pregnancy?
   (a) Positive pregnancy test (sensitive radioimmunoassay method)
   (b) Outlining the fetus (Leopold's maneuvers)
   (c) Perception of fetal movements by the examiner
   (d) Ballottement
   (e) Intermittent uterine contractions (Braxton Hicks sign)

7. Which one of the following causes of abortion is most clearly associated with losses in the second trimester?
   (a) Abnormal chromosomes
   (b) Anomalous or pathologic uterus
   (c) Localized anomaly of embryo
   (d) Abnormal placentation/defective trophoblast
   (e) None of the above

8. The patient was in her 10th gestational week and she began to complain of crampy pain, gush of clear fluid followed by minimal vaginal bleeding. On examination, her uterus was compatible with dates with respect to size and the cervix was dilated to about 1-cm to 2-cm size. What type of abortion listed below is the most likely diagnosis?
   (a) Inevitable abortion
   (b) Threatened abortion
   (c) Incomplete abortion
   (d) Missed abortion
   (e) Hydatidiform mole

9. Which one of the following entries is more effective in distinguishing between a missed abortion and hydatidiform mole?
   (a) Disappearing symptoms and signs of pregnancy
   (b) Dark brown turbid vaginal drainage
   (c) Presence of consumption coagulopathy
   (d) Presence of cystic ovaries
   (e) Ultrasonic snowstorm pattern in the uterus

10. Which one of the following entries is best in identifying a high-risk case of trophoblast disease that may require more aggressive initial therapy?
    (a) Duration of disease prior to onset of chemotherapy of more than 4 months
    (b) Initial HCG titers over 100,000
    (c) Cerebral metastases
    (d) Hepatic metastases
    (e) All of the above

11. Three weeks postpartally following a normal term delivery, the patient developed persistent vaginal bleeding, uterine subinvolution, and bilateral cystic ovaries. The most likely diagnosis is:
    (a) Hydatidiform mole
    (b) Choriocarcinoma
    (c) Retained placental fragments
    (d) Pelvic inflammatory disease
    (e) Pelvic hematoma

12. Which one of the following types of ectopic pregnancy is more often associated with delayed rupture and marked hemorrhage?
    (a) Ovarian implantation
    (b) Interstitial tubal implantation
    (c) Isthmic tubal implantation
    (d) Ampullary tubal implantation
    (e) Infundibular tubal implantation

13. A multipara stated that in the first trimester of pregnancy she experienced sudden pain and sensation of syncope, which subsided, but subsequently in the second and third trimesters, she has been experiencing gastrointestinal symptoms, painful fetal movements, and now at term, attacks of false labor without bleeding. A probable diagnosis is:
    (a) Abdominal pregnancy
    (b) Abruptio placentae with concealed hemorrhage
    (c) Placenta previa
    (d) Silent uterine rupture with contained broad ligament hematoma
    (e) Multiple gestation with impaired circulation in one twin

14. Which one of the following obstetric situations would you least likely associate with the complication of consumption coagulopathy?
    (a) Abruptio placentae
    (b) Rupture of the uterus
    (c) Placenta previa
    (d) Amniotic fluid embolus
    (e) Missed abortion

15. If a laboring patient you have been examining and following suddenly ruptures her

membranes and develops minimal vaginal bleeding and fetal distress in the absence of increased pain or uterine tone, hypotension, tachycardia, oliguria, or other local or systemic sign or symptom, which of the following underlying clinical conditions would you suspect?

(a) Ruptured umbilical cord vessel
(b) Cervical laceration
(c) Marginal abruptio placentae
(d) Silent uterine rupture
(e) Change of low implantation to placenta previa where cervix dilates

16. Based on your clinical impression from question 15, which one of the following methods of investigation would provide the best means of establishing the diagnosis?

(a) Pelvic sonogram (placental localization)
(b) Check urine for blood indicative of bladder trauma
(c) Speculum examination of the lower generative tract
(d) Kleihaur smear
(e) "Double setup" examination

17. Abruptio placentae is a complication of one or more obstetric conditions listed below. Which entry below is most likely responsible?

(a) Chronic hypertension
(b) Diabetes mellitus class D
(c) Chronic nephritis
(d) Preeclampsia–eclampsia
(e) All of the above

18. The least likely cause of postpartal hemorrhage is which one of the following potential etiologies?

(a) Uterine atony
(b) Laceration or hematoma; ruptured varix
(c) Retained placentae or membranes
(d) Ruptured uterus, prolapsed uterus, or inversion of uterus
(e) Blood dyscrasia

19. Clinical signs and symptoms during labor characterized by cessation of uterine contractions, fetal distress with rapid disappearance of fetal heart sounds, regression of a previously engaged presenting part, hypovolemic shock, and external or concealed hemorrhage suggest which one of the following complications?

(a) Ruptured uterus
(b) Abruptio placentae
(c) Abdominal pregnancy (or intraligamentary)

(d) Heterotopic pregnancy (*in utero* gestation in addition to an ectopic gestation
(e) Placenta accreta (or placenta with rupture through the wall by the myometrial trophoblast)

20. A 20-year-old primigravida had a normal pregnancy until the 37th gestational week, when she developed a rise in the systolic blood pressure of 40 and a rise in diastolic pressure of 20. The other findings were hyperreflexia, proteinuria of 3 g/24 hours, urinary output of 100 ml/24 hours, and mild edema of the face and hands. There was no tachycardia, fever, pulmonary edema, anasarca, epigastric pain, CNS irritability, or cloudy sensorium. Her past medical history was totally unremarkable. Apparently, the fetal growth and development was normal and the uterus was compatible with dates, and there was no evidence of fetal distress. Which one of the following therapeutic approaches is the best?

(a) Force fluids to flush the kidneys but restrict the salt intake substantially.
(b) Administer diuretics to correct edema and minimize risk of pulmonary edema.
(c) Administer Digoxin to minimize the risks of congestive heart failure (along with prescribed rest regimen).
(d) Administer apresoline (hydralazine) to minimize the risks of intracranial hemorrhage.
(e) Admit the patient immediately to the hospital for evaluation *without any* ambulatory treatments.

21. The patient under discussion in question 20 was given intravenous fluids and magnesium sulfate intravenously. Which one of the following findings reflects most acutely upon the dose level and timing of $MgSO_4$ administrations?

(a) Lowered blood pressure in the first 30 minutes after administration
(b) Decreased variability of the fetal heart on the heart rate monitor
(c) Reduction in urinary output to 500 ml/24 hours
(d) Increase in proteinuria to 4 g/24 hours
(e) Absent knee jerks

22. The physiological action of hydralazine is best represented by which one of the following responses?

(a) All of the actions below
(b) Reflex tachycardia

(c) Increases renal flow

(d) Increased cardiac output

(e) Smooth muscle relaxant

23. Which one of the following statements about twins is correct?

   (a) Monozygotic twinning is a recessive autosomal trait inherited from the female descendants of mothers of twins.

   (b) Monochorionic placentas are *always* monozygotic.

   (c) Divisions occurring in a single ovum before the differentiation of the trophoblast at day 5 or before result in single placentas with one chorion.

   (d) Monochorionic placenta with vascular communications of the artery-to-artery or vein-to-vein are the most serious fetal risks.

   (e) The so-called fetus acardiacus is a fetal teratomatous tumor arising in the gonad that resembles a parasitic second twin.

24. Which one of the following categories of multiple pregnancy constitutes the gravest hazard to the fetuses?

   (a) Monochorion diamniotic placenta

   (b) Dichorionic diamniotic placenta

   (c) Dichorionic fused placenta

   (d) Velamentous insertion of the cord

   (e) Monoamniotic monochorionic placenta

25. Which one of the following entries pertaining to the progress of labor and eventual outcome represents the best response to the question of which major factor(s) is or are involved?

   (a) The passage

   (b) The powers

   (c) The passenger

   (d) The placenta

   (e) All of the above

26. Most female pelves are morphologically of which type?

   (a) Gynecoid

   (b) Android

   (c) Anthropoid

   (d) Platypelloid

   (e) Mixed

27. What is the most common dysfunction leading to abnormal progress in labor?

   (a) Soft-tissue dystocia

   (b) Hypotonic labor

   (c) Dystonic labor

   (d) Hypertonic labor

   (e) None of the above

28. Oxytocin stimulation of dysfunctional labor has its greatest usefulness in certain types of clinical symptoms. Which one of the following entries is the best response relative to indication for this approach to management?

   (a) Hypertonic labor

   (b) Dystonic labor

   (c) Reverse peristalsis

   (d) Segmental tetanic contracture

   (e) None of the above

29. Which one of the following mechanisms of normal labor in vertex presentation is an abnormal occurrence before the fetal head reaches the perineum?

   (a) Engagement

   (b) Extension

   (c) Descent

   (d) Internal rotation

   (e) Flexion

30. The patient has a septic abortion associated with anaerobic organisms with a gram-negative bacteremia. She was treated with ampicillin and chloramphenicol. After 3 days of some clinical improvement, she began to experience fatigue, pallor, and tachycardia, and when blood counts were evaluated she had a pancytopenia. There was an alarmingly low red count of 1 million mm^3 red blood cells and these were slightly macrocytic; the icteric index was low. A bone marrow study revealed normal hemosiderin on stained smear but the marrow was fatty with few red cells, white cells, or megakaryocytes. The likely diagnosis is:

   (a) Iron deficiency anemia

   (b) Folic acid deficiency anemia

   (c) Pernicious anemia

   (d) Aplastic anemia

   (e) Drug-induced anemia

31. An 18-year-old female with primary amenorrhea had normally developed secondary sex characteristics. On workup she failed to have withdrawal bleeding after the progestational challenge or cyclic conjugated estrogen–progesterone administrations. Workup revealed a normal 46 XX karyotype. An intravenous pyelogram revealed an anomalous urinary tract on the left. On pelvic examination, a morphologic defect was discovered. What do you suspect it is (indicate one of the following conditions)?

   (a) Testicular feminization

   (b) Asherman's syndrome

   (c) Müllerian agenesis

   (d) Transverse vaginal septum

   (e) None of the above

32. A 30-year-old patient with secondary amenorrhea, galactorrhea, and hyperprolactinemia is likely to have which one of the following disorders?
    (a) Hypothalamic amenorrhea
    (b) Disorder of the pituitary gland (adenoma)
    (c) Ovarian disorder (ovarian steroid defect)
    (d) Breast disorder (response to chronic suckling)
    (e) Disorder of genetic constitution with uterine or lower generative tract defect

33. Which one of the following statements is the best response concerning the majority of testosterone produced in the normal female?
    (a) Testosterone in the circulation arises from direct ovarian secretion.
    (b) Testosterone in the circulation arises from direct secretion from the adrenal gland.
    (c) Testosterone in the circulation arises from peripheral conversion, mainly from the reduction of androstenedione.
    (d) A major fraction of secreted ovarian androgens is synthesized in the stroma.
    (e) All of the above are correct.

34. Which one of the following statements is the best response concerning conditions associated with a steady state of estrogen stimulation that leads to irregular endometrial shedding characteristic of dysfunctional uterine bleeding?
    (a) Continuously proliferating endometrium may outgrow its blood supply.
    (b) The persistence of acid mucopolysaccharides causes a loss of nutrients by preventing depolymerization and diffusion of these substances.
    (c) Asynchronous development of the glands, stroma, and blood vessels.
    (d) Overdevelopment of Golgi-lysosomal complex capable of releasing excessive amounts of hydrolytic enzymes.
    (e) All of the above are correct.

35. A 25-year-old patient developed dysuria, frequency, urgency, chills, fever, malaise, lower abdominal pain, yellow vaginal discharge, and marked pelvic tenderness. Which one of the following simple procedures is most likely to establish the diagnosis?
    (a) Gram stain of cervical smear
    (b) Wet preparation of vaginal discharge
    (c) Nickerson's medium culture of vaginal discharge
    (d) Papanicolaou smear
    (e) Urine culture

36. Which one of the following causes of vaginitis is the best response to the clinical problem of vaginal burning, pruritus, and dyspareunia in association with a thin, often watery, bubbly, frothy white to yellowish vaginal discharge, erythematous mucosa, petechial hemorrhages, and "strawberry" spots?
    (a) *Trichomonas vaginalis*
    (b) Monilial vaginitis
    (c) Atrophic vaginitis
    (d) Nonspecific vaginitis
    (e) Early cervical carcinoma

37. Which one of the following is the best response to the question of theories of etiology and mechanism of dissemination in endometriosis?
    (a) Tubal reflux (Sampson theory)
    (b) Coelomic metaplasia
    (c) Vascular dissemination
    (d) Lymphatic dissemination
    (e) All of the above

38. The patient is a 35-year-old who has aborted twice at the 18th gestational week and she has complained of severe dysmenorrhea, hypermenorrhea, some increased vaginal discharge, and spotting intermenstrually. On pelvic examination the uterus was slightly irregular, firm, and enlarged to an 8-week gestational size. The impression is that she has a leiomyomatous uterus. What type of uterine tumor is associated with these types of clinical presentations?
    (a) Submucous leiomyoma
    (b) Intramural leiomyoma
    (c) Subserosal leiomyoma
    (d) Intraligamentary leiomyoma (or parasitic)
    (e) None of the above

39. What are the basic infertility screening procedures? Which entry below represents the best answer?
    (a) Semen analysis
    (b) Evaluation of ovulatory function
    (c) Tubal patency tests
    (d) The postcoital examination
    (e) All of the above

40. The important causes of female infertility include the following factors:
    (a) Tubes and peritoneum
    (b) The ovaries
    (c) The cervix
    (d) The uterine fundus
    (e) All of the above in descending order of relative importance

41. If the basic tests in the infertility workup are uninformative, which one of the following special investigations is likely to be most rewarding?
    (a) Tests for sperm allergy
    (b) Skull roentgenogram for sella turcica
    (c) Buccal smear (chromosomal analysis)
    (d) Laparoscopy
    (e) Hysteroscopy

42. Which one of the five leading reversible methods of contraception is the most effective?
    (a) Oral contraceptives (the pill)
    (b) Barrier contraception with jelly
    (c) The intrauterine device (IUD)
    (d) Condom and foam
    (e) Postovulatory rhythm

43. Which one of the complications is least likely to be associated with the use of the IUD?
    (a) Breakthrough vaginal bleeding
    (b) Hypermenorrhea
    (c) Dysmenorrhea
    (d) Endometrial cancer
    (e) Pelvic infection

44. Which one of the following entries is the best response to the question of positive colposcopic findings in the cervix?
    (a) White epithelium
    (b) Punctuation
    (c) Mosaic structure
    (d) Abnormal vessels
    (e) All of the above

45. A high-risk microinvasive cervical lesion requiring special surgical attention involves which one(s) of the following histopathologic features? Mark the entity which represents the best response.
    (a) Microinvasive lesion of more than 3 ml to 5 ml in depth
    (b) Deep cell nests
    (c) Confluence of nests of cells
    (d) Lymphatic or vascular involvements
    (e) All of the above findings

46. A 52-year-old woman who had never been able to conceive presented with anorexia, weight loss, nausea, abdominal discomfort, bloating, fullness, and increasing tightness of the clothes. She was 1 year postmenopausal, and there had been no vaginal bleeding. She had a positive family history of gynecologic cancer. On pelvic examination, it was possible to feel a pelvic mass. The suspicion of a malignancy should focus upon which one of the following sites?
    (a) Ovary
    (b) Tube
    (c) Endometrium
    (d) Cervix or vagina
    (e) Nongynecologic organ

Based on your knowledge that a certain pattern of urine loss often characterizes a particular type of underlying defect or disorder, please match the following items (47–49 and 50–52) by writing the appropriate letter (a, b, or c).

47. Genitourinary fistula	(a) Slightly delayed loss after coughing
48. Neurogenic bladder	(b) Continuous urine loss
49. Detrustor dyssynergia	(c) Precipitous voiding

50. Irritable bladder syndrome	(a) Without conscious voiding action losses with increased abdominal pressure
51. Urethral deformity	(b) Dribbling upon standing after emptying the bladder
52. Stress incontinence	(c) Loss with urge

Recognizing that flexible clinical policies and some degree of controversy exist about the selection of proper definitive procedures in the management of early cervical neoplasia, please choose your preference of therapeutic modality listed in the right column (a–d) for each of the cervical lesions indicated in the left column.

53. Mild to moderate dysplasia	(a) Radical hysterectomy with pelvic lymphadenectomy
54. Severe dysplasia	
55. Carcinoma *in situ*	(b) Extrafascial hysterectomy with or without excision of vaginal cuff
56. Microinvasion, less than 3 mm, nonconfluent; absence of lymphatic or vascular channel invasion	(c) Intrafascial hysterectomy without excision of vaginal cuff
57. Microinvasion, 3 mm to 5 mm, confluent; vascular and lymphatic invasion	(d) LEEP and curettage

Please assign to each statement below, the proper letter based on the following key (pertains only to question 58):

(a) If only 1, 2, and 3 entries are best answers
(b) If only 1 and 3 are best answers

(c) If only 2 and 4 are best answers

(d) If only 4 is the best answer

(e) If some other combination is best

58. (1) The superimposition of preeclampsia is the most common hazard of hypertensive disease.

    (2) Preeclampsia superimposed on chronic hypertensive disease manifests itself by a subtle rise in blood pressure, and the appearance of edema or substantial proteinuria is relatively uncommon.

    (3) When preeclampsia develops in association with hypertension, it is likely to be earlier than in normal pregnancy.

    (4) Control of blood pressure by antihypertensive drugs has been highly effective in reducing the incidence of preeclampsia and in reducing perinatal mortality.

Please indicate the single best answer to the following question.

59. Which of the following anaerobic bacteria is the most likely species to be encountered clinically when serious pelvic infections develop?

    (a) Fusobacteria (gram-negative bacillus)

    (b) Clostridia (gram-positive bacillus)

    (c) Peptostreptococci (gram-positive coccus)

    (d) *Actinomyces* (gram-positive bacillus)

    (e) *Bacteroides fragilis* (gram-negative bacillus)

Please match the rather classic clinical lesions on the left with the corresponding venereal diseases.

60. Destructive vulvar ulceration, nodal masses, and proctocolitis

61. Nontender, raised, firm, indurated papules with a raised border

62. Tender, irregular, serpiginous ulcerations, soft erythematous, grayish or yellowish necrotic exudate

63. Autoinoculation, beefy granulations, keloidlike depigmented scars, superficial ulcerations

    (a) Granuloma inguinale

    (b) Chancroid

    (c) Primary syphilis (chancre)

    (d) Lymphogranuloma venereum

    (e) Condylomata acuminata

64. Multiple and flesh-colored pinkish papillary or sessile growths on mucous membranes or perineum

The presence or suspicion of one venereal disease requires multiple tests to exclude others. Please match the relatively standard tests itemized on the left with the appropriate letter.

65. Diploid human fibroblast culture; cytologic changes in Pap smear

66. Culture purulent discharge (cervix) on modified Thayer-Martin medium. agar; culture anus

67. Gram stain material at base of ulcer (Giemsa stain) to detect *H. Ducreyi* bacillus

68. Biopsy granulation tissue (Wright and Giemsa stains) to detect Donovan bodies

69. Positive chlamydial complement fixation test; Frei test

    (a) Lymphogranuloma venereum

    (b) Herpesvirus 2

    (c) Gonorrhea

    (d) Chancroid

    (e) Granuloma inguinale

Please associate the following venereal diseases with their recommended treatment. Discount the fact that resistant organisms may be present and that alternative therapy may be required.

70. Gonorrheal cervicitis

71. Primary syphilis

72. Lymphogranuloma venereum

73. Chancroid

74. Granuloma inguinale

    (a) Doxycycline

    (b) Sulfasoxazole

    (c) Ceftriaxone

    (d) Tetracycline

    (e) Benzathine penicillin G

75. Which one of the following antepartal methods of assessing fetal jeopardy is most

valuable in programming clinical management in patients with Rh incompatibility?

(a) Obstetric history
(b) Determination of maternal antibody titers
(c) Spectrophotometric screening of amniotic fluid
(d) Chemical assay of amniotic fluid bilirubin
(e) Rh genotype test to determine zygosity of the father

Specific anatomic and functional changes occur at the several phases of the menstrual cycle in synchronized events involving glandular, vascular, and stromal components of the endometrium. Please match the following:

76. Shallow endometrium with desquamation and collapse of the supporting matrix representing a transitional state bridging exfoliative and growth stages

77. Saw-tooth glands; vacuoles, stromal edema; coiled spiral vessels; tortuous distended gland lumina

78. Shrinkage of endometrial height; diminished blood flow and venous drainage; vasodilation, rhythmic vasoconstriction and relaxation of spiral arterioles; ischemia; white-cell migration; interstitial red cells, tissue disorganization

79. Continuous epithelial lining; unbranched spiral vessels; peripheral extension of gland epithelium pseudostratification, mitoses; loose, synctial-like stroma; increasing endometrial height

(a) Endometrial breakdown
(b) Preparation for implantation
(c) Proliferative phase
(d) Menstrual endometrium
(e) Secretory phase

80. Engorged subepithelial capillaries and spiral vessels; large, polyhedral stromal cells in superficial endometrium; lacelike edematous stroma; coiled spiral vessels; exhausted, dilated glandular ribbons of stratum spongiosum compressed gland necks

81. Among DES-exposed young females with gross structural changes in the vagina or cervix, which one of the following abnormalities is most likely to interfere with thorough evaluation and ultimately require surgical attention because of associated symptoms or worrisome epithelial changes, and potential of subsequent reproductive losses?

(a) Transverse ridges, complete or incomplete bands of tissue in the proximal part of the vagina
(b) Peaked, roughened anterior cervical lip (cock comb shape)
(c) Cervical collar or hood
(d) Hypoplastic cervix or eccentrically located cervical os
(e) Pseudopolyps of the cervix

82. Which one of the following genital organs originates from the involvement of two distinct embryologic structures?

(a) Ovaries
(b) Tubes
(c) Uterus
(d) Vagina
(e) External genitalia

Among apparently healthy women who suffer from abnormal or absent menstrual function, disturbances within the hypothalamic-pituitary-ovarian axis may be classified broadly according to three major faults. Please match the resultant clinical expressions with the appropriate defect noted in questions 83, 84, and 85.

83. Ovarian failure
84. Central failure
85. Anovulatory dysfunction

    (a) Hypogonadotropic hypogonadism
    (b) Asynchronous gonadotropin and estrogen production
    (c) Hypergonadotropic hypogonadism

86. Among the various presenting symptoms of patients with ovarian malignancy, which one of the following manifestations is the most common?
    (a) Abnormal vaginal bleeding
    (b) Gastrointestinal symptoms
    (c) Abdominal distention or discomfort
    (d) Weight loss
    (e) Urinary complaints (pressure frequency)
87. Which one of the following surgical procedures designed to restore reproductive function in the presence of tubal and pelvic peritoneal disease enjoys the overall greater chance of success?
    (a) Salpingolysis
    (b) Fibrioplasty
    (c) Partial resection and reanastomosis
    (d) Tubal implantation
    (e) Tubal bypass (Estes procedure and replacement operations)
88. Which one of the following chemotherapeutic agents has documented activity and enjoys considerable popularity as the traditional drug of choice as initial adjuvant therapy in ovarian malignancy?
    (a) Cyclophosphamide
    (b) Actinomycin D
    (c) Methotrexate
    (d) Adriamycin
    (e) Melphalan
89. Roughly what percentage of patients with metastatic epithelial ovarian cancer will benefit from treatment with an alkylating agent?
    (a) Less than 10%
    (b) 25% to 49%
    (c) 50% to 74%
    (d) 75% to 89%
    (e) More than 90%
90. The best prognosis in endometrial adenocarcinoma occurs in Stage Ia. Which ones of the following features are characteristic of the early lesions?

    (a) If only 1, 2, and 3 entries are best answers
    (b) If only 1 and 3 are best answers
    (c) If only 2 and 4 are best answers
    (d) If only 4 is the best answer
    (e) If some other combination is best
    (1) The disease is confined to the corpus of the uterus.
    (2) The uterus sounds to less than 8.0 cm.
    (3) The histologic appearance is that of a well-differentiated tumor.
    (4) Endocervical curettings are positive for tumor but not the ectocervix.

91. Endometrial cancer is now considered to be the most common female pelvic malignancy with respect to the presence of associated conditions and epidemiologic variables. Which one(s) of the following entries and possible etiologic factors have been identified? *Note:* Please use the same key presented in question 90.
    (1) Long-standing endogenous or exogenous estrogen exposure, particularly estrone
    (2) Obesity and increased tissue conversion of androstenedione to estrone
    (3) Diabetes mellitus or hypertension
    (4) Endometrial polyps, adenomyosis, or leiomyomata
92. Which one of the following vulvar diseases is *not* one of the circumscribed or diffuse "white lesions"?
    (a) Hypertrophic dystrophy (lichen simplex chronicus or neurodermatitis)
    (b) Atrophic dystrophies (lichen sclerosus et atrophicus)
    (c) Mixed vulvar dystrophies
    (d) Intraepithelial cancer
    (e) Extramammary Paget's disease
93. In considering the hormonal interrelationships in lactation, which one of the following agents is primarily involved in milk ejection rather than breast preparation, initiation of lactation, or maintenance of lactation?
    (a) Drop in serum estrogen and progesterone
    (b) Oxytocin
    (c) Prolactin
    (d) Placental lactogen
    (e) Thyroxine
94. Certain anatomic considerations of the cervix must be taken into account in obtaining materials for diagnostic study. Which one of the following statements is *least* likely to be correct?
    (a) The early lesions of the cervix are usu-

ally associated with the squamocolumnar junction.

(b) The portio vaginalis, which is most visible and easiest to biopsy, is not the area of greatest interest in diagnosing early carcinoma.

(c) As metaplasia develops in columnar epithelium, tongues of stratified squamous epithelium may extend from the endocervical canal onto the portio vaginalis.

(d) The squamocolumnar junction is always within the distal 2 cm of the endocervical canal.

(e) Surgical biopsies taken properly should attempt to include intact and adequate epithelium from the endocervical canal in the specimen.

95. Critical pelvic dimensions, assuming an average-sized fetus, include all of the following:
(a) Diagonal conjugate greater than 12.5 cm
(b) Obstetric conjugate (anteroposterior of the inlet) greater than 10.0 cm
(c) Transverse of the midpelvis of greater than 9.0 cm
(d) Sum of the posterior sagittal and bi-tuberous of more than 15.0 cm

Please match each of the following pelvic architectures with the *best* statement concerning its *most likely clinical presentation:*

96. Inlet dystocia
97. Midpelvic dystocia
98. Outlet dystocia
99. Gynecoid pelvis
100. Android pelvis
101. Anthropoid pelvis

(a) Rare, as an isolated finding
(b) Occiput posterior arrest
(c) Few labor problems
(d) Marked by a floating presentation
(e) Deep transverse pelvic arrest
(f) The most common pelvic limitation

102. The predispositions of dizygotism include all of the following except:
(a) A recessive autosomal trait via the male descendants
(b) Stopping oral contraceptives
(c) Artificial ovulation induction
(d) Greater maternal height or weight
(e) Advanced maternal age

103. All of the following are associated with an enhanced rate of major structural abnormalities in the offspring except:
(a) Monozygotic multiple gestation
(b) Battledore placenta
(c) Two-vessel cord
(d) Advanced maternal age
(e) Small-for-gestational-age fetus

ANSWERS TO MULTIPLE-CHOICE QUESTIONS

1. c	27. b	53. e	79. c
2. d	28. e	54. c	80. b
3. e	29. b	55. b	81. a
4. c	30. d	56. b	82. d
5. a	31. c	57. a	83. c
6. c	32. b	58. b	84. a
7. b	33. c	59. e	85. b
8. a	34. e	60. d	86. c
9. e	35. a	61. c	87. a
10. e	36. a	62. b	88. e
11. b	37. e	63. a	89. c
12. b	38. a	64. e	90. a
13. a	39. e	65. b	91. a
14. c	40. e	66. c	92. e
15. a	41. d	67. d	93. b
16. d	42. a	68. e	94. d
17. e	43. d	69. a	95. c
18. e	44. e	70. c	96. d
19. a	45. e	71. e	97. f
20. e	46. a	72. a	98. a
21. e	47. b	73. b	99. c
22. a	48. c	74. d	100. e
23. b	49. a	75. c	101. b
24. e	50. c	76. d	102. a
25. e	51. b	77. e	103. b
26. e	52. a	78. a	

Rypins' Clinical Sciences Review, 16th Edition,
edited by Edward D. Frohlich. J. B. Lippincott
Company, Philadelphia © 1993.

5

Pediatrics

Margaret C. Heagarty, M.D.
Director of Pediatrics, Harlem Hospital Center

Professor of Pediatrics, College of Physicians
and Surgeons, Columbia University
New York, New York

Children, by definition, are growing, developing, and vulnerable organisms. This simple, if obvious, fact differentiates pediatrics from other areas of medicine. Although the field shares many concepts and approaches with all of medicine, it also requires special knowledge, skills, and attitudes. Since any attempt to summarize all of pediatrics in a single essay is manifestly impossible, this chapter will focus on those aspects of the field that are unique or particularly important to the general physician.

GROWTH AND DEVELOPMENT

The hallmark of any professional concerned with the health and welfare of children resides in a profound understanding of and interest in children's growth and development.

Growth

Growth is defined as the process by which the human body increases in size as a result of an increase in the size or the number of the body's cells. Children do not grow at the same rate throughout childhood. The most rapid period of growth occurs during the embryonic and fetal period, during which the fetus grows from a single cell at conception to about 3,300 g (7.5 lbs) at birth. Although infants obviously grow in size, the actual rate of growth actually decreases during the first 3

years of life. From the age of 3 years until the onset of puberty, children's rate of growth remains relatively steady; at puberty their growth rate again increases.

WEIGHT

The normal infant gains about 1 ounce (30 g) a day for the first 5 to 6 months of life. Thus, normal infants are expected to double their birth weight by 5 to 6 months of age. During the second 6 months of life infants gain 3 to 4 ounces (90–120 g) a week; the birth weight usually triples by 1 year of age. After the first year weight gain is relatively steady and averages about 4 to 6 pounds (2–3 kg) each year. At about 2.5 years the birth weight is quadrupled. The following formulas provide a method of estimating average weights in children:

3 to 12 months of age (weight in pounds) =
age in months + 11
2 to 12 years (weight in pounds) =
age in years × 5 + 18

HEIGHT

Growth in stature progresses less rapidly than weight. The average newborn measures about 20 inches (51 cm) in length. The length increases about 10 inches (25 cm) in the first year of life. The birth length usually doubles by 4 years of age and triples by 13 years of age. On average, a child gains about 3 inches (7.6 cm) in height annually between the ages of 2 and 5 years. The eventual adult height can be approximated by doubling the value of the child's height at about 2 years of age. An estimate of the height of children between the ages of 2 and 12 years can be calculated using the following formula:

$$\text{height in inches} = \text{age in years} \times 2 + 32$$

HEAD CIRCUMFERENCE

In addition to weight and height, several other measurements are routinely used to determine a child's growth status. The head circumference, which parallels the rapidly growing central nervous system, should be included as part of the physical examination of all infants. The head circumference is obtained by measuring the head in its widest diameter, including the most prominent part of the occiput through the area just above the supraorbital ridges of the forehead. During the first year of life the head circumference normally increases by about 4 inches (10 cm). In general, a normal 7-month infant has a head circumference of 17 inches (43 cm); a 19-month-old child has a head circumference of 19 inches (48 cm); and a 5-year-old has a head circumference of about 20 inches (51 cm).

BONE AGE

Since the ossification centers of the bones form at different and predictable ages, roentgenographic examination of the hands and feet provides an estimate of the child's bone age. Five ossification centers are usually present at birth, the calcaneus, cuboid, talus, the distal end of the femur, and the proximal end of the tibia. Until the age of 6 years, with the aid of the following formula, a roentgenograph of the wrist will assist in the determination of the child's bone age:

age in years + 1 = number of ossification
centers in the wrist

GROWTH CHARTS

Serial measurements of these parameters of growth in populations of normal children has provided the clinician with standards against which to measure the individual child. Several growth charts have been developed for this purpose. The most commonly used, which was prepared by the United States National Center for Health Care Statistics, presents height, weight, and head circumference growth curves for children of different ages and sex.

Because these growth curves have been derived from a cross section of children of different social classes and ethnic backgrounds living in the United States, they represent only an approximation of normal growth. For that reason repeated measures of a child's growth are more useful than any single set of measurements plotted on a derived growth curve. Over time a child should follow the same pattern on a growth curve. Any significant deviation from this pattern suggests serious organic disease or a noxious environmental influence.

Development

Development may be defined as a continuous, progressive, and sequential process by which a child's level of function becomes more complex. This gradual progression of function, which reflects the gradual maturation of the central nervous system, proceeds in a cephalocaudad, proximodistal direction. Although the child's developmental process is assessed clinically at discrete points in time, in fact, the process continues throughout life in a general sequence and pattern that does not vary a great deal among normal children. For the purposes of assessment this developmental process can be classified into categories of gross motor, fine motor, language, and social development. Gross motor developmental tasks include those that involve the large muscle groups of the trunk and extremities; fine motor tasks involve those of the small muscles of the body, specifically, the hands; language development refers to the growth of language and communicative skills; social development is defined as that involving interpersonal and social skills.

Just as significant deviation in growth can signal serious disease or environmental problems, so, too, does a significant deviation in a child's developmental progress indicate a serious problem. A vari-

TABLE 5-1. Developmental Milestones: Gross Motor Development

ACTIVITY	AGE
Sits with support	3–4 mo
Sits alone	7–8 mo
Stands alone for a few seconds	12–13 mo
Walks unassisted	12–15 mo
Climbs on furniture	24 mo
Walks up the stairs one step at a time	24 mo
Rides tricycle	36 mo

TABLE 5-2. Developmental Milestones: Fine Motor Development

ACTIVITY	AGE
Grasp reflex	At birth
Intentional reaching	4–5 mo
Palmar grasp	6–8 mo
Princer grasp	9–10 mo
Builds a six-block tower	24 mo
Builds a three-block bridge	36 mo
Reproduces a cross with a crayon	36 mo

TABLE 5-3. Developmental Milestones: Language Development

ACTIVITY	AGE
Indistinct throaty noises	3–5 wk
Cooing	10–12 wk
Single and multiple syllables	6–8 mo
Two-word phrases	24 mo
Three-word sentences	36 mo
Six- to seven-word sentences	48 mo

TABLE 5-4. Developmental Milestones: Social Development

ACTIVITY	AGE
Social smile	4–6 wk
Smiles at self in mirror	6 mo
Responds to "no"	8 mo
Becomes frightened with strangers	8–10 mo
Knows own gender	24–30 mo
Plays in parallel	24–36 mo

ety of screening developmental tests are available to assist the clinician in tracking a child's development over time. However, physicians caring for children should have a working knowledge of the common developmental milestones and the ages at which they are expected in normal children. Common developmental milestones from infancy to the preschool period are summarized in Tables 5-1 through 5-4.

NUTRITION

Because adequate nutrition is a prerequisite for normal growth and development in children, physicians must not only understand the physiologic requirements of the growing child but must also be able to translate these requirements into a diet consonant with the prevailing culture of the child and family. The basic requirements of any diet include water and calories in the form of carbohydrate, fat, and protein as well as minerals and vitamins.

Water Requirements

Water requirements vary directly with the body's metabolic rate. Although the water requirements for infants are much larger per unit of body weight than for those of adults, in fact, the requirements when calculated in relation to the infant's caloric intake are virtually identical to those of adults. At basal conditions obligatory water requirements are about 100 ml/100 calories metabolized. However, the daily fluid requirements for infants represent about 10% to 15% of their body weight, while requirements for adults represent only about 2% to 4% of total body weight.

Water balance in children varies with fluid intake, age, maturity of the kidney, diet and solute load, body temperature, and respiratory rates.

Low-birth-weight infants require a higher fluid intake than full-term infants. Newborn infants with hyperbilirubinemia treated with phototherapy also have increased fluid requirements.

Perhaps most important, under ordinary circumstances the thirst mechanism, regulated by the central nervous system, controls an adult's or a child's water intake. Since infants cannot actively seek water, their daily water requirements must be provided. In general, infants to the age of about 1 year require between 150 ml and 160 ml of water per kilogram of body weight. The requirements for older children can be calculated using the following formula:

$$\text{ml/kg} = 125 - (5 \times \text{years of age})$$

Infants and toddlers are particularly vulnerable to dehydration, usually caused by fluid loss from the vomiting and diarrhea of infectious gastroenteritis.

Caloric Requirements

The daily caloric requirements for children vary with their age, stage of growth, activity level, and basal metabolic needs. The average caloric requirements for infants during the first year of life is about 100 to 120 kcal/kg of body weight. During the succeeding 3 years of life these requirements decrease about 10 kcal/kg each year. During the growth spurt of adolescence the daily caloric requirements again increases. These average requirements represent only an approximation of a child's needs; the most accurate method of determining an individual child's caloric requirements resides in a careful determination of the child's growth pattern over time. Deficits or excesses in caloric intake will be reflected in the child's growth pattern. Details of the physiology and metabolism of the average daily requirements of carbohydrate, fat, protein, minerals, and vitamins are provided in Table 5-5.

INFANT FEEDING

Breast feeding is the preferred method for feeding most infants. Human milk has many advantages; it is available in an uncontaminated form so that the danger of gastrointestinal infections is reduced. It contains bacterial and viral antibodies, including secretory IgA, as well as macrophages, all of which may protect the infant against infection. Human milk contains more calories, more carbohydrates, and less protein than cow's milk. Moreover, the protein in breast milk is more easily digested because it produces a smaller, softer curd to be acted upon by gastrointestinal enzymes. In short, human milk is the complete food that provides the infant with almost all the nutrients required for the first 6 to 12 months of life.

The iron stores in full-term infants as well as the absorption of iron from breast milk are sufficient for the first 6 months of life. Beyond that age supplemental iron should be added to the diet through the gradual introduction of iron-containing solid food. Since breast milk does not contain sufficient vitamin D to prevent nutritional rickets in children not regularly exposed to sunlight, breast-fed infants should receive 400 IU of vitamin D daily. Since the fluoride content of human milk is also low, breast-fed infants should also receive 0.25 mg of fluoride daily. Some drugs (laxatives, anticoagulants, radio-

active agents, atropine, quinine, nicotine, caffeine, and tetracyclines) are transferred in varying amounts from the maternal circulation to breast milk. Oral contraceptives, steroids, diuretics, and most sedatives should also be prescribed cautiously because of the danger of maternal transfer to breast milk.

Although the merits of breast feeding seem obvious, most infants in the United States continue to be fed commercially prepared infant formulas. Most of these preparations are based upon cow's milk that has been treated so that the protein is somewhat more digestible. Most of the butterfat has been replaced with vegetable oil; thus these formulas contain a higher level of polyunsaturated fatty acids than human milk. All of these commercial formulas are fortified with vitamins and most are fortified with iron. The most commonly used of these commercial preparations are isocaloric; that is, they contain 20 calories per ounce.

Formulas based on evaporated milk, a concentrated form of cow's milk available in cans, was at one time the most common form of cow's milk formula in this country. With the appearance of easy-to-use commercially prepared infant formulas, the use of evaporated milk had declined dramatically. Nevertheless, an evaporated milk formula remains an inexpensive and safe cow's milk formula for healthy infants. Because evaporated cow's milk contains a higher solute load than human milk, it is usually diluted to decrease the effects of a high solute load on an immature infant kidney. Sugar is added to increase the formula's caloric content to the level of 20 calories per ounce.

Most newborns, either breast- or bottle-fed, must be fed at 2- to 3-hour intervals. As the infants become older, the intervals between feedings lengthen. By 6 to 8 weeks of age most infants will have established a feeding schedule so that they can sleep as long as 6 hours during the night. By 5 to 6 months of age most infants can be fed 6 to 8 ounces of formula three to four times a day.

Since infants require about 110 calories per kilogram of body weight and since the usual formula contains 20 calories per ounce, the physician can readily estimate the total amount of formula needed for any infant. Milk intake should never exceed 32 ounces (1 quart) of milk per day.

The introduction of solid food into the diet should be delayed until the infant's developmental level (5 to 6 months) is such that the infant can sit with support, has good head control, and can accept the spoon. Iron-fortified cereals are usually recommended as the first solid food to be introduced.

TABLE 5-5. Average Daily Nutritional Requirements for Infants and Children

AGE	CALORIES	PROTEIN (g)	VITAMINS A (IU)	D (IU)	C (mg)	MINERALS Fe (mg)	Ca (mg)
0–6 mo	115/kg	2.2/kg	1,386	400	35	10	360
6–12 mo	105/kg	2.0/kg	1,320	400	35	15	540
1–3 yr	1,300	23	1,320	400	45	15	800
4–6 yr	1,700	30	1,750	400	45	10	800
7–10 yr	2,400	34	2,310	400	45	10	800

(Adapted from Recommendations of the Food and Nutrition Board, National Academy of Science National Research Council, Revised, 1980)

Vitamin Imbalances

While details of the physiology and metabolism of vitamins is provided elsewhere, certain clinical syndromes caused by vitamin deficiency or excess are of particular importance to the physician caring for children.

VITAMIN D DEFICIENCY

The syndrome of nutritional vitamin D deficiency or *rickets* is characterized by growth failure; delayed closure of an infant's cranial fontanelles; *craniotabes,* or thinning of areas of calcification in the skull, causing a crackling yielding sensation with pressure; widening of the distal ends of the long bones and ribs, caused by abnormal ossification of the epiphyseal plates; bowing and distortion of the lower extremities; and fractures.

These clinical signs and symptoms of rickets are found in children with inadequate intake, impaired absorption, or impaired metabolism of vitamin D, calcium, or phosphorus. In addition to nutritional deficiency of vitamin D, rickets is also found in children with severe chronic renal failure, chronic liver disease, or those with certain metabolic inborn errors of metabolism that cause impairment of either absorption of vitamin D or retention of calcium or phosphorus.

Nutritional rickets is relatively rare in the United States because most milk and many foods are fortified with vitamin D; however, infants who are exclusively breast-fed into the second year of life are at risk for the disease. Thus, all breast-fed infants should receive vitamin D supplementation. Children of families adhering to certain cultural diets that proscribe vitamin D–fortified milk are also at risk for the development of rickets.

Treatment of nutritional rickets includes therapeutic doses of vitamin D as well as appropriate changes in the child's basic diet.

HYPERVITAMINOSIS D

Excess amounts of vitamin D cause a toxic syndrome characterized by anorexia, growth failure, constipation, polyuria, polydipsia, soft-tissue calcification, and elevated serum levels of calcium. The treatment of *hypervitaminosis D* involves the removal of excess vitamin D from the diet.

VITAMIN C DEFICIENCY

Scurvy, or vitamin C deficiency, relatively rare in the United States, is found in children who have not received regularly at least 35 mg of vitamin C in their diet. Vitamin C deficiency, which causes a defect in the formation of collagen, in its classic form is characterized by growth failure, swollen, painful joints, bleeding of the mucous membranes, spongy, friable gingiva with loosening of teeth and impaired healing of wounds. The diagnosis of scurvy is usually confirmed by typical findings of the distal shaft of the long bones, particularly the knee, on x ray.

Treatment of this condition includes 100 mg to 200 mg of ascorbic acid given orally or parenterally. Children with scurvy rapidly improve with the addition of vitamin C.

VITAMIN K DEFICIENCY

Typically vitamin K deficiency occurs in the presence of disorders of gastrointestinal malabsorption, when the bacterial flora of the gastrointestinal tract has been disrupted by the prolonged administration of antibiotics, in patients treated with vitamin K antagonists (coumarin and the like), and transiently in the newborn period. The condition is characterized by bleeding and a prolonged prothrombin time. Therapy for vitamin K deficiency involves the parenteral administration of the vitamin.

VITAMIN A DEFICIENCY

Vitamin A deficiency is very uncommon in children with a varied diet but may be found in those with gastrointestinal malabsorption syndromes or certain metabolic disorders. Classically, the condition is characterized by loss of dark adaptation and night blindness and eventual blindness; growth failure; mental retardation; and a variety of lesions involving hyperkeratosis of the skin and mucous membranes. Treatment involves the addition of therapeutic doses of vitamin A.

HYPERVITAMINOSIS A

Hypervitaminosis A, in which children receive chronically high doses of vitamin A, is characterized by growth failure, irritability, bone pain, hair loss, skin eruptions, and elevated levels of vitamin A. Acute ingestion of toxic amounts of vitamin A (more than 300,000 IU) may result in infants in irritability, bulging fontanelles, nausea, vomiting, drowsiness, and increased intracranial pressure. These conditions are treated by correcting the diet in terms of vitamin A.

THE CARE OF THE NEWBORN

Scientific advances in our understanding of the physiology of sick and well newborns have transformed the clinical management of these children. Such techniques as electronic fetal monitoring, ultrasonography, methods for determination of acid–base balance, phototherapy for hyperbilirubinemia, exchange transfusions, the use of respirators in the newborn and techniques of hyperalimentation, have developed over the past 20 years. In addition, the development of regional perinatal centers at which high-risk women and newborns have access to tertiary medical care have substantially improved perinatal and infant mortality rates in this country.

PREGNANCY AND ITS EFFECTS ON THE FETUS

Since the mother and fetus represent a single physiologic unit, any serious maternal disease or condition can affect the fetus. Maternal exposure to certain infectious agents, chemicals, drugs, or radiation may predispose to the development of serious abnormalities in the fetus. A summary of the environmental hazards to the fetus is provided in Table 5-6.

Toxemia of Pregnancy

The syndrome of maternal hypertension, edema, oliguria, and proteinuria, a common cause of intrauterine growth retardation, results in a vasculitis that involves the placenta and produces chronic intrauterine hypoxia. A chronically hypoxic fetus does not tolerate labor well and may develop intrapartum fetal distress, meconium aspiration, and birth asphyxia. Infants of mothers who develop seizures because of eclampsia are very vulnerable to intrauterine asphyxia or fetal death.

Maternal Diabetes Mellitus

Maternal diabetes mellitus, especially if poorly controlled, is associated with the delivery of infants with abnormally high weights. However, women in whom the vascular complications of diabetes are well advanced tend to deliver small infants with intrauterine growth retardation. Possibly because of the effects of uncontrolled maternal hyperglycemia during the first trimester of pregnancy, infants of diabetic mothers also have an increased incidence of congenital birth anomalies.

TABLE 5-6. Environmental Factors and Their Effects on the Fetus

FACTORS	EFFECTS
Chronic diabetes mellitus	Low birth weight, respiratory distress syndrome, macrosomia, hypoglycemia, hypocalcemia
Hypoparathyroidism	
Chronic	Hyperparathyroidism
Primary	Neonatal tetany
Thyroid disorders	
Hyperthyroidism	Hyperthyroidism (if untreated), low birth weight
Hypothyroidism	Hypothyroidism, CNS defects, prematurity
Chronic cardiac or renal disorders	Low birth weight
Infectious diseases	
Rubella	Cataracts, deafness, CNS defects, cardiac anomalies
Cytomegalovirus	Microcephaly, hydrocephaly, cardiac lesions, chorioretinitis
Toxoplasmosis	Microcephaly, seizures, chorioretinitis, hydrocephaly
Syphilis	Depends on the timing of exposure (i.e., first, second, or third trimester)
Malnutrition	Unless severe, may have no effect upon the fetus. Severe or prolonged maternal malnutrition may affect fetal CNS development.
Radiation	Increased risk of malignancy, CNS malformations
Maternal use of drugs	
Narcotics (heroin, methadone, etc.)	Small-for-gestational-age infants, withdrawal symptoms, irritability, seizures
Sedatives	Irritability, tremulousness
Phenytoin	Cleft lip and palate, congenital heart disease, CNS and skeletal abnormalities, failure to thrive
Aspirin	Hemorrhage, salicylate toxicity
Anticoagulants	Hemorrhage
Antimicrobials	
Streptomycin	Deafness
Tetracycline	Bone and dental abnormalities
Sulfonamides	Kernicterus at low bilirubin levels
Quinine	Deafness
Anticancer agents	Multiple anomalies, intrauterine growth retardation
Antihypertensives	Nasal stuffiness, hypothermia
Corticosteroids	Possible cleft palate
Sex hormone	Virilization of female, feminization of male
Radioactive thyroid	Goiter
Lead, mercury	Multiple anomalies
Alcohol	Low birth weight, characteristic facies
Tobacco use	Low birth weight

Infants of diabetic mothers are several times more likely to develop the respiratory distress syndrome (see the following section) than those of normal mothers. Finally, these infants are at considerable risk for the development of neonatal hypoglycemia in the first few days of birth. The symptoms of this condition include irritability, lethargy, poor feeding, temperature instability, and convulsions. Neonatal hypoglycemia is associated with a significant increase in the incidence of neurologic deficits.

LABOR AND DELIVERY AND THEIR EFFECTS ON THE INFANT

Prolonged Rupture of the Membranes

Prolonged rupture of the membranes (PROM) prior to delivery (usually longer than 18–24 hours) is associated with an increased risk of maternal chorioamnionitis and may lead to neonatal sepsis. While this risk is relatively low, the mortality of neonatal sepsis is high. For this reason some obstetricians consider PROM an indication for immediate delivery by induction or cesarean section. However, if the membranes rupture early in the third trimester of pregnancy, the risks of prematurity and its complications must be weighed against the risk of intrapartum infection.

Premature Labor

The management of women in premature labor remains one of the most difficult tasks for the obstetrical and neonatology team. Such drugs as magnesium sulfate or sympathomimetic agents (ritodrine, isoxsuprine, or tolbutamide) have been used in attempts to suppress uterine contractions; however, their value has not been conclusively established. Glucocorticoids are commonly administered to women in premature labor in an attempt to decrease the newborn's risk for the development of the respiratory distress syndrome. The evidence for the efficacy and safety of these drugs is reassuring, but confirmatory data about their use are not yet available. Many obstetricians advocate cesarean section as the method of delivery for premature infants as a way to avoid the dangers of neurologic damage due to trauma and birth asphyxia during labor.

Intrapartum Asphyxia

Electronic fetal monitoring during labor permits the demonstration of patterns of prolonged fetal bradycardia, periodic fetal cardiac decelerations or alterations in rate, or variability of the fetal cardiac rate, which may signal fetal distress or intrapartum asphyxia. Sampling of capillary blood from the fetal scalp permits the determination of fetal pH; a pH of less than 7.25 demonstrates a significant degree of fetal acidosis usually caused by fetal hypoxia. The presence of meconium in the amniotic fluid is also a sign of fetal distress or asphyxia. These signs of distress and asphyxia require the prompt delivery of the fetus.

THE NORMAL NEWBORN

The normal newborn has a large head, a round ruddy face, and a relatively small jaw. The chest is round and the abdomen prominent. The arms and legs are short in proportion to the length of the trunk.

The average newborn in the United States weighs about 3,300 g, with a normal range of between 2,500 g and 4,250 g. The average length is about 51 cm, with a range between 46 cm and 56 cm. The head circumference is on average about 35 cm, with a range of 32 cm to 35 cm.

Neonatal Anatomy and Physiology

The newborn's anatomy and physiology show certain developmental immaturities important in their care and management.

SKIN

The newborn's skin is anatomically immature; the epithelial layer is relatively thin and the sweat and sebaceous glands are incompletely developed. Several benign skin lesions are common. For example, *capillary hemangiomata,* "stork bites," which are bluish-red areas in the skin found commonly at the nape of the neck, the bridge of the nose, and the eyelids. These lesions, which fade and disappear with time, require no therapy; and *mongolian spots,* bluish-black discolorations found in the area of the sacrum and back in Oriental and black children, also fade with time and require no therapy.

CARDIORESPIRATORY SYSTEM

Respiratory Changes. At birth the infant's cardiorespiratory system undergoes enormous changes that allow the newborn to take the first breath and to convert from the fetal to the adult cardiovascular system within minutes. Prior to birth the airways are filled with fetal lung fluid, which contains surfactant, a phospholipid substance produced by lung pneumocytes during the third trimester of pregnancy. At birth, fetal lung fluid is quickly removed and replaced by an equal volume of air. Surfactant remains to line the air fluid interface of the alveoli and to reduce the surface tension that opposes lung expansion. Without pulmonary surfactant, airway resistance is enormous; a residual volume of air cannot be maintained and severe atelectasis develops. This atelectasis is the cause of the respiratory distress syndrome described below.

Cardiovascular Changes. The changes in the cardiovascular system are equally dramatic. The fetal circulation is maintained by specific pressure relationships between the right and left sides of the heart. In the fetal circulation the right-sided pressure (pulmonary) exceeds the left-sided pressure (systemic) so that blood flows from right to left through the foramen ovale and the ductus arteriosus. This right-sided pressure elevation depends on pulmonary vascular resistance caused by pulmonary arteriolar vasoconstriction. In contrast, left-sided pressure remains low in the fetal circulation because of the low resistance of the placental circulation.

At birth these relationships reverse. With the clamping of the umbilical vessels, left-sided (systemic) pressure rises sharply, while the pulmonary arterial pressure drops as the lungs expand with air. As the Po_2 rises, a prostaglandin-mediated pulmonary vasodilatation dramatically increases pulmonary blood flow. The elevated left arterial pressure closes the foramen ovale; the ductus arteriosus closes in response to a prostaglandin-mediated vasoconstriction. While these fetal vascular shunts (the foramen ovale and the ductus arteriosus) close functionally at birth, transient cardiac murmurs may be heard in the first few days of life because of delays in their structural closure. Most of these murmurs disappear within the first few weeks of life.

HEMATOPOIETIC SYSTEM

Hemoglobin. The newborn's red blood cells contain hemoglobin F, which during fetal life binds and transports oxygen at lower pressure levels than the hemoglobin found in adult red cells. The fetal total oxygen capacity is also improved by an absolute increase in hemoglobin levels to between 15 g/dl and 20 g/dl. This high level of hemoglobin falls rapidly so that by 2 to 3 months of age the normal infant's hemoglobin is at a level of 9 g/dl to 13 g/dl. This normal fall in hemoglobin (physiologic anemia) is caused by a decreased production of red blood cells by the bone marrow, is self-limiting, and requires no treatment.

IMMUNOLOGIC SYSTEM

The neonatal immunologic system is immature; the cellular immune responses of chemotaxis, opsonization, phagocytosis, and killing are reduced. The newborn's humoral response is antigenically inexperienced and depends on maternal IgG antibodies that cross the placenta. IgM and IgA do not cross the placenta. Maternal IgG antibodies gradually disappear from the infant's circulation over the first 3 to 12 months of life. By 3 to 6 months of age, the infant's own humoral immune system begins to function. Since IgM does not cross the placenta, the newborn is particularly vulnerable to gram-negative infections, which are usually managed by this class of antibodies.

RENAL SYSTEM

The neonatal renal system is also immature; the glomerular filtration rate is about one sixth of adult values, the proximal tubules have a lower threshold for bicarbonate resorption, the kidney's concentrating capacity is about half of an adult's function, and the excretion of inorganic phosphates and sulfates is limited. This renal immaturity makes newborns particularly vulnerable to the development of metabolic acidosis, especially those on a cow's milk formula, which contains a high solute load.

Most newborns void within the first 24 hours of life. The normal newborn, who requires about 150 ml/kg of water daily has a highly variable urinary output. By 2 weeks of age the average neonate excretes about 200 ml of urine daily.

GASTROINTESTINAL SYSTEM

The neonatal gastrointestinal system also exhibits several developmental immaturities. Since most gastrointestinal enzymes are present, the infant digests carbohydrates, fats, and proteins efficiently. However, pancreatic amylase is absent in the newborn; hence, starches are digested somewhat less well.

Meconium, a viscid greenish-black material found in the newborn's gastrointestinal tract, consists of a mixture of mucus, sloughed epithelial cells, bilirubin, and amniotic fluid. Infants usually pass meconium within the first 6 hours of life. Over the first 4 to 5 days meconium disappears from the bowel movements and is replaced by the yellowish stools of the milk-fed infant.

The neonatal liver is relatively immature and under certain circumstances will show functional insufficiencies. For example, the liver is responsible for the conjugation and excretion of bilirubin. The newborn liver regularly shows immaturity of the enzymes of conjugation, particularly glucuronyl

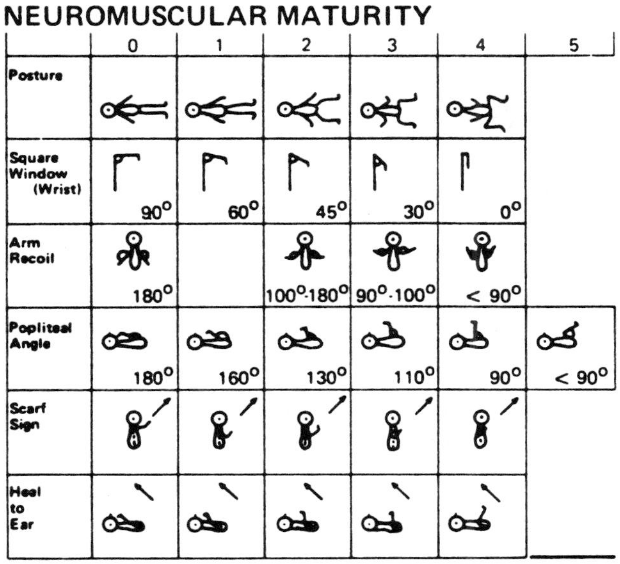

NEUROMUSCULAR MATURITY

PHYSICAL MATURITY

	0	1	2	3	4	5
SKIN	gelatinous red, transparent	smooth pink, visible veins	superficial peeling &/or rash, few veins	cracking pale area, rare veins	parchment, deep cracking, no vessels	leathery, cracked, wrinkled
LANUGO	none	abundant	thinning	bald areas	mostly bald	
PLANTAR CREASES	no crease	faint red marks	anterior transverse crease only	creases ant. 2/3	creases cover entire sole	
BREAST	barely percept.	flat areola, no bud	stippled areola, 1–2 mm bud	raised areola, 3–4 mm bud	full areola, 5–10 mm bud	
EAR	pinna flat, stays folded	sl. curved pinna, soft with slow recoil	well-curv. pinna, soft but ready recoil	formed & firm with instant recoil	thick cartilage, ear stiff	
GENITALS Male	scrotum empty, no rugae		testes descending, few rugae	testes down, good rugae	testes pendulous, deep rugae	
GENITALS Female	prominent clitoris & labia minora		majora & minora equally prominent	majora large, minora small	clitoris & minora completely covered	

MATURITY RATING

Score	Wks
5	26
10	28
15	30
20	32
25	34
30	36
35	38
40	40
45	42
50	44

Apgars _____ 1 min _____ 5 min

Age at Exam _____ hrs

Race _____ Sex _____

B.D. _____

LMP _____

EDC _____

Gest. age by Dates _____ wks

Gest. age by Exam _____ wks

B.W. _____ gm. _____ %ile

Length _____ cm. _____ %ile

Head Circum. _____ cm. _____ %ile

Clin. Dist. None _____ Mild _____

Mod. _____ Severe _____

Fig. 5-1. Assessment of gestational age, University of Cincinnati. (Ballard J, Kazmaier K, Driver M: A Simplified Assessment of Gestational Age, Pediatric Research, 1977, 11, p 374)

transferase, so that most infants are mildly jaundiced in the first few days of life. This "physiologic" jaundice approximates an average of about 6.5 mg/dl by the third day and falls to less than 2 mg/dl by the first week of life.

CENTRAL NERVOUS SYSTEM

The myelination of the central nervous system, incomplete at birth, continues throughout infancy. Most of the growth of the nervous system is complete within the first 2 years of life.

The normal newborn exhibits a variety of primitive reflexes that persist through the first few months of life. The Moro, or startle, reflex, in which the infant rapidly extends and then flexes the arms and legs in response to a sudden change in position or a loud noise, disappears by 3 to 6 months of life. The rooting, the grasp, and the tonic neck reflexes disappear within the first 6 to 12 months of life.

Classification of the Newborn

APGAR SCORE

The Apgar score, a technique of assessment of a newborn's general condition is based on assessment of the cardiac rate, respiratory effort, muscle tone,

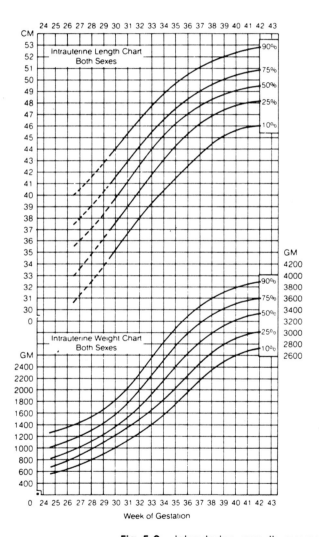

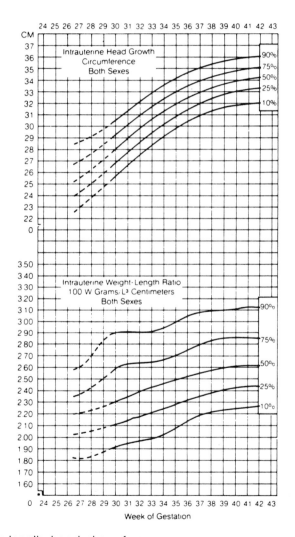

Fig. 5-2. Intrauterine growth curves for length, head circumference, and weight for singleton births in Colorado. (Lubchenco L, Hansman C, Dressler M, et al: Intrauterine Growth in Length and Head Circumference as Estimated from Live Births at Gestational Ages from 26 to 42 Weeks, Pediatrics, 1966, 37, p 403. Copyright American Academy of Pediatrics, 1966)

reflex irritability, and color within 1 and 5 minutes of birth. Two points are awarded for each of these items; an Apgar score of 8 to 10 represents a normal newborn. The 5-minute Apgar score is considered a more accurate predictor of the infant's prognosis.

GESTATIONAL AGE

While gestational age can be calculated from the mother's report of the date of her last menstrual period, these histories are frequently inaccurate. Systems based on physical and neurologic signs found on examination of the newborn have been devised to estimate gestational age. A commonly used version of these scoring systems for gestational age is found in Figure 5-1.

By definition, *full-term infants* are those born between 37 and 42 weeks of gestation, *postterm infants* are those born after 42 weeks of gestation, and *preterm infants* are those of less than 38 weeks gestation.

Low-birth-weight infants (less than 2,500 g) may represent either preterm gestations (less than 38 weeks) or infants suffering from intrauterine growth retardation. Intrauterine growth retardation may be caused by abnormalities of the fetus itself, maternal malnutrition, placental abnormalities, maternal chronic disease, and multiple or twin births.

A growth chart that displays the standard for weight and length and head circumference for infants of a variety of gestational ages is provided in Figure 5-2. *Appropriate-for-gestational-age (AGA) infants* fall within the 10th and 90th percentiles for their gestational age. *Small-for-gestational-age (SGA) infants* rank below the 10th percentile for their gestational age. These infants are more vulnerable to perinatal asphyxia, meconium aspiration, pneumothorax persistent fetal circulation, hypoglycemia, and polycythemia. *Large-for-gestational-age (LGA) infants* rank above the 90th percentile for their gestational age. These infants frequently develop hypoglycemia, polycythemia, and neurologic complications. Neonatal mortality rates decline steadily as the gestation approaches 40 weeks but again increase in LGA infants.

DISEASES OF THE NEWBORN

Since newborns can suffer from a wide variety of diseases and conditions, a detailed description of all their possible problems is beyond the scope of this discussion. A review of the serious and prominent symptoms and their causes will provide the general physician with a clinical approach to this age group.

Respiratory Distress and Cyanosis

Respiratory distress and/or cyanosis in the newborn suggests the presence of one of several serious diseases. Hypoxemia in a newborn resulting in visible cyanosis suggests either serious cardiac or respiratory disease. If on physical examination cyanosis is suspected, an arterial blood gas determination must be obtained to establish the presence of hypoxemia. A normal infant achieves a Po_2 of 50 to 70 torr within several hours of birth.

RESPIRATORY DISTRESS SYNDROME

Respiratory distress syndrome, also called hyaline membrane disease, is a disease of preterm infants caused by a deficiency of surfactant in the distal airways which results in severe atelectasis and poor lung compliance. About 20% of infants of 28 to 32 weeks' gestation develop this condition.

Respiratory distress syndrome presents shortly after birth with tachypnea, nasal flaring, grunting, intercostal, subcostal, and supraclavicular retractions, and cyanosis. On chest x ray a typical diffuse ground-glass opacity is found in the lung fields.

The disease that tends to worsen in the first 12 to 24 hours can have a mortality as high as 60% to 75% in untreated infants. However, advances in management of this condition has improved this prognosis.

The therapy for respiratory distress syndrome, which is largely supportive, includes assisted respiratory support, particularly with continuous positive airway pressure (CPAP), meticulous control of the blood pressure, careful monitoring, correction of acid–base balance, and nutritional support. Recently in some centers surfactant has been added to the therapy of respiratory distress syndrome.

Two complications, bronchopulmonary dysplasia (BPD) and retinopathy of prematurity (ROP) are found in increased incidence in these infants. *Bronchopulmonary dysplasia* (BPD), found in infants who for a variety of reasons have required prolonged oxygen or assisted ventilated therapy, is characterized by pulmonary edema and atelectasis, which progresses over time to chronic pulmonary fibrosis and emphysema. *Retinopathy of prematurity,* a major cause of blindness in children, is also found in preterm infants who require prolonged high-level oxygen therapy at birth. The immaturity of the premature infant's retina in combination with relative periods of hyperoxia often necessary for the small infant's survival seems to be cause of this condition.

CONGENITAL HEART DISEASE

Congenital heart disease is usually classified as cyanotic or acyanotic. *Cyanotic heart disease,* which often involves more serious lesions, usually presents itself within the first few days of life. The most common cyanotic cardiac lesion of the newborn is transposition of the great vessels. Newborns with cyanotic congenital cardiac defects usually present with cyanosis, poor feeding, and a degree of respiratory distress, which is less than that found in infants with the respiratory distress syndrome or other primary pulmonary conditions. Cardiac murmurs are usually but not invariably present.

Acyanotic congenital cardiac lesions do not usually present until the infant is several weeks old. Indeed, milder acyanotic lesions may not become symptomatic until childhood or later.

Neonatal Jaundice

Jaundice appears in newborns when the serum bilirubin exceeds 5 mg/dl. Elevated levels of bilirubin can be the result of increased hemolysis of red blood cells, of immature liver function, or of congenital obstructions of the biliary system.

HEMOLYTIC JAUNDICE

A classification of the common causes of hemolytic jaundice in newborns is given in Table 5-7. The most common form, *isoimmune hemolysis,* is caused by incompatibilities between the mother's and infant's red blood cells. Hemolysis results from the destruction of fetal and neonatal red blood cells by maternal antibodies of the IgG class that cross the placenta during pregnancy. These maternal antibodies develop as a result of maternal exposure to foreign red-cell antigens of a blood group or Rh type. This maternal sensitization occurs during a fetal–maternal transfusion during current or prior pregnancies or from mismatched blood transfusions.

Erythroblastosis fetalis or Rh incompatibility occurs when an Rh-negative mother has an Rh-positive infant. The level of hemolytic anemia found in these infants varies, but severely affected infants are born with severe anemia, jaundice, and even signs of congestive heart failure. The incidence of Rh hemolytic disease of the newborn has been reduced dramatically with the use of potent anti-Rh antibodies given to the Rh-negative mother immediately after the birth of an Rh-positive infant.

ABO incompatibility occurs when the mother and infant have an incompatibility of the major blood groups. This form of isoimmune hemolysis is usually less severe and less likely to require clinical intervention.

KERNICTERUS, PHOTOTHERAPY, AND EXCHANGE TRANSFUSIONS

In newborns high levels of indirect bilirubin from any cause, if untreated, will result in the development of kernicterus, permanent neurological damage, and death. For that reason a variety of techniques have been developed to control hyperbilirubinemia in the neonate.

Phototherapy, the use of ultraviolet lights, depends on the absorption of radiant energy by the indirect bilirubin molecule to make it water soluble and to allow its further metabolism and excretion by the kidney.

If the level of indirect hyperbilirubinemia cannot be controlled by phototherapy, *exchange transfusions* of the infant are required. The level of hyperbilirubinemia for which an exchange transfusion is necessary varies with the birth weight and condition of the infant. In general, premature infants with an indirect bilirubin of 15 mg/dl or more and full-term infants with levels of over 20 mg/dl are considered candidates for exchange transfusion.

NEONATAL SEPSIS

Neonatal infections, both congenital or acquired, are common causes of jaundice in the newborn. The incidence of neonatal sepsis, which varies from 1 to 9 per 1,000 live births, is higher among infants from the lower socioeconomic classes and infants of low birth weight.

TABLE 5-7. Causes of Hemolytic Jaundice in the Newborn

Isoimmune hemolysis	ABO, Rh, minor blood group incompatibility
Enzyme defects	G6PD, pyruvate kinase deficiency
Red-cell membrane defects	Hereditary spherocytosis, vitamin E deficiency
Hemoglobinopathies	Thalassemia syndromes

Acquired Infections

Virtually any bacteria can cause sepsis in the neonate; however, the usual causative agents are those found in the maternal vaginal or gastrointestinal tract. The pattern of bacterial causes of neonatal sepsis has varied over the years. In the past Group A β-hemolytic streptococcus and *Staphylococcus aureus* have been major causes of infection in the newborn, but more recently Group B β-hemolytic streptococci have become a major problem. In addition, because of the immaturity of the immune system, neonates are especially vulnerable to infections with such gram-negative organisms as *Escherichia coli*.

Neonatal sepsis may present with a fulminant course resulting in death within hours, or it may present with vague, nonspecific symptoms. A variety of symptoms may signal the presence of sepsis, including lethargy, poor feeding, jaundice, temperature instability, respiratory distress or periods of apnea, abdominal distention, hypotonia, and altered cry. In the late stages of the disease, infants will present with shock, coma, sclerema, purpura and respiratory and/or renal failure.

Since neonatal sepsis is commonly associated with more localized forms of infection, the presence of sepsis should alert the clinician to the possibility of meningitis, pneumonia (particularly in infants with respiratory distress syndrome), osteomyelitis, urinary tract infection, and necrotizing enterocolitis. Thus, in the face of symptoms and signs of possible sepsis, a complete evaluation including examination of the spinal fluid is required.

However, because no laboratory or radiographic finding is rapid or reliable enough to substitute for clinical judgment and because of the urgency of the situation, the treatment of neonatal sepsis is regularly begun before a causative organism is identified. Broad antibiotic coverage to deal with both gram-negative *(E. coli)* and gram-positive (group B streptococcus or *Staph. aureus*) organisms is commonly employed until a definitive bacteriologic diagnosis can be made.

Congenital Infections

The TORCH syndrome represents a group of congenitally acquired infections, which present with similar symptoms and signs in the neonate. The TORCH acronym refers to:

T = toxoplasmosis
O = "other" (*e.g.,* syphilis, coxsackie virus, malaria, and varicella)
R = rubella
C = cytomegalic inclusion disease
H = hepatitis B and herpes simplex

Unlike the other congenital infections, herpes and hepatitis are usually acquired during or immediately after birth rather than during the pregnancy. The clinical features of the TORCH syndrome include intrauterine growth retardation, jaundice, hepatosplenomegaly, anemia, purpura, chorioretinitis, pneumonia, myocardiopathies, and moderate to severe neurological symptoms. Seizures, microcephaly, deafness, and mental retardation are not uncommon sequelae of these infections.

The diagnosis of TORCH infections depends on viral cultures and/or serologic testing. Since many of the antibodies responsible for seroconversion are transmitted placentally from mother to fetus, serologic diagnosis usually requires the demonstration of a rising serologic titer over several weeks. The cytomegalovirus, herpes, and rubella virus can be cultured from urine or mucous secretions. The *Treponema pallidum* of syphilis can be demonstrated on dark field microscopy of secretions.

Women who are hepatitis B surface antigen positive (HBsAG-positive) and particularly those who are also hepatitis Be antigen positive (HbeAG-positive) can transmit the infection to their infants at birth. These infants can also become chronic carriers of the disease. For that reason it is important that all pregnant women are screened at delivery for the presence of the HB antigen. Infants of hepatitis BsAG positive women should be given hepatitis B immune globulin within 12 hours of birth. They should also be given hepatitis B vaccine within 12 hours of birth and again at 1 month and 6 months of life.

The management of these congenital infections varies with the organism. Penicillin is used to treat congenital syphilis; a combination of sulfadiazine and pyrimethamine is used to treat congenital toxoplasmosis; cytosine arabinoside or acyclovir has been used with limited success in the treatment of herpes. No specific therapy is available for the treatment of congenital rubella or cytomegalovirus infections.

DISEASES OF CHILDREN

Since children are not miniature adults but growing and developing organisms, the diseases of childhood vary considerably from those of adults. Although a full description of the gamut of diseases of children is clearly beyond the scope of this chapter, certain diseases and conditions are sufficiently important or unique to warrant inclusion in this summary of pediatric medicine.

Growth Retardation

Failure to thrive and growth retardation are among the most common presenting symptoms of serious disease in children. *Failure to thrive* is a term usually reserved for infants who show significant deviations in growth; the term *growth retardation* is usually reserved for older children. While the causes of growth retardation are legion, the differential diagnosis of this symptom should include consideration of the following categories of diseases.

1. Endocrine disorders: hypopitituitarism caused either by congenital structural pituitary defects, destructive lesions of the pituitary, such as craniopharyngiomas, or by idiopathic or functional defects in pituitary function; ovarian agenesis or Turner's syndrome found in girls with a 45, XO chromosome pattern and characterized by short stature, primary amenorrhea, webbed neck, and cubitum valgum; precocious puberty of a variety of etiologies, which leads to premature closure of the epiphyseal lines and eventual short stature as adults.
2. Malnutrition: starvation because of poverty or other forms of environmental deprivation; gastrointestinal malabsorption associated most commonly with cystic fibrosis as well as other less common forms of malabsorption.
3. Metabolic disorders: virtually any inborn error of metabolism results in failure to thrive or growth retardation.
4. Congenital cardiac lesions: cyanotic cardiac lesions always present with failure to thrive as a prominent presenting symptom. Moreover, acyanotic lesions, such as severe ventricular septal defects, can present with failure to thrive as a presenting symptom in the early months of infancy.
5. Congenital skeletal disorders, including osteogenesis imperfecta, achrondrodystrophy, and congenital anomalies of the spine, result in growth retardation.
6. Neurologic disorders, especially those that cause severe central nervous system damage and those associated with severe mental retardation, are also associated with growth failure.
7. Familial or genetic short stature is found in children whose families have a history of short stature, who are otherwise healthy, and in whom laboratory studies of growth are normal.
8. Constitutional delay in growth or puberty is found in adolescents with delayed onset of puberty. This delay in onset of puberty represents a normal variation in the timing of the event. These adolescents eventually attain normal adult height.

Metabolic and Endocrine Disorders

Inborn errors of metabolism is a term used to describe a group of genetically transmitted conditions that result in an alteration or interference with the normal biochemical mechanisms of the body. More than 100 of these relatively rare conditions have been described, most of which involve amino acid metabolism. While rare, these diseases if not detected and treated promptly will result in serious damage, especially to the central nervous system.

Microtechniques using capillary blood have been devised that permit screening of newborns for the presence of many of these metabolic disorders. Throughout the United States metabolic screening of newborns while in the hospital nursery is required by law.

CONGENITAL HYPOTHYROIDISM

Newborn screening programs have established an incidence of congenital hypothyroidism at a level of 1 in 3,800 to 4,000 live births. Females are more commonly affected than males. About 90% of children with congenital hypothyroidism have congenital structural lesions of the thyroid. In addition, congenital hypothyroidism may be caused by congenital pituitary lesions, maternal intake of radioiodine during pregnancy, thyrotropin or thyroxine unresponsiveness, and the defective synthesis of thyroxine.

Infants with congenital hypothyroidism may be asymptomatic at birth. Classically the disease presents with a history of prolonged neonatal jaundice, feeding problems, constipation, and mottling of the extremities. On physical examination a child with congenital hypothyroidism will have growth failure with height more seriously affected than weight, developmental delay and general hypotonia, coarse facial features, a flattened nasal bridge, a large coarse, protruding tongue, a hoarse cry, and a protruding abdomen and umbilical hernia. The diagnosis is established by measurement of T_4 and triiodothyronine (T_3) and confirmed by thyroid-stimulating hormone (TSH) assay.

Untreated, these children become mentally retarded, but early diagnosis and replacement therapy with thyroid can do much to prevent this mental retardation.

CONGENITAL ADRENAL HYPERPLASIA

Congenital adrenal hyperplasia, an inborn error of metabolism in the biosynthesis of adrenal corticoids, is inherited as an autosomal recessive trait. While five different enzymatic defects in the synthesis of adrenal corticoids have been described, 95% of the cases are caused by a deficiency in 21-hydroxylase. The second most frequent cause of the disease, caused by a deficiency in 11-β-hydroxylase, is especially common in children of North African Jewish ancestry. In all forms of the disease the deficiency in cortisol production causes an increased secretion of ACTH, which leads to adrenal hyperplasia and the excess production of intermediary metabolites of cortisol.

Salt-losing Form (Adrenal Hyperplasia). About one third to one half of children with the 21-hydroxylase defect will present with metabolic symptoms of adrenal insufficiency. These "salt losers" present in the first few months of life with failure to thrive, vomiting and diarrhea, dehydration leading to vascular collapse and death, low-serum sodium, and chloride with high-serum potassium and blood urea nitrogen.

Non-salt-losing Form (Adrenal Hyperplasia). In *males* the disease presents as premature isosexual precocity often, but not always, within the first 6 months of life. Enlargement of the penis, scrotum, and prostate; deepening of the voice; and the appearance of pubic hair in young children are all clinical signs of the virilization typical of the disease.

In *females* congenital adrenal hyperplasia causes pseudohermaphroditism, evident at birth. The degree of virilization may vary from mild clitoral hypertrophy and labial fusion to true ambiguous genitalia. Hence it is critical that all newborns with ambiguous genitalia are carefully investigated immediately to ensure that a correct sex is assigned and that proper therapy is instituted promptly.

JUVENILE DIABETES MELLITUS

Type I (juvenile-onset) diabetes, a familial, chronic disorder of carbohydrate, protein, and fat metabolism, results from an absolute inadequate amount of endogenous insulin. The most common metabolic or endocrine disorder of children, Type I diabetes has a prevalence of about 1.9 in 1,000 schoolchildren.

The disease usually presents in the preschool or early school years or during adolescence. Classically children with diabetes present with rapid weight loss, fatigue, polyuria, polydipsia, and polyphagia. However, the first manifestation of the disease often is with the abrupt onset of impending or overt diabetic ketoacidosis.

The treatment of diabetes in children includes the daily administration of insulin (oral hypoglycemic agents should not be used in the treatment of juvenile diabetes), dietary management, and social support and health education for the child and parents in the management of this chronic disease.

PHENYLKETONURIA

Phenylketonuria is an inborn error of metabolism in which the enzyme, phenylalanine hydroxylase, required to metabolize phenylalanine, an essential amino acid, is absent. The disease is inherited as an autosomal recessive trait with a general incidence of about 1 in 10,000. It is somewhat less common in blacks and more common in Ashkenazi Jews. Phenylketonuria is one of the conditions that can be detected by newborn screening, but the screening test should not be performed until the infant has had several feedings containing phenylalanine.

Children with phenylketonuria appear normal at birth but gradually develop fair skin, light hair, and eczematoid or seborrheic dermatitis, growth retardation, and seizures. If the disease is untreated, severe mental retardation will result; thus, any delay in the diagnosis and treatment of phenylketonuria will worsen the degree of mental retardation. The treatment consists of dietary manipulation in which phenylalanine is eliminated from the diet.

GALACTOSEMIA

Galactosemia, an inborn error of carbohydrate metabolism, is the result of a deficiency of the enzyme, galactose-1-phosphate uridyl transferase. The absence of this enzyme causes a gradual and toxic accumulation of galactose in all body tissues. The disease is inherited as an autosomal recessive.

Infants with galactosemia appear normal at birth, but begin to develop symptoms when fed milk containing galactose. While the onset of symptoms is variable, typically infants present with vomiting and diarrhea, jaundice, failure to thrive, hepatosplenomegaly, and cataracts. Children with untreated galactosemia develop cirrhosis and severe mental retardation.

The disease, which should be considered in any infant with these symptoms, can be diagnosed tentatively by the demonstration of a reducing substance in the urine using the Clinitest technique. The definitive diagnosis is made by chromatography or enzyme assay.

The treatment of galactosemia involves the removal of galactose from the diet. Soy-based formulas are used to replace galactose milk–based formulas.

Hematologic Disorders

Although the hematologic disorders in childhood are many and varied, most are relatively rare. However, a few conditions are important or unique enough to be included in this summary.

IRON DEFICIENCY ANEMIA

Iron deficiency anemia, the most common hematologic disease in children, results from an absolute deficit in the body's iron stores. Prematurity is a major cause of this anemia. Since the storage of fetal iron occurs in the third trimester of pregnancy, premature infants may be born with insufficient iron stores and require iron supplementation during infancy. Infants of multiple births (*e.g.,* twins), may also receive insufficient iron stores during fetal life and thus require extra iron supplementation. Sick newborns who suffer fetal or neonatal blood loss are also at risk for the development of iron deficiency anemia. By far the most common cause of iron deficiency anemia is a deficient intake in dietary iron. Since cow's milk contains no iron, infants who receive most of their calories from milk are likely to become iron deficient between the ages of 8 to 24 months. Finally in the United States adolescent girls who are prone to experiment with fad diets may be iron deficient; this dietary iron deficiency combined with the loss of iron through menstruation can result in a serious iron deficiency.

A child with iron deficiency may have few symptoms or may present with increased fatigue, decreased exercise tolerance, anorexia, and increased irritability. On examination, only pallor of the skin and mucous membranes may be evident. However, children with severe iron deficiency may present with signs of congestive heart failure, tachycardia, hemic murmurs, and cardiac dilatation.

Iron deficiency anemia is treated with iron usually in the form of ferrous salts. Dietary counseling and careful follow-up are also important parts of the management of this condition.

CONGENITAL HEMOLYTIC ANEMIAS

Hemolytic anemias occur when the life span of the red blood cell is shortened. These conditions are characterized by anemia, reticulocytosis, hyperplasia of the bone marrow, and elevations of indirect bilirubin. Two forms of hemolytic anemia are particularly important in children.

Sickle-Cell Anemia. Sickle-cell anemia is a chronic hemolytic anemia caused by the presence of a structural substitution of valine for glutamic acid in the sixth position of the β-polypeptide chain of hemoglobin. Sickle-cell hemoglobin, transmitted as a recessive trait, is found in the heterozygous condition in about 8% of the black population of the United States. Sickle-cell anemia, the homozygous form of the trait, is found in about 1 in 600 blacks in the United States.

Children with sickle-cell trait have between 35% and 40% of total hemoglobin in the form of hemoglobin S. This level of hemoglobin S is not sufficient for the development of any physical abnormalities, symptoms, or anemia.

In children with sickle-cell anemia, the hemoglobin contains about 90% hemoglobin S and 2% to 10% hemoglobin F, and a normal amount of hemoglobin A2. The red blood cells contain no hemoglobin A. Children with sickle-cell anemia present with characteristic signs of chronic hemolytic anemia, including reticulocytosis, intermittent indirect hyperbilirubinemia, in addition to moderate or severe anemia. Children with sickle-cell anemia also have episodes of pain caused by the occlusion of capillaries and small blood vessels by the distorted sickled red blood cells resulting in microinfarctions. Occasionally a child with sickle-cell disease will suffer an infarction of the brain, resulting in serious brain damage due to sickling in vessels supplying the central nervous system. They are also prone to serious bacterial infections, particularly pneumococcal and *Salmonella* infections because of an impairment in splenic function as well as a deficiency in serum opsonins. Finally, infants and young children with sickle-cell disease may develop an acute splenic sequestration in which for unknown reasons blood pools acutely in the spleen. Children with acute splenic sequestrations may rapidly go into vascular shock; immediate blood transfusions may be indicated.

The treatment of children with sickle-cell anemia

involves the management of the acute episodes with antibiotics, hydration, and transfusions when necessary. Most authorities recommend the administration of the pneumococcal vaccine at the appropriate age and daily prophylactic penicillin as methods for the prevention of serious pneumococcal infections in these children.

Thalassemia. Thalassemia (Cooley's anemia) is a chronic congenital hemolytic anemia found in children of Italian or Mediterranean descent. Transmitted as an autosomal recessive trait, it is caused by the presence of increased amounts of hemoglobin F, resulting in a decreased life span of red blood cells, increased hemolysis, and severe chronic hypochromic, microcytic anemia.

Thalassemia minor, the heterozygous form of this disease, is characterized by mild to moderate anemia. Children with this mild form of the disease are usually asymptomatic.

Children with thalassemia major, the homozygous form, present with failure to thrive, pallor, jaundice, splenomegaly, and a typical facies which develops over time as a result of bone marrow hyperplasia in the skull and face. The only treatment for thalassemia major is regular and frequent blood transfusions. A variety of chelation techniques using desferoxamine have been developed in attempts to prevent or ameliorate the hemosiderosis that is the inevitable complication of transfusion therapy.

IDIOPATHIC THROMBOCYTOPENIA

Idiopathic thrombocytopenic purpura, which usually occurs in children between the ages of 2 and 8 years, usually presents after a minor viral illness with the abrupt onset of petechiae and/or purpuric skin lesions. The total platelet count is low and the hematocrit and hemoglobin may be low. Bone marrow examination reveals a normal or increased number of megakaryocytes; the other elements of the bone marrow are normal. The condition remits within a few weeks or months in most children without therapy. Some authorities suggest the use of corticosteroids or intravenous gamma globulin for the treatment of this disease, particularly if it is severe.

HENOCH-SCHÖNLEIN PURPURA

Henoch-Schönlein, or anaphylactoid, purpura (HSP) is a nonthrombocytopenic purpura of unknown cause and is more common in children than adults. The disease usually occurs in children between the ages of 2 and 8 years and is more common in boys than girls. The condition commonly affects the skin, kidneys, and gastrointestinal tract. Children with HSP present with skin lesions that have a distinctive peripheral distribution over the legs, arms, and buttocks. The lesions, which are erythematous and maculopapular, may become petechial or purpuric. Children may also have colicky abdominal pain, which may be accompanied by gross or occult gastrointestinal bleeding. Occasionally these children may develop an acute intussusception secondary to edema and hemorrhage in the intestinal wall. Microscopic hematuria and other signs of nephritis as well as arthritis of the large joints, especially the knees and ankles, may also be present.

The prognosis of Henoch-Schönlein purpura is excellent. Most children recover within a few weeks or months. However, those with signs of renal involvement may develop persistent renal disease.

In general, the treatment of this condition is symptomatic and supportive. Children with severe forms of the disease may require corticosteroid therapy.

HEMOPHILIA

Factor VIII deficiency, or classical hemophilia, a disease transmitted by the sex-linked mode of inheritance, causes about 80% of all cases of hemophilia. Factor IX, or Christmas disease, also transmitted by the sex-linked mode, represents about 15% of the cases of hemophilia. Both diseases vary in clinical severity.

Children with hemophilia present in early childhood with easy bruising, the formation of large hematomas after trivial trauma and prolonged bleeding at surgery. On laboratory evaluation they will have abnormal partial thromboplastin time (PTT), prothrombin consumption, and thromboplastin generation tests. The treatment of hemophilia involves the replacement of the missing clotting factors with concentrated forms of these factors.

With the appearance of acquired immunodeficiency syndrome (see Diseases of the Immune System, below), it has been discovered that significant numbers of children with hemophilia have been infected by the HIV virus as a result of contamination by the virus in the blood used to prepare their replacement therapy. With the recent widespread screening of all blood donations for the presence of this virus, this threat to these children should be corrected. Recently new Factor VIII concentrates have been developed using the monoclonal antibody techniques. These forms of the concentrates have the advantage of safety in regard to infectious agents but are also more expensive at the present time.

Malignancies

Malignant disease is the principal medical cause of death, following accidental injury and poisoning, in the 1- to 14-year-old age group. Leukemias, lymphomas, and other malignancies of the hematopoietic system account for 50% of all neoplasms in childhood. Tumors of the central nervous system, kidney adrenal, and bone tumors comprise most of the other malignancies in children. Carcinoma is rare in childhood.

LEUKEMIA

Acute leukemia, a disease characterized by the uncontrolled proliferation of immature white blood cells, is usually classified according to the type of white blood cell involved. *Acute lymphatic leukemia* accounts for about 80% and *acute granulocytic leukemia* accounts for about 15% of all cases of leukemia in children. The peak incidence of the disease occurs between the ages of 3 and 6 years. Children with trisomy 21, or Down's syndrome, have an increased incidence of leukemia.

Children with leukemia present with a history of increased lethargy, irritability, fatigue, fever of unknown origin, easy bruising, and weight loss. On physical examination pallor, ecchymoses, petechiae, generalized lymphadenopathy, splenomegaly, and hepatomegaly may be found. The diagnosis is made by examination of the blood smear and bone marrow for the presence of typical immature white blood cells.

Therapy involves specific chemotherapy with antineoplastic agents. The prognosis of these diseases has improved substantially during the past 20 years. Currently 90% of children will have a period of remission, and fully 50% survive beyond 5 years.

TUMORS OF THE CENTRAL NERVOUS SYSTEM

Two thirds of central nervous system tumors in children are located infratentorially and present as symptoms referable to the cerebellum. Hence children with these tumors typically present with ataxia, uncoordinated movements of the arms and legs, projectile or nonprojectile vomiting, and papilledema.

Astrocytomas of the cerebellum, which account for 25% of these tumors generally occur in children between the ages of 6 and 9 years. These are rather slow-growing malignancies that may first be manifested by the appearance of a unilateral ataxia accompanied by a tilting of the head toward the side of the tumor. Prompt surgical removal results in about a 90% long-term survival.

Medulloblastomas, which account for 20% of intracranial tumors in children, tend to be located in the vermis of the cerebellum. They are more common in boys than girls with a peak incidence between the ages of 2 and 6 years. Surgical removal accompanied by irradiation constitutes the therapy for these lesions. Recently chemotherapy has been added to this therapeutic regimen. Despite this combined therapy the prognosis of this tumor is guarded.

Gliomas of the brain stem constitute about 15% of cerebral tumors. Those located in the fourth ventricle are usually ependymomas.

Supratentorial tumors present with symptoms depending on their location. Those of the hypothalamus and/or optic chiasm will present with growth failure, polyuria, polydipsia, somnolence, atrophy of the genitals, and irregular defects in the temporal portion of the visual fields. Tumors in the region of the pineal body may produce sexual precocity, especially in males. If the midbrain is involved there may be difficulty in upward gaze and loss of the pupillary reflex.

NEUROBLASTOMA

Neuroblastoma, malignancy of the sympathetic nervous system, may appear where this tissue is found in the body, but most often arise from the adrenal gland or from the thoracic or abdominal sympathetic chain. Neuroblastoma is a tumor of childhood; 90% have been identified by the age of 10 years.

The presenting symptoms depend on the location of the tumor. Since the tumor commonly arises in the abdomen, the usual presenting sign is a firm, nontender abdominal mass. Occasionally neuroblastoma will present as a unilateral exophthalmos with proptosis, periorbital swelling, and ecchymoses caused by metastasis of the tumor to the eye.

Since these tumors produce elevated levels of catecholamines, a 24-hour urine analysis for vanillylmandelic acid (VMA) is used as an adjunct to the diagnosis. The definitive diagnosis is made by surgical biopsy. Treatment for these tumors include surgery, chemotherapy, and irradiation. The prognosis for neuroblastomas varies with the stage of the disease, cellular type, age, and sex of the child.

WILMS' TUMOR

Wilms' tumor, or nephroblastoma, the most common renal tumor of children, occurs in the first 3 years of life. It is usually unilateral, but in 10% to 15% of patients the tumor may be bilateral. Children with this malignancy typically present with an abdominal mass that is asymptomatic and that does not usually cross the midline. Hypertension is present in 30% to 60% of patients. Several congenital anomalies, including genitourinary anomalies, hemihypertrophy, and sporadic aniridia are associated with Wilms' tumor.

The diagnosis is made by intravenous pyelogram, which will demonstrate an intrarenal mass. Therapy includes surgical removal of the primary tumor. The addition of chemotherapy and/or irradiation depends on the stage of the tumor. The prognosis of Wilms' tumor has improved dramatically with newer forms of chemotherapy and depends on the stage of the disease, the age of the child (children under 2 years have a better prognosis), and the size of the tumor. The overall 5-year survival rate now approaches 60%.

HISTIOCYTOSIS

Histiocytosis X is a term used to describe a group of relatively rare diseases characterized by proliferation of the cells of the reticuloendothelial system at one or more sites in the body. Three patterns of this disease have been described.

Letterer-Siwe syndrome is found in infants and primarily affects soft tissue with minimal or no bony involvement. Seborrheic dermatitis, generalized lymphadenopathy, leukopenia, and thrombocytopenia are common clinical findings. This form of the disease is rapidly progressive and often fatal. *Hand-Schüller-Christian syndrome* is characterized by defects in membranous bone, exophthalmos, and diabetes insipidus. Pulmonary infiltrates, seborrhea of the scalp, and mild hepatomegaly are also prominent features of the syndrome. *Eosinophilic granuloma* is characterized by usually solitary cysts of one or more bones. Almost any bone can be involved, but the skull, pelvis, and extremities are common sites for these lesions.

Since the etiology of this family of conditions has not been determined, therapy is not definitive. Steroids, chemotherapy, and irradiation are used in the treatment of the progressive forms of the disease.

Neurologic Disorders

The immaturity and vulnerability of the central nervous system of newborns and infants make it imperative that the general physician is skilled in the diagnosis and management of conditions likely to result in irreversible neurologic damage to the developing brain. Almost any serious disease or condition has the potential for damage to the central nervous system. Birth asphyxia, inborn errors of metabolism, genetic disorders, meningitis and encephalitis, trauma, and chronic lead intoxication or other environmental agents are among the common causes of serious neurologic disorders in childhood.

SEIZURE DISORDERS

Major motor seizures, petit mal seizures, and temporal lobe seizures are not unlike those found in adults, but two types of seizure disorders are peculiar to infants and children and deserve special attention.

Febrile Seizures. *Febrile seizures,* the most common cause of seizures in children, are generalized tonic–clonic seizures that occur most commonly in infants between the ages of 6 and 36 months with a peak incidence at 18 months. There is often a family history of febrile seizures. These episodes are usually of short duration and often occur in the face of a rapid rise in temperature to hyperpyrexic levels (104° F).

After immediate control of the seizure, the physician's first priority should be in diagnosis of the cause of the fever. Since meningitis can present with seizures and fever, many physicians elect to perform a lumbar puncture to exclude this possibility in all children with first febrile seizures.

Many children with a single febrile seizure will never have another, but about one third will have repeated febrile seizures and about 2% to 3% will develop nonfebrile seizures or idiopathic epilepsy later in childhood. Children with a family history of seizures, focal seizures or neurologic symptoms, and prolonged duration of the febrile seizure are more likely to develop afebrile seizures.

Myoclonic Epilepsy of Infancy. *Myoclonic epilepsy* is a condition that presents in infancy as episodes in which the infant's head suddenly drops to the chest, the thighs flex on the abdomen, and the arms adduct and flex on the chest. The individual episodes are brief but may be extremely frequent, following one another in rapid succession. The electroencephalogram shows a characteristically disorganized pattern termed "hypsarrhythmia." Infantile myoclonic epilepsy is associated with moderate to profound mental retardation.

MENINGITIS

Meningitis, bacterial infection of the central nervous system, is one of the more common serious infections of children. The presentation of the disease varies with the age of the child. The classic signs of this infection include fever, irritability or lethargy, headache and vomiting, seizures, and nuchal rigidity with a positive Kernig and Brudzinski sign. Infants with meningitis commonly do not exhibit a Kernig or Brudzinski sign, and fever, irritability, lethargy, and bulging of the anterior fontanelle may be the only signs of meningitis. The diagnosis is made by examination of cerebrospinal fluid. The spinal fluid of a child with bacterial meningitis will contain white blood cells, usually leukocytes, a decreased level of sugar, and an elevated protein level. Gram stain of the fluid may reveal the causative organisms. Culture of the spinal fluid may permit the diagnosis of the specific agent. In general a very low spinal fluid sugar and a very elevated protein are serious prognostic signs.

In the newborn period meningitis is commonly caused by *E. coli*, Group A β-hemolytic streptococcus, or Group B β-hemolytic streptococcus. *Hemophilus influenzae, Streptococcus pneumoniae,* and *Neisseria meningitidis* are the agents responsible for 95% of bacterial meningitis in children over the age of 2 months.

The long-term sequelae of meningitis include hydrocephalus, hearing loss, seizures, speech or developmental delay, and mental retardation. As many as 10% to 20% of children with meningitis may have neurodevelopmental sequelae.

Since these three organisms account for most bacterial meningitis in children, a regimen of broad-spectrum antibiotics is usually instituted until a definitive bacteriologic diagnosis can be made.

DEVELOPMENTAL AND MENTAL RETARDATION

Mental retardation may be defined as below-average general intellectual functioning that originates during the developmental period and that is associated with impairment of adaptive behavior. About 3% of the general population is retarded. Of this total 70% are mildly retarded or educable. This group will function at about the fifth-grade level and as adults can manage unskilled or semiskilled occupations. Twenty-five percent are moderately retarded or trainable, will be able to dress themselves, feed themselves, and be toilet trained. As adults they can function in a sheltered workshop setting. Only about 5% are so severely retarded that they are totally dependent and require custodial care. A classification of the major causes of mental retardation is provided in Table 5-8.

Chromosomal Abnormalities. Abnormalities in the number and structure of the chromosome complement are associated with clinical syndromes characterized by multiple congenital anomalies and mental retardation. *Trisomies* are genetic conditions in which an extra chromosome is present in all body cells.

Down's syndrome (trisomy 21), the most common of these conditions, is associated with an extra chromosome 21. Trisomy 21 is associated with advancing maternal age but is also found in offspring of younger mothers as a result of a translocation of the genetic material rather than the simple addition of an extra chromosome. Thus these children will have the stigmata of trisomy 21 but will have a normal number (46) of chromosomes.

Children with trisomy 21 have typical facies with prominent epicanthal folds, small nose, prominent tongue, and small head with flattened occiput. They have poor muscle tone and coordination, short stubby feet with a widened space between the first and second toes, and short stubby hands with an incurved fifth finger and a palmar crease (a single line that extends across the breadth of the palm). They will all exhibit growth and developmental retardation, but children with the translocation

TABLE 5-8. Major Causes of Mental Retardation

  I. Chromosomal abnormalities
    A. Trisomies, Down's syndrome
 II. Degenerative neurologic diseases
III. Inborn errors of metabolism
IV. Infections of the central nervous system
    A. Congenital infections
    B. Postnatal infections
 V. Congenital anomalies
    A. Hydrocephalus, microcephaly
VI. Toxic agents
    A. Lead intoxication
VII. Trauma, hypoxia
    A. Perinatal hypoxia
    B. Birth trauma
    C. Head injury

form of the condition are generally less retarded than those with trisomies.

Several other congenital anomalies including congenital heart disease, usually defects in the septum of the heart, and duodenal atresia and imperforate anus are also associated with Down's syndrome. Acute leukemia is also more prevalent in these children.

Congenital Anomalies. Several congenital anomalies are associated with mental retardation. *Microcephaly,* an abnormally small head, usually indicates the presence of severe retardation in the growth of the brain with resulting severe mental retardation. Any insult that limits central nervous system growth can cause microcephaly. *Hydrocephaly,* the result of excess accumulation of cerebrospinal fluid, presents as rapid enlargement of an infant's head. The two types of lesions may cause hydrocephaly. Obstructive hydrocephaly is caused by a blockage within the ventricular system of the brain that prevents the normal circulation of spinal fluid. Communicating hydrocephaly is caused by a blockage located in the subarachnoid space that prevents the reabsorption of spinal fluid by the arachnoid villi but that permits the ventricles to communicate with the spinal subarachnoid space. Hydrocephalus may be associated with a variety of genetic disorders or be caused by a wide variety of insults to the brain.

Meningomyeloceles are congenital malformations of the vertebral column and the spinal cord in which the cord and the meninges herniate through a bony defect in the spine. This anomaly, usually located in the lumbar sacral region, can cause severe neurologic deficits. Paralysis of the legs, bladder, and bowel dysfunction and obstructive hydrocephalus are common in this condition. Meningomyeloceles are relatively common with an incidence of about 1 in 1,000 live births; the appearance of the lesion varies with ethnic background and is relatively uncommon in African-Americans.

Cerebral Palsy. *Cerebral palsy* is a term used to describe a neurologic syndrome characterized by impairment of motor function. One of the most common neurologic syndromes of childhood, the term usually connotes static, nonprogressive lesions of the central nervous system or the spinal cord. The disorder is usually classified as spastic, extrapyramidal (choreoathetosis), atonic, and mixed types. Although cerebral palsy is associated with mental retardation and seizure disorders, many children with this neurologic syndrome have normal intelligence.

Pulmonary Disorders

Although the diagnosis and management of many of the pulmonary disorders of children resemble those of older patients, some are unique or of greater importance to the physician caring for children.

CONGENITAL ANOMALIES

Choanal atresia, the most common congenital anomaly of the nose, consists of a bony or membranous obstruction between the nasal passage and the upper airway. The diagnosis is made by the inability to pass a catheter into the nasopharynx of a newborn.

Tracheoesophageal fistula is a congenital anomaly involving the esophagus and the trachea. In its most common form, the proximal portion of the esophagus is atretic and the distal portion connected to the trachea by a fistula. Within the first few hours of life in newborns with a maternal history of polyhydramnios who have excessive pharyngeal secretions, choking, and coughing or cyanosis when fed by mouth. The treatment of this condition represents a surgical emergency.

INFECTIONS

Infections of the pulmonary tract are one of the most common causes of illness in children. Several are particularly important in pediatrics.

Otitis media is characterized by inflammation and the accumulation of purulent fluid in the middle ear. Although acute otitis media is often viral in etiology, the most common bacterial causes include *Hemophilus influenzae, Streptococcus pneumoniae,* and Group A β-hemolytic streptococcus. The child with acute otitis media usually presents with a history of a viral upper respiratory infection, fever, otalgia, and irritability. On examination a red, bulging tympanic membrane that does not move with pneumatic otoscopy is observed. The children will also have a mild conductive hearing loss. Since the causative agent is rarely known, empirical therapy with a broad-spectrum antibiotic is usually prescribed.

Acute epiglottitis, a *Hemophilus influenzae* infection of the larynx and the epiglottis, represents a severe and life-threatening pediatric emergency. Usually found in children between the ages of 2 and 7 years, it presents with significant fever and general signs of toxicity; the acute onset of stridor, hoarseness, drooling; and significant respiratory distress.

The pharynx of a child with these symptoms should not be examined unless the examiner is prepared to intubate or perform a tracheostomy immediately; stimulation of the posterior pharynx may cause immediate laryngeal obstruction and respiratory arrest.

Bronchiolitis, a viral infection of infants and small children, usually occurs during the winter and early spring. Respiratory syncytial virus is the most common cause. A child with this condition presents with a history of a viral upper respiratory infection followed by the abrupt onset of respiratory distress and wheezing. On examination, tachypnea, tachycardia, prolonged expirations, and wheezing are found. In severe cases, cyanosis and prostration may be present.

The treatment of bronchiolitis is largely supportive; in young infants, the disease may be so severe as to require mechanical ventilation for respiratory failure.

CYSTIC FIBROSIS

Cystic fibrosis is a multisystem inherited disease characterized by abnormalities of the body's exocrine glands. Its basic cause is unknown, but the trait is probably transmitted as an autosomal recessive. Uncommon in black children, it has a general prevalence of about 1 in 2,500 children of central European ancestry. The disease varies in its severity; about half of the children with the condition will present during infancy.

The child with cystic fibrosis commonly has symptoms of failure to thrive, recurrent pulmonary infections with chronic cough, large, foul-smelling bowel movements, and occasionally rectal prolapse or nasal polyps. Cirrhosis of the liver and diabetes may develop in those who survive to adolescence.

The diagnosis of cystic fibrosis is based on the presence of an elevated amount of sodium and chloride in the sweat (>60 mEq/liter) and evidence of chronic pulmonary disease, or documented pancreatic insufficiency or a positive family history of the disease.

The management of cystic fibrosis involves the use of oral pancreatic enzymes to enhance gastrointestinal absorption, supplemental water-soluble multivitamins, vigorous antibiotic therapy for pulmonary infections, physical therapy to promote postural drainage of respiratory secretions, genetic counseling, and support of the child and family in coping with this chronic disease.

Cardiovascular Disorders

With the marked reduction in the incidence of rheumatic fever in the United States, congenital heart disease has become the most common serious cardiac problem in children.

CONGENITAL HEART DISEASE

Congenital heart disease is often classified as cyanotic or acyanotic. ***Tetralogy of Fallot,*** the most common type of cyanotic congenital heart disease, consists of pulmonary stenosis or atresia, ventricular septal defect, dextroposition of the aorta that overrides the septal defect, and right ventricular hypertrophy. In most instances children with this lesion are not cyanotic at birth but present with failure to thrive and tachypnea and cyanosis on feeding and exercise within a few weeks to months of life.

Ventricular septal defect, the most common congenital cardiac lesion, is usually but not always a solitary lesion. The severity of symptoms varies with the size of the defect. The murmur of ventricular septal defects is a typically loud systolic murmur heard best along the left sternal border and often associated with a thrill.

Congenital cardiac lesions are associated with a variety of chromosomal abnormalities, genetic conditions, maternal disease, and congenital infections. The lesions of congenital heart disease are often very complex and require expert consultation and often cardiac catheterization for definitive diagnosis.

Congestive heart failure can be caused by a variety of conditions. Children in cardiac failure usually present with tachycardia and tachypnea, anorexia and failure to thrive, poor exercise tolerance, pallor or cyanosis, hepatomegaly, and edema.

RHEUMATIC FEVER

Rheumatic fever is a systemic disease that represents a nonsuppurative complication of β-hemolytic streptococcal infections. The signs and symptoms of rheumatic fever are discussed elsewhere. However, chorea is a symptom of rheumatic fever more frequently found in children than adults. It is more common in females and is usually found in the age range of 5 to 16 years. The symptoms of chorea include aimless and involuntary movements that may be associated with increased emotional lability and speech dysfunction.

Rheumatic fever is more common in children of lower socioeconomic class, in which the crowded housing conditions predispose to the rapid spread of streptococcal infections. The incidence of rheumatic fever has declined dramatically in the United States over the past 30 years.

Gastrointestinal Disorders

The gastrointestinal tract is the first organ system of the newborn to share the contribution of the mother and society. In fact, one of the initial tensions that the newborn experiences is that of hunger, with relief derived from feeding and having the nipple placed in its mouth. It is the necessity that brings mother and infant together, and it is no surprise that love and eating soon become synonymous.

CONGENITAL ANOMALIES

Pyloric stenosis is a condition caused by hypertrophy of the pyloric sphincter, resulting in partial obstruction of the stomach. It is more common in first-born males and tends to be familial. Typically this condition presents in the first week or two of life with projectile vomiting, failure to thrive, and dehydration. On examination a small mass located about midway between the umbilicus and the costal margin at the lateral border of the right rectus muscle may be palpated. Peristaltic waves that begin at the left costal margin and pass toward the midepigastric region may also be observed. On laboratory evaluation hypochloremic alkalosis may be found. The prognosis of pyloric stenosis is excellent with surgical correction of the lesion.

Congenital aganglionic megacolon, or Hirschsprung's disease, is a rare congenital anomaly in which the autonomic nervous system's innervation of the colon is interrupted. The condition is familial and more common in boys. Infants with the disease may present with a history of difficulty or delay in passing meconium, persistent or recurrent diarrhea, and severe infection or perforation of the bowel. Older children with the disease present with a history of chronic constipation present since birth, an absence of the urge to defecate, marked abdominal distention, fecal abdominal masses, and the absence of feces in the rectum.

The diagnosis is made by barium enema and by biopsy of the involved segment of the colon. Surgical resection of the involved colon is required for therapy.

INFECTIONS

Acute gastroenteritis with severe diarrhea and vomiting is one of the most frequent causes of death in children in the underdeveloped countries. With the improvement in sanitation and nutrition in the industrialized countries, the mortality from gastroenteritis has been reduced markedly. Viral agents, particularly rotovirus, represent the most common causes of gastroenteritis. *Salmonella, Shigella, Campylobacter,* and *Staphlococcus* are the common bacterial causes of gastroenteritis in children. The management of acute gastroenteritis depends on its severity and the presence of dehydration and acidosis. Most children with this disease can be managed on an outpatient basis with manipulation of the diet and careful fluid intake. Children with significant dehydration require hospitalization and parenteral therapy.

Acute appendicitis is the most common condition requiring abdominal surgery in children. After the first 18 to 24 months of life, the signs and symptoms of acute appendicitis resemble those of older patients. In the child younger than 2 years the diagnosis can be very difficult to make, and for that reason the diagnosis is often delayed until the appendix has ruptured and classic signs of acute peritonitis have developed.

Intussusception, a condition in which one portion of the intestine telescopes or invaginates on another, causes symptoms of acute intestinal obstruction. It is found most commonly in children under the age of 2 years, is slightly more common in boys, and has been associated with an antecedent adenovirus infection. Typically, children with an intussusception present with a history of the abrupt onset of crampy abdominal pain, vomiting, and the passage of blood and mucus in the stool ("current jelly stools"). On examination they are usually prostrate and listless; manifest a flat and flaccid abdomen, which becomes distended as the obstruction worsens; and have a tender abdominal mass.

An intussusception may be reduced using the hydrostatic pressure of barium into the gastrointestinal tract by rectum; however, if this maneuver is not successful, immediate surgical intervention is required.

Renal Disease

Congenital renal defects should be considered in all situations in which renal function is impaired. Congenital hydronephrosis and hydroureter are frequently associated with congenital anomalies of the lower gastrointestinal tract. Posterior urethral valves are significant causes of hydronephrosis in boys.

Acute glomerulonephritis, characterized by the acute onset of edema, hypertension, and hematuria, is one of the nonsuppurative complications of β-hemolytic streptococcal infections. Streptococcal infections of the skin, as well as pharyngitis, are found commonly to have preceded the onset of glomerulonephritis. The specific pathologic mechanism of acute streptococcal nephritis is not completely understood, but it is generally agreed that the condition represents an antigen–antibody reaction to certain strains of streptococcus. Laboratory evaluation of children with this disease will reveal hematuria, azotemia, elevation of the antistreptolysin O antibody, and decreased levels of complement. The disease usually has a relatively benign course, most children recovering completely within 8 to 16 weeks. A small percentage of children develop chronic renal disease.

Idiopathic nephrotic syndrome of childhood is a disease of unknown etiology characterized by the gradual onset of edema, proteinuria, hypoproteinemia, and hyperlipidemia. About 80% of children with nephrosis have "minimal change" disease, a term used to describe the relative lack of findings of light microscopy of renal biopsy material. This prognosis for this group of children is excellent with steroid therapy. The remaining 20% of children with nephrosis have a variety of histologic findings on renal biopsy, often do not respond to therapy satisfactorily, and have a more guarded prognosis.

Diseases of the Immune System

HUMORAL IMMUNITY

An infant is born with a fairly well-developed capacity for humoral immune response, but with little preformed antibody. Maternal IgG antibodies are transferred across the placenta, but these antibodies disappear within the first 6 to 12 months of life. IgM and IgA antibodies do not cross the placenta, and although the newborn is capable of producing these antibodies if stimulated, they are generally at quite low levels in the healthy infant. IgM antibodies are thought to have particular protection against gram-negative bacteria, which may explain the newborn's susceptibility to these infections. IgM is also the first type of antibody formed in response to infection, so that IgM levels

can be used as index of prenatal or perinatal infections.

Children with deficiencies of immunoglobulins, especially IgG and IgM, present with repeated and serious bacterial infections (otitis media, pneumonia, meningitis, etc.). These children are less susceptible to most viral infections. Hypogammaglobulinemia may be congenital, acquired, or transient.

CELLULAR IMMUNITY

T lymphocytes, thought to be dependent on the thymus for their function, serve to protect the body against viruses, fungi, such chronic bacterial infections as tuberculosis and brucellosis, and tumors. They are also primarily involved in the rejection of organ transplants.

DiGeorge's syndrome is a congenital condition characterized by thymic hypoplasia, neonatal tetany, congenital heart disease, abnormal facies, and cellular immunity defects.

Severe combined immunodeficiency disease (SCID) involves deficiencies in both T and B cells and is thought to be due to a deficiency in a common lymphocyte stem cell. The disease may be transmitted as a sex-linked or an autosomal recessive trait.

Acquired immunodeficiency syndrome (AIDS) is found in infants and children either who are born to women infected with the human immunodeficiency virus, or who have received blood or blood products contaminated by the virus.

In general the disease seems to present in one of several patterns: young infants who present with overwhelming and often lethal sepsis; infants with failure to thrive, generalized lymphadenopathy, hepatosplenomegaly, persistent monilial infections, and recurrent bacterial or opportunistic infections, particularly *Pneumocystis carinii pneumonitis;* and infants and young children with a progressive leukoencephalopathy, which results in a gradual loss of developmental milestones and deterioration of neurologic function.

The management of the disease includes vigorous therapy of infections, attention to nutrition, and support for the family and child. For some children treatment with intravenous gamma globulin on a monthly basis seems to protect them from serious bacterial infections. AZT therapy is also used for the treatment of AIDS in children.

Three other immune deficiency syndromes deserve mention. The *Wiskott-Aldrich syndrome* is a sex-linked recessive disorder characterized by repeated infections, eczema, and thrombocytopenia. *Ataxia telangiectasia* is an autosomal recessive disorder characterized by progressive ataxia, telangiectasia, and a mixed cellular and humoral deficiency. ***Chronic granulomatous disease*** (CGD) is a genetic condition that is usually sex-linked recessive and that is characterized by a dysfunction of the body's polymorphonuclear leukocytes. Children with this condition present with repeated infections, local lymphadenopathy, and hepatosplenomegaly.

PREVENTIVE PEDIATRICS

The physician who cares for children must not only provide direct, curative medical care but must also be involved in the prevention of disease and disability. Since children are growing and developing, the physician's focus on prevention will vary with the child's age.

Accidents and Poisonings

Accidental ingestions are common in two age groups. Children under the age of 6 years, especially toddlers, are particularly susceptible to accidental ingestions. As part of well child care, physicians should regularly inquire about the family's storage of household products and drugs and constantly warn parents about the dangers of accidental ingestions.

Lead poisoning continues to be a serious hazard for many children in the United States. The major sources of lead continue to be dust and plaster in old housing that has been painted with lead-based paints. Since the symptoms of lead poisoning can be very subtle, routine screening for lead intoxication is recommended for all children residing in areas in which they might be exposed to excessive amounts of lead. The treatment of chronic lead poisoning includes removal of the child from the environment containing lead. In children with significantly elevated lead levels chelation therapy with CaEDTA is required.

Automobile accidents, both pedestrian and vehicular, continue to be the most common cause of death in children in the United States. Physicians should do everything possible to make certain that

TABLE 5-9. Recommended Schedule for Immunization of Healthy Infants and Children*

RECOMMENDED AGE†	IMMUNIZATION‡	COMMENTS
2 mo	DTP, HbCV,§ OPV	DTP and OPV can be initiated as early as 4 wk after birth in areas of high endemicity or during epidemics
4 mo	DTP, HbCV,§ OPV	2-mo interval (minimum of 6 wk) desired for OPV to avoid interference from previous dose
6 mo	DTP, HbCV§	Third dose of OPV is not indicated in the U.S., but is desirable in other geographic areas where polio is endemic
15 mo	MMR,‖ HbCV#	Tuberculin testing may be done at the same visit
15–18 mo	DTP,**·†† OPV‡‡	(See footnotes)
4–6 yr	DTP,§§ OPV	At or before school entry
11–12 yr	MMR	At entry to middle school or junior high school unless second dose previously given
14–16 yr	Td	Repeat every 10 yr throughout life

* For all products used, consult manufacturer's package insert for instructions for storage, handling, dosage, and administration. Biologics prepared by different manufacturers may vary, and package inserts of the same manufacturers may change from time to time. Therefore, the physician should be aware of the contents of the current package insert.

† These recommended ages should not be construed as absolute. For example, 2 months can be 6 to 10 weeks. However, MMR usually should not be given to children younger than 12 months. (If measles vaccination is indicated, monovalent measles vaccine is recommended, and MMR should be given subsequently, at 15 months.)

‡ DTP = diphtheria and tetanus toxoids with pertussis vaccine; HbCV = Haemophilus b conjugate vaccine; OPV = oral poliovirus vaccine containing attenuated poliovirus types 1, 2, and 3; MMR = live measles, mumps, and rubella viruses in a combined vaccine; Td = adult tetanus toxoid (full dose) and diphtheria toxoid (reduced dose) for adult use.

§ As of October 1990, only one HbCV is approved for use in children younger than 15 months (see Infections).

‖ May be given at 12 months of age in areas with recurrent measles transmission.

Any licensed *Haemophilus b* conjugate vaccine may be given.

** Should be given 6 to 12 months after the third dose.

†† May be given simultaneously with MMR at 15 months.

‡‡ May be given simultaneously with MMR and HbCV at 15 months or at any time between 12 and 24 months; priority should be given to administering MMR at the recommended age.

§§ Can be given up to the seventh birthday.

(From Report of the Committee on Infectious Diseases, 22nd ed. Chicago, IL: American Academy of Pediatrics, 1991, p 17. Copyright American Academy of Pediatrics, 1991) parents obtain car seats for transporting infants and young children in automobiles and that they establish the habit of using seat belts for all members of the family.

Vaccines

An important aspect of prevention in pediatrics lies in the use of vaccines now available to prevent many of the common communicable diseases that in the past accounted for much of the mortality of childhood. The current recommended schedule of immunizations during childhood is provided in Table 5-9. Revisions are, of course, made from year to year as new information and new vaccines become available.

For clean, minor wounds a booster dose of tetanus toxoid is not needed for a fully immunized child at the time of injury unless more than 10 years has elapsed since the last tetanus immunization. For contaminated wounds a booster dose should be given if more than 5 years has elapsed since the last dose.

Pneumococcal vaccines are recommended for high risk groups such as children with sickle-cell anemia or children with asplenia from any cause. Passive immunization with gamma globulin or special immune serum globulin can be used to prevent or ameliorate a variety of viral diseases.

QUESTIONS IN PEDIATRICS

Essay Questions

List 10 causes of respiratory distress in a newborn.

What is the expected approximate weight and length/height of a 6-month-old? A 12-month-old? A 4-year-old?

Outline the recommended immunization schedule for a normal child.

List the major causes of growth failure.

What are the expected signs and symptoms of the adrenogenital syndrome in boys? In girls?

What are the signs and symptoms of intussusception?

List the signs and symptoms of cystic fibrosis.

Contrast the signs and symptoms of acute glomerulonephritis and the nephrotic syndrome.

Compare the signs and symptoms of neuroblastoma and Wilms' tumor.

What is histiocytosis X?

What is Down's syndrome? List the signs and symptoms.

What are the advantages of breast feeding?

Define *small-for-gestational-age*, *appropriate-for-gestational-age*, and *large-for-gestational-age*.

What is the most common cause of death in children?

What is the pathophysiology of Rh incompatibility?

Clinical Cases

Read the following cases carefully and do not quickly jump to conclusions. Answer in five words or less and give only one diagnosis unless you are requested to provide more. Make your diagnoses as specific as possible.

A 4-hour-old infant develops generalized seizures. What are the most likely causes?

A 5-month-old boy has been constipated since birth. He goes 4 to 5 days without a bowel movement. Physical examination is normal except for the presence of an umbilical hernia and fecal masses in the abdomen. Formula changes have been to no avail. What are the probable diagnoses?

A 1-day-old infant has been unable to retain any feeding, but vomits bile-stained material. What are the possible diagnoses?

A 1-day-old infant becomes cyanotic with each feeding. What are the likely diagnoses?

A 6-month-old presents with failure to thrive. The infant has been hospitalized twice for pneumonia. What are the possible diagnoses?

A 2-year-old girl presents with unilateral exophthalmus. What is the likely diagnosis?

A 9-year-old girl is seen with a 7-hour history of vomiting, fever, and periumbilical pain. She has a cold and has had one diarrheal stool. List the three most common diagnostic possibilities.

A 5-month-old infant with a head circumference of 42 cm has been previously well until he began convulsing 4 hours ago. The medical student listed the following diagnoses to be considered: (1) microcephaly, (2) hydrocephaly, (3) doliocephaly, (4) menigitis, (5) tetany. Which is the most likely diagnosis?

A 2-year-old boy presents with the abrupt onset of fever, cough, and purpura. List three common diagnostic possibilities.

A 2-year-old girl presents with a history of several hours of crampy abdominal pain and bloody stools. She appears lethargic and listless. A mass is palpated in her abdomen. What is the most probable diagnosis?

Multiple-Choice Questions

1. Jaundice in the newborn may be caused by:
   (a) Hepatitis
   (b) ABO blood group incompatibilities
   (c) Congenital spherocytosis
   (d) Gallstones

2. The adrenogenital syndrome in early childhood:
   (a) Occurs only in males
   (b) May result from an autosomal recessive trait
   (c) May cause virilization
   (d) May cause hypernatremia

3. Meningitis in children is most frequently caused by:
   (a) *Staphylococcus aureus*
   (b) *H. influenzae*
   (c) *N. meningococcus*
   (d) *Streptococcus pneumoniae*

4. The common cyanotic congenital cardiac lesions include:
   (a) Ventricular septal defect
   (b) Atrial septal defect
   (c) Tetralogy of Fallot
   (d) Transposition of the great vessels

5. An infant with frequent pulmonary infections may have:
   (a) Cystic fibrosis
   (b) Hypogammaglobulinemia
   (c) Chronic granulomatous disease
   (d) All of the above

6. Sickling of red blood cells occurs:
   (a) In 8% of the black population
   (b) Only in sickle-cell anemia, not in sickle-cell trait
   (c) In thalassemia and sickle-cell trait occurring together
   (d) In congenital spherocytosis

7. Vomiting in the newborn can be caused by:
   (a) Malrotation and volvulus
   (b) Intestinal atresia
   (c) Meconium ileus
   (d) Sepsis
   (e) All of the above

8. Children with juvenile diabetes:
   (a) Usually have an abrupt onset of symptoms
   (b) May be treated with oral hypoglycemic agents
   (c) Need not be concerned with the degenerative complications of the disease
   (d) Have marked variations in their insulin requirements

9. A 2-year-old can:
   (a) Ride a tricycle
   (b) Climb on furniture
   (c) Walk up stairs one step at a time
   (d) Know own gender

10. Breast-fed infants should receive supplemental:
    (a) Vitamin D
    (b) Fluoride
    (c) Iron
    (d) Vitamin K

11. The congenital rubella syndrome includes:
    (a) Cataracts
    (b) Deafness
    (c) Congenital cardiac disease
    (d) Microcephaly
    (e) All of the above

12. The TORCH infections include:
    (a) Toxoplasmosis
    (b) Syphilis
    (c) Rubella
    (d) All of the above

13. Newborns may be particularly susceptible to gram-negative infections because they have:
    (a) Low levels of IgM
    (b) High levels of IgM
    (c) Maternal IgG
    (d) No IgG

14. Sex-linked inherited diseases include:
    (a) Hemophilia
    (b) Cystic fibrosis
    (c) Sickle-cell anemia
    (d) Galactosemia

15. The most common anemia in children is:
    (a) Sickle-cell anemia
    (b) Thalassemia
    (c) Iron deficiency
    (d) Congenital spherocytosis

16. Congenital nephrosis is characterized by:
    (a) Hypertension
    (b) Elevated ASLO titer
    (c) Albuminuria
    (d) Hypoproteinemia

17. The most common cause of death in children in the United States is:
    (a) Malnutrition
    (b) Malignancy
    (c) Accidents
    (d) Congenital defects

18. The average caloric requirements for infants during the first year of life are:
    (a) 80 to 90 kcal/kg
    (b) 100 to 120 kcal/kg
    (c) 120 to 130 kcal/kg
    (d) 90 to 100 kcal/kg

19. Neuroblastomas may present with:
    (a) Abdominal masses
    (b) Unilateral exophthalmus
    (c) Hematuria
    (d) Lowered VMA levels
20. Nephroblastomas are:
    (a) Sometimes bilateral
    (b) Associated with hemihypertrophy
    (c) Associated with aniridia
    (d) All of the above
21. Children with nutritional rickets are likely to have:
    (a) A prolonged history of breast feeding
    (b) Growth failure
    (c) Craniotabes
    (d) All of the above
22. Iron deficiency anemia is commonly found in:
    (a) Premature infants
    (b) Adolescent boys
    (c) Infants fed with whole milk
    (d) Adolescent girls
23. Acute epiglottitis:
    (a) Is a condition caused by the respiratory syncytial virus
    (b) Is a condition caused by *H. influenzae*
    (c) Is a benign infection requiring only supportive therapy
    (d) Is a life-threatening infection
24. The cardiac lesions of the tetralogy of Fallot include:
    (a) Aortic stenosis
    (b) Pulmonary stenosis
    (c) Atrial septal defect
    (d) Ventricular septal defect
25. A child with pyloric stenosis usually presents:
    (a) Over the age of 6 months
    (b) With growth failure
    (c) With seizures
    (d) With hypocloremic alkalosis

ANSWERS TO MULTIPLE-CHOICE QUESTIONS

1. a,b,c	**8.** a,d	**15.** c	**22.** a,c,d
2. b,c	**9.** b,c,d	**16.** c,d	**23.** b,d
3. b,d,e	**10.** a,b	**17.** c	**24.** b,d
4. c,d	**11.** e	**18.** b	**25.** b,d
5. d	**12.** d	**19.** a,b	
6. a,c	**13.** a	**20.** d	
7. e	**14.** a	**21.** d	

Rypins' Clinical Sciences Review, 16th Edition, edited by Edward D. Frohlich. J. B. Lippincott Company, Philadelphia © 1993.

6

Public Health and Community Medicine

Richard H. Grimm, Jr., M.D. M.P.H., Ph.D.*

Associate Professor, Division of Cardiovascular
Diseases, Department of Internal Medicine and
Division of Epidemiology, School of Public Health,
University of Minnesota School of Medicine
Minneapolis, Minnesota

To the medical student just finishing 4 years of school, eager to start an internship, where he or she can finally take on real patients, the arena of public health holds little charm. To these students (and most practicing doctors) the primary focus is *individual patient care;* after all, isn't this what 2 years of didactic work and 2 years of clinical apprenticeship point toward? During the years of clinical education, mentors emphasize establishing a differential diagnosis and, by exclusion and deductive reasoning, arriving at the diagnosis. Little attention is paid to selecting the appropriate treatments and assuring adherence to those treatment(s), even less to achieving adequate follow-up and continuity of care.

Practicing physicians rightfully focus on diagnosis and individual patient care as their main concern; however, much is lost by not including the public health perspective as well. The conditions physicians diagnose frequently are preceded by years or even decades of exposures that caused the disease,

* The author of this revised chapter would like to credit the original author, Charles M. Wylie, M.D., Dr. P.H. and to recognize his colleagues who reviewed and contributed to the chapter. They include John Flack, M.P.H., M.D.; Mark Kjelsberg, Ph.D.; and John Nyman, Ph.D. Finally, the author would like to acknowledge Jeanne Clark, Ph.D., who provided valuable editorial assistance.

which may have existed for many additional years in the subacute nonsymptomatic state. Although it is gratifying to make the correct diagnosis of the end-stage disease, what then follows is frequently the sad realization that treatment at this point is often at best palliative and, at worst, harmful. Including a public health perspective would allow physicians to get more involved in much earlier stages of the process and actually help prevent disease from developing. Since the early stage of disease begins in the community, the community is the appropriate focus of this involvement.

In addition to diagnosis, contemporary physicians must also be able to evaluate and select appropriate treatments. Medical treatments have a significant potential for harm, so careful evaluation of new therapies is needed. A primary tool for evaluating new therapies is the randomized clinical trial. Physicians need to understand the design, method, and analysis of such trials in order to properly evaluate the results. Community medicine has evolved to bridge the gap between clinical medicine and public health. It concerns itself with people and patients within the community. This chapter covers basic concepts of public health and community medicine in order to provide a perspective vital not only to those who expect to devote themselves to research in prevention and treatment of disease in large popula-

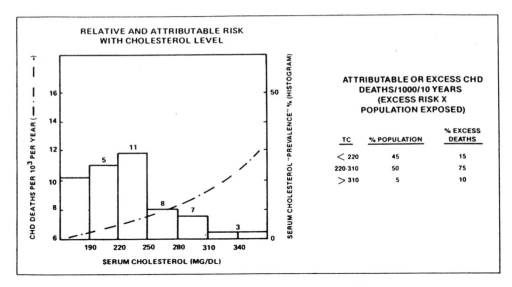

Fig. 6-1. Serum cholesterol. (Blackburn H: Coronary Risk Factors—How to Evaluate Them, Eur J Cardiol, 1975, 2, p 252)

tions but to those whose focus is the practice of individual patient care.

For most physicians who see only individual patients it is difficult to appreciate the potential for prevention in community-based interventions. Physicians assume that to prevent disease in a patient, major changes in lifestyle (*e.g.,* smoking cessation and weight loss) are necessary for the patient to benefit. They grow skeptical that these changes are possible after seeing the difficulties many patients and families undergo in trying to make major lifestyle changes.

They doubt that moderate changes in behavior will be able to lower risk significantly and justify the disruptions and considerable effort made by the patient to make these changes. They may be aware, for example, that the difficult task of cutting sodium intake by 50 mEq, or about one third, might result in a 2 to 3 mmHg reduction in diastolic pressure, an improvement that seems small when compared to a 10 mmHg reduction achieved more easily with drugs. Most physicians are not enthusiastic about prevention when observations of the individual provide their sole basis for judgment.

However, a different view begins to arise when a major contribution of public and community health, the ***population perspective,*** is taken into account. This way of looking at prevention includes trends that can be detected in the community as a whole. It is true that high-risk patients in the population, persons with severe hypertension, hypercholesteremia, and so forth, have the greatest absolute risk for contracting disease. However, most of the actual cases

of disease that occur (*e.g.,* heart attacks and strokes) are found in those at average or above-average but not necessarily abnormal risk by our conventional medical standards. Thus, if this very large, lower-risk population can change its distribution of the risk factor only slightly, then the amount of disease that is prevented in the community is substantial. This is shown for serum cholesterol in Figure 6-1. Another example would be physicians working with patients to lower sodium and weight along with community health efforts by schools, mass media, and volunteer organizations to achieve a significant change in blood pressure in the community as a whole. If only a small change in average blood pressure is achieved (~2 mmHg systolic), then a substantial percentage of cases of stroke and heart attack could be prevented. If physicians can begin to take into account both the individual patient and population perspective, they can expect to improve greatly their ability to prevent and treat the patient population they see.

HEALTH STATISTICS

Health has been defined in many ways. Most people think of health as the absence of disease; however, it is less than precise to define something by what it is not. The World Health Organization (WHO) defined health in 1948 as "a state of complete physical, mental, and social well-being, and not merely the absence of disease or infirmity."

Clear definition is the first step in measurement; setting limits that should tell us whether people fall between or outside them. Measurement then goes further, to indicate more precisely that part of a scale in which subjects fall. Most devices used to measure public health come from the fields of health statistics and epidemiology.

Since the population is the base for most health statistics, complete enumeration of the population is important. In the first year of each decade, the U.S. Census Bureau conducts a national census to provide this information. The estimates made for intermediate years are sufficiently reliable for the purposes of most research.

Population trends in the United States differ from those in the developing countries where the path toward population stability continues to be difficult. These countries adopt in a matter of years the life-saving techniques that the more advanced countries took decades to acquire. Family planning activities are adopted more slowly. Thus, in most developing countries birth rates have not fallen far enough to compensate for a more rapid fall in death rates. No form of life can continue to multiply without eventually coming to terms with its environment. Thus the rate of human population growth must inevitably slow down and level off; the major unknowns are when, at what levels, and with what cost to the public health this will occur. Figure 6-2, based on predictions regarded as reasonable in the mid-1980s, suggests that the world population will continue to expand through the first half of the 21st century.

In contrast to population figures, which form the denominators of most health statistics, vital facts such as births, morbidity, and deaths form the numerators. Registration of births and deaths by the departments of health of the various states is required throughout the United States. The attending physician is responsible for filing birth certificates

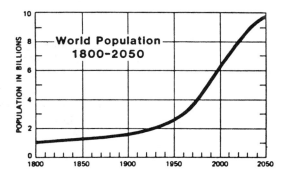

Fig. 6-2. Estimates of the world population in billions, 1800 to 2050.

with the local registrar, and the funeral director is responsible for filing death and stillbirth certificates.

In the internationally agreed-upon form of the death certificate, Part I emphasizes the underlying cause of death as determined by the certifying physician. Because many older patients who die have multiple diseases, the way in which physicians select the underlying cause of death may have an important effect on reported time trends in death rates. There is good evidence that certain swings in death rates in recent decades relate more to changes in diagnostic habits of physicians than to true changes in incidence of diseases. To compensate for variations in medical fashion, the United States is beginning to attempt to record and analyze all causes on the certificate rather than the underlying cause alone.

Death Certification

For more than 50 years the United States has had mandatory standardized certification of all deaths. It is the physician's duty to fill out death certificates and ascribe an immediate cause of death as a consequence of a specific disease. Figure 6-3 shows a standard-format death certificate used by all states with some modification. Death certificates are collected locally and forwarded to state health departments, which keep them and develop summary data. Death certificates are coded for specific diseases by nosologists, using a standard International Classification of Diseases System (ICDS). Data tapes from state health departments are sent to the National Center for Health Statistics (NCHS), where national summary data is compiled and periodically published. Today death certification is virtually 100% complete in the United States, Canada, and Europe; however, most developing countries do not have adequate systems for certifying deaths, and data from such countries should not be viewed as accurate.

Although death certification is very useful and allows us to track disease incidence and prevalence over time, there are problems with validity. Studies comparing autopsy death ascertation with death certifications show that only about 10% of deaths are autopsied. There is some discrepancy between death certification and autopsy; for example, cardiovascular diseases tend to be somewhat overestimated by death certification compared to autopsy, whereas cancer deaths are more accurately reflected. Nevertheless, the system works well to reflect change of disease incidence over time and to serve as an early warning system for new disease

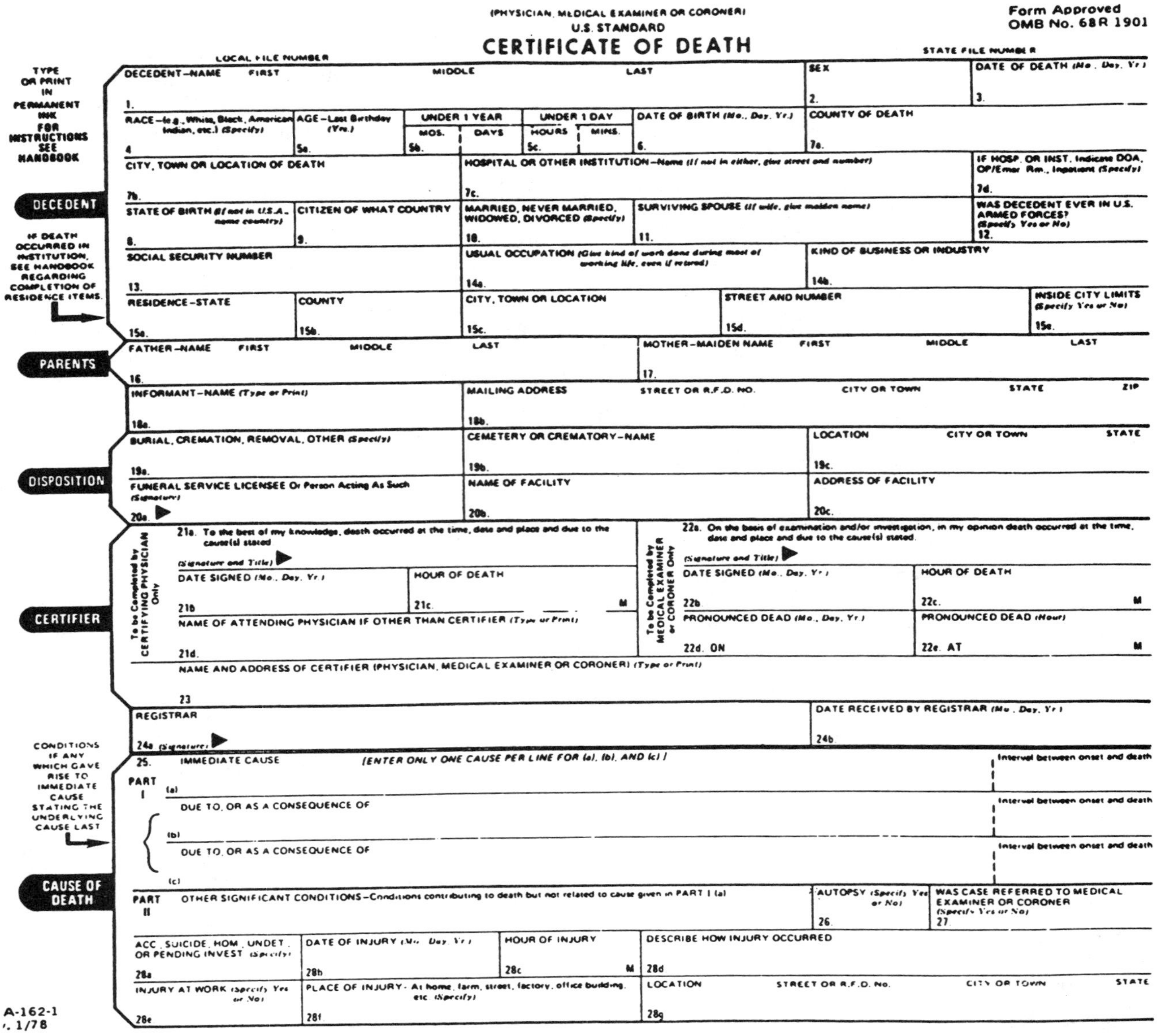

(PHYSICIAN, MEDICAL EXAMINER OR CORONER)
U.S. STANDARD
CERTIFICATE OF DEATH

Form Approved OMB No. 68R 1901

LOCAL FILE NUMBER — STATE FILE NUMBER

TYPE OR PRINT IN PERMANENT INK. FOR INSTRUCTIONS SEE HANDBOOK

DECEDENT: DECEDENT—NAME FIRST MIDDLE LAST 1. | SEX 2. | DATE OF DEATH (Mo., Day, Yr.) 3. | RACE—(e.g., White, Black, American Indian, etc.) (Specify) 4. | AGE—Last Birthday (Yrs.) 5a. | UNDER 1 YEAR MOS. DAYS 5b. | UNDER 1 DAY HOURS MINS. 5c. | DATE OF BIRTH (Mo., Day, Yr.) 6. | COUNTY OF DEATH 7a. | CITY, TOWN OR LOCATION OF DEATH 7b. | HOSPITAL OR OTHER INSTITUTION—Name (If not in either, give street and number) 7c. | IF HOSP. OR INST. Indicate DOA, OP/Emer. Rm., Inpatient (Specify) 7d. | STATE OF BIRTH (If not in U.S.A., name country) 8. | CITIZEN OF WHAT COUNTRY 9. | MARRIED, NEVER MARRIED, WIDOWED, DIVORCED (Specify) 10. | SURVIVING SPOUSE (If wife, give maiden name) 11. | WAS DECEDENT EVER IN U.S. ARMED FORCES? (Specify Yes or No) 12. | SOCIAL SECURITY NUMBER 13. | USUAL OCCUPATION (Give kind of work done during most of working life, even if retired) 14a. | KIND OF BUSINESS OR INDUSTRY 14b. | RESIDENCE—STATE 15a. | COUNTY 15b. | CITY, TOWN OR LOCATION 15c. | STREET AND NUMBER 15d. | INSIDE CITY LIMITS (Specify Yes or No) 15e.

IF DEATH OCCURRED IN INSTITUTION, SEE HANDBOOK REGARDING COMPLETION OF RESIDENCE ITEMS.

PARENTS: FATHER—NAME FIRST MIDDLE LAST 16. | MOTHER—MAIDEN NAME FIRST MIDDLE LAST 17. | INFORMANT—NAME (Type or Print) 18a. | MAILING ADDRESS STREET OR R.F.D. NO. CITY OR TOWN STATE ZIP 18b.

DISPOSITION: BURIAL, CREMATION, REMOVAL, OTHER (Specify) 19a. | CEMETERY OR CREMATORY—NAME 19b. | LOCATION CITY OR TOWN STATE 19c. | FUNERAL SERVICE LICENSEE Or Person Acting As Such (Signature) 20a. | NAME OF FACILITY 20b. | ADDRESS OF FACILITY 20c.

CERTIFIER: To be Completed by CERTIFYING PHYSICIAN Only — 21a. To the best of my knowledge, death occurred at the time, date and place and due to the cause(s) stated. (Signature and Title) | DATE SIGNED (Mo., Day, Yr.) 21b | HOUR OF DEATH 21c. M | NAME OF ATTENDING PHYSICIAN IF OTHER THAN CERTIFIER (Type or Print) 21d.

To be Completed by MEDICAL EXAMINER or CORONER Only — 22a. On the basis of examination and/or investigation, in my opinion death occurred at the time, date and place and due to the cause(s) stated. (Signature and Title) | DATE SIGNED (Mo., Day, Yr.) 22b. | HOUR OF DEATH 22c. M | PRONOUNCED DEAD (Mo., Day, Yr.) 22d. ON | PRONOUNCED DEAD (Hour) 22e. AT M

NAME AND ADDRESS OF CERTIFIER (PHYSICIAN, MEDICAL EXAMINER OR CORONER) (Type or Print) 23

REGISTRAR 24a (Signature) | DATE RECEIVED BY REGISTRAR (Mo., Day, Yr.) 24b

CAUSE OF DEATH: 25. IMMEDIATE CAUSE (ENTER ONLY ONE CAUSE PER LINE FOR (a), (b), AND (c).) | Interval between onset and death
PART I (a) DUE TO, OR AS A CONSEQUENCE OF (b) DUE TO, OR AS A CONSEQUENCE OF (c)

CONDITIONS IF ANY WHICH GAVE RISE TO IMMEDIATE CAUSE STATING THE UNDERLYING CAUSE LAST

PART II OTHER SIGNIFICANT CONDITIONS—Conditions contributing to death but not related to cause given in PART I (a) | AUTOPSY (Specify Yes or No) 26. | WAS CASE REFERRED TO MEDICAL EXAMINER OR CORONER (Specify Yes or No) 27

ACC., SUICIDE, HOM., UNDET., OR PENDING INVEST. (Specify) 28a | DATE OF INJURY (Mo., Day, Yr.) 28b | HOUR OF INJURY 28c M | DESCRIBE HOW INJURY OCCURRED 28d | INJURY AT WORK (Specify Yes or No) 28e | PLACE OF INJURY—At home, farm, street, factory, office building, etc. (Specify) 28f | LOCATION STREET OR R.F.D. No. CITY OR TOWN STATE 28g

A-162-1 ... 1/78

Fig. 6-3. Standard-format death certificate.

developments such as influenza outbreaks and AIDS.

Two indices are often used to describe the frequency of a disease in the population. The first is the ***incidence rate,*** which is the number of new cases of the disease occurring over an interval of time in the population; it is often adjusted for the age, race, and gender distribution of the specified population so that figures from relatively young and relatively old groups can be compared. The second is the ***prevalence ratio,*** which is the number of cases of the disease population present at one point or cross section in time. Both these rates are usually expressed as cases per 100,000 population. These figures again are often made specific for age, gender, and race. The longer the duration of illness, the greater the number of cases in the population at any point in time. Thus, a high prevalence ratio may reflect a high incidence rate, a long duration of illness, or both. The prevalence ratio reflects a community photograph of disease at one moment in time. When illness is rare, the larger prevalence ratio is more easily understood and studied than the smaller incidence rate.

Generally, cause of death should be reported in accordance with the disease classification developed by the International Statistical Classification of Diseases, Injuries, and Causes of Death, which is distributed by the WHO. The ninth revision of this publication, first used in the United States for 1979 death statistics, produced some artificial changes in death rates between 1978 and 1979. Such changes in classification of causes of death must be taken into account when interpreting the significance of death rates. In addition to providing important data on health problems, the death certificate is used for legal purposes such as the settlement of estates and insurance claims.

The mortality statistics compiled from the death registrations are usually expressed as rates:

1. The ***crude death rate*** is formed by the number of deaths in a calendar year per 1,000 population

at the middle of that year. After having fallen rapidly between 1930 and 1950, the crude death rate for the United States changed little in the 1950s and 1960s and fell again in the 1970s. In the United States, in 1987, the rate was 8.7/1,000 (Fig. 6-4). Crude death rates in the United States reflect the pattern of deaths primarily in the older population, and in each year they also show a seasonal pattern, with winter highs and summer lows (Fig. 6-5). Crude death rates fall more swiftly in the developing countries, however, where older age groups form a smaller proportion of the total population. In the United States, death rates also fall more steeply when adjusted for the increasing age of the total population (Fig. 6-4).

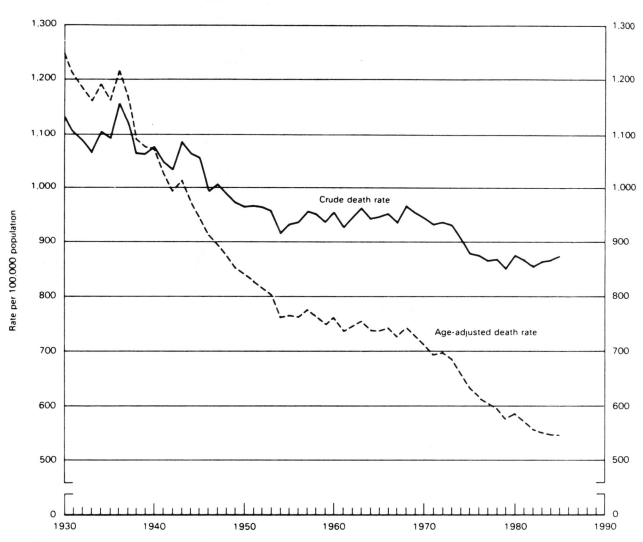

Fig. 6-4. Crude and age-adjusted death rates per 100,000 U.S. population, 1930 to 1985. The crude rate hides part of the fall in deaths since it does not adjust for the expanding elderly population.

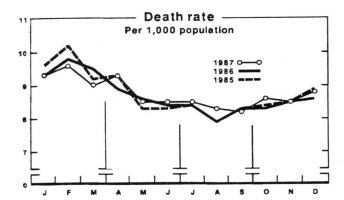

Fig. 6-5. Seasonal change in crude death rates per 1,000 U.S. population, by month of calendar years 1985, 1986, and 1987.

2. Specific death rates are calculated for certain groups because the crude death rate is much affected by age, gender, race, and marital and socioeconomic differences in the population being studied. One example is the age-specific death rate, which is formed by the number of deaths in a specific age group in a given year per 1,000 population at that specified age.

In any given year, however, age-specific rates are low until age 30, after which they rise markedly into older ages. A population with a high proportion of elderly persons has a high crude death rate. To compare mortality in the same country in different years, standardized procedures are used to correct for changing age distributions. These calculations produce an *age-adjusted death rate,* which falls more steeply for the United States than the crude death rate does (see Fig. 6-4). At every age, the adjusted rates have fallen since 1900.

At almost every age, mortality in women is now lower than in men; this is not the case in most developing countries, where complications of childbirth occurring under adverse conditions raise the mortality rates of women in the reproductive ages.

Death rates in the United States are higher in men than in women for coronary heart disease, chronic obstructive lung disease, lung cancer, and accidents. One major area in which death rates are similar in men and women is diabetes mellitus, which has been higher in women in past decades. Age-specific death rates have fallen more for women than for men in the United States and more for whites than for blacks. Socioeconomic factors and perhaps inferior health care among blacks are believed

to be partly responsible for this latter difference.

Specific death rates are also developed for gender, race, marital status, and other factors. At each age, for example, death rates among the married population are lower than among the unmarried population; this finding is partly explained by the likelihood that persons who marry are already more healthy than those who do not, but other factors may play a part.

Disease-specific death rates are widely used in most developed countries. Each rate is the number of deaths from a given disease during the year per 100,000 population. Until the 1980s, the rates were based on the diagnosis that the attending physician stated to be the underlying cause of death. The death rate for a particular disease was assumed to reflect the size of the threat to public health from that condition.

3. The *infant mortality rate* is the number of deaths among children under 1 year of age in a given year per 1,000 live births in the same year. Rates for blacks are consistently higher than rates for whites. The infant mortality rate was once regarded as a good (and perhaps the best) measure of the effectiveness of public health programs, which caused the rates to fall rapidly. It was sensitive to many changes in society, including improvements in health care.

However, now it seems likely that reductions in infant mortality exaggerated the effectiveness of environmental health, communicable disease, and maternal and child health programs in former years. They do not reflect well our current efforts to treat patients with chronic disease, mental illness, and other problems of the older population. Infant mortality rates are lower in many other developed countries than they are in the United States. It seems clear that certain differences are real and not caused artificially by the way in which data are reported. Nevertheless, it is difficult to separate the effect of improved medical care from that of socioeconomic improvements and nutritional advances. The neonatal death rate, part of the infant mortality rate based on deaths occurring in the first 4 weeks of life, is now viewed by some as the better measure of health care effects. Thus, the debate over the value of infant mortality rates in assessing the health of populations has been vigorous in the United States.

4. The *maternal mortality rate* is determined by the number of deaths from puerperal causes in

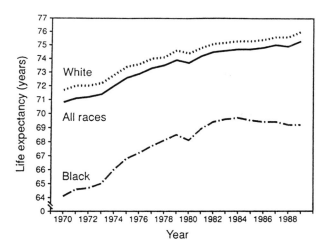

Fig. 6-6. Life expectancy at birth, by year of birth, and by race—United States, 1970 to 1989. (MMWR, 1992, 41, p 124)

a given year per 1,000 live births in the same year. Like the infant mortality rate, this rate is falling more slowly than before in the United States and is considerably higher for nonwhites than for whites. Hypertensive disease of preg-

nancy forms the largest single cause of maternal death.

The leading causes of death have changed radically since 1900. At the beginning of the century, infections such as tuberculosis, influenza, and pneumonia were the dominant causes of death. Currently, noninfectious chronic diseases are dominant, with cardiovascular disease and cancer being the major causes of death, making up approximately 50% and 22% of all causes of death, respectively. Those who set priorities for disease control programs for society, however, must also consider the average age of death and the likelihood of success in disease prevention when setting policies for public health.

Another commonly used measure of health is *life expectancy*. Although the average expectation of life is sometimes advocated as a "positive" measure of health—the higher the figure, the better the public health—life expectancy is basically determined by the death rates of the population involved. The lower the subsequent death rates, the higher will be the expectation of life. It is hard to argue convincingly that the expectation of life measures something different from the force of mortality. Figure 6-6

TABLE 6-1. Abridged Life Table, United States, 1981

AGE INTERVAL	PROPORTION DYING	OF 100,000 BORN ALIVE		STATIONARY POPULATION		AVERAGE REMAINING LIFETIME
Period of Life between Two Exact Ages Stated In Years (1)	Proportion of Persons Alive at Beginning of Age Interval Dying During Interval (2)	Number Living at Beginning of Age Interval (3)	Number Dying During Age Interval (4)	In the Age Interval (5)	In This and All Subsequent Age Intervals (6)	Average Number of Years of Life Remaining at Beginning of Age Interval (7)
$x + x + n$	$_nq_x$	l_x	$_nd_x$	$_nL_x$	T_x	e_x
All races						
0–1	0.0119	100,000	1,194	98,965	7,417,771	74.2
1–5	0.0024	98,806	236	394,675	7,318,806	74.1
5–10	0.0015	98,570	144	492,463	6,924,131	70.2
10–15	0.0015	98,426	146	491,822	6,431,668	65.3
15–20	0.0045	98,280	447	490,386	5,939,846	60.4
20–25	0.0061	97,833	598	487,689	5,449,460	55.7
25–30	0.0064	97,235	624	484,615	4,961,771	51.0
30–35	0.0068	96,611	655	481,489	4,477,156	46.3
35–40	0.0090	95,956	859	477,770	3,995,667	41.6
40–45	0.0134	95,097	1,277	472,503	3,517,897	37.0
45–50	0.0219	93,820	2,053	464,288	3,045,394	32.5
50–55	0.0344	91,767	3,161	451,424	2,581,106	28.1
55–60	0.0521	88,606	4,617	432,110	2,129,682	24.0
60–65	0.0776	83,989	6,521	404,395	1,697,572	20.2
65–70	0.1141	77,468	8,837	366,109	1,293,177	16.7
70–75	0.1648	68,631	11,309	315,778	927,068	13.5
75–80	0.2335	57,322	13,386	253,613	611,290	10.7
80–85	0.3450	43,936	15,158	181,171	357,677	8.1
85 and over	1.000	28,778	28,778	176,506	176,506	6.1

shows that life expectancy at birth has slowly risen in recent decades. It is consistently higher for women than for men, and the gap continues to widen.

Professionals interested in disease prevention and health promotion have been concerned that disease and death have been overemphasized as measures of public health. For this and other reasons, age-specific death rates are used to calculate the likelihood of surviving and the average years of life remaining at any given age. The results of these life table calculations are illustrated in Table 6-1, based on the death rates occurring in the United States in 1980. More detailed life tables form the statistical basis for the work of life insurance companies. The same methods produce figures that guide the charges and viability of health insurance plans and health maintenance organizations (HMOs). Few physicians need to develop their own life tables, but many need to understand the basis of the figures (particularly those in columns 2 and 7 in Table 6-1) to ensure financial and organizational survival of the settings in which they work.

Morbidity Reporting

Reportable diseases are those that by law must be reported to health authorities. The list varies from state to state and from time to time according to the importance attributed to a given disease. Such reporting, if incomplete, gives a distorted picture of the frequency of disease in communities, Moreover, the incidence of many disease groups that do not usually kill people, such as the mental illnesses and the arthritides, are underrepresented in death rates. Attempts to require the reporting of noninfectious diseases have had some success, with cancer registries being the most common example.

The United States National Health Survey is trying to correct these deficiencies of reporting through the use of interviews of a nationwide sample of households; other NHS surveys include medical examinations to provide clinical information that is not obtainable from interviews. These surveys now provide good information on many nonfatal conditions in the U.S. population.

EPIDEMIOLOGY

Epidemiology may be the most important public health field to community medicine; it also represents the closest link to clinical medicine. Epidemiology is the study of disease as it manifests itself in a *population*. As the word *epidemiology* implies, it

has its roots in the study of infectious disease epidemics and efforts to understand the causes and means to prevent them. Epidemiology is characterized by the population perspective and rates of disease occurrence in the population. Whereas clinical medicine's focus is on the individual cases, epidemiology is concerned also with the denominator, or the persons in the population who do not get the disease. In comparing biologic, genetic, and environmental characteristics between cases and noncases, risk factors can be identified and hypotheses formulated about causation. Once causes are identified, prevention becomes a possibility. Prevention can then be tested experimentally by using the clinical trial.

Some basic epidemiologic concepts originate from the field of infectious diseases. They suggest that the frequency of many diseases may be explained on the basis of a host (the susceptible person) interacting with an agent (the factor causing the disease) and with the environment (including its psychosocial, biologic, and other aspects). Also from the infectious disease field comes the concept of an incubation period, the time between exposure to an etiologic agent and the onset of disease. A third concept is that of herd immunity; this concept emphasizes the notion that populations will stop spreading infectious disease even before they are fully immunized against the condition. For example, in a population in which 70% of persons are immune to an infection, the person-to-person spread may never become established because the infectious agent reaches many individuals who do not transmit the disease. The proportion of the population that produces herd immunity varies with the infectivity of the agent and with the size and social behavior to the community. The phenomenon of herd immunity makes it unnecessary to have 100% participation in some immunization programs; it is customary, however, to aim at as close to that level as possible. Epidemiologic concepts and methods can be applied to accidents, poisonings, measurements, attitudes, and, indeed, to any observable characteristic of people. Epidemiologic studies ideally involve all cases with a given characteristic or disease in a defined population, and information is collected on the unaffected as well as affected persons. Such studies often develop rates (or ratios) in which the numerator represents those with the characteristic under study, and the denominator represents the total population, both the affected and unaffected.

Often the first clues to the etiology or the mode of transmission of disease come from field observations and lead to confirmatory observations in the clinic and the laboratory. For example, a number of carcinogenic substances, such as asbestos, uranium-bearing ores, and cigarette smoke, have been identified by observation of the excessive frequency of cancer among those exposed to the agent. Sometimes the situation is reversed, and field study confirms or changes the conclusion of clinical or laboratory studies.

Besides the infectious diseases, contemporary epidemiology concerns itself with chronic diseases, especially cardiovascular diseases, cancer, and AIDS, for these are the epidemics of our modern age. Clinical epidemiology is a relatively new field, which is closely tied to academic clinical medicine. This field applies epidemiologic design and methods to clinical research.

The primary methods of epidemiologic research are the following:

1. *Observational Studies.* Usually these are large prospective studies in which many measures or exposures are carried out at a point in time in a defined population, and then the population is systematically followed at regular intervals for years or decades. In the observational study there is no attempt made to intervene or change any factors. Follow-up involves reassessment of the measures of interest and also ascertainment of which individuals in the population develop the disease. Prevalence and incidence rates can be calculated for specific diseases, and risk of becoming *a case* based on baseline exposure is examined. A well-known example of an observational study is the Framingham Heart Study, which began in 1949 and involved measuring numerous factors (*e.g.,* blood pressure, blood cholesterol, cigarette smoking, etc.) in 5,200 residents of this Massachusetts community. Participants have been followed every 2 years for more than 40 years. This study and 15 similar observational studies also done in the United States have contributed much of what is now known about cardiovascular risk factors. For example, those people with serum cholesterol in the upper quintile or 20th percentile of the population were three times more likely to develop heart disease in the ensuing years compared to those in the lowest quintile. An example of observational study data formatted for risk by serum cholesterol level is shown in Figure 6-7. Observational studies have contributed greatly to understanding of disease occurrence and causation in the cardiovascular field and also in other areas, such as cancer and infectious disease.

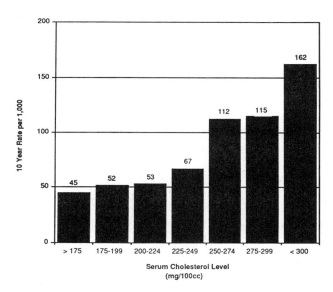

Fig. 6-7. Relationship of serum cholesterol and first coronary event in men 30 to 59. (Data on serum cholesterol and risk from several observational studies—The Pooling Project.) (Blackburn H: The American Heart Association Heartbook, A Guide to Prevention and Treatment of Cardiovascular Diseases, p 5. Dallas, 1980. Reproduced with permission. © *Heartbook, A Guide to Prevention and Treatment of Cardiovascular Diseases,* 1980. Copyright American Heart Association.)

2. *Case Control Studies.* The case control study is another method useful in epidemiology for exploring differences between those who get a disease and those that do not. Unlike the observational study, case control studies identify people who already have a disease, for example, lung cancer. Case control studies are especially useful with diseases that are rare because recruiting enough persons with rare diseases is prohibitively expensive and logistically impossible. Identification of cases is often done from hospital admission records or disease registries. Potential exposures such as cigarette exposure, alcohol intake, and so forth are then catalogued for the cases. The cases are matched to control groups, usually for age, gender, and sometimes for other factors, such as education or income. Exposures are ascertained in control groups. The groups are then compared to see what exposures are different in control groups compared to cases. For example, cases of lung cancer have a higher cigarette exposure compared to control groups. The ratio of the exposures in cases to control groups is called the **ODDS ratio.** For example, if smoking is 10 times more prevalent in lung cancer cases, compared to control groups, the

odds ratio is 10. Case control studies are useful in generating hypotheses about factors that cause a disease; however, they cannot prove causation because the timing of the exposure is usually not known. Also, it is difficult in case control studies to identify proper control groups. Control groups selected from the community are generally more useful than those from hospitals.

3. *Clinical Trials.* The most sophisticated of epidemiologic methods is the clinical trial. In the clinical trial the risk factor is actively changed or manipulated in one group and left unchanged or standard care is used in a comparison or control group. The disease incidence in both groups is tracked over time, and if the study is positive, a reduction in disease incidence compared to control subjects is observed in the treated group. The clinical trial is the best method of investigation for establishing causation. Clinical trials, however, are time-consuming and expensive, so they are generally carried out on widespread diseases with important social and economic impact.

4. *Meta-analysis.* Availability of resources and size of samples often limit the ability of any individual observational study or clinical trial to answer the study question definitively. Conclusive studies generally require very large

study groups and are, therefore, very expensive. Smaller studies have much less statistical power, and frequently the outcomes of such studies indicate no evidence for benefit when a larger study would have shown benefit (Type II error).

Meta-analysis examines scientific questions by pooling results of similar studies to create a data set much larger than any single study. For each separate study the number of persons in the intervention group who develop the disease are termed the *observed* events and they are contrasted with the *expected* events, assuming treatment does nothing. Calculation of the expected outcome, therefore, is based on the combined events, disease in the intervention groups and disease in the control groups. If the intervention and treatment group are no different, it would be expected that the observed minus the expected rate would vary randomly around zero. This assumption can be tested using standard statistical tests. An example of a recent major meta-analysis is shown in Figure 6-8. The question under study is whether lowering blood pressure with drugs will prevent the occurrence of strokes and coronary heart disease. In this meta-analysis, 14 studies with similar aims and event ascertainment are pooled. Observational studies would predict that a 5 to

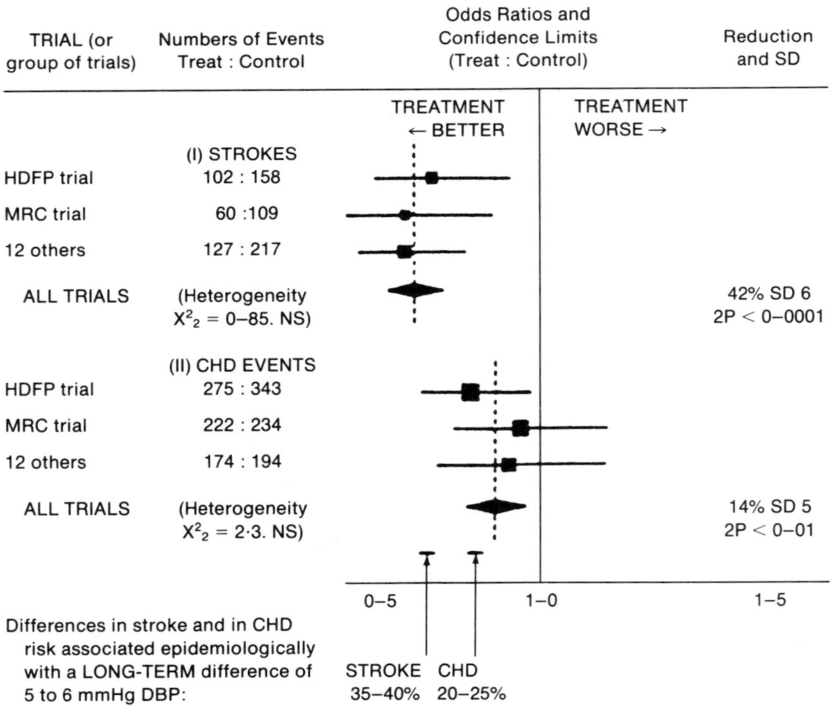

Fig. 6-8. Reduction in the odds of stroke and of CHD in the HDFP trial, the MRC trial, and in all 12 other smaller unconfounded randomized trials of antihypertensive therapy (mean DBP difference 5 to 6 mmHg for 5 years). (Collins R, Peto R, McMahon S, et al: Lancet, 1990, 335, p 833)

6 mmHg difference in diastolic pressure between treatment and control should result in a 35% to 40% reduction in stroke and a 20% to 25% reduction in coronary heart disease (CHD). The meta-analysis shown in the figure illustrates that the observed reduction in stroke from the pooled studies was 42%, close to predicted, but the reduction in CHD was only 14%, considerably less than predicted. This meta-analaysis involves pooling 14 studies with nearly 37,000 patients. Any of the studies taken individually would be far too small and lack power in observing this outcome. Meta-analysis is a powerful technique for analyzing data across studies.

Epidemiologic Reasoning

Establishing causation is an illusive but highly desirable goal in epidemiology and medicine. Once causation is established, change is often possible and the disease may be prevented. Causality is usually established using large-scale clinical trials. Causation can be inferred from epidemiologic data by applying the following criteria (see Table 6-2):

1. *Strength/Independence.* Does the suspect factor have a strong relationship to the disease and is it working directly to influence the disease, or is it merely associated with another factor that is a more direct cause? For example, it has been observed that sugar consumption and CHD are strongly related. However, it is also true that high sugar consumers have heavier fat intakes. When one examines CHD in sugar consumers who have lower fat intake, no elevation is found. Therefore, one can conclude that sugar consumption is not independently associated with CHD; rather, it reflects a surrogate measure of fat consumption, which is independently associated with CHD.

2. *Graded or Dose Response.* Is the suspect factor related to graded or dose response to the disease? In other words, if one increases the expo-

sure, does the disease risk increase? Factors not related to the disease in a graded fashion are probably not causative.

3. *Temporality.* Does the exposure *precede* the development of the disease? Only factors that precede the development of the disease are possible causes of the disease. For example, high blood cholesterol precedes the development of CHD; however, low blood cholesterol usually follows the development of cancer. In other words, high blood cholesterol causes CHD; cancer probably causes low blood cholesterol. In the former, cholesterol is the *cause* of the disease; in the latter, the *consequence* of the disease.

4. *Specificity.* Is the risk factor suspected of causing the disease specific for the disease or is it also associated with many other diseases? Again, high blood cholesterol is specific for risk of developing cardiovascular disease. Low blood cholesterol is associated not only with cancer death, but also death from stroke, cirrhosis, lung diseases, and so forth. Low blood cholesterol is nonspecific and so is probably not a cause of these diseases.

5. *Consistency.* Has the factor under examination as a cause of the disease also been found to be related to the disease in other similar studies? Factors that are consistently related to the disease across a number of studies involving different populations are more likely to be causative. Furthermore, factors that are found to be related to the disease in some studies but not others are suspect. Again, high blood cholesterol as a risk factor for heart disease has been consistently shown in many studies carried out all over the world, whereas low blood cholesterol as a cause of cancer risk has not been found in several studies.

6. *Congruence.* Are there other fields of investigation that support the relationship? For example, are there animal studies that manipulate the factor and find an association with the disease? Are there clinical studies consistent with the finding? Those factors that are congruent or "hold together" with other fields of investigation are more likely to be causative.

7. *Biologic Plausibility.* Is there a biologic mechanism known or hypothesized whereby the risk factor may cause the disease? Biologic plausibility is a powerful force in inferring causation. An example of this is HDL cholesterol. For years it was observed that a minor fraction of blood lipids, the high-density lipoprotein cho-

TABLE 6-2. Epidemiologic Factors for Inferring a Causal Relationship

Strength/Independence
Dose response
Temporality
Specificity
Consistency
Congruence
Biologic plausibility

lesterol, was *inversely* related to CHD risk. This fact was essentially ignored until a biologic mechanism was proposed whereby HDL cholesterol could act as the elimination mechanism of the body for excess cholesterol. Once this mechanism was proposed, decreased HDL cholesterol was further investigated and later accepted as a major causative factor for cardiovascular diseases.

These several criteria are useful not only in epidemiology but also in interpreting clinical studies and in clinical medicine. They provide a systematic construct to infer the likelihood of causation without conducting an expensive intervention trial.

EVALUATING DIAGNOSTIC TESTS

The physician today is faced with an almost continuous introduction of new diagnostic tests. New tests are frequently highly technical and expensive. It is important that new tests be evaluated against established tests to determine their practical value and cost-effectiveness.

A frequent approach to this evaluation is to establish the sensitivity and specificity of the new test against the established or "gold standard" test. The "gold standard" is currently the best test used to establish the presence of the disease.

Two kinds of errors are commonly made when a new test is conducted. If a test is negative when done on a patient known to have the disease, it is called a *false-negative.* If a test is positive and the patient does not have the disease, this is referred to as a *false-positive.* A test that is positive on patients with the disease is a *true-positive,* and a negative test in a person free of the disease is a *true-negative.* These values are used to determine the sensitivity and specificity of a test. *Sensitivity* is defined as the proportion of positive tests in patients who have the

disease or:

$$\frac{\text{True-Positives}}{\text{True-Positives} + \text{False-Negatives}}$$

Specificity is defined as the proportion of correct assessments in persons without the disease or:

$$\frac{\text{True-Negatives}}{\text{True-Negatives} + \text{False-Positives}}$$

The *predictive value* of a test is the percentage of true positives of all the positives:

$$\frac{\text{True-Positives}}{\text{True-Positives} + \text{False-Positives}}$$

A theoretical example is provided in Figure 6-9, which shows congestive heart failure (CHF) and the test cardiomegaly with a cardiothoracic ratio of ≥ 0.5 on standard chest x ray. Note in the example that the predictive value of the test is moderate (72%) because this test has a large number of false-positives associated with it.

Some diagnostic tests can detect the presence of disease long before the patient becomes clincally ill (*e.g.,* positive HIV test versus AIDS). Frequently, it is beneficial to detect disease early, especially if treatments are available that will cure the disease (*e.g.,* mammography and breast cancer). Such tests are frequently used to screen the population to detect early disease. It is very important with screening tests to establish the sensitivity, specificity, and predictive value of the test.

MEDICAL STATISTICS

The word *statistics* conjures all kinds of negative images and seems to be a concept remote from the diagnosis and treatment of patients. Most of us were exposed in the first year or two of medical school to an obligatory statistics or public health course in one

Fig. 6-9. Diagnostic sensitivity and specificity for diagnosing congestive heart failure (CHF) by chest x ray.

	PATIENTS WITHOUT CHF	PATIENTS WITH CHF
NEGATIVE TEST Normal X-ray	True Negative (TN) 1033	False Negative (FN) 50
POSITIVE TEST (increased cardio-thoracic ratio)	False Positive (FP) 104	True Positive (TP) 273

$$\text{Sensitivity} = \frac{\text{TP}}{\text{TP} + \text{FN}} = \frac{273}{273 + 50} = .85$$

$$\text{Specificity} = \frac{\text{TN}}{\text{TN} + \text{FP}} = \frac{1033}{1033 + 104} = .91$$

$$\text{Predictive Value} = \frac{\text{TP}}{\text{TP} + \text{FP}} = \frac{273}{273 + 104} = 72\%$$

of a variety of formats in some of the least appreciated of all medical school courses. The material seems remote from patient care, the "real" mission of medical school. Only later, during internship and residency when we find ourselves late at night in the hospital library, desperately trying to interpret the relevant studies that deal with critically important clinical decisions about treatment, can biostatistics be appreciated. This section presents basic concepts on medical statistics that all physicians should know.

Physicians who care for patients are constantly stating hypotheses and forming opinions on diagnosis and treatments based at least in part on clinical experience. Relying only on clinical experience to make such decisions is extremely hazardous because of its inevitable bias and random associations. Clinical research is essential to guiding treatment decisions, and medical statistics is the primary tool for separating what is a real difference from random variation.

BIOLOGIC VARIABILITY

Biologic measures (variables) in medicine are not set at specific levels, rather they change constantly, moving up or down around an average or mean. This is true of blood pressure, pulse, temperature, or any biologic measure. Fortunately, the distance in which this movement occurs is measurable and predictable according to the standard deviation. Understanding this inherent variability of biologic measures is the crux of biostatistics.

TESTING HYPOTHESES

Stating a hypothesis is an important first step in beginning a scientific investigation. Theoretically, hypotheses are stated in the null form, which holds that the treatment is the same as a placebo or an alternate treatment. In practice, however, hypotheses are thought of as stating that a new treatment is better or worse than a placebo or an established therapy. Clearly stating the hypothesis to be tested is a crucial step, which will later determine the study design and approaches to analyses.

Two types of errors can be made in testing the hypothesis. One error is that when the study is finished, one will observe a difference between treatments when a difference really does not exist. This is called a *type I,* or *alpha, error.* Type I errors may be due to study bias or to random variation in the data. To ensure that this error does not occur, the random variation in the data and alpha level is set in designing the trial. Generally alphas are set at 0.05,

which means that with the size sample in the study group, one would expect to see a significant difference by chance in only one of 20 similar experiments (5%). This alpha value corresponds to the "p values" considered statistically significant (usually at a $p < .05$ value). This means that the difference between treatments will be accepted as statistically significant only when the chance of biologic variation indicating a false-positive result is very low ($<5\%$).

The *type II error,* though little known or appreciated, is also important. A type II error is the error of stating that two treatments are identical when a true difference actually exists. Type II errors are also called *beta (β) errors.* Beta errors in designing the study are usually set at 0.90 or 0.80. This means that when the study outcome shows no difference, 90% of the time this will truly indicate no difference. The *power* of a study is related most significantly to the type II error; power is the likelihood that no type II error exists. The power of a study is highly related to the sample size of study; the larger the sample size, the greater the power. Power is also related to the precision with which the crucial variable can be studied and to the size of the treatment effect. The larger the treatment effect and the more precise the measures, the greater the power. Medical literature is filled with small studies that report no effect of certain treatments but that have little power because of the presence of type II error. Larger sample size studies carried out later frequently show an effect to be present. Insufficient power is a major problem in clinical studies. However, specific statistical tests have been developed that test whether treatments are different, and tests are available to examine differences in average or mean change and also for categorical variables.

REGRESSION TO THE MEAN

All factors measured in biology and medicine change constantly, moving up or down around an average value. Thus, we take frequent measures of blood pressure, where several measures over time vary, and cholesterol, which varies less and need not be measured as often. Individuals experience this variability, as do study groups and even whole populations. We have already discussed how this variability influences inferences in clinical trial results. It also influences how one interprets individual patient responses. An important statistical and clinical phenomenon that results from this pattern of variability is called *regression to the mean.* Regression to the mean is defined as the tendency for measures that are initially taken from persons selected above or below the mean of the group to become more like the mean on subsequent measures. For example, we can take a hypertensive group defined as ≥90 mmHg selected from a group or population with a mean or average blood pressure of 75 mmHg. On repeat measurement of this group of hypertensives, all or almost all of them will be *lower* than they were on the first measurement. They will have regressed toward the population mean. This phenomenon, which may at first seem like an esoteric statistical concept, has great practical clinical significance as well as significance for interpreting the results of studies. Frequently, apparently favorable changes in studies that are credited to specific treatments are actually attributable to regression to the mean. Clinically, the concept is also useful. For example, it may explain the phenomenon of "white coat hypertension," the observation that some hypertensives' blood pressures are higher in the doctor's office. Regression to the mean is the tendency for abnormal laboratory values to be normal on repeat measurements.

Regression to the mean can be minimized or eliminated by doing multiple measures over time and averaging those measures to arrive at the values used for purposes of record, either clinical management or scientific study. Figure 6-10 shows the relationship of repeated measures of cholesterol and the tendency for regression to the mean as well as showing how the approximate additional measures better the true value. It is an important concept to be aware of since it will always operate if cutpoints are set as they commonly are in clinical management and clinical studies.

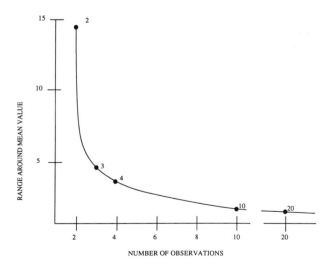

Fig. 6-10. Effect of repeated observations on precision of measurement.

ADMINISTRATION OF HEALTH SERVICES

Good administration of public health services should ensure that individuals needing health care will receive it promptly and effectively, using measures that are readily accepted and understood by consumers. The nature of public health programs has changed markedly over the years. The earliest efforts were to prevent the introduction and the spread of infection by quarantine of ships or infected communities and isolation of infectious cases. As knowledge grew concerning infectious disease, the control of water supplies, milk, and many other foods was found to be necessary. Control of the disposal of human, household, and industrial wastes also was found to improve the health of the people, as did improvements in housing.

In some parts of the world, government became involved in control or eradication of disease carriers, such as certain species of insects. Particularly in the United States and Western Europe, social reforms have taken place in which public health has been an important issue. Governments have become greatly interested in maternal and child welfare, in aid to the physically handicapped, and in special disease problems such as tuberculosis, venereal disease, cancer, cardiovascular disease, and mental illness. Indeed, rehabilitation, the early detection of chronic illness, and the assurance of continuity of medical care are becoming touchstones of modern public health. The rising cost and better distribution and financing of personal health services have also become leading concerns of the U.S. government in the 1980s and 1990s.

Whereas previously the emphasis of public health administration was on the establishment of basic public health services, now there is equal emphasis on the better use of existing services and the development and evaluation of new programs. In theory, new developments in public health should reduce the need for individual action (such as regular visits to the dentist) and motivate larger numbers of individuals to participate in voluntary programs. These developments have changed materially the character of government organization for the protection of the public health. The impersonal mass approach through environmental controls is being complemented by the financing of personal health services and by controlling the rising cost of health care.

Federal Health Services in the United States

The political structure and beliefs of the United States have guided the historical development of its public health services. A national government formed by a federation of the member states possesses only those powers delegated to it by the sovereign states. Article I of the Constitution of the United States provides for the federal government interest in the general welfare and gave some basis in authority for the development of national health services. The Constitution also delegated power to the federal government specifically for interstate and foreign quarantine.

In 1980, Congress created the Department of Health and Human Services (HHS), combining some of the federal agencies involved in health care services and regulation. Many health activities remain in other departments of the national government such as the extensive health efforts of the Veterans Administration, the armed forces, the Occupational Safety and Health Administration (OSHA), and the Environmental Protection Agency (EPA).

UNITED STATES PUBLIC HEALTH SERVICE

The Public Health Service is one of the principal federal agencies concerned with public health. Originally formed to provide health care to sailors in the merchant marine, its functions now include interstate and international quarantine, research and demonstration programs, advice on technical matters, and the loan of personnel to other agencies with health services. A significant impact on health services is made through financial support to state and local health agencies for the expansion and improvement of their programs.

HEALTH CARE FINANCING ADMINISTRATION

Established in 1977, the Health Care Financing Administration is the federal agency responsible for Medicaid and Medicare, both launched in 1966. It also guides the activities of PROs, which monitor length of stay and quality of hospital care through peer review efforts. Medicaid and Medicare now form about two thirds of the total federal budget on health.

STATE AND LOCAL HEALTH ORGANIZATIONS

The state government is the sovereign power in the United States. In theory, the national and local governments possess only those powers delegated to them by the states. In practice, however, financial strength has given the federal government more influence in the development of state and local health programs than might otherwise have occurred.

Health laws differ greatly among the 50 states. Some have extensive, detailed health legislation; in others, only broad principles are laid down, and special laws are enacted as urgent needs are recognized. All states make some provision for a board of health or a comparable body with advisory and legislative functions.

In most states, the state health officer is a physician appointed by the governor with the advice of the state board of health. The state health officer's qualifications, duties, and compensation are usually specified by law. In the early years of the state health departments, control of communicable disease was the first objective, followed by environmental sanitation, dealing with water supply, and the safe disposal of wastes. In recent years some states have created environmental protection agencies that have taken over most environmental services. They correspond to the EPA and to the OSHA on the national level.

Other responsibilities of state health departments are maternal and child health services, the recording of health statistics, medical and hospital care for special groups, and certain long-term care and rehabilitation services. Most state health departments have a division of local health services to provide grants-in-aid to local communities and to advise local health departments. Most local health services are maintained by cities or counties, while the state delegates authority and often provides funds to the local community for developing the program. Local health departments give direct services, such as water purification and the supervision of sewage disposal, and a wide range of clinical services. Sparsely populated areas have only limited public health services, and in a few states the state health department directly provides local health services to its residents.

VOLUNTARY HEALTH AGENCIES

A voluntary health agency is formed by a group, the members of which wish to pursue a common interest; membership is voluntary, and the agency is independent of the state. Although the United States is reputed to be a nation of joiners, probably less than 20% of its population participate actively in its 100,000 voluntary health agencies. Such associations have become more common as society has grown more complex and activities more numerous. In situations of rapid social change, voluntary associations are considered to be important as a means of achieving new goals, raising new funds, or providing new labor.

Ideally, the voluntary health agency is more sensitive than the government to the changing needs of society; many agencies have initiated health programs that were later assumed by government. In recent years, however, as many voluntary agencies have become more stable and conservative, government agencies have become increasingly innovative. As the vitality of voluntary health agencies has decreased, public resistance has risen against giving funds for health activities over and above the taxes paid to government. It is now accepted policy to have voluntary associations carry out public functions, such as payment for medical and hospital care and professional licensure; thus, some voluntary agencies, such as Blue Cross/Blue Shield, receive increasing support from government funds.

Voluntary health agencies take many forms. First, there are the large group of agencies that focus on specific diseases (*e.g.,* American Cancer Society) or specific organs (*e.g.,* American Heart Association), or on specific populations or techniques (*e.g.,* Planned Parenthood). These agencies concentrate more on health education and less on service. More service-oriented are agencies such as hospitals, group practice clinics and HMOs, and visiting nurse associations. HMOs are medical groups that contract with an enrolled population to provide complete health services, preventive and curative, inpatient and outpatient, in return for an annual payment per enrollee. A third group includes the funding associations, such as the Robert Wood Johnson or Kellogg foundation, which distribute funds to nonprofit groups for service, research, and educational activities. Planning and coordinating associations, such as community councils, form a fourth group of voluntary agencies. A fifth and influential group is composed of the professional associations, such as the American Medical Association, which are concerned with setting standards for and licensing the profession, and with public and professional education and legislation related to the beliefs and activities of the profession. State and local medical societies also guide most PROs, even though federal funds support their reviews of hospital care. Last but not least, some academic institutions may be included that are concerned with the research and teaching of health professionals.

Voluntary health associations can help stimulate social change and mediate between population groups and government. They help communities set priorities in health and influence the decisions of local government. They create interest and consensus among their members but also induce stresses between one organization and another. If this conflict results in improved health services for a reasonable expenditure of funds, the results will be helpful to society. However, the way one views voluntarism must be based on intuition, social values, and personal opinion rather than on scientific findings since to date no conclusive research exists to settle the question.

HIGH-PRIORITY AREAS OF PROBLEM AND TREATMENT

Prevention and treatment are not mutually exclusive activities, although a number of health services tend to approach them in that fashion. Today, part of the effort to control rising costs of treatment involves raising the priority of preventive services. In contrast to the brief preventive measures such as immunizations, much prevention in the future will be long term, continuous, and aimed at improving the individual's knowledge about disease and health-related behavior patterns. The following sections cover what will be high-priority areas of prevention in the coming years.

Hypertension

One of the most prevalent of all cardiovascular risk factors, hypertension affects about one fourth of the U.S. adult population, more than 65 million people. It is a major risk factor for stroke and coronary heart disease, heart failure, and renal disease. The prevalence of hypertension rises with age and is higher in the black and elderly populations. Diastolic blood pressure increases with age until the mid-50s and systolic blood pressure continues to increase with age during the entire aging process. The result is that older people have much more isolated systolic hypertension. It is now well established that drug treatment of isolated systolic hypertension is highly effective in preventing total stroke and CHD and cardiovascular disease (CVD) (Fig. 6-11). Systolic blood pressure is more and more a concern in all hypertensives regardless of age and is the driving force causing risk. New guidelines suggest active lowering of systolic pressure in older as well as younger hypertensives.

Blood pressure is continuously related to CVD risk. Hypertension, or high blood pressure, is arbitrarily defined as ≥ 140 or ≥ 90 mmHg systolic and diastolic. This level classifies approximately one in four adults for special attention. Although the etiology of hypertension is recognized to be multifactorial, involving a complex interplay of genetic

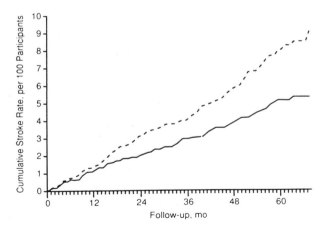

Fig. 6-11. Cumulative fatal plus nonfatal stroke rate per 100 participants in the active treatment (solid line) and placebo (broken line) groups during the Systolic Hypertension in the Elderly Program. (SHEP: JAMA, 1991, 265, pp 3255–3264. Copyright 1991, American Medical Association.)

susceptibility and environmental and hormonal factors, certain risk factors have been clearly established. These risk factors are obesity, dietary sodium intake, alcohol intake, and physical activity. Treatment of high blood pressure should initially involve nondrug therapy to achieve weight loss, sodium and alcohol reduction, and increased physical activity. Treatment in many patients also involves using active drug therapy selected from many classes of agents currently available. Thiazide diuretics have been especially impressive in preventing stroke but have been somewhat disappointing in preventing CHD. Other major classes of drugs include beta blockers, calcium channel blockers, alpha blockers, and angiotensin-converting enzyme inhibitors. More and more therapy is tailored to fit individual risk factor profiles of the hypertensive patient since the presence of other risk factors in the hypertensive, such as hyperlipidemia, cigarette smoking, and diabetes mellitus, greatly add to the risk. In the last 15 years, age-adjusted death rates from stroke and CHD have fallen dramatically in the United States; this remarkable result is no doubt due in part to the much improved identification and treatment of patients with high blood pressure.

Acquired Immunodeficiency Syndrome (AIDS)

The first AIDS cases were diagnosed in the United States in the early 1980s. Reported cases were primarily found in male homosexuals, IV drug users, blood transfusion patients, and hemophiliacs, and the transmission pattern suggested an infectious etiology. In 1984, the human immunodeficiency virus (HIV) was isolated and established as the agent of transmission. Screening tests for AIDS antibodies were developed to assist the identification of asymptomatic carriers. The HIV virus is a retro virus that has a long incubation period of several years. The virus severely impairs the immune system and creates susceptibility to a variety of infections. Major concomitant diseases are *Pneumocystis carinii* and Kaposi's sarcoma. In 1990, it was estimated that 1 to 2 million Americans were infected with the AIDS virus, and AIDS cases have steadily increased each year (Fig. 6-12). The virus has been isolated from all body fluids, including blood, semen, saliva, tears, urine, breast milk, and cerebrospinal fluid. Major routes of transmission are (1) sexual contact, (2) IV drug use, (3) blood transfusions, and (4) perinatal contact of a fetus with an infected mother. In 1990, 135,000 cases of full-blown AIDS had been reported. Of the reported cases, 66% are male homosexuals, 18% IV drug users, 7% male homosexuals and IV drug users, 1% hemophiliacs, 2% recipients of transfusions, 2% heterosexual, and 3% unknown. Heterosexual transmission is a small percentage of the total incidence, but it is increasing at the fastest rate.

AIDS patients are high utilizers of health care. Hospital admissions are usually for opportunistic infectious diseases. Already in many large U.S. cities, AIDS is the number-one cause of death in men ages 25 to 44. The AIDS epidemic is much worse in many developing countries, especially those in Central and East Africa.

The most common modes of transmission for AIDS are semen and blood, and a widespread AIDS

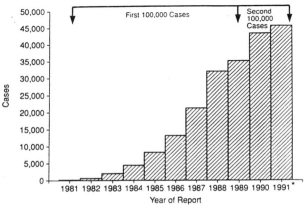

Fig. 6-12. AIDS cases, by year of report—United States, 1981 to 1991. (MMWR, 1992, 41, p 28)

education program aimed at promoting "safe sex" is under way. This program aims at persuading people to avoid high-risk sexual behaviors such as anal sex and promiscuity, and encourages the use of condoms. Treatments for clinical AIDS have been limited, but AZT has been shown to be effective in palliative treatment and also in prolonging remissions in AIDS patients. Other promising agents have been developed, which are currently being evaluated against AZT. It is hoped that immunizations can be developed against AIDS, but such a vaccine is probably years away from being a reality. In 1991, health education and prevention are the best hope to stem the spread of the AIDS virus.

Family Planning

Family planning is based on the voluntary decisions and actions of individuals who wish to reduce unintended fertility or to correct infertility. This effort may or may not be compatible with national population policy, but it helps individuals and couples decide for themselves about reproduction. In recent decades in the United States, patterns have changed, and many women are waiting until their 30s and 40s to begin families. In addition, more single women are having children. Family size has fallen as employed women have fewer children, and the total fertility rate is declining.

Contraceptive practices have also changed. Sterilization has become more common among married women. The pill remains popular with unmarried women, and the use of condoms by unmarried men is rising. Teenagers continue to exhibit high rates of unintended pregnancy, high abortion rates, and low use of contraceptive methods. Teenage pregnancies are associated with increased risks of maternal morbidity and mortality, with high rates of serious neurologic impairment in infants, and with an increased proportion of low-birth-weight infants. Moreover, unwanted pregnancies impose psychological and social costs that may be lifelong. Thus, sexually active teenagers remain an important target group for family planning services.

On the other hand, millions of couples are infertile, unable or unlikely to have children. One fourth of these couples are childless. Proportionately more black than white couples are infertile. Since the technology for improving fertility is less advanced and less available than that for contraception, the possibility of success of organized efforts to lessen infertility seems less likely. Most infertility visits are to private medical sources in the United States, and proportionately fewer blacks and other minorities

have access to and use of these sources. Unfortunately, in recent years policy debates have focused on the ethics and financing of abortion and less on family planning.

Pregnancy and Infant Health

Since 1960, maternal and infant death rates have fallen steadily in the United States. The rate of fall was 5% to 6% per year in the 1970s but less than 3% per year in the 1980s. Black and unmarried mothers account for a proportionately high percentage of low-birth-weight-infants, who sustain higher-than-average infant mortality rates despite costly improvements in neonatal intensive care. Black infant mortality rates remain at nearly double that of white infants (Table 6-3). A recent development that impairs access to quality care for all patients is the tendency of physicians and hospitals to withdraw from high-risk obstetrical care for marketplace and malpractice reasons.

The success of programs for pregnancy and infant health depends partly on other health programs, such as programs for environmental control, nutrition, and communicable disease. Mortality and morbidity rates range markedly between different population groups and geographic regions. Cigarette smoking during pregnancy is associated with birth weights that are 150 g to 200 g lower than average. Maternal drinking is one of the most common causes of mental retardation. Untreated diabetes in mothers is a potent risk factor for congenital anomalies in infants. Congenital anomalies, the highest cause of infant death, seem equally common in black and white infants (Table 6-4). Most other causes of infant death, such as the respiratory distress syndrome and infections, are more common in blacks. Most deliveries now take place in a hospital, where the newborns are also screened for the early detection of phenylketonuria (PKU) and hypothyroidism.

Breast feeding has been shown to prevent both malnutrition and obesity in infants. Moreover, it may provide the infant short-term immunity from

TABLE 6-3. Infant Mortality Rates by Race, Specified Years (Deaths Age 0–1 Year/1,000 Live Births)

YEAR	WHITE	BLACK	BLACK/WHITE RATIO
1950	26.8	43.9	1.64
1960	22.9	44.3	1.93
1970	17.8	32.6	1.83
1980	11.0	21.4	1.95
1983	9.7	19.2	1.98

TABLE 6-4. Top Ten Causes of Infant Mortality, by Race, United States, 1983 (Deaths/100,000 Live Births)

RANK	CAUSE	ALL	RACE BLACK	WHITE
1	Congenital anomalies	240.0	246.2	241.9
2	Sudden infant death syndrome	145.8	259.0	124.4
3	Respiratory distress syndrome	101.2	159.4	92.1
4	Disorders related to short gestation and low birth weight	91.6	228.3	66.5
5	Maternal complication	39.9	73.7	34.4
6	Intrauterine hypoxia and birth asphyxia	32.9	56.0	29.1
7	Accidents and adverse effects	26.3	45.6	23.0
8	Infections specific to the perinatal period	23.9	36.7	21.7
9	Newborn affected by complications of placenta, cord, and membranes	23.9	16.9	11.6
10	Pneumonia and influenza	21.1	47.6	16.0

some infectious diseases. Breast feeding more than doubled to 53% by 1980, rising more swiftly in white mothers than black mothers. On the more technical side, diagnostic ultrasound has become more frequent in obstetrics, and electronic fetal monitoring is used on half or more mothers in labor. Rates of cesarean section deliveries have been rising. It is unclear how much of these high-tech and surgical approaches are medically indicated and how much are carried out because of malpractice and economic reasons.

High-quality and readily accessible prenatal care can decrease the risk of low birth weight and other complications. The preventive services recommended in prenatal care are summarized in Table 6-5; they include screening tests for the early detection of Down's syndrome and open neural tube defects before the 20th week. For the normal infant, services advised are shown in Table 6-6, with related services discussed under Immunization.

Genetic Screening

Screening is a systematic process that separates those who probably have abnormalities from those who probably do not. Through early detection, screening may lead to prompt treatment before advanced damage has occurred. More recently, genetic screening has evolved as a systematic search for persons of certain genotypes to detect those at risk for genetically transmitted diseases.

Fetal screening and prenatal diagnosis are usually performed by analyzing fetal cells present in amniotic fluid obtained by amniocentesis. The most common indication for amniocentesis is a maternal age of 36 or older, in which case Down's syndrome is the most common abnormality found in the fetus. Less common is a neural tube defect, usually accompanied by elevated serum alpha fetoproteins.

The overriding issue in prenatal diagnosis is the controversy over abortion, which is the sole method of preventing the birth of an impaired child. Inadequate access to and insufficient understanding of amniocentesis cause lower-income populations to be underserved by the recently developed technology.

Newborn screening focused largely on inborn errors of metabolism identifies serious genetic disease at birth. PKU screening is mandatory in most states, since the low phenylalanine diet prevents serious mental impairment when begun in the first weeks of life. Testing for hypothyroidism has also become a frequent newborn screening test.

Screening of adults is also more often considered now in order to identify individuals who are heterozygous for a gene for a serious recessive disease and who may therefore produce impaired offspring. Tay-Sachs disease and sickle-cell trait have been the disorders most often considered for large-scale carrier screening. Few other diseases are common enough to justify widespread programs to screen for carriers.

The challenge to society in genetic screening has been to provide good genetic counseling and follow-up to all who may benefit. In addition, debates continue on the best ways to ensure confidentiality of finding, freedom of choice about treatment, and how to avoid misunderstanding and stigmatization of those with positive tests.

Surveillance and Control of Infectious Diseases

In the early 1900s, programs of communicable disease control relied on isolation and quarantine. The discovery that many new cases result from contact with asymptomatic carriers of the organism greatly reduced confidence in such methods. The new control measures have resulted from better knowledge

TABLE 6-5. Preventive Services for the Pregnant Woman and Fetus

SERVICES		INITIAL VISIT*	SUBSEQUENT VISITS†
History	General medical	●	
	Family and genetic	●	
	Previous pregnancies	●	
	Current pregnancy	●	●
Physical examination	General	●	
	Blood pressure	●	●
	Height and weight	●	●
	Fetal development		●
Laboratory examinations	VDRL	●	
	Papanicolau smear	●	
	Hemoglobin/hematocrit	●	
	Urinalysis for sugar and protein	●	●
	Rh determination	●	
	Blood group determination	●	
	Rubella HAI titer	●	
	Amniocentesis (for women over 35)‡		
Counseling with referrals as necessary and desired	Nutrition during pregnancy	●	●
	Nutrition of infant, including breast feeding	●	●
	Cigarette smoking	●	●
	Use of alcohol, other drugs during pregnancy	●	●
	Sexual intercourse during pregnancy	●	●
	Signs of abnormal pregnancy	●	●
	Labor and delivery (including where the mother plans to deliver)	●	●
	Physical activity and exercise	●	●
	Provisions for care of infant	●	●
	In response to patient concerns	●	●

Labor and delivery§

Postpartum visit (including family planning counseling and referral, if desired)

* Initial visit should occur early in the first trimester.

† Subsequent visits should occur once a month through the 28th week of pregnancy; twice a month from the 29th through the 36th week; and once a week thereafter.

‡ If desired, amniocentesis should be performed at about the 16th week for women who are over 35 or who have specific genetic indications.

§ Although not a "preventive" service, labor and delivery should be included in a package of pregnancy-related services.

of the sources and modes of transmission of disease and from improved methods of treatment. However, the evolution of new pathogens and the development of resistance in existing pathogens continue to challenge our control measures.

Infections continue to plague the Third World countries. Each infectious disease is now reported for individual illnesses or organisms. The total reported cases of infectious disease are invariably fewer than the true incidence due to underreporting. Infectious diseases are a common cause of visits to physicians' offices and for absences from work and from school. Moreover, nosocomial infections, acquired in patient care facilities, affect millions of persons each year in the United States.

The spread of an infection rises directly with the number of existing cases, the number of susceptible persons, and a *transmission parameter*. The latter rises with ease of transmission and relates to season, probability of contracting the infection, duration of infectivity, and frequency of subclinical infection. If a single case introduced into a real-life population causes no new infections, no epidemic will occur. In most developed countries, for example, cases of measles stop reproducing when 94% of the population has become immune. Producing this level of immunity is regarded as feasible in the United States and Canada, where national elimination of measles is the officially adopted objective for measles control efforts.

A significant infectious disease problem in the 1990s has been the reemergence of high-risk diseases such as drug-resistant tuberculosis. This phenomenon is mostly due to the increased number of

TABLE 6-6. Preventive Services for the Normal Infant

	SERVICES	BIRTH VISIT	SECOND VISIT*	SUBSEQUENT VISITS†
History and physical examination	Length and weight	●	●	●
	Head circumference	●		
	Urine stream	●		
	Check for congenital abnormalities	●		●
	Developmental assessment			●
Procedures	PKU screening test		●	
	Thyroxin T_4		●	
	Vitamin K		●	
	Silver nitrate prophylaxis	●		
Immunizations	Diphtheria			●
	Pertussis			●
	Tetanus			●
	Measles‡			
	Mumps‡			
	Rubella‡			
	Poliomyelitis			●
Parental counseling, with referrals as necessary and desired	Infant nutrition and feeding practices (especially breast feeding)		●	●
	Parenting		●	●
	Infant hygiene		●	●
	Accidental injury prevention (including use of automobile restraints)		●	●
	Family planning and referral for services		●	●
	Child care arrangements		●	●
	Medical care arrangements		●	●
	Parental smoking, use of alcohol, and drugs		●	●
	Parental nutrition, physical activity, and exercise		●	●
	In response to parental concerns		●	●

* Second visit should occur within 10 days or before leaving the hospital.
† Four health visits the rest of first year or enough to provide immunizations.
‡ Measles, mumps, and rubella immunizations occur at 15 months.

persons immunologically compromised because of AIDS. The challenge of this decade will be to develop new drugs and techniques for dealing with these diseases.

Immunization

During the past three decades, vaccination programs have facilitated declines of 98% or more in the incidence of measles, mumps, rubella, diphtheria, and polio. An intense worldwide vaccination program resulted in the global eradication of smallpox. It is estimated that measles will soon be eliminated as an indigenous disease in the continental United States.

As preventable infections become less frequent, the rare adverse effects of immunization have been increasingly publicized. A major source of this adverse publicity was an increased risk of Guillain-Barré syndrome caused by the influenza vaccine given in 1976; the vaccines of subsequent years have not resulted in similar risks, but the public reaction has not subsided entirely. The risk of lawsuits for compensation of those injured by immunization have hampered these preventive services and considerably raised the price of the vaccines. Thus, a maintenance system is needed to deliver routine immunization services without financial barriers in all health care settings. Medicare and Medicaid have agreed to cover the cost of influenza and pneumonia vaccines to older patients so long as the health care providers and institutions do not charge for them.

Education and information tend to be more acceptable to the public and less controversial than governmental legislation and regulation. Thus, we continue to debate how strongly we should enforce existing school immunization programs that have created immunization levels for most areas of the United States to levels that are the envy of other developed countries. Lowered levels of immunization in the United Kingdom, despite its national health service, relate partly to the greater reluctance among the British to use legal measures to get them done. In recent years, the frequency of tetanus has moved markedly into older age groups. Case fatality ratios for tetanus are greater than 50% in persons older than 60 years; about half of all persons at these ages lack the protective antibody against tetanus toxin. Since many patients have not received a primary series of either tetanus or diphtheria toxoids, all adults should complete a series with the combined vaccine. Booster doses are then given every 10 years.

Influenza can infect the elderly as well as younger persons with chronic cardiopulmonary disability, often resulting in hospitalization and complications. Antibody to the virus antigens reduces attack rates and the severity of infection. Because of the frequent change in the antigens, however, the most recent vaccine must be used, usually available in the fall. In 1987, only about 20% of the high-risk population had been immunized, creating continued annual health problems for the American population.

During an epidemic of influenza type A, amantadine helps kill the virus in individuals who have not received influenza vaccine. Amantadine is highly effective in preventing influenza type A in nonimmunized persons, but side effects such as insomnia, dizziness, and personality changes may occur.

Sexually Transmitted Diseases

The primary targets of prevention programs for sexually transmitted diseases (STDs) used to be gonorrhea and syphilis. The spectrum expanded in the 1970s to include trichomoniasis, genital herpes, hepatitis, genital warts, and others. An addition in the 1980s, acquired immunodeficiency syndrome (AIDS), was reviewed above.

Identification and surveillance of STDs have been particularly difficult because of high carrier rates in asymptomatic persons. Moreover, diagnostic tests are expensive, and the national reporting systems have been weak. Women and children bear an inordinate share of STD complication: pelvic inflammatory disease, sterility, ectopic pregnancy, infant pneumonia, fetal and infant deaths, and mental retardation. Like other infections, STDs dispropor-

tionately affect the poor. Stronger financial support and adequate specialized clinics and programs are required to control and prevent these diseases.

More sustained and effective health education programs must aim at high-risk groups. Legislation that decreased classroom education in STDs caused a rise in teenage venereal disease; when the legislation was rescinded, the disease trends reversed. In the most common of all STDs in the United States, trichomoniasis caused by *Chlamydia trachomatis,* the high cost and difficulty of detection has resulted in recommending the treatment of presumptive cases despite the lack of confirmation of diagnosis; 70% of such cases have no symptom. Condoms, when properly used during sexual activity, are the best-known measure to avoid acquiring or transmitting many of the STDs.

Occupational Health

Occupational health is concerned with all factors that influence the health and productivity of working people. A wide variety of occupational hazards pose significant risks to health. Within the federal government, the National Institute for Occupational Safety and Health (NIOSH) estimates that 10 million persons are injured, 3 million severely, while at work each year. About 70,000 injuries result in permanent impairment. Of nontraumatic illness, skin diseases account for the highest proportion of occupational illness.

In recent years, hospitals and medical groups have begun to deliver occupational health programs to smaller industries. More physicians have become better trained in the diagnosis and treatment of occupational illness. These steps have been motivated as much by the need to improve revenue of delivery programs as to improve occupational health in society.

Occupational health physicians and labor unions have been particularly active in prevention and treatment of diseases that arise either in the course of employment or as a result of work. However, in the last decade employers have also become interested in workplace health promotion programs. When health care costs begin to encroach on profits, employers become more interested in self-help and self-care programs for employees. Growth of the for-profit health care sector, with its continuing need to contain costs, is also changing the way of providing health programs and facilities at the workplace.

Both governmental and private health programs at the work site are likely to emphasize prevention and improved health, morale, and job satisfaction. These programs also attempt to promote safety and control accidents, and to reduce risks to health such as smoking, hypertension, poor nutrition, and occupational stress. When effective, these programs should improve health and productivity and control health care costs. However, scientific studies are scarce that confirm that the benefits of work-site health promotion activities outweigh the costs. Positive studies will enhance even more employers' adoption of health promotion programs.

Within the federal government, NIOSH conducts research and recommends standards for toxic substances used in industry; implementing that information, OSHA promulgates standards and inspects industries to ensure compliance. Recently, OSHA has tried to streamline its efforts, eliminating many factors that weaken occupational safety and health programs. State and local systems for recognizing and preventing occupational health and safety hazards must also be developed and improved.

Toxic Agents and Radiation

For decades concern has grown over the condition of the environment and its effect on health and quality of life. In 1970, the federal EPA was created and began to set national air, water, and other pollution standards. In 1976, the Toxic Substances Control Act identified the need to control the risk of exposure to 65,000 commercial chemicals, about which we have good information on health hazards for only 2%. In 1980, a federal act known as Superfund recognized the need to clean up thousands of hazardous waste sites in America. To date only a fraction of these sites have been cleaned up.

Low-level ionizing radiation occurs naturally and also comes from medical x rays. Much higher doses of radiation are known to be carcinogenic, mutagenic, and teratogenic. Most Americans are exposed to 200 mrem or less of ionizing radiation per year. In the 1980s a naturally occurring radioactive gas called *radon* has been recognized as potentially dangerous to health.

The regulatory agencies, EPA and OSHA, need to hire better-trained professionals to enforce the many laws that control the use and disposal of hazardous substances in the environment. Moreover, we may have to withhold new chemicals from use until industry can demonstrate safety. Unfortunately, epidemiologic studies of human populations can demonstrate harm, but they rarely arrive at precise dose–response relationships. The permissible exposure levels must reflect real-life multiple exposures, the history of previous exposure, individual susceptibilities, and the changing effects with increasing age. Safety standards must, therefore, be negotiated between interest groups.

Pharmaceutical and biologic hazards also deserve full attention. We have yet to resolve the conflicting social goals of increased consumption, industrial expansion, and adequate health protection in the United States. Because the balance is complex, we cannot depend on mechanistic decision making using simple cost-benefit analysis. Unfortunately, the political stresses involved in the public environment debates discourage all but the most insensitive and the most dedicated professionals from becoming involved.

Accident Prevention and Injury Control

In the United States, accidents rank fourth as a cause of death; they lead in causing death up to the age of 44 years. Motor vehicle accidents cause about half of all accidental deaths. Among the elderly, where accidents cause a proportionately lower incidence of death and disability, the combination of osteoporosis with falls has raised interest in the prevention of hip fractures.

Among those dying in motor vehicle accidents, about half involve the use of alcohol by one or both the drivers. Accident patients treated in hospital emergency rooms also include significant numbers with alcohol detected in their blood, including more than half of those injured in fights or assaults. Of course, many accidents do not result in death. Injury without death is one of the leading causes of visits to physicians' offices. Personal and social maladjustment are common among accident repeaters. Thus, it becomes clear the host factors such as alcohol abuse are important in determining the incidence of accidents.

Technologic changes such as improved automobile design, and passive measures such as window guards for apartment buildings have been most effective in preventing injuries. Regulatory measures such as building codes, fire codes, reduced highway speed limits, and the reduced availability of handguns through licensing have also been effective. Economic incentives are also a potentially strong source of improved prevention. These incentives include low insurance rates for documented safe drivers, higher taxes on cigarettes and alcohol, and lower life insurance rates for those who use no alcohol or cigarettes. The field of injury control, therefore, involves a complex variety of measures. They can be expedited further if physicians use their social consciences as well as their therapeutic techniques.

Dental Health and Fluoridation

Periodic surveys of dental health problems indicate that the nation's dental health has improved in recent decades in the United States. The prospects for further prevention of dental problems continue to be encouraging. The use of fluoride at optimal levels before and after the eruption of permanent teeth has reduced the amount of dental caries by more than one half.

Dental caries had been a disease problem of massive proportions. Even in the 1990s, low-income children have many more untreated decayed teeth than high-income children. Fluoride, in the water supply of the majority of the United States population, delays the onset of dental caries and reduces the need for treatment by dentists. Prepayment for dental care through dental insurance has become a job-related benefit of many employees in recent years.

Half of all caries develop in the pits and grooves of the chewing surfaces of teeth, where the fluoride seems to be least effective. Dental sealants are plastic resins that are applied to these surfaces to prevent further decay. These sealants appear to be very effective, but many dentists have been slow to use them, possibly because of unfamiliarity and concerns about future economic consequences.

Smoking

Cigarette smoking causes much preventable illness and death and is, in fact, the chief, single, avoidable cause of death in our society. Cigarette smoking causes 85% of lung cancer in the United States and is linked to cancer of the larynx, mouth, pancreas, and bladder. It is the principal cause of chronic obstructive lung disease, and it is a major risk factor in coronary heart disease, stroke, and peripheral vascular disease.

Smoking by mothers slows fetal growth and raises the risk of spontaneous abortion and fetal and neonatal death. The danger to adult health of living with a smoker is now well established and has caused significant social concern. Smoking also contributes to death and injury from fires and burns. Finally, the benefit of quitting smoking is clearly established; the overall mortality of ex-smokers after 15 years of cessation is similar to that of nonsmokers, and for cardiovascular disease, mortality is cut in half after only 1 to 2 years' postcessation.

Even in the face of these known health hazards, many smokers find it difficult to give up this powerful addiction. Key strategies in the cessation of smoking include facilitating the individual's decision to quit, using a self-guided cessation program, and participating in an organized group program with social support. Cessation methods have included behavior modification, aversive conditioning, biofeedback, hypnosis, acupuncture, nicotine gum, and nicotine patches. Smoking cessation efforts in the United States have been very successful. Many adults have successfully quit smoking using these methods. About half of middle-aged men who ever smoked have quit, as well as 26% of the U.S. adult population smokers. The prevention of smoking in young people is also very important in advancing public health. National efforts are under way to prohibit or limit smoking in public places, and many states have passed aggressive antismoking legislation and are now working to prohibit sales of cigarettes to minors.

Misuse of Alcohol and Drugs

Misuse of alcohol and other drugs is a major health hazard in America and the Western world. Both the toxic effect and the increased risk of injury and death while under their influence constitute their medical consequences. The personal, family, social, and occupational consequences of alcohol and drug addiction are disasterous. Other abused drugs include the illicit drugs such as heroin or cocaine and legal drugs used for nonmedical purposes. Tranquilizers, barbiturates, and amphetamines have been among the most abused prescription drugs. The effect sought is primarily a dulling of normal emotional feelings and appropriate processing of those feelings.

Regulatory measures have been the nation's primary tool to reduce these problems. For example, federal legislation has sought to induce states to adopt 21 years of age as the minimum drinking age in the United States; such legislation restricts a portion of highway construction funds until the state has passed the desired laws. Educational programs have also been tried, including special information programs for high-risk populations, including physicians themselves. In one national program, hospital emergency rooms report admissions for abuse. In recent years, alcohol combined with other drugs has been a leading cause of both admissions and deaths in emergency rooms. Alcohol and drug abuse is a major risk for physicians and health care workers. Treatment programs with good success rates based on the "twelve-step" program are now widely available. Identification of the addiction problem by the patient, family, and friends, and active involvement in treatment are essential to controlling this progressive disease.

Nutrition

In recent years, the focus of nutritional science has moved from curing deficiency diseases to searching for relationships between diet and chronic disease and to investigating the role of diet in promoting health. Increased public awareness about these relationships now causes patients to ask for sophisticated nutritional advice from their personal physicians. The U.S. public has recently decreased its intake of fat, whole milk, eggs, beef, and pork. The risk of developing premature coronary heart disease is greater when blood cholesterol levels exceed 200 mg/dl. Many dedicated patients seek the advice of physicians in their attempts to reduce their cholesterol to this level. New guidelines for reducing cholesterol levels are found in Tables 6-7 and 6-8.

Obesity, an excess of adipose tissue, raises the risk of hypertension, high-serum cholesterol levels, diabetes, and certain cancers such as those of the breast and colon. Other evidence suggests that foods rich in vitamin A may reduce the risk of cancer. Inadequate nutrition is associated with poor pregnancy outcome, and iron and folic acid deficiency still occur in pregnant women.

TABLE 6-7. Initial Classification and Recommended Follow-up Based on Total Cholesterol*

Classification, mg/dl	
<200	Desirable blood cholesterol
200–239	Borderline—high blood cholesterol
≥240	High blood cholesterol
Recommended follow-up	
Total cholesterol, <200 mg/dl	Repeat within 5 years
Total cholesterol, 200–239 mg/dl	
Without definite CHD or two other CHD risk factors (one of which can be male sex)	Dietary information and recheck annually
With definite CHD or two other CHD risk factors (one of which can be male sex)	Lipoprotein analysis; further action based on LDL cholesterol level
Total cholesterol ≥240 mg/dl	

* CHD indicates coronary heart disease; LDL, low-density lipoprotein.
(Arch Intern Med, 1988, 148, pp 36–69)`

TABLE 6-8. Classification and Treatment Decisions Based on LDL Cholesterol*

Classification mg/dl		
<130	Desirable LDL cholesterol	
130–159	Borderline high-risk LDL cholesterol	
≥160	High-risk LDL cholesterol	
	Initiation Level, mg/dl	Minimal Goal, mg/dl
Dietary treatment		
Without CHD or two other risk factors†	≥160	<160‡
With CHD or two other risk factors†	≥130	<130§
Drug treatment		
Without CHD or two other risk factors†	≥190	<160
With CHD or two other risk factors†	≥160	<130

* LDL indicates low-density lipoprotein; CHD, coronary heart disease.
† Patients have a lower initiation level and goal if they are at high risk because they already have definite CHD, or because they have any two of the following risk factors: male sex, family history of premature CHD, cigarette smoking, hypertension, low high-density lipoprotein (HDL) cholesterol, diabetes mellitus, definite cerebrovascular or peripheral vascular disease, and severe obesity.
‡ Roughly equivalent to total cholesterol level of <240 mg/dl or <200 mg/dl.
§ As goals for monitoring dietary treatment.
(Arch Intern Med, 1988, 148, pp 36–69)

At times the profit-making marketplace may play as large a part in improving nutrition as the health services. Thus, livestock practices have developed to produce leaner meat, a step that reduces intake of saturated fat. Useful technologic measures have included fortifying bread and developing new products that are lower in fat, cholesterol, and sodium. As the 1990s progress, it seems likely that physicians will play an increasingly important role in getting their patients to make important nutritional changes.

Physical Fitness and Exercise

Physical fitness relates significantly to our ability to perform effectively our usual work, household chores, sports, and dance. Forty percent of American adults regularly exercise or play sports. Physical activity is recommended at least 3 days a week, lasting at least 20 minutes a session. The sessions should be sufficiently intense to use a minimum of 300 kcal and must be continued regularly to maintain the training effect.

The time that adults spend on vigorous activity has increased since the 1970s. It seems likely, however, that an individual commitment to improve physical fitness is needed to spur this activity. Certain demographic groups, including women, the elderly, inner-city and rural residents, and persons from low-income groups show low participation in exercise and should be particularly encouraged by physicians to take advantage of its benefits.

The rhythmic use of large muscle groups does reduce the risk of coronary heart disease and slows the loss of calcium in postmenopausal women. Physical activity also modestly helps in controlling hypertension, improves lipid profile, and increases the effect of insulin in patients with insulin-dependent diabetes mellitus. The antidepressant effect of exercise is well known. Long-term studies have strongly suggested that regular sustained physical activity consisting of 2,000 kcal of energy expenditure per week will help prevent cardiovascular disease. This is a level similar to walking 3 miles daily.

Older Adults

Achievements in disease prevention and treatment in recent decades have raised the duration of life of many adults who would formerly have died because of heart disease, strokes, cancer, and other major causes of death. The expanding survival rate has changed the nation's demography. The proportion of the population aged 65 years and older has increased markedly. Among that group, those aged 85 and older form the fastest growing segment of the population. Life expectancy has increased less for men than for women, who form an increasing majority of older age groups, so much so that discussants commonly infer that the "problem" of aging is particularly a "problem" of women. These changes by gender have had significant implications for the economics and health of the United States, and the expanding survival rate generally has influenced many political decisions about organizing and financing contemporary health care in the United States.

In the 1980s, the population of those persons who are 65 and older formed 12% of the total population, with about 150 women for every 100 men. Proportionately more men still have a spouse living. Thus, men are more often cared for at home and less often admitted to nursing homes. At any one time, about 5% of those aged 65 and older are in nursing homes, with most residents being women. About 30% of the elderly live alone and have little opportunity to discuss their health problems with a family member. Such persons become more dependent on their family physician for advice and help. Visiting nurses who deliver care in homes find that most of their clients are women; when called to help a disabled man living with his spouse at home, the nurse will usually find a more severely disabled male who has been able to stay at home because of the physical help given by his spouse. Thus, the demography of the elderly plays an important role in health care needs.

In both sexes in the elderly, the major causes of death have fallen. Diseases of the heart and cerebrovascular diseases have steeply fallen in recent decades, probably because of better lifestyles and detection. In contrast, the cancers have fallen less, partly because of an increase in lung cancer in women who have increased their cigarette smoking habit in recent decades.

Among the elderly, the causes of impaired function differ from the causes of death. Thus, the arthritides affect 44% of those aged 65 and older, with women more often and more seriously impaired than men of the same age. While rarely causing admission to hospital, the arthritides result in many visits to physicians and about 16% of all disability days spent in bed. Deafness and impaired visual acuity are also major losses of function; they diminish quality of life but rarely cause death.

Older persons smoke less than younger age groups because cigarette smokers do not often survive into old age and because smokers tend to quit as they age. Of the 16% who smoke, there is good evidence that health improves after quitting. Older persons tend to exercise less regularly than younger groups. Scalds from hot water lead in causing burns in the elderly. Osteoporosis and easily fractured hips are potential causes of impairment and death; they may be reduced in elderly women in the coming decades because of improvements in nutrition and in pharmacologic and surgical treatment modalities.

Even at a late age, behavior may be changed to improve health and alleviate discomfort. Prevention efforts are not wasted on older patients.

Ethnicity

Race is a commonly used descriptor in medicine. It is frequently used to describe individual patients during bedside rounds or in other medical settings and enjoys widespread use as a descriptor of groups of individuals. The meaning of race is elusive and is rarely defined, though the ubiquity of its continued use suggests that there is a least some implied understanding of what race means. There is no accepted scientific definition of race, although racial classifications are based largely on phenotypic differences, most notably skin color. A common perception exists that racial classifications are founded in biologic differences that legitimize genetic classification or partitioning humans into subspecies. The rationale for this paradigm is severely flawed.

Race is deeply intertwined with socioeconomic conditions, including income, housing, nutrition, exposure to violent crime, and other lifestyle variables. Disentangling their influence from that of race is extremely difficult. While numerous examples of racial differentials in disease occurrence can be cited, the interaction of environmental exposures with genetic factors must always be considered. Perhaps no disease process has been the subject of such intense speculation about the cause(s) of the observed racial differences as hypertension, a condition that has been observed to occur at a younger age in blacks than in whites. Several environmental exposures such as obesity and physical inactivity are known to be associated with hypertension, conditions that are more prevalent in blacks, particularly in black women, than in whites. Moreover, irrespective of race, because blood pressure increases with age, the lifetime risk of becoming hypertensive exceeds 75%. Despite the presence of these environmental factors, genetic factors have sometimes been deemed responsible for the hypertension differential between blacks and whites. However, recent data from national surveys indicate that between 1960 and 1980, the age-specific black-white blood pressure differential has narrowed considerably, a fact, given the timeframe of its occurrence, that is much more consistent with changing environmental exposures than genetic evolution. Hypertension is also associated inversely with socioeconomic standing in both blacks and whites; therefore, it should not be surprising that some of the blood pressure differential present between blacks and whites relates to the well-documented differences in income that likely translate into different lifestyle exposures. Finally, race differentials in disease occurrence are not static; thus, one racial group may have higher disease rates at one point but, relative to another race, lower disease rates at another. Breast cancer is an example of such a flip-flop in disease rates between blacks and whites.

Why has medical research been so focused on racial comparisons? First, there are clear race differentials in disease rates that merit explanation, such as in the case of hypertension. However, the problem has not been that race differences have been reported but that unconvincing reasons are sometimes given for the observed differences. Moreover, when genetic factors are invoked to explain racial differences in disease rates, an aura of inevitability is cast on potentially preventable and/or modifiable disease processes. It can also be argued that genetic explanations for race differentials in disease have been detrimental because of the selective use of such explanations in diseases with a significant social stigma; the acquired immunodeficiency syndrome (AIDS) and other sexually transmitted diseases serve as notable examples. When this occurs, the definition of strategies to prevent and/or treat the disease in question becomes marred. Such explanations tend to ignore the fact that race is only one variable by which individuals or groups can be classified, and the influence of other factors that may be associated with race that are more logical explanations of disease differences are sometimes not taken into account. Even if possible confounders are taken into account, and mathematical models cannot fully explain black-white differences, the imprecision of such models are seldom mentioned.

When race differentials in disease are observed, the most likely explanation for an excess in one racial group relative to another relates to environmental influences. Among American blacks there is a tremendously diverse genetic gene pool, which spans the continent of Africa, the Caribbean, and Central/South America and includes whites. Among whites, a wide genetic diversity also exists. Thus, it is hardly surprising that race does not equal genetic homogeneity—because of genetic heterogeneity within ill-defined racial groups—and that genetic factors are unlikely to explain racial differences in disease occurrence at the population level. The notion of race as a means of providing a biologic framework for classifying humans is a concept that is likely flawed and should be reconsidered.

Health Behavior

If we understand current health behavior, we may become more effective in persuading people to improve this behavior. One might expect that the use of health services depends primarily on the frequency of disease or discomfort suffered by individuals or groups. This expectation, however, proves to be only partly true. For the many preventable or treatable conditions that are more common in lower-income groups, persons at greatest risk use health care and take preventive measures less often than those at lower risk.

Compared with higher-income groups, the poor have higher infant mortality rates, a higher incidence of infectious disease, and a higher prevalence of untreated dental disease. However, almost all surveys show that the poor have lower utilization rates of preventive and ambulatory health care. Within each poverty level, blacks usually show lower utilization rates than whites.

Hospital admission rates are high, both for the poor and nonpoor, but the former have longer durations of stay. Such findings suggest that the poor delay longer before seeking care, and when admitted they have developed more serious illness. This interpretation is confirmed by the finding that for almost every diagnostic group, death is a more frequent outcome among the lower-income patients admitted to hospital.

How can these observations be explained? The vast literature on health services utilization describes possible approaches:

1. The *economic approach* studies the impact of financial barriers to seeking health care. In the United States, the arrival of Medicare and Medicaid in 1966 raised hospital discharge rates for those 65 years and older and temporarily increased length of stay. In contrast, for those under 65 years, hospital discharge rates fell while little change occurred in length of stay. These factors suggest that the under-65 age group faced higher prices than before the introduction of Medicare. Moreover, even when financial barriers are eliminated, wide variations still occur among income and ethnic groups. The factor of education is believed to perpetuate the lower use rates among the poor, even in countries with a national health service where significant financial barriers do not exist.

2. The *sociodemographic approach* analyzes utilization rates for various easy-to-identify groups. Such studies show that utilization of hospital and physician care tends to be higher for women than for men of the same age, income, and education, particularly in the middle decades of life. The problem with this approach is that it offers no explanation of the reason why differences exist, nor does it explain all the wide variations that occur within similar groups.

3. The *geographic approach* studies the association between geographic proximity of services to clients and utilization rates. The existing studies suggest that geographic convenience has slight or moderate importance.

4. The *social–cultural approach* studies cultural values, norms, beliefs, and lifestyles. This approach focuses, for example, on the differences between "middle-classness," which is deemed to show the desired or ideal norms, and working or "lower-classness." The so-called culture of poverty is believed to be partly responsible for the low utilization rates of elective and preventive health care among low-income groups. At most ages, however, the higher incidence of symptoms among the poor causes a higher frequency of physician visits by low-income families.

5. The *organization approach* emphasizes elements of the health delivery system that foster or impede utilization. Some studies suggest that large organizations, in order to survive financially, may neglect clients in greatest need of health care but with least ability to pay for it. Other critics say that the delivery system has been so arranged as to maximize the convenience of health care providers, with less attention given to the needs of consumers. Further aspects of health services organizations will be reviewed later in this chapter.

6. The *social–psychologic approach* emphasizes motivation, individual perceptions, and learning. Using this approach, one group of investigators suggests that a number of conditions seem important in inducing patients to seek and follow professional health advice. (a) The individual must believe that he or she is suffering from an illness or must be liable to develop an illness of serious consequence. (b) The individual must believe that the illness can be prevented, controlled, or cured. (c) The individual must be sufficiently "future-oriented" to justify taking immediate action to ward off health threats that are far in the future. (d) The individual's social group—family, friends, peers—must approve of the professional health care system. (e) The individual must be willing to overcome whatever obstacles exist to obtaining health care. (f) The individual must be willing to follow professional advice.

This list of factors is likely to change with further research but highlights the many attitudes that health educators must consider as they try to improve health behavior. Clearly, conveying information about health and disease is not sufficient to motivate patient behavior. However, as we develop more effective ways to foster these essential attitudes, we will become more effective in improving health behavior and advancing human health.

ECONOMIC ASPECTS OF HEALTH CARE

Health care has a number of characteristics that distinguish it from other types of services and commodities. First, health care may produce external benefits; thus, health care includes many procedures that benefit society as well as the individual who receives the service. Second, besides being a consumption commodity, something that we use up and spend money on, health care is partly an investment good; dollars spent on health care now may raise future productivity and return the same dollars with interest. Third, certain health services have a collective value when used by one person, and there is no decrease in availability to others. For example, when one person consumes fluoridated water, an abundance remains to give the benefits of fluoridation to other drinkers. The large dollar investment needed—such as for water and sewer systems, or for the buildings and personnel to provide hospital or nursing home care—also applies to many health services.

The amount in dollars that individuals are willing to pay for preventive measures tends to be below its true value to society; generally the individual does not care to pay for the additional benefits to society or for intangible future benefits. When the income of the average American family doubles, its demand for preventive care more than doubles while that for curative care rises less. However, low-income families give priority to treatment when ill, and they regard as luxurious and postponable the preventive measures that are also indicated for continued good health. Thus, the argument is strong that government funds should support a number of health services and should, in particular, be funneled into preventive health services. The political controversy over the appropriate area for government funds has been in the support of curative care. Science does not guide the development of a consensus on this point, and future decisions will arise politically.

In recent years the costs of medical care have risen more steeply than other costs in the United States, particularly in the field of hospital care. The main reasons for the rise in hospital costs have been the following:

1. Hospitals used to require many employees to work long hours at low wages. Since the 1960s, they have closed the gap in wages and working conditions between themselves and other industries.

2. Technical and scientific advances have increased the complexity of hospital care. Rarely does an improvement replace a step that was more expensive; most often the innovation forms an extra step to improve the quality of care.

3. Hospitals make intensive use of human services; they have not raised their productivity as fast as has the economy at large.

4. Some educational and training programs cost more than the value of the benefits obtained. Part of inpatient hospital charges finance the training of nurses and physician residents.

5. With insurance and subsidies, consumers face a price for health care that is below the true cost of providing it, causing consumers to purchase more than they otherwise would.

An increasing amount of money spent on health services comes from health insurance plans, sometimes described as third-party payments. Persons with hospital insurance have higher rates of inpatient hospital use than those without insurance. However, there has been evidence to suggest that those without insurance have greater, rather than less, need for hospitalization. The government-financed Medicare program helped reduce this problem for those aged 65 years or older but did not eliminate it. The debate on nationwide compulsory health insurance focuses on the need for better coverage of other groups as well.

With third-party payments, rising prices cause less individual protest and less change in use than when the individual pays directly for care. Thus, the price of a health service does not relate so inversely to its consumption as does price in other fields. Other rationing devices tend to develop when the price mechanism is not effective. Waiting lists for services develop, and registration at outpatient clinics may become unpleasant, partly to discourage a rapid return of patients. These deterrents have a different impact on different groups; price deters high-income patients less than low-income ones; long waiting times deter the unemployed less than those eager to return to the job they hold.

Federal legislation in 1982 detailed a payment-per-case system for general hospital care of Medicare inpatients. Each patient is placed into 1 of 470 mutually exclusive classes called *diagnosis-related groups (DRGs)*. Based partly on the principal diagnosis, complications, and treatment procedures used, the assigned DRG leads to the "appropriate" payment for care, which is unchanged whether the stay is short or long. Intended to control costs without weakening quality, the actual effect of widely using DRGs has been to discharge patients more quickly at a more seriously ill stage.

Health Care Facilities

The system of health care facilities can be pictured as forming a bridge that carries the individual seeking help to the health worker who provides that service. The system also provides the necessary equipment and technology to make the service as effective as possible.

There never will be a single best system of health care. The way in which personal health services and facilities are organized depends mainly on factors outside the control of health professionals. The most prominent characteristics of the existing system of health care facilities are its scientific complexity and the difficulty it has in responding to the conflicting demands of high quality versus lower cost.

Although there is no ideal pattern of organization, the goals to be aimed at are clearer now than they were in the past. The health care facilities should be organized so that they produce health services that are:

1. Readily accessible, with no socioeconomic or geographic barriers that discriminate among population groups
2. Adequate in quantity, providing enough of each necessary service
3. Comprehensive, covering the range of needed services, and facilitating continuity of care
4. Effective, reaching their stated goals, which will become more ambitious as techniques improve
5. Efficient, reaching their goals with a reasonable degree of economy
6. Of good quality, satisfying the consumer as well as the producer of health services

What steps should be taken toward meeting these goals? Only partial and political answers to this question exist; the solutions chosen depend largely on the judgment of those who have power to decide about community health problems. The push for efficiency requires frequent reconsideration of alternative ways to reach goals. The current diversity of ownership and facilities makes it difficult to plan as a community to improve accessibility to health services. Fragmentation of care has been common in a system with extensive specialization. Continuity of care now depends on the individual patient's being able to find his way to the appropriate points of the health care system at the right time. We particularly need to integrate into the system those facilities that provide long-term care, rehabilitation, and mental health services. The developing HMOs may facilitate integration for younger and middle-aged clients. Lack of funding has posed problems to HMOs serving the elderly.

Also needed are further alternatives to institutional care. Many patients now admitted to institutions may be cared for in the future by day hospitals, home care programs, geriatric day care centers, hospice care programs, and outpatient clinics. The efforts of health insurance and government funding programs to speed institutional discharge may speed the development of these alternatives. Such alternatives may not thrive, however, if they are intended primarily to control cost of care rather than to improve quality of care for the patient population.

ACUTE GENERAL HOSPITAL

In the forefront of the U.S. health care facilities is the acute general hospital, whose orientation has always been toward the treatment of existing diseases. At times its policymakers have paid lip service to health promotion and disease prevention, but rarely have these activities been regarded as higher than public relations efforts. Recently, a number of smaller general hospitals have found their financial viability in danger, and efforts have been made to broaden the hospital activities. Hospital survival relates most strongly to providing sickness care, of good quality, with a reasonable amount of efficiency. Such cost-control efforts as the DRGs in Medicare have probably raised the cost of each patient-day but have also speeded the discharge of patients so that total cost per stay is lower.

In 1986 about 140 patients were discharged from acute general hospitals per 1,000 population. The 1986 discharge rate is a new low in hospital discharge rates since Medicare began in 1966. In the acute general hospital, length of stay for both sexes has also been falling. Evidence is accumulating that some hospital patients may have serious health difficulties because of "premature" discharge; this is particularly true of older patients who may proceed to poorly staffed nursing homes. In addition, the probability rises that further contractures of hospital stay will not reduce its cost but may merely squeeze into the shorter stay an avalanche of activities that succeed each other too swiftly to produce optimal benefit to patients.

Health Care Personnel

Since 1970 the number of people employed in health care has nearly doubled. In that period, physician-population ratios have increased about 40%, without much improvement in the regional variation in the supply of physicians. Thus, physicians continue to be most abundant in the Northeast and are most scarce in the South. Community hospitals continue to be the largest employers of personnel in health care. Despite increases in physician-population ratios, two thirds of consumers interviewed in health surveys still believe that they get no advice from physicians about improving their health habits.

The physician, who will continue to dominate among providers of health care, is the major topic of this section. The classic ideal of an authoritative but nurturing physician who provided complete medical care to several generations of the family may never have been so common as nostalgia suggests. Whether common or not in the past, this ideal cannot survive in the face of changing patient demands and the wide expansion of medical knowledge.

Much of the medical profession's strength is based on the legally supported monopoly of practicing physicians. This monopoly operates through a system of licensing, which gives physicians the privilege to hospitalize patients and the right to prescribe drugs and order laboratory tests that are otherwise virtually inaccessible to the layperson. In the 1990s, the economic and political autonomy of physicians varies from country to country and has varied in the United States at different times. More constant is their scientific autonomy, because even the most socialized countries leave the medical profession fairly free to develop its special area of knowledge and to determine which practices are scientifically acceptable. Similarly, almost everywhere, the medical profession has remained free to control the technical instruction of medical students.

PROFESSIONAL CONTROL AND AMBULATORY CARE

Ambulatory health care is provided to those who are not inpatients in institutions. The providers range from hospital emergency room personnel to private practitioners and voluntary free clinics. The earliest group practices in the United States formed in rural areas in the late 1800s. Although initially opposed by medical societies, they became more numerous in the 1900s. Their advantages included shared operational costs, professional management, more flexi-ble hours, greater economies of scale, and probably lower hospital admission rates. A Health Maintenance Organization Act in 1973 encouraged a wider concern for prepaid comprehensive care delivered to a known population. In today's competitive marketplace, physician groups called Preferred Provider Organizations (PPOs) focus more on minimizing charges to consumer groups, without much concern for the effect of cost control on quality of care.

Although administrative arrangements change, the average annual number of visits to physicians peaked above 5 per person in the 1970s and diminished through 1980. As one would expect, the frequency of consulting physicians in 1980 was lowest for those whose functional status was good. At every age, an increased loss of function was accompanied by more frequent visits to physicians, averaging 12 per person or higher when a major activity was lost.

Like those in most professions, physicians control their own performance in private practice. In isolated, solo practice, quality of ambulatory care rests solely on the physician's motivation, capacity, and conscience. In urban areas, even solo practitioners usually belong to a colleague network; by referring patients to each other, practitioners can observe one another's performance; and by being economically and technically interdependent, physicians can influence one another.

Group practices and HMOs increase the opportunity for physicians to observe and influence one another's performance. In this increasingly common arrangement, physicians from several specialities collaborate and pool their earnings, which are divided among them according to some prearranged plan. Most groups function on a fee-for-service basis, but a number operate a health insurance program in which patients receive all the services they need for a fixed annual fee. Convenience for the physicians and improved accessibility of care for their patients are the basic motivating factors in the formation of group practices; the physicians' improved ability to monitor one another's performance is a secondary benefit to both patient and doctor, stated less openly as an objective of group practice.

FORMAL AND INFORMAL ORGANIZATION

The national, state, and local medical associations make up the formal organization of physicians. These associations do only part of the job of ensuring high-quality care by setting minimum standards and the basic core of training required for licensing, by publishing new knowledge and by educating the practitioners.

At least equally important is the informal structure of the profession. As mentioned above, most physicians in urban areas join a network of colleagues who have common interests, including improved professional satisfaction and reasonable financial survival. The networks probably interact little with one another, and their standards and practices differ from one another. One basic control mechanism is the informal boycott—practitioners refuse to refer patients to those practitioners of whom they disapprove. This practice may or may not change the physician's performance; sometimes it merely pushes him or her outside a network of high standards into the company of those with lower standards.

INDIVIDUAL PHYSICIAN BEHAVIOR

Once physicians were seen as powerful, wise, and charismatic, possessing knowledge about human beings denied to other mortals. For social, administrative, and therapeutic reasons, recent decades have seen a reaction against this view in favor of seeing the physician as one of many professionals providing health care in society. Acceptance of the newer view is slow in gaining physicians themselves but is more widespread among administrators, politicians, and consumers in the United States.

The physician's behavior will reflect the adaptation to the medical role as he or she sees it. For example, the physician may prefer to treat critically ill patients where he or she can rely mainly on biological knowledge and technical skills, largely ignoring the patient as a person. In a crisis, the physician is active and the patient passive. In an acute but less desperate situation, the physician guides while the patient cooperates, with the latter knowing what goes on and exercising some judgment. The third relationship is that of mutual participation, whereby the physician helps the patient to help himself or herself; this mode is particularly useful in chronic disease and disability. This last role is closest to the modern view of physicians, particularly since the technical knowledge and skills of other health professionals can also help the patient with chronic disease. Therefore, the treatment of both chronically ill and elderly patients tends not to appeal to many physicians because if reinforces the reaction against the "physician-on-a-pedestal."

Today the high costs of medical care and the fact that about two thirds of Americans are without health care coverage has placed much strain on the health care system. There is much public and political pressure to overhaul it. Several models are being proposed, which range from supplemented private insurance to the staff models of Canada and the United Kingdom. Change is no doubt inevitable. Physicians should be centrally involved in this restructuring so that quality can be maintained as costs are controlled.

QUESTIONS IN PUBLIC HEALTH AND COMMUNITY MEDICINE

Review Questions

When do health problems become public health problems? Discuss the value and limitations of your answer.

Explain health in terms of what it is and what it does. Discuss the good and bad points of the WHO definition, and give an alternative description of health that more closely approaches our real-life activities in health promotion and disease control.

Discuss three important factors that influence population size in the Third World countries.

What factors affect time trends in the crude death rates of the United States? If crude death rates are slowly rising while age-specific rates are falling slowly in a given developed country, what is the most likely explanation for this contrast?

What are the differences between incidence and prevalence, and how do they relate to each other?

Can infant mortality rates remain level in a country that is truly improving its health services? Justify your answer.

Discuss one well-established method of reducing the incidence and prevalence of a major chronic disease in the United States.

From the economic viewpoint, how does health care differ from other goods and services appearing in the marketplace?

When is a test result valid but not reliable? Under what circumstances would you continue to use such a test?

What is the desirable objective of good health services administration?

Why has it been easier to eradicate smallpox than measles from the United States?

Discuss two factors that confuse cause-and-effect discussions in occupational medicine.

Define *regression to the mean*. Explain how regression to the mean must be taken into account in interpreting the results of treatment benefits in clinical trials.

When a nutritional factor participates in causing illness, how can we best change eating habits in individuals?

Review the current status and possible changes that may occur in the medical profession in the United States.

How do governmental health agencies differ from voluntary health agencies? Contrast in terms of two important differences.

Suggest 10 different areas that deserve high priority in prevention in the coming years. Review in detail the procedures that would be part of the preventive effort in one high-priority area.

Should family planning and population control services be subsidized by government in a developed country? Justify your answer.

List the seven criteria for inferring causation from epidemiologic data. Describe for a major risk factor (*e.g.*, cholesterol, smoking, blood pressure) how these criteria can be applied to what is known about risk for cardiovascular disease.

Multiple-Choice Questions

Choose the best answer for each question. Answers are at the end of this chapter.

1. The group of "physician extenders" now being trained and studied in the United States includes such personnel as:
   (a) Nurse practitioners
   (b) Licensed practical nurses
   (c) Occupational therapists
   (d) Physical therapy assistants

2. A questionnaire mailed to 1,000 adult women asked about the presence or absence of joint stiffness. Of these women, 500 returned the questionnaire, and 100 stated that they had stiff joints. The appropriate rate for the prevalence of stiff joints would be:
   (a) 100/1,000, provided the questionnaires are correctly answered
   (b) 100/500, provided the nonrespondents are similar to the respondents
   (c) 500/1,000, provided women with stiff joints are likely not to reply
   (d) None of the above

3. Epidemiologic studies of hepatitis have been more productive than those of diabetes mellitus in orienting prevention programs because:
   (a) The causes of hepatitis are more easily controlled by antibiotics than the causes of diabetes.
   (b) Hepatitis is more accurately diagnosed than diabetes.
   (c) It is easier to classify hepatitis cases by the causal agents than it is to classify diabetes cases.
   (d) Hepatitis has more risk factors associated with it than diabetes does.

4. Japanese migrants to Hawaii develop more cancer of the colon than Japanese who live in Japan. This difference is best explained by the following:
   (a) Migrants from a country may differ from those remaining in the country
   (b) Hawaii may have environmental carcinogens that are absent in Japan
   (c) Japanese living in Hawaii may eat different foods from those eaten by Japanese living in Japan
   (d) All of the above factors may play a part

5. In recent decades, the U.S. public has come to believe that health care is a human right. The response of government to this demand has been mainly at the federal level primarily because:
   (a) State and local governments have no authority to respond
   (b) Many state governors disagree with the "human right" view
   (c) Local government officials have neither the training nor the experience to respond
   (d) Federal government officials are more sensitive to public demands
   (e) Financial resources are most abundant at the federal level

6. When a measurement, such as blood pressure level, leads to a diagnosis of disease or no disease, the cutoff point between the two groups may be defined:
   (a) By statistical means, such as two standard deviations from the age-specific average
   (b) By clinical means, such as the level at which symptoms and complications become more frequent
   (c) By prognosis, such as an elevated risk of future disease
   (d) By any of the above means, depending on the purpose of the cutoff point

7. A small study attempted to guide health plan-

ners as to whether death certificates for esophageal cancer form a useful guide to the frequency of that disease. Its findings were:

Diagnosed before death	74
Confirmed at autopsy	53
Not confirmed at autopsy	21
First diagnosed at autopsy	22

Indicate which of the following statements is/ are correct:
   (a) 22/74 of individual cases were missed before death.
   (b) The false-positive diagnoses before death about balance the false-negatives.
   (c) Autopsies are essential to obtain the approximate population frequency.

8. The average expectation of life at birth:
   (a) Rises with improvements in health
   (b) Falls as death rates increase
   (c) Is higher for U.S. females than males
   (d) Has all of the above characteristics

9. The legal requirement that physicians report selected diseases:
   (a) Has succeeded particularly for mental illnesses
   (b) Gives an incomplete picture of disease incidence
   (c) Has been used mainly for noninfectious conditions
   (d) Has slowed the control of infectious disease

10. Epidemiologic studies of disease usually involve:
   (a) Both the sick and healthy populations
   (b) Discarding the clinical knowledge of disease
   (c) Emphasizing the cases of advanced disease
   (d) Relating local cases to the national population

11. The frequency of much infectious disease can best be explained by:
   (a) Host factors
   (b) Characteristics of the infectious agent
   (c) Environmental factors
   (d) Interaction of all of the above

12. A clinical trial is ''double blind'' when:
   (a) The subjects know that they belong to the control group.
   (b) The investigators do not understand the pathology of the condition.
   (c) Neither observer nor subject knows to which group the subject belongs.
   (d) All of the above conditions are met.

13. In an epidemic of food poisoning, the contaminated food must:

   (a) Be eaten by all cases
   (b) Have been avoided by all who remained well
   (c) Be consumed by most cases and by few of the well
   (d) Be characterized by none of the above

14. In the United States, the Public Health Service is:
   (a) A federal agency with many public health functions
   (b) The agency using about two thirds of the federal health budget
   (c) The guide for the activities of PROs
   (d) A federal agency responsible for Medicare and Medicaid

15. The prevention and better control of hypertension involves:
   (a) Obesity control, reduced salt and alcohol intake, and increased physical activity
   (b) A lifetime of antihypertensive treatment in established cases
   (c) More extensive screening for elevated blood pressure in employees
   (d) All of the above steps

16. Maternal and child health activities usually include:
   (a) Use of Medicare funds for immunizations
   (b) The supervision and care of mothers and children
   (c) The early detection and treatment of atherosclerosis
   (d) All of the above measures

17. The delivery of routine immunizations could be widened by:
   (a) Eliminating charges for these procedures
   (b) Funding preventive measures through government subsidies
   (c) Offering vaccines free to physicians who do not charge their patients for immunizations
   (d) All of the above steps

18. Identifying the environmental causes of disease is complicated because:
   (a) The period may be short between exposure and disease onset.
   (b) Clear data are usually available, but overlooked, that reveal the association.
   (c) Many agents may contribute to the same disease.
   (d) All of the above reasons play a part.

19. The Health Care Financing Administration is a:
   (a) Voluntary agency that funds health care
   (b) Philanthropic association, such as the Rockefeller Foundation

(c) Professional association that funds health administrators

(d) Federal agency responsible for Medicare and Medicaid

20. Randomization into a clinical trial is best characterized by which of the following?
    (a) Group assignment is unknown to the participant.
    (b) There is an equal chance of group assignment
    (c) Group assignment is unpredictable.
    (d) Group assignment is sequential.

21. Which of the following best describes the population perspective on disease prevention in the community?
    (a) To most efficiently prevent disease, only high-risk individuals (*e.g.,* hyperlipidemics, hypertensives) should be treated.
    (b) Lowering risk factors by a substantial amount in high-risk patients and patients with clinical disease will achieve the best results in preventing the disease.
    (c) Lowering the population mean level of the risk factor (*e.g.,* blood cholesterol, blood pressure) by only a small percent will shift the entire population distribution of the risk factor and prevent the most disease.
    (d) It is not possible for populations to change their risk levels significantly.

22. What is the "gold standard" in research for evaluating the efficacy of new therapies?
    (a) Case control study
    (b) Case history
    (c) A prospective observational study
    (d) Clinical trial

23. Case control studies are useful for:
    (a) Studying diseases that are rare
    (b) Generating causal hypotheses
    (c) Estimating risk for an exposure
    (d) All of the above

24. Which of the following is the most efficient and least costly method of establishing benefit of a treatment?
    (a) Prospective clinical trial
    (b) Case control study
    (c) Prospective observational study
    (d) Meta-analysis—pooling results of several clinical trials

25. Which of the following is not one of the seven epidemiologic criteria used for inferring causation?
    (a) Sensitivity
    (b) Independence

(c) Specificity
(d) Temporality

26. What term is used to describe the ratio of true-positive tests to all tests that are positive (true-positives plus false-positives)?
    (a) Sensitivity
    (b) Predictive value
    (c) Specificity
    (d) Congruence

27. Which of the following statements in a clinical trial evaluating a new treatment best describes the meaning of the term "p < .05"?
    (a) The outcome is statistically significant and therefore clinically important.
    (b) A type II, or beta, error has likely occurred.
    (c) One must reject the alternative hypothesis.
    (d) If a similar experiment was carried out repeatedly, one would expect the observed result to occur less than 5% of the time by chance, given the variability of measures in the study.

28. A study's statistical *power* is related to:
    (a) The type II, or beta, error
    (b) The treatment difference from control
    (c) Sample size
    (d) All of the above

29. In a study, hypertensives with diastolic blood pressures above 95 mmHg were selected as subjects. These patients were randomized to two new dietary treatments: (1) potassium supplementation and (2) calcium supplementation. Baseline diastolic blood pressure was 102 mmHg. After 6 weeks the groups' diastolic blood pressure fell by -12 ± 5 (standard error of difference) in the potassium group and by -11 ± 4 in the calcium group. What is the most likely explanation for the favorable reduction in blood pressure?
    (a) Potassium and calcium both are equally effective in lowering blood pressure.
    (b) Neither is effective. Regression to the mean can explain the drop in blood pressure.
    (c) Placebo effect has occurred.
    (d) Errors were made in blood pressure measurement.

30. Which of the following drugs taken during pregnancy is the most common cause of mental retardation in the United States?
    (a) Alcohol
    (b) Cocaine
    (c) Heroine
    (d) Amphetamines

31. What is the most likely explanation for the

increased incidence of certain diseases in African-Americans versus whites?

(a) Race-related genetic differences
(b) Inherent susceptibility of races to different diseases
(c) Differences in access to health care
(d) Environmental and socioeconomic differences

32. In 1992, what disease in many U.S. cities was the most common cause of death in men ages 25 to 44?

(a) AIDS
(b) Cancer
(c) Hypertensive stroke
(d) Drug overdose

ANSWERS TO MULTIPLE-CHOICE QUESTIONS

1. a	**9.** b	**17.** d	**25.** a
2. b	**10.** a	**18.** c	**26.** b
3. c	**11.** d	**19.** d	**27.** d
4. d	**12.** c	**20.** c	**28.** d
5. e	**13.** c	**21.** c	**29.** b
6. d	**14.** a	**22.** d	**30.** a
7. b	**15.** d	**23.** d	**31.** d
8. d	**16.** b	**24.** d	**32.** a

Rypins' Clinical Sciences Review, 16th Edition,
edited by Edward D. Frohlich. J. B. Lippincott
Company, Philadelphia © 1993.

7

Psychiatry

Gordon H. Deckert, M.D., F.A.C.P.
David Ross Boyd Professor, Department of
Psychiatry and Behavioral Sciences,
University of Oklahoma Health Sciences Center
Oklahoma City, Oklahoma

Ronald S. Krug, Ph.D.
David Ross Boyd Professor and Interim Chairman,
Department of Psychiatry and Behavioral Sciences,
University of Oklahoma Health Sciences Center
Oklahoma City, Oklahoma

Psychiatry is a science and a medical specialty. As a science, it seeks to understand disorders of the psyche (mind). The term *mind* is part of a psychological language reference system, along with such concepts as personality, anxiety, ego, neurosis, and so forth. The organ of the mind is the brain. The term *brain* is part of a physiological language reference system, along with such concepts as neurotransmitters, the limbic system, higher cortical functions, and so forth. Psychiatry employs both language systems. As a medical specialist, a psychiatrist seeks to study, diagnose, treat and prevent mental, emotional, behavioral, and psychophysiological disorders, and adverse psychological responses to illness. While these five areas of major concern overlap, most students of the field distinguish between them.

A given person, his mind, emotions, behavior, and soma (body) are influenced by many factors—so many that it becomes difficult to define the limits of psychiatry. There are various language models for describing human behavior, multiple theories to facilitate understanding, and even a variety of medical nomenclatures. No wonder the student may find all this perplexing. Nonetheless, despite these difficulties and differences, there is considerable agreement as to the major clinical entities and their management.

Mental illness is ubiquitous. The Institute of Medicine of the National Academy of Sciences, summarizing recent epidemiologic studies, states that approximately 25% to 30% of visits to ambulatory care medical facilities are attributed directly to mental illness. The majority of these visits relate to the manifestations of anxiety and depression. At any one time, as many patients with mental illnesses occupy hospital beds as do all other patients combined, even though the number of patients resident in state and county mental hospitals has decreased over the last several decades. Rates of admission and discharge, however, have increased at mental hospitals. In the United States, approximately one in ten individuals will be hospitalized in a psychiatric hospital for mental illness. Many others are admitted to general hospitals. One person in every three or four will seek specific medical assistance for a mental disorder. Increasing numbers of patients are being seen in community mental health centers and hospital emergency rooms. These figures and statements do not even include patients with psychosomatic illnesses, or those who present with psychological response to disease. Virtually *every* disease has accompanying psychological consequences. No wonder, then, that studies indicate that 75% to 90% of all patients present with psychological factors playing some role in their discomfort. Add to this the increasingly recognized problem of compliance, that is, the relatively low percentage of patients who follow their prescribed medical regimen. Consider the mounting interest in prevention. One can understand the current resurgence of interest in psychiatry. Undergraduate and graduate medical curricula have placed increasing emphasis on neurobiology, behavioral sciences, psychiatry, psychological medicine, and behavioral medicine. This, in turn, is reflected nationally on certification, licensure, and speciality examinations.

Practicing physicians frequently work with patients who **somatize,** that is, focus on their body, tend to ignore or deny psychological dimensions to their illness, and resist efforts at psychological intervention. Less well recognized is another group of patients who **psychologize,** that is, who tend to ignore their body or the possibility of illness in their body and resist appropriate biological intervention. The physician by education, training and role is potentially in a unique position to help both groups of patients. Ideally, a physician has a biological and a psychological perspective and the capability to understand, manage and treat "disease."

Psychiatry in the United States has undergone a major change in its diagnostic nomenclature. The *Diagnostic and Statistical Manual of Mental Disorders of the American Psychiatric Association* (DSM-III R) is officially in use. Therefore, the language and outline of DSM-III R will be followed in this section. Where necessary, comparable terms will be placed in parentheses so the student can correlate this material with the various headings used by many psychiatric texts still in print.

HISTORY

Humans are curious about themselves. They have always attempted to explain their behavior, including that behavior called mental illness. Humans have had a tendency to ascribe the phenomena of mental illness to supernatural causes, especially to possession by some outside influence. Nonetheless, many early Greek physicians, including Hippocrates, taught that mental illness resulted from natural causes, and both Hippocrates and his near

contemporary in India, Susruta, held a rather sophisticated view of psychosomatic processes. After the death of the Roman physician, Galen, in 200 A.D., a gradual return of primitive attitudes in the West culminated in demonology and the persecution and execution of so-called witches. This practice was much more pervasive in parts of Europe than is generally recognized. In the late 15th and early 16th centuries, conservative estimates put the figure of executions to approximately 100,000 in Germany and a similar number in France. *Malleus Maleficarum* (The Witch's Hammer) published by two Dominicans, Sprenger and Kramer, has had a profound influence on Western medicine. Medicine's separation of mind from body during this time was perhaps inevitable given the theology of the day. Thomas Aquinas spoke for his culture when he argued that the soul could not be sick. During this era, advances in medical psychology were found primarily in the Moslem world, especially among Arab physicians.

The first effective answer to demonology was *De Praestigüs Daemonum,* by Johann Weyer (1515–1588), often called "the father of psychiatry." Two centuries later in 1792, Philippe Pinel struck the chains from the mental patients in the Bicetré in France. His contemporary, Benjamin Rush, a physician and a signer of the Declaration of Independence, was considered the father of American psychiatry because of his efforts for the mentally ill in Philadelphia.

During the 19th century, French and German psychiatrists, especially Emil Kraepelin (1855–1926), applied descriptive and statistical methods to clinical studies and elaborated a classification of personality disorders and mental illness. This classification influences ours today. Later, Eugene Bleuler revised the Kraepelinian concept of dementia praecox and introduced the term *schizophrenia.*

Paralleling the development of desciptive psychiatry was an increasing understanding of psychological mechanisms. Many scholars trace a sequence of ideas from Paracelcus (1493–1541) to Franz Anton Mesmer (1733–1815) to James Braid (1795–1860), who coined the term *hypnosis,* and Jean Martin Charcot (1825–1893) among others to the first giant in dynamic psychiatry, Sigmund Freud (1856–1939). His concepts of the unconscious, the ego, id, and super ego, defense mechanisms, and neurotic conflict have become an integral part of psychiatric thought. Some of these terms are now used on an everyday basis by the public as well. His emphasis on early life experiences as a determinant of later behavior was one stimulus among many for the increasing interest in psychological growth and development. Piaget's study of the development of the intellect is one example. Modification of Freudian psychoanalytic theory to include broader sociological and cultural influences is perhaps most prominently evident in the work of Erik Erikson.

More recently, a series of discoveries involving the brain, its neurophysiology and neurochemistry, have brought biology into modern psychiatry, along with descriptive (phenomenological), psychological, sociological, and cultural approaches. Today, when examining a given patient, the physician must be capable of thinking and working within these multiple frameworks of understanding human behavior, whether the behavior in question is molecular or molar. The term *biopsychosocial* is often used in this context.

EVALUATION

Concepts

When evaluating patients, certain critical concepts are essential to facilitate a complete diagnosis and a positive therapeutic outcome.

THE UNIFIED MIND, BRAIN, AND BODY

Modern clinicians in their thinking and in their approach to patients avoid the historical mind/brain/body trichotomy still inherent in our language system. They function from the thesis of empirical parallelism. With any human event, there is the component that is experienced, for example, any phenomenal event of seeing, hearing, thinking, wishing, and so forth. This **subjective** experience can be communicated to another with words. The other component of the event is that **observed** by those others outside the event. When these observations are consensually validated, we tend to call the evidence objective. An example is a neurophysiological or neurochemical response in the brain. By the parallelism thesis, these two components are not separate events, nor does one cause the other. A given thought does not cause a given neurophysiological response, nor does the neurophysiological event cause the thought. There is instead a single unitary event. In parallel, empirically, what I experience, you observe; what you experience, I observe.

This concept when applied to the clinical setting has very practical consequences. For example, we

will recognize that what the patient experiences is not necessarily what we see. What we see, the patient may not experience. The question of whether the patient's problem is a physical illness or an emotional illness is seen as an increasingly useless and potentially destructive dichotomous question. Only patients can experience their distress or declare their dis-ease. It is not the physician's task to decide whether someone is sick. The physician's task is to help the patient understand the disease process, and given that understanding, to help the patient with appropriate intervention. The mind/brain/body trichotomy can no longer be supported by the weight of scientific evidence. Physics has understood this for several decades. It is puzzling that biology and medicine have lagged so far behind. To hold this view, as unfortunately many physicians still do, is to risk inefficiency, ineffectiveness, and even harm to the patient.

MULTIPLE ETIOLOGY

Any event (or constellation of events) labelled disease is multiply determined. More often than not in medical practice it is no longer useful to assume that for a given effect there is a given cause. Rather, we deal with multiple causality, multiple factors, and multiple determinants in any disease process. Hence, multiple interventions at multiple levels are usually required.

THE INDIVIDUAL VERSUS STIMULUS–RESPONSE SPECIFICITY

These two concepts originate in physiology, but their theoretical scientific underpinnings derive from the fields of chaos and quantum mechanics, respectively. **Individual response specificity** states that before one can predict the response of a given human to a given stimulus, one must first understand the individual. Or, given a particular response, one can postdict the events leading to that response only by knowing the individual organism. Only in the individual is there a specific response to a specific stimulus. More often than not, this applies to the practice of medicine with most patients most of the time. The **stimulus–response specific assumption** states that a lawful, predictable relationship exists between the stimulus and the response; therefore, one can predict the response by simply knowing the stimulus or postdict the stimulus by knowing the response. Knowledge about a particular, unique individual is not required. A light falling on the eye will constrict the pupil. This model is very efficient and powerful when applicable. It has been and continues to be a valuable model in the development of scientific medicine. However, many physicians attempt to use this model, often unknowingly, when it simply does not apply. Understanding and distinguishing between these two models and knowing when one is more applicable than another is critical to the day-by-day, even moment-by-moment, practice of medicine. When employed appropriately, these two complimentary concepts shape the priorities of the doctor/patient interaction and enhance accuracy of evaluation and effectiveness of intervention.

Purpose

Although seemingly almost self-evident, it is useful nonetheless to keep in mind the various purposes of the interviewing–evaluating process. These may be outlined as follows:

1. To give patients the opportunity to express and share their distress
2. To observe and to elicit data
3. To establish rapport, an effective working relationship
4. To develop understanding of the disease in question *and* the patient with the disease
5. To exchange information with the patient
6. To develop a working contract and an intervention strategy and to effect implementation of that strategy

Process

A prerequisite for an effective evaluation process is an understanding of the doctor/patient relationship and a skill in developing that relationship. Another is in knowing how to utilize certain communication styles when interviewing. Finally, a fairly thorough knowledge of the phenomenology of mental processes is required. Given all the above, the interaction with a patient may proceed.

INTERVIEWING PRIORITIES

Usually the encounter begins with the patient and the physician confronting each other visually. Very early in the encounter, often with a glance, the physician determines whether or not there is an immediate medical emergency (*e.g.,* cardiac standstill). Next, observing the patient's behavior, the clinician makes a fairly early and accurate judgment

as to whether the patient is oriented. Evidence for the possibility of an organic mental disorder should have a major influence on the remaining interaction. Also relatively early in the interview, a skilled clinician can usually determine whether or not there may be a profound thought disorder by carefully listening to the patient's speech. In the overwhelming number of instances, there is no immediate medical emergency, the patient is oriented and does not demonstrate a thought disorder of psychotic proportions. In short, the physician has another "brain" with which to work. Then should come the question, "What is it that I would like to know next?" From the principle of individual response specificity, comes the answer, "I would like to know something fairly reliable about this particular individual." The royal road to understanding a given individual at a given moment is to conduct an inventory of that individual's primary emotions.

IDENTIFYING THE PRIMARY EMOTIONS AND OBTAINING CONGRUENCE

Let's take a specific example. A male family physician in an office setting introduces himself to his next patient and notes that she is in no acute medical distress and seems oriented. She appears to be in her mid-30s, is neatly and well dressed, is sitting on the edge of her chair with one foot ahead of the other and greets him with wide open eyes. She licks her lips and says at the height of inspiration, "I'm certainly glad to see you." Many physicians in this situation would then say something like, "Thank you. Well, what brings you to see me?" But a more efficient and a more effective response is something of the order, "Yes. Do you feel anxious?" With this the patient responds, "Frankly, Doctor, I'm more than anxious. I'm scared to death. A week ago, while riding my horse, I hit my head on the limb of a tree. I felt a little dazed but not anything else and I went on with the ride, but several days later I started having headaches unlike any kind of headaches I've ever had in my life and I'm worried that maybe I have a subdural hematoma like my younger sister had after an automobile accident."

This patient looks anxious or fearful. The physician wonders if she feels anxious. He structures his response accordingly. Indeed, through her words, it is clear; she feels anxious and fearful. In short, the objective and subjective evidence, the behavioral and the verbal evidence, are *congruent*. Psychologically healthy individuals in trusting situations "look how they feel and feel how they look." Also when patients are congruent, they characteristically have a very good idea why they are feeling the way they are feeling. If this information is not volunteered, the physician can ask and the answer usually can be taken at face value. This particular patient volunteers this information in a direct and succinct manner.

The first step, then, in an interview process, is to ask oneself questions about the patient's primary emotion: Do I hear words indicating that the patient is aware of this emotion? Do I see evidence that portrays this emotion? In short, is the patient congruent? If the patient presents objective evidence, for example, of anger, one must attempt to determine whether the patient is aware of feeling angry. If the patient states that he or she is feeling a particular way in the absence of objective evidence for that particular emotional state, the effective interviewer notes that discrepancy and often draws the attention of that incongruity to the patient. Patients with neurotic conflict tend to be incongruent in one fashion or another. Patients' words and behaviors often suggest the particular defense mechanisms whereby they either hide their feelings from others or hide their feelings from themselves. Such patients usually are not completely aware of the factors that precipitate the feeling as experienced or portrayed. However, this was not the case with our example.

ESTABLISHING CONSENSUS REGARDING THE STRESS

Once congruence is established, the patient and the physician usually can come to an agreement as to what may account for the distress fairly quickly. However, with many patients this can be difficult. They have been trained or have trained themselves not to show their distress or even to be aware of it. Usually, this is accomplished through the elaboration of a neurotic personality. Accompanying this structure is usually a lack of accurate awareness of the constellations of events, past and present, leading to the disease in question. In contrast, this patient, a genital character (psychologically healthy, nonneurotic), looks anxious, feels anxious, and knows why she is anxious and is ready to work toward a solution with the physician. The physician's response might be, "Your anxiety is understandable. From what you have told me so far, a subdural hematoma, while possible, is unlikely." Consensus is established. When effective physician interviewers are studied, they then tend to verbally summarize their understanding of the patient's *visit* before proceeding to the next step. (Please note that

this summary is not a summary of the present illness, and it is more than a restatement of the chief complaint!)

MAKING A CONTRACT

At this point in the process, effective physicians usually obtain the patient's *chief expectation.* In our example, the physician might say, "I take it you're here to get to the bottom of these different kind of headaches you're having." The patient nods and says, "Yes, indeed!" What follows is an explicitly stated understanding of how the two of them will work together to solve the problem, what length of time will be required for more detailed history taking, physical examination, the possibility of laboratory studies, and so forth. When this is accomplished, through an exchange of information, a decision is made as to the nature of the problem. This allows the final step in the process of a therapeutic interaction.

DEVELOPING A STRATEGY FOR INTERVENTION AND IMPLEMENTATION

The physician's particular knowledge of disease processes will be very helpful to the patient at this point. The patient's special knowledge of himself or herself, in turn, can be very helpful to the physician, as together they develop a strategy of intervention and create a specific plan for implementation. Each, then, proceeds to fill their particular role in that plan.

National competency examinations are paying increased attention to the measurement of interpersonal skills. By attending to the five process steps outlined above, a candidate may answer a whole series of questions on such examinations. (See the examples at the end of the chapter.) But more important, patient outcome research increasingly points to this particular sequence as enhancing therapeutic outcome. Training and practice are required for any physician to become an accurate diagnostician and an effective therapist, especially when the physician is working with the many patients who resist the process.

Structure

In the context of the doctor/patient interaction and during the process of effective interviewing as outlined above, the clinician keeps in mind an historical outline. During and after the interview, the physician organizes this history into a particular format. In the practice of psychiatry and behavioral medicine, the structural outline of a usual medical history is perfectly appropriate and will not be detailed here. The chief complaint or the presenting complaint is significant and usually easily obtained, but again, for effective interviewers, it is not their first concern. In the preceding example, if the physician's first response or inquiry was toward the chief complaint, the patient would undoubtedly have presented her headaches. Typically what would follow would be a whole series of questions and answers regarding the specific nature of the headaches. By paying attention first to the patient's emotional state, the patient volunteered very salient information, after which there can be the necessary medical interrogative interview and in *less* time and with a *better* outcome. In addition to the presenting complaint, information is gathered regarding the history of the presenting illness and the past personal and family medical history.

Especially when psychological factors seem particularly significant to the patient's problem or to the doctor/patient interaction, it is frequently very helpful, even necessary, to obtain a more detailed personal, familial, and social history. Special attention should be paid to growth and development issues, the history of present and past family relationships, an education and work history, and a history of leisure activities. Patients' descriptions of themselves as persons and patients' descriptions of their significant others as personalities are often of special value.

Also in the context of the interview process and while obtaining a history, a mental status examination is conducted. This is sometimes called the psychological or mental status examination. Various authors arrange the content somewhat differently; however, the following outline is presented since meaningful diagnostic implications can be drawn from dysfunction reflected in the various groupings.

1. Sensorium
   Consciousness: level and stability
   Orientation: four spheres of person, time, place, and situation
   Memory: immediate, recent, and remote
   Attention and concentration
   The first letters of these variables spell the *mnemonic* (memory aid) COMA, which is particularly meaningful since dysfunction in any of these four areas should alert the physician to a possible organic condition.

2. Thought process
   Production rate
   Continuity
   Dysfunctions of thought process have implications for the major psychotic-proportion affective and thought disorders, as well as organic brain syndrome.

3. Thought content
   Relationship to reality (autism or delusions)
   Concept formation: relative abstractability
   Intelligence
   Insight and judgment
   Characteristic topics
   These parameters are disrupted mostly in the major thought disorders, but also in affective psychotic conditions and organic brain syndromes.

4. Perceptions
   Hallucinations
   Illusions
   Dysfunction in perception should always alert the physician to possible organic substrates.

5. Emotional regulation
   Subjective and objective evidence for emotional states and relative congruence
   Ambivalence
   Appropriateness to thought content
   Disruptions here can accompany any major psychotic condition, especially thought disorders, but most commonly the problem lies within the realm of anxiety or depression spectrum disorders.

6. Relevant somatic functioning
   Sleep
   Appetite
   Weight
   Sexual functioning
   These are vegetative behaviors that, when dysfunctional in a syndrome complex, usually accompany affective disorders.

Some aspect of a physical examination is required for evaluation purposes in most, but not all, instances in a medical setting. Indeed, on many occasions a rather thorough physical examination is very much in order even if the patient presents primarily with what seems like an emotional or mental problem. This is particularly true if one suspects an organic mental disorder or a psychosomatic illness. Also in some patients, certain illnesses mimic conversion hysteria, just as conversion hysteria often mimics certain medical problems.

Evaluation Beyond History, Mental Status, and Physical Examination

INVOLVEMENT OF FAMILY, FRIENDS, AND OTHER HEALTH PROFESSIONALS

Perhaps next in significance to the evaluation of the patient is interviewing one or more members of the patient's family or friends. Their view of the problem can be extraordinarily valuable; their involvement with strategies for intervention may be crucial. This is especially true for children. A review of the patient's past medical records is also too frequently overlooked as is direct contact with other health professionals with whom the patient has worked.

PSYCHOLOGICAL TESTS

In some instances, formal psychological testing is helpful.

LABORATORY TESTS

When certain nosological entities are suspected, specific roentgenographic or laboratory tests are often indicated. These are covered under the various diagnostic headings in the clinical chapters.

ELECTROENCEPHALOGRAPHIC EXAMINATION

The electroencephalogram (EEG) is a recording of the electrical activity of the brain. Leads are attached to the scalp, and the brain waves are recorded. The amplitude of normal brain activity is from 20 μV to 70 μV.

Brain waves vary from 1 to 50 cycles/second. The most conspicuous activity is *alpha,* 8 through 13 cycles/second, especially seen in recordings from the occipital region. This rhythm tends to disappear when the eyes are opened, or when the subject is tense, engaged in mental activity, or experiencing considerable anxiety. In the normal waking population, *theta* activity is also seen, ranging from 4 to 7 cycles/second. *Delta* activity refers to waves under 4 cycles/second. Delta activity is very unusual in a normal waking person. When seen it suggests sleep, delirium, or diffuse brain damage. When slow wave activity seems to be localized over one area of the brain, it may suggest a space-occupying lesion. Fast activity beyond 13 cycles/second is called *beta* activity. Sudden bursts of high-voltage disordered activity different from background rhythm of paroxysmal nature are frequently seen in patients with epilepsy. Random activity from recordings over the temporal lobe is reported with increased frequency in patients with temporal lobe epilepsy, but many patients without any pathology whatsoever also show occasional spiking in these areas. Some patients with temporal lobe epilepsy have normal EEGs. A characteristic pattern is often seen with petit mal epilepsy, that is, a pattern of 3 cycles/second spike and wave activity (spike and dome pattern).

It is often stated that the EEG is not of particular value in psychiatry. While this may be true generally with the traditional recording techniques, sophisticated measurements involving computer analysis are making it clear that certain psychiatric illnesses are accompanied by dysrhythmias of one kind or another. Most of this work is still experimental and does not as yet have wide diagnostic or therapeutic application.

IMAGING STUDIES

Of increasing significance in psychiatry are the various imaging technologies—that is, computerized tomography (CT), magnetic resonance imaging (MRI), and positive emission transaxial (PET) scans.

NOSOLOGY

Disorders Usually First Evident in Infancy, Childhood, or Adolescence

MENTAL RETARDATION

Mental retardation is defined as lower than average general intelligence with resulting deficits or impairments in adaptive behavior. The four subtypes—mild, moderate, severe, and profound—have prognostic implications. Milder cases often are not diagnosed until scholastic difficulty is noted in grade school. They may attain a sixth-grade performance level. The moderate group is also educable, perhaps to the fourth-grade level. The severe are trainable to some degree. The profound require custodial care.

From 1% to 3% of the population of the United States is mentally retarded. The term *primary* designates those instances where no specific etiology can be identified or reasonably postulated. This constitutes the largest group, approximately 30% of the patient population. They usually have no other symptoms. There may be family history. All others are referred to as *secondary.* Perinatal infections, especially viral, and early childhood encephalitides cause about 20% of cases. Prematurity and birth trauma may account for another 20%. Causes may be categorized under **prenatal** factors, for example, phenylketonuria, Gaucher's disease, cretinism, Hurler's syndrome (gargoylism), and Down's syndrome (mongolism). About 10% of persons who are mentally retarded suffer from mongolism. **Perinatal** factors are a second category, for example, prematurity, birth injury, kernicterus. Examples of **postnatal** factors include viral meningoencephalitis, lead poisoning, and malnutrition. Sociocultural factors may play a role. Emotional problems and environmental deprivation may result in a picture sometimes called pseudo-mental retardation, a particularly important diagnosis to make. Prevention of retardation should be a special concern of all health professions. Treatment should focus on etiologic factors whenever possible. In the main, treatment means bringing appropriate support to the family and to the child, with particular attention to special classes in school or appropriate institutional or custodial care to those instances of profound retardation.

ATTENTION-DEFICIT HYPERACTIVITY DISORDER

Attention-deficit hyperactivity disorder is characterized by inattention, for example, having difficulty concentrating on school work; impulsivity; and, sometimes, hyperactivity. Onset is before age 7. The diagnosis should not be made unless symptoms have been present for at least 6 months. Parents report excessive activity and short attention span. Similar reports come from teachers. Present thinking about etiology points to central nervous system maturational factors interacting with environmental stresses. Treatment is directed toward parental counseling, education, environmental manipulation, and usually medication with methylphenindate or pemoline.

CONDUCT DISORDERS

The diagnosis of conduct disorder may be made in patients under 18 when there is a repetitive and persistent pattern of conduct for at least 6 months in which the basic rights of others are either ignored or violated. The behaviors may be **aggressive,** for example, physical violence against property or persons, theft, or **nonaggressive,** for example, a recurring and chronic tendency to violate rules, or lying. Another important distinction is whether the disorder is of the **undersocialized** or **socialized** variety. The undersocialized group fails to establish normal bonds of affection with others. In the socialized variety, there is evidence of emotional bonding or attachment to others, frequently to peers, often with considerable loyalty to the peer group (this variety previously was called group delinquent reaction). This disorder commonly is found in the slums of our large cities where security and self-esteem are found in antisocial acts supported by peers. Etiology relates primarily to faulty parental attitudes, poor child-rearing practices, emotional conflicts, and a variety of sociocultural factors. Intervention follows accordingly.

ANXIETY DISORDERS

The **separation anxiety disorder** is characterized by manifestations of excessive anxiety clearly relating to separation from a significant person to whom the child feels attached. Symptoms should be present for at least 2 weeks before this diagnosis is made.

The **avoidant disorder** (withdrawal reaction) of childhood or adolescence is characterized by persistent shrinking from contact with strangers, often to the degree that social functioning with peers may not occur. Usually there are satisfying relationships with family members. For diagnosis, symptoms should persist for 6 months.

The **overanxious disorder** involves symptoms of anxiety for at least 6 months. There is a generalized and persistent worry regarding future events or past behaviors or competence and generalized tension and self-consciousness. If the symptoms are present for a relatively short period of time and relate to a specific stress, the diagnosis of an **adjustment reaction** is usually more appropriate. Here, the symptoms persist and tend to be symptomatic of an underlying neurotic disorder. Various psychological and counseling techniques are indicated. Antianxiety medication generally should be avoided except in special cases and for brief periods of time.

EATING DISORDERS

Pica refers to the eating of nonnutritive substances repeatedly for at least one month.

Bulimia nervosa refers to recurrent episodes of binge eating of large quantities of food, often with termination by self-induced vomiting, repeated attempts to lose weight by severely restrictive diets or purging through laxatives, marked weight fluctuation, awareness that the eating pattern is abnormal, and a fear of being unable to stop, an overconcern about body shape and weight together with depression and self-deprecatory thoughts. This group is to be distinguished from those with anorexia nervosa.

Anorexia nervosa, more common in adolescent girls than boys, presents with all of the physiological findings of what is essentially self-induced starvation. The syndrome is not related to a known physical illness. The diagnosis should be considered when there is weight loss of at least 15% of the original body weight, a refusal to maintain body weight over a minimum normal for the age and height, and when there is an intense fear of becoming obese or a disturbance of body image. These patients may report feeling fat when objectively they are almost emaciated. Many feel quite energetic and may even engage in body-building exercises. Amenorrhea is common. Without effective intervention, there is significant mortality to this syndrome. Hospitalization may be necessary as a life-saving procedure. Intervention is often complicated because there is a tendency on the part of the patient and the family to deny the presence of serious psychological difficulties. With therapy severe conflicts regarding dependency and sexuality usually become apparent. No medication, to date, has been shown to be consistently effective.

STEREOTYPED MOVEMENT DISORDERS

Tics are to be distinguished from choreiform, dystonic, and athetoid movements. They are characterized as recurrent, involuntary, repetitive, purposeless movements. The patient is able to suppress the movement voluntarily for minutes to hours. A tic disorder may be subclassified either as *transient,* that is, at least a month but no more than a year, or *chronic.* The syndrome is usually thought to be psychogenic in origin, and hence counseling and psychotherapy are indicated.

A separate syndrome, relatively rare, is *Tourette's disorder.* The tics involve multiple muscle groups. There are frequently vocal tics as well, sometimes with compulsive and stereotyped coprolalia. Here also the movements may be suppressed for minutes to hours and symptoms vary in intensity over weeks to months. The criteria for diagnosis include the presence of symptoms for more than a year. Organic pathology of the central nervous system has consistently been suspected as playing a role in this disorder. To date, there is no reliable effective treatment, although recently haloperidol has been reported to be helpful in some cases.

OTHER DISORDERS WITH PHYSICAL MANIFESTATIONS

Stuttering is a syndrome for which there is considerable controversy regarding etiology and treatment. However, in some cases psychological factors clearly play a role and psychological intervention is effective. In others such is not the case.

Functional enuresis and *functional encopresis* are not due to a physical disorder by definition. They are manifested by the repeated, involuntary voiding of urine by day or night or the voluntary or involuntary passage of feces. One or both may be present. There should be a history of at least one event per month in children over age 4 or 5 for this diagnosis. Eighty to ninety percent of children are dry, that is, not enuretic by age 4½. By age 18, the percentage of enuretics in the general population drops to about 2%. With enuresis there is a growing opinion that causation in many cases may relate more to maturational or developmental factors than to classic psychodynamic considerations. Encopresis is much less common. When these symptoms appear transiently in essentially healthy young children in response to a specific stressful life event, the diagnosis of an *adjustment reaction* is more appropriate.

Sleepwalking and *sleep terrors* occur during non-REM (*r*apid *e*ye *m*ovement) periods of sleep, in contrast to nightmares. Nightmares have psychological significance but sleep terrors relate more to maturational lags in central nervous system (CNS) development than to psychodynamic factors, and reassurance and counseling to parents are in order.

PERVASIVE DEVELOPMENTAL DISORDERS

The child with *infantile autism* seems within his own world and out of reach. He lacks responsiveness to other people. There is a gross deficit in language development. Responses to environment are bizarre. Onset is before age 3. There is considerable controversy about etiology but a recent emphasis is on biological factors. Normal siblings are common. Patterns of interaction seen between parents and such children probably relate more to the parents' reaction to the frustration of dealing with such a child and should ordinarily be viewed in that context rather than seeing the interaction as pathogenic for the syndrome.

Pervasive development disorder is the current term for a group of patients whom earlier would have been called childhood schizophrenia. However, there is an absence of delusions, hallucinations, or marked loosening of association. What is seen is marked impairment in social relationships with lack of appropriate affective responsivity and poor verbal and nonverbal communication skills. Both of these diagnostic categories are relatively uncommon.

SPECIFIC DEVELOPMENTAL DISORDERS

Specific developmental disorders are to be distinguished from inadequate schooling, impaired vision or hearing, mental retardation, or infantile autism. The deficit may relate specifically to arithmetic or to spoken language. With language the problem may be primarily expressive or receptive or relating to articulation. Another category are those with a deficit related to the written or printed language. This is often called *dyslexia.* It tends to occur in children who have average or better than average intellectual endowment and achievement in non-language-related subjects. There are few if any positive signs on classical neurologic examination, and these are of the so-called "soft" variety. The diagnosis may be suspected by teachers. It should also be considered by physicians in children who may present with a variety of psychophysiological, behavioral, and emotional symptoms but symptoms that develop secondary to the stress of attempting to cope with what has heretofore been an unrecognized problem by peers, parents, and teachers. Learning disorders are quite common. What happens to these children depends on the support they get from their family, the kind of remedial help they receive from their school, plus their own capacity to learn coping techniques to compensate for the specific deficit.

OTHER ISSUES

Most children and adolescents that present to health professionals with psychological problems do *not* fall into one of the above categories. First, there are *age-appropriate behaviors* that are of concern to parents for whom educational techniques and reassurance are indicated. Examples include the expected stranger anxiety of 8 months, the oppositional behaviors of the 18- to 36-month-old toddler, the transient phobias of the 4- or 5-year-old and the insecurity and identity issues of early adolescence.

Second, many responses in children are most appropriately diagnosed as *adjustment disorders* in response to such environmental stresses as illness, hospitalization, surgery, divorce of parents, birth of siblings, loss of a playmate, difficulty in school, and so forth. These symptoms tend to be transient, especially when given support in a system by concerned others. The symptoms may be regressive to earlier behaviors such as thumb-sucking or wetting the bed. Or, depending on the age, the symptoms may be manifested as a conduct disturbance of one

kind or another or that group of symptoms that have been called neurotic traits.

Persistent neurotic behaviors with evidence for psychopathology in children or adolescents should be diagnosed as one of the neurotic disorders to be outlined and described later in this chapter. Schizophrenia essentially indistinguishable from that seen in young adulthood in onset can also develop in late childhood and early adolescence. Finally, many symptoms presented by children fall into the psychophysiological disorder category now categorized under *psychological factors affecting physical condition.*

Other issues of considerable concern to child psychiatry are such psychological problems as maternal deprivation, child abuse, the cultural aspects of delinquent behavior, and substance abuse in children and adolescents.

Organic Mental Disorders

SYNDROMES

A group of brain syndromes of organic etiology or presumed organic etiology are fairly well defined and recognizable. Each has multiple possible etiologies. These syndromes will be described first. We will then discuss more specific disorders linked to more specific etiologies.

Delirium. Delirium develops over a relatively short period of time, usually hours or days, and tends to fluctuate over the course of the day. Symptoms include clouding of consciousness, disorientation, memory impairment, frequent perceptual disturbances such as illusions or hallucinations, speech which may be incoherent, a disturbed sleep–wakefulness cycle, and either increased or decreased psychomotor activity. With this syndrome, as with all those that follow, from history, physical examination or laboratory tests, there is reason to believe that a specific organic factor may be etiologically related to the disturbance. Delirium is to be differentiated from acute schizophrenic illness. In general, acute visual hallucinations should suggest a delirium. Auditory hallucinations are more characteristic of schizophrenia. The type of thinking disorder typical of schizophrenia tends to be absent with organic delirium. Clouding of consciousness, typical of delirium, is absent in schizophrenia.

Dementia. With dementia, in contrast to delirium, there is not a clouding of consciousness, and symptoms usually develop over a longer period of time. There is evidence for loss of intellectual ability, memory difficulties (especially for recent memory), impairment of abstract thinking with substitution of concrete thinking, and impairment of judgment. Emotional lability is common. Other disturbances of higher cortical function such as aphasia, apraxia, and agnosia may be present. Often a personality change that tends to be an accentuation of premorbid personality traits is noted. Especially in elderly individuals, severe depression may be confused with dementia and vice versa. It is critical that this differential is made, since depression with treatment tends to have a better prognosis.

Amnestic Syndrome. With the amnestic syndrome, there is both short-term memory impairment and long-term memory impairment but in the absence of clouding of consciousness, as in delirium, and in the absence of general loss of major intellectual functions, as in dementia.

Organic Delusional Syndrome. In the absence of clouding of consciousness and loss of intellectual abilities and prominent hallucinations, delusions are the prominent clinical feature.

Organic Hallucinosis. Persistent or recurring hallucinations are the predominant feature.

Organic Mood Syndrome. Most prominent here is a mood disturbance, either of the manic or depressive variety.

Organic Anxiety Syndrome. This syndrome is characterized by either panic attacks or generalized anxiety. There is evidence of a specific organic factor etiologically.

Organic Personality Syndrome. This syndrome is characterized by a marked change in behavior or personality. Here, as with the organic hallucinosis and affective syndromes, there is absence of clouding of consciousness, as in delirium, and absence of significant loss of intellectual abilities, as in dementia.

Intoxication. This term is used when a substance-specific syndrome develops following the recent ingestion of that substance. Maladaptive behaviors such as disorientation, impaired judgment, and belligerence result from the impact of the substance on the central nervous system. Intoxication has many features comparable to delirium.

Withdrawal. This refers to the development of a substance-specific syndrome following the cessation of that substance or reduction of intake of that substance when previously used by the individual to induce a state of intoxication. Clinical features are similar to delirium or to other of the various organic syndromes.

DISORDERS

Alzheimer's Disease, Pick's Disease (Senile Dementia, Presenile Dementia). While this disease may begin at any age, it usually develops insidiously later in life. The final features are usually that of dementia but the disorder may begin as an amnestic syndrome. The dementia may be accompanied by delirium, delusions, or depression. From 5% to 15% of persons over 65 have dementia of this category. Throughout the world this disorder results in one of our most significant medical and sociologic problems. The precise etiology is unknown. In some families, there is a hereditary factor, which probably involves chromosome 21. The transmitter acetylcholine has been implicated in some studies. Neuronal degeneration occurs, producing amyloid deposits and neurofribrillary tangles. Early in the illness, the patient may be aware of losing previous capacity and may react to this loss with grief or depression. However, later in the course of the illness, patients often show little indication of being aware of their problem.

Multi-infarct Dementia. Most of the statements made above apply to this category of dementia as well. The syndrome is secondary to multiple infarcts. Symptoms may appear over a short period of time and not so insidiously as with Alzheimer's. Diagnosis is made by history and course and later by pathologic findings. Imaging studies are useful for diagnosis. Arteriosclerotic dementia is a diagnosis that is being used less and less as evidence increases that these so-called cases, when closely examined, tend to be either Alzheimer's disease or multi-infarct dementia.

Disorders Induced by Alcohol. Alcohol can produce the whole spectrum of organic brain syndromes described above. In addition to the very common *alcohol intoxication,* there is also *alcohol idiosyncratic intoxication,* in which there is a marked behavioral change with behavior atypical of the person when not drinking but behavior secondary to an ingestion of an amount of alcohol insufficient to induce intoxication in most individuals. The *alcohol withdrawal syndrome* (delirium tremens) is well known and may or may not be accompanied by delirium. The syndrome develops within 1 week of withdrawal and is characterized by a course tremor of hands or tongue, frequently nausea and vomiting, weakness, anxiety, depressed mood or irritability, orthostatic hypotension, and various signs of autonomic hyperactivity. While withdrawal may be limited to these symptoms, a delirium may be superimposed as may seizures. This illness without vigorous medical treatment has significant mortality. *Alcohol hallucinosis* may be confused with an acute schizophrenic illness. On withdrawal from alcohol, usually within 48 hours, there are vivid hallucinations, predominantly auditory. In contrast to delirium tremens, there is no clouding of consciousness. The *alcohol amnestic disorder* (blackouts) is a pathognomonic indicator of alcohol dependency. Prolonged, heavy ingestion of alcohol may also result in *dementia*.

Disorders Induced by Other CNS-Active Agents. *Barbiturates* may result in intoxication and withdrawal syndromes with or without delirium. The same can be said of almost any similarly acting sedative including the benzodiazepines. *Opioid intoxication* is usually accompanied with pupillary constriction and a change in mood, that is, euphoria, dysphoria, or apathy. *Opioid withdrawal* is characterized by pupillary dilation, lacrimation, rhinorrhea, piloerection, sweating, diarrhea, yawning, mild hypertension, tachycardia, insomnia, and fever. *Cocaine intoxication,* in addition to physical symptoms and signs of hyperactivity of the autonomic nervous system, often includes symptoms of psychomotor agitation or elation with elements of grandiosity or hypervigilance. *Amphetamines* or similarly acting sympathomimetic agents can result in intoxication, delirium, and withdrawal. The intoxication is similar to that of cocaine. The delirium and especially the accompanying delusional disorder may be very similar to an acute schizophrenic illness with rapidly developing persecutory delusions as a prominent feature. Withdrawal is characterized by depressed mood, disturbed sleep, and increased dreaming. *Phencyclidine* or similarly acting agents may result in intoxication or delirium. The *hallucinogens* may produce an hallucinosis or a delusional disorder or an affective disorder. Perceptual changes are characteristic of the hallucinosis with synesthesias, hallucinations, illusions, depersonalization, or merely the report of subjective intensification of perceptions, all occurring in a state of full wakefulness and alertness. Again, physiologic symptoms and signs, mainly of hyperactivity within the autonomic nervous system, frequently accompany this disorder. *Cannabis intoxication* is characterized by tachycardia, euphoria or apathy, a sensation of slowed time, and a subjective intensification of perceptions. Physical symptoms and signs often include increased appetite, dry mouth, and conjunctival injection. Cannabis can also result in a delusional disorder but one that does not persist beyond 6 hours following cessation of its use. Many other substances can produce intoxication and withdrawal, including *caffeine* and *tobacco* in sufficient doses.

Disorders Secondary to Other Etiologies. In addition to multi-infarct dementia and arteriosclerotic dementia, circulatory disturbances can result in a variety of organic brain syndromes. Acute cerebral infarction may include a deliriumlike syndrome in addition to focal signs. Bilateral lesions of the hippocampus may result in an amnestic syndrome. Any hypoxic state, whatever the etiology, can accentuate delirium or superimpose upon dementia an increased confusionlike state. Of particular interest are the confusional states following cardiac surgery.

In the category of metabolic and endocrine disorders, delirium is a feature of hepatic, uremic, and hypoglycemic encephalopathies, as is diabetic ketoacidosis. Symptoms of anxiety and emotional instability, even delirium, may accompany acute intermittent porphyria. Endocrine disorders, whether involving the thyroid, the parathyroid, or the adrenal gland can be accompanied by changes in personality and impairment of mental functions and memory. Myxedema may mimic depression or early dementia.

Huntington's chorea, although relatively rare, is a hereditary disorder characterized by choreiform movements and dementia that begins in adult life.

Normal-pressure hydrocephalus may be characterized by a progressive dementia. These patients have enlarged ventricles but normal cerebrospinal fluid pressure. There may be associated gait disturbances.

Brain trauma can present acutely as a delirium and over time a Korsakoff-like syndrome showing elements of amnesia and confabulation. Delayed sequelae, depending upon the nature of the trauma, and whether the trauma is repetitive, can result in the whole spectrum of brain syndromes.

Infections of the CNS or systemic infections frequently include features of delirium. If the CNS infection is more chronic, a dementia can result, the classic example being the general paralysis of the insane secondary to syphilis (dementia paralytica). Neuropsychiatric complications in patients with acquired immunodeficiency syndrome (AIDS) are common and of increasing concern.

Organic brain disorders may be associated with intracranial neoplasia.

Certain organic brain disorders may be associated with epilepsy. Following a grand mal seizure, the patient's confused state has features of delirium. Temporal lobe seizures may be difficult to differentiate from dissociative reactions. Some epileptics between seizures may show brief, interseizure psychotic episodes. The majority of these occur in cases of psychomotor epilepsy.

TREATMENT

Treatment of the organic brain syndromes should focus on the underlying etiology. The more specific medical treatments will not be reviewed here. But beyond this, certain guidelines regarding general management can be made.

With delirium in particular, general medical support measures are indicated—fluids, electrolyte balance, nutrition, and so forth. Sedatives and all other nonvital drugs should be discontinued. Precautions against suicide should be considered. Human contacts with others, especially friends, should be encouraged. Friends and personnel can be extremely helpful in providing reassuring, orienting verbal input. When the patient is awake the light should be on in the room. Avoid mechanical restraints if at all possible. Urge the patient to accept their hallucinations as bad dreams. If medication becomes necessary to manage agitated or aggressive destructive behavior, avoid barbiturates, and consider haloperidol 5 mg to 10 mg orally or intravenously or chlorpromazine beginning 10 mg orally three times a day, gradually increasing the dose, being attentive to the possible development of hypotension. Chlordiazepoxide is often helpful with alcohol withdrawal syndromes.

With the dementias, in addition to instituting a specific treatment aimed at a known etiology, general treatment should be focused on consulting with the patient's family, providing a protected physical and social environment, maintaining activity, and avoiding social isolation, physical isolation or immobilization. Appropriate supportive psychotherapeutic and environmental maneuvers can sometimes result in dramatic improvement. Again, depression can be superimposed on a dementia or be confused with it. Any medical illness can intensify the symptoms of dementia. Some patients with "dementia" improve dramatically when unnecessary medications are withdrawn or inappropriately high doses of medication are reduced.

Substance Abuse

Clinically, indicators of alcoholism (alcohol dependence) include a steady increase in alcohol intake or drinking sprees, solitary drinking, early morning drinking, and occurrence of blackouts. Operationally, an individual may be considered an alcoholic if he cannot stop the consumption of alcohol despite the fact that his drinking is clearly causing physical illness or repeated difficulty for him with his employer, his family, or the police. Two types of alcoholism have been characterized: type I, with passive dependent or anxious personality traits, having its onset usually after age 25; and type II, with antisocial traits with its onset before age 25. Multiple therapeutic approaches are utilized, including alcohol treatment programs in hospital and community settings, psychotherapeutic intervention in selected patients, the use of conditioned reflex treatment involving disulfiram (Antabuse), Alcoholics Anonymous, and other group therapies or support systems. Initially, denial is a major mechanism seen in most alcoholics. Many are experts in self-destruction and are skilled in manipulating their environment to provide a continuing source of alcohol. Many physicians have severe countertransference problems with these patients. Nonetheless, if the illness is viewed as a chronic one and intervention is persistent, the prognosis for many can be quite good.

The abuse and dependence on different drugs varies from time to time and from country to country. Many addicts state they take drugs to experience euphoria or to feel "normal" or to overcome states of depression. Narcotic addicts have a wide range of personality characteristics, but many are described as immature, impulsive, and emotionally unstable. Treatment programs, as with alcohol treatment programs, are multifaceted. Addicts Anonymous is modeled after Alcoholics Anonymous. Substitute programs in which, for example, methadone is substituted for heroin, are widely used but still seen by many as experimental and subject to increasing criticism in recent years. In the clinical setting, nalorphine (Nalline), an antagonist, may be used to test for evidence of readdiction. A current trend for individuals who abuse drugs is involvement with more than one agent.

Schizophrenic Disorders

Schizophrenia is one of the psychoses. A salient feature is a defect in reality testing that may be manifest in the schizophrenic's relationship to self, to the objects in the world, or to others. Bleuler distinguished between primary and secondary symptoms. The primary or fundamental symptoms include disturbances in associations (e.g., loosening, blocking, neologisms), disturbances in affect (disharmony or incongruity between ideas and emotion), ambivalence (multiple and contradictory feelings of extreme degree), and autism (preoccupation with self). Secondary or accessory symptoms include hallucinations, delusions, and bizarre behavior.

Modern criteria emphasize the thought disorder. The disorder may be so profound that speech is incoherent. Examination more commonly reveals tangentiality, loosening of association, or poverty of content of speech. A mixture of autistic and concrete thinking is common. This may be accompanied by blunted or inappropriate affect. Disorganized behavior is common. Delusions are bizarre in content. They may be somatic, grandiose, religious, nihilistic, or persecutory. Hallucinations, especially auditory hallucinations, may be evident. When one or more sets of these symptoms are accompanied by deterioration of previous level of functioning, whether relating to taking care of self, relating to significant others or to educational activities or work, and when these signs have been present for at least 6 months, the diagnosis is warranted. Differential diagnoses include the organic mental disorders and manic–depressive illness. The full-blown illness may be preceded by a prodromal phase with symptoms including social isolation or withdrawal, impairment in role functioning, peculiar behavior, impairment in personal hygiene, affect disturbances, thought disturbances manifested by vague, digressive, circumstantial or metaphysical speech, bizarre ideation, or magical thinking, and unusual perceptual experiences, which may not be diagnosable as clear hallucinations. Similar symptoms are seen in remission with or without treatment.

The currently recognized subtypes follow.

DISORGANIZED TYPE (HEBEPHRENIA)

In addition to the clinical picture outlined above, this relatively uncommon type shows blunted, inappropriate, and especially silly affect. Systemized delusions are characteristically absent and speech is frequently incoherent. Prognosis tends to be poor.

CATATONIC TYPE

Here the schizophrenia is determined by any of the following: catatonic stupor, catatonic negativism, catatonic rigidity or posturing, and catatonic excitement. Onset is often acute. Introjection is a common defense mechanism. Prognosis is relatively good.

PARANOID TYPE

The most common of the differentiated schizophrenias, the paranoid type, is dominated by persecutory or grandiose delusions or hallucinations with persecutory or grandiose content. Projection is a prominent defense mechanism.

UNDIFFERENTIATED TYPE

The category of "undifferentiated" is utilized when the criteria for schizophrenia are met, but when one of the above three differentiations is not in evidence.

RESIDUAL TYPE

The diagnosis of residual type is utilized when there has been the history of at least one previous episode of frank schizophrenia but on the present occasion, the clinical picture does not present prominent psychotic symptoms although there is continuing evidence of illness.

Schizophrenia constitutes the largest group of severe behavioral disorders in our culture. About 1% to 3% of the population are affected. It is seen most commonly in lower socioeconomic groups, especially in areas of high mobility and social disorganization. One explanation for the prevalence in these groups is the "downward drift" hypothesis, which essentially states that schizophrenic patients move toward such a lower socioeconomic categorization. Onset is usually in persons between 20 and 40 years of age although onset may be earlier. It is unusual for a first episode to appear after age 45. Long-term studies suggest that there is not a separate category of childhood schizophrenia and that schizophrenia in childhood or adolescence simply represents the earlier appearance of schizophrenic illness.

The etiology of schizophrenia is unknown. There is evidence for both a genetic component and a biochemical component. Various studies suggest left hemisphere dysfunction, a subgroup of patients with dilated ventricles, a high state of dopamine activity, especially with acute illness, and conversely a low state of dopamine activity in others, especially those with chronic illness. Psychodynamic formulations are many but currently focus on a disturbance of ego with an inability to differentiate between self and object and unusual sensitivity to sensory input. Psychoanalytic theory views the logic of schizophrenia as primary process thinking and sees similarity to the associative patterns present in dreams and in fantasies, especially those of imaginative children.

Two broad categories of schizophrenia have been proposed: *process* schizophrenia, a variety in which the illness begins at a younger age and progresses slowly, seemingly inevitably toward a final state of deterioration, and *reactive* schizophrenia, which begins temporally in relationship to a traumatic event and is often of acute onset. The latter seemingly has a better prognosis. In fact, if a patient is hospitalized for less than 3 months with the first illness, the remission rate is at least 75%. If the patient has been hospitalized for over 2 years, the remission rate is approximately 1% to 2%.

Treatment is empirical. Hospitalization during the acute illness is often required. Although difficult to obtain, the development of a trusting doctor/patient relationship that can be maintained over time seems particularly important whereby the physician, so to speak, becomes an auxiliary reality tester for the patient and helps the patient in a growing-up process. The absence of a familial or community support system seems to trigger exacerbation of illness and rehospitalization. Today, every schizophrenic patient should also be given an adequate trial of pharmacologic treatment, usually one of the phenothiazines.

Other Psychotic Disorders

Some patients who are psychotic do not present with the full picture of schizophrenia, but show persistent persecutory delusions or delusions of jealousy with emotion and behavior appropriate to the content of these delusions but without prominent hallucinations. There is no evidence of organic mental disorder nor are the criteria for the manic–depressive syndrome present. If the illness is of at least 2 months' duration, the diagnosis *paranoid disorder* is made.

The diagnosis *schizophreniform disorder* according to modern evidence and thought is the appropriate appellation for patients who present with the symptoms of schizophrenia but in whom the illness, while lasting more than 2 weeks, has been present less than 6 months. Since many patients with such an acute illness recover without recurrence, labelling such individuals as schizophrenics is inappropriate. Frequently this disorder is in reaction to an acutely stressful life event. Patients with a borderline personality seem particularly subject to such responses.

Some patients seem to have a mixture of schizophrenia and a major affective disorder with symptoms such that neither diagnosis can clearly be made. For some clinicians, the diagnosis *schizoaffective disorder* is utilized. There is controversy as to whether such a category is warranted or not.

Affective Disorders

The principle and characteristic feature of the affective disorders is a disturbance of mood, especially depression, but mania or hypomania, anxiety, and anger may be present as well. These patients may be psychotic.

MAJOR AFFECTIVE DISORDERS

A *manic episode* is characterized by a distinct period of an elevated or expansive or irritable mood. Duration is at least of 1 week. In addition to the mood disturbance, there are frequently several or more of the following: increase in activity or physical restlessness; increased talkativeness; flight of ideas or at least the subjective experience that thoughts are racing; inflated self-esteem to the point of grandiosity; seemingly decreased need for sleep; distractability; and an excessive involvement in activities that have a high potential for painful consequences, such as buying sprees, sexual indiscretions, and so forth. In some patients, this may be accompanied with psychotic features, that is, impairment in reality testing with delusions, hallucinations, or bizarre behavior. Many patients with a manic episode do not present with psychotic features.

A *major depressive episode* is characterized by dysphoric mood or anhedonia (loss of interest or pleasure in usual activities and pastimes). The patient may describe the mood as depressed, sad, down in the dumps, irritable. A sense of helplessness and hopelessness is very common as is guilt and such accompanying emotional states as anxiety and anger. These symptoms should be present nearly every day for a period of at least 2 weeks. They are accompanied by several of the following: poor appetite and significant weight loss or, in some patients, increased appetite with significant weight gain; insomnia or, in some patients, hypersomnia; psychomotor agitation or retardation; loss of interest in usual activities or decrease in sexual drive; loss of energy, a sense of fatigue; feelings of worthlessness, self-reproach with excessive or inappropriate guilt; complaints of diminished ability to think or concentrate; recurring thoughts of death or suicidal ideation or a history of a suicide attempt.

There may be psychotic features with delusions and hallucinations. When the subjective experience of depression is particularly severe, when the depression is particularly worse in the morning and often accompanied by early morning awakenings as well as psychomotor retardation or agitation and significant anorexia or weight loss, and profound guilt, the term *melancholia* is often used.

Bipolar Disorder (Manic–Depressive Illness). Patients in this category over time show features cyclically of both manic episodes and depressed episodes. In some individuals, depressive episodes predominate and in others manic episodes predominate. In a smaller percentage, the episodes are intermixed, rapidly alternating every few days.

Major Depression (Unipolar, Endogenous). Patients with this type of affective disorder meet the requirements of a major depressive episode as described above but have never had a manic episode.

More than one half of patients with bipolar disorders become ill prior to age 30. Unipolar onsets reach their peak in the 40s. Bipolar disorders are equally predominant in men and women. Manic episodes typically begin more suddenly than depressive episodes and may last from a few days to months but tend to be briefer in duration than depressive episodes. In some patients, perhaps 20%, the course seems chronic. Epidemiologic evidence suggests that about 20% of females and 10% of males will have a depressive episode sometime in life with hospitalization required in about 6% of females and 3% of males.

The precise etiology of this disease is unknown. There is good evidence that the illness is familial and for some there is a genetic component, especially those with bipolar illness. There is also evidence of a disturbance in those neurotransmitter systems especially utilizing the catecholamines.

Depending on the severity of the illness, treatment may involve electroshock therapy (EST), drug therapy, or psychotherapy. Electroshock is particularly efficacious in a high percentage of patients with depression. Most clinicians utilize EST after an unsuccessful trial of drug intervention. Phenothiazines, especially haloperidol, may be initially useful in manic states. Lithium, however, is the treatment of choice in bipolar disease, especially to effect prevention of manic episodes. Lithium may also be useful in the treatment of some patients with recurring unipolar depression. However, a full trial of an antidepressive tricyclic drug is the treatment of choice for major depression. Psychotherapy is *extremely* difficult and is usually disappointing if there is the expectation of significant improvement in mood or energy level. However, studies do show that patients can show significant improvement in self-esteem and in their interpersonal relationships. Also the relationship established with the physician facilitates psychopharmacologic intervention.

OTHER AFFECTIVE DISORDERS

Cyclothymic Disorder (Cyclothymic Personality). Some patients present with a history of numerous periods in which symptoms characteristic of both depressive and manic syndromes are present but not of such severity to meet the criteria of either a major depressive or manic episode. These episodes are also separated by periods of normal mood that may last for months. While some patients may proceed over time to frank bipolar illness, many do not and these tend to be viewed as individuals who have developed this personality disorder in response to psychologic factors.

Dysthymic Disorders (Depressive Neurosis). Current criteria for this diagnosis require at least a 2-year history of symptoms characteristic of a depressive syndrome most of the time but not of such severity to meet the criteria for a major depressive episode. There may be periods of normal mood lasting for a few days to a few weeks. There are clearly no psychotic features. This diagnostic entity is more common than bipolar or unipolar disease in primary care settings. While some patients benefit from antidepressant medication, many do not. In fact, some seem even worse. Psychotherapy is the usual mode of treatment. In recent years, careful studies evaluating the effectiveness of psychotherapy show distinct benefit compared to control groups, and in some studies psychotherapy alone shows better outcome than psychotherapy plus antidepressant medication. Psychotherapy seems particularly helpful when the depression has been triggered by an identifiable life stress. The term *reactive depression* is often used in this instance. A careful study of these patients often suggests a vulnerability to certain kinds of stress, especially loss, through earlier life events and the elaboration of a particular character structure. Introversion is a common defense mechanism. Some patients' complaints especially in primary care settings, are primarily somatic. If treatment is focused only on the somatic complaints, improvement at best is only transitory. The underlying depression must be recognized and treated. Some clinicians see these patients as suffering from a *depressive equivalent.*

Many, maybe most, patients in ambulatory primary care settings whose complaints suggest depression do *not* represent patients who fall into *any* of the above diagnostic categories. Many patients who speak of themselves as depressed have experienced losses and are responding appropriately with grief. We are speaking here of **uncomplicated bereavement.** Therapy facilitating the grief work is the physician's major responsibility. Others are responding to an identifiable stressor, often a loss, in a maladaptive way, and the diagnosis **adjustment disorder with depressed mood** is appropriate. Here again, psychotherapeutic intervention is indicated and rarely psychopharmacologic. Finally, a number of physical conditions may be accompanied by depression, including carcinoma of the lung, carcinoma of the head of the pancreas, myxedema, and so forth. Certain drugs can precipitate a depressive syndrome (*e.g.,* reserpine). The appropriate diagnosis in these instances is an **organic affective disorder,** and such patients should be treated accordingly. Again, in older individuals depression may mimic or accompany dementia.

All in all, depression is one of the most common complaints bringing patients to physicians. Some studies indicate that it is *the* most common complaint. Other studies suggest anxiety, and still others, depending on the season, list upper respiratory complaints. A final reminder—depression should alert the physician to evaluate the risk for suicide.

Anxiety Disorders

This nosological category and several that follow represent disturbances or disorders that previously have been called the psychoneuroses. These disorders do not show gross disturbances of reality testing nor severely antisocial behavior and in the main are determined by environmental factors. The factors in part are in the present, those precipitating stresses that immediately precede an exacerbation of psychoneurotic symptoms. These factors also relate to the past when environmental influences acting on the infant or the child produced a defect in personality development, leaving the person vulnerable to the later elaboration in adult life of neurotic patterns of response. To a degree, the childhood experience for all of us becomes the paradigm for all experiences that follow.

Key to understanding psychoneurosis is the concept of conflict, conflict that may be partially conscious but that is predominately unconscious. An individual must be carefully evaluated to determine what, in fact, represents a significant conflict and

beyond that, a conflict related to a neurotic disorder. Conflict tends to develop around the issues of dependency, aggression, sexuality, or some mixture thereof. Subjective and objective evidence for emotions during the evaluation frequently suggests the nature of the conflict, especially those emotions experienced or displayed when discussing significant present situations reminiscent of past events and those linked to the exacerbation of neurotic symptomatology.

PHOBIC DISORDERS (PHOBIC NEUROSIS)

With phobic disorders, repression followed by isolation and displacement are characteristic defense mechanisms. In some patients, the neurotic response evolves from those conflict issues typical of a child from age 3 through age 6 years. Premorbidly an avoidant or compulsive personality is common. Phobias have a higher prevalence rate than *any* other disease.

Agoraphobia. These patients have a marked fear of and thus avoid being in public places from which there may be no immediate escape. They usually restrict their normal activities to the point that avoidance behavior dominates their life. To venture forth is to experience overwhelming incapacitating anxiety. One group of patients have a history of severe panic attacks while another group do not. In the group with panic attacks especially, the panic attacks often occur without evidence of there being a particular understandable situational stress related to a particular underlying conflict. The individual's response to these panic attacks is to become increasingly phobic. Management of the panic attacks with imipramine together with appropriately structured psychotherapy may be the treatment of choice for this particular group.

Social Phobia. These patients experience a persistent, irrational fear of and a desire to avoid a situation in which they are exposed to possible scrutiny by others. The patient recognizes that the fear is excessive or unreasonable but feels powerless to effect change.

Simple Phobia. Here the irrational fear is of an object or a situation other than being away from home (agoraphobia) or anxiety regarding social situations (social phobia). Fear of animals, heights, and close spaces are examples. Again, the patient recognizes that the fear is excessive or unreasonable. Therapy may include dynamic psychotherapy, the technique of reciprocal inhibition, or behavioral therapy employing some schedule for desensitization.

ANXIETY STATES (ANXIETY NEUROSIS)

Panic Disorder. With this disorder the patient presents with a history of distinct panic attacks, which occur in the absence of a life-threatening situation or marked physical exertion. The patient describes subjective awareness of anxiety, apprehension, or fear and usually reports several or more physical symptoms, which are in the category of the typical psychophysiological manifestations of anxiety, such as dyspnea, palpitations, sweating, trembling, and so forth. For a subgroup of patients, there is a family history, a genetic factor probably is present etiologically, and management of the panic attacks requires pharmacologic intervention. Psychotherapy, itself, does not stop the attacks in this group of patients.

Generalized Anxiety Disorder. This disorder is characterized by the manifestations of anxiety either consistently present or frequently recurring. The patient may report a subjective awareness of this anxiety, using such expressions as fear, afraid, apprehension, worry, and so forth; or describe feeling constantly on the alert, dreading some unknown and unidentified danger or tragedy; or report various of the psychophysiological manifestations of anxiety (*e.g.*, sweating, feeling cold, clammy hands, lightheadedness, or a combination of these various groups of symptoms). Patients who report the physiologic manifestations of anxiety may deny feeling apprehensive, anxious, or fearful. Other patients who describe overwhelming fear and anxiety may not in fact look fearful or anxious to the physician. Psychotherapeutic intervention will be different for the different subgroups described. However, even when the patient feels anxious and reports the symptoms of anxiety and appears anxious to the physician, the patient rarely understands the basis for the anxiety, or if he or she does link it to a particular situation or event, the linkage does not make sense to him or her. Anxiety is an extraordinarily common complaint of patients in primary care ambulatory settings. This disorder is to be distinguished from normal fear of real life-threatening situations or from an adjustment reaction manifested by anxiety. Certain illnesses mimic this disorder (*e.g.*, hyperthyroidism, mitral valve prolapse syndrome, pheochromocytoma); however, the description of the symptoms by these patients are qualitatively different (*e.g.*, they describe their symptoms as feeling *as if* they were afraid). Repression and denial are common defense mechanisms. Some hold that the neurotic personality structure (often a histrionic personality) and the neurotic symptoms frequently date to those conflicts and issues typical of children ages 4 through 7. Psychopharmacologic agents if used should be used judiciously and then for only brief periods. Some form of psychotherapy ordinarily is the treatment of choice.

Obsessive–Compulsive Disorder (Obsessive–Compulsive Neurosis). Obsessions or compulsions become a significant source of distress to the individual to a degree that they interfere with social or role functioning. These patients are particularly distressed in knowing their symptoms are irrational. Reaction formation, undoing, and overintellectualization are typical defense mechanisms. The premorbid personality sometimes is a compulsive personality, which in many patients dates to particular responses to conflicts and issues of childhood typical of ages 1½ to 3. Frequently the patient presents behaviorally as a clean, neat, overly polite individual who speaks in a rather controlled and guarded fashion. While subjective awareness of anxiety and sadness may be present, there is typically an absence of evidence for anger. In fact, many patients either take pride in the infrequency of their experiencing anger or express considerable fear of it. Psychotherapy is often the treatment of choice, but the course may be quite long and difficult. Recent reports implicate the serotonin transmitter systems and antiserotonin agents may reduce symptoms.

POSTTRAUMATIC STRESS DISORDER

The recently recognized syndrome of posttraumatic stress disorder seems to merit a separate diagnostic category. In response to a specific recognizable stressor that would tend to evoke symptoms of distress in almost anyone, these patients, however, *continue* to reexperience the trauma. This is manifest through either recurring dreams, or intrusive recollections of the event, or subjective sensations that the event is occurring again, triggered in association to an environmental or thought stimulus reminiscent of the trauma. Examples of typical stressors include accidents, combat, surgery, deaths, and so forth. In addition, these patients report a numbing of responsiveness to the external world manifest by marked diminished interest in previously significant activities and subjective feelings of detachment or estrangement from significant others. There are frequently exaggerated startle responses, sleep disturbances, guilt about surviving when others have not, trouble concentrating, avoidance behavior toward activities that might trigger recollection of the event, and intensification of symptoms by exposure to events that symbolize the traumatic occurrence. Some form of psychotherapy is the preferred treatment, together with group therapy. Prognosis is usually good with early intervention.

Somatoform Disorders

SOMATIZATION DISORDER (BRIQUET'S SYNDROME)

Briquet's syndrome is characterized by multiple somatic complaints not adequately explained by physical disorder, injury, or side effects of medication or drugs. These patients typically report that they have been sickly all or a good part of their life. Complaints include symptoms that might fall into the conversion or pseudoneurologic category (*e.g.*, loss of voice, double vision, muscle weakness, difficulty urinating), gastrointestinal symptoms (*e.g.*, abdominal pain, nausea, bloating), female reproductive symptoms (*e.g.*, painful menstruation, menstrual irregularity, severe vomiting through pregnancy), psychosexual symptoms (*e.g.*, pain during intercourse, sexual indifference, lack of pleasure during intercourse), pain (*e.g.*, in back, joints, extremities), and cardiopulmonary symptoms (*e.g.*, shortness of breath, palpitations, dizziness). Current diagnostic criteria require at least a dozen of such symptoms and a history of several years' duration beginning before age 30. There may be a genetic disposition to this disorder. There is often a family history of a similar syndrome, especially in female relatives, or antisocial behavior, especially in male relatives, or alcoholism. A history of multiple trials of medications without significant change in symptomatology is common. Pharmacotherapy seems to have little value. These patients are very resistent to treatment.

CONVERSION DISORDER (HYSTERICAL NEUROSIS, CONVERSION TYPE)

Conversion disorder is characterized by an involuntary psychogenic loss or disorder of function often suggesting a physical illness. Symptoms typically are limited to impairment of motor or sensory functions (*e.g.,* blindness, paresthesia, paralysis), but also may involve the autonomic system to a lesser degree. Symptoms characteristically begin and end suddenly. Often symbolic of an underlying conflict, the symptoms solve, so to speak, the underlying dilemma. In psychodynamic terms, this is called the ***primary gain***. A ***secondary gain*** is often superimposed, such as avoiding some unpleasant

activity, obtaining additional attention from significant others, avoiding responsibility, and so forth. Many patients give the impression of being naive, behave in a seductive fashion toward the examiner, or may seem strangely indifferent or aloof to their symptomatology (*la belle indifference*) and yet under certain circumstances demonstrate poor emotional control. These patients are frequently misdiagnosed as malingerers by the general medical profession. Repression, denial, and dissociation are common defense mechanisms. It is not unusual for a patient to have few if any memories prior to age 6 years. A premorbid histrionic character is common, frequently with an underlying sexual conflict reminiscent of the Oedipal conflict of ages 4 through 7 years. Psychotherapeutic intervention may be dramatically successful especially early in the course of the illness. Hypnotherapy may be especially helpful in some patients. If symptoms have been present for months or years, therapy becomes difficult.

PSYCHOGENIC PAIN DISORDER

Here the predominant feature is severe, prolonged pain, often inconsistent with the anatomic distribution of the nerves, in the absence of organic pathology or when there is organic pathology the pain is grossly in excess of what would be expected from findings. Psychological factors are judged to be etiologically involved in the genesis of the pain. Some clinicians would see this syndrome as being a variation of a conversion disorder. Except for the symptom presentation, many of the statements made above would apply to this category as well.

Some of these patients develop a ***chronic benign pain syndrome*** (a term used by many authors). Patients with chronic depression constitute another major group. Many utilize multiple medications in large doses. Some in fact are addicted. An intensive multidisciplinary treatment approach is required with individual, group, and family therapy and a conservative approach toward pharmacotherapy. This syndrome is attracting increasing attention for many reasons, one of which is that a high percentage of resources from the health arena is devoted to this group of patients.

HYPOCHONDRIASIS (HYPOCHONDRIACAL NEUROSIS)

The predominant disturbance here is an unrealistic interpretation of physical signs or sensations as abnormal, leading the patient to a preoccupation with the fear of having or the belief in having a serious disease, a disease that tends in their view to go unrecognized by family and physicians. The malady causes considerable social and occupational impairment, tends to persist despite medical reassurance that no such disease exists, and often becomes the central theme around which the family is organized. In this manner control and attention are obtained simultaneously. Patients, therefore, tend to have serious conflicts in the area of dependency and aggression. Considerable psychotherapeutic skill is needed in working with this group of patients.

Dissociative Disorders (Hysterical Neurosis, Dissociative Type)

Subgroups in this category include psychogenic amnesia, psychogenic fugue, multiple personality, and depersonalization disorder (depersonalization neurosis). All are predominately psychogenic in origin. *Amnesia* refers to the sudden inability to recall important personal information that is too extensive to be explained by forgetfulness. A *fugue* is characterized by the assumption of a new identity by the patient, often traveling away from home or usual place of work with inability to recall the past. During a fugue a patient may seem to behave normally to the casual observer. *Multiple personality* is defined as the existence within a given individual of two or more distinct personalities, each of which predominates at a particular time. Many statements made about patient characteristics, etiology, and treatment under the conversion disorder apply to this group as well. Patients with multiple personality usually have a very complex personality structure and considerable psychotherapeutic skill is required for a successful outcome. They often have a history of severe and recurrent abuse as a child, physical and/or sexual. Frequently, that history becomes evident only during therapy.

Patients with a *depersonalization disorder* respond to neurotic conflicts in such a manner that they experience parts of their bodies as not belonging to them or greatly expanded or changed in size or shape, or they may experience themselves as unreal, phony, in a fog, and so forth. The experience is often transient and in response to a meaningful life event but usually not recognized as such by the patient. When severe, patients may seem psychotic. Symptoms of derealization may or may not accompany the depersonalization, that is, the sensation or feeling that the surround is strange or unreal. Depersonalization is also experienced

with sleep deprivation, and by individuals under severe and prolonged stress, *e.g.,* tortured prisoners of war.

Psychosexual Disorders

Current nosology categorizes psychosexual disorders into the *gender identity disorders,* including trans-sexualism and gender identity disorder of childhood; the *paraphilias,* including fetishism, tranvestism, zoöphilia, pedophilia, exhibitionism, voyeurism, sexual masochism, sexual sadism; and the psychosexual dysfunctions. Ego-dystonic homosexuality is also considered a psychosexual disorder by some, though no longer included in DSM-III R. Ego dystonia refers to the fact that the individual is uncomfortable with and does not want a particular set of symptoms. In this instance, the patient wishes not to be a homosexual in terms of fantasy, sexual arousal, or overt behavior. Behaviors that are ego syntonic do not cause subjective distress.

More commonly, the disorders seen in medical practice are as follows. Categories include *inhibited sexual desire.* Here, the patient reports a persistent and pervasive inhibition of sexual interest. Often the patient does not experience this as a source of personal distress; the report of distress comes from the partner. Next is *inhibited sexual excitement or arousal.* Here, the patient reports sexual interest, but for males there is partial or complete failure to attain or maintain erection throughout the sexual act and for females the partial or complete failure to attain or maintain the lubrication and swelling response of sexual excitement throughout the act. *Inhibited female orgasm* relates to a recurring and persistent pattern of delay or absence of orgasm, although there has been normal sexual excitement. *Inhibited male orgasm* is similarly defined. *Premature ejaculation* refers to ejaculation occurring before the individual wishes it because of an inability to bring reasonable voluntary control of ejaculation to the sexual act. Obviously the term *reasonable control* requires clinical judgment. This diagnosis is probably made too frequently by both physicians and their patients. A patient may insist that he is a premature ejaculator, yet upon careful inquiry the length of time or the number of sexual thrusts during intercourse is at or above average. *Functional dyspareunia* refers to pain during intercourse of psychogenic origin. This diagnosis also is made too frequently. Discomfort may occur because the penis is inserted before the female has reached the plateau phase; communication between partners solves this problem. Foreplay may take place with the patient exclusively on her back and introital lubrication does not take place given the slant of the vagina. In some women, with deep penetration, penile thrusting impinges on the cervix, causing pain; here a change in position of intercourse effects a solution. For all these circumstances, educational counseling is indicated. Major psychogenic factors may not be playing a role. *Functional vaginismus* refers to voluntary spasm of the musculature of the outer one third of the vagina hindering or preventing insertion. In some patients, this is essentially a conversion reaction. In others it has become a learned response. Psychotherapy is probably the treatment of choice for the former group, behavior therapy for the latter group.

All of the diagnostic categories under psychosexual dysfunction are disturbances not caused exclusively by organic factors. In fact psychogenic factors predominate. Anxiety regarding the sexual act or hostility between partners is the typical psychodynamic picture. Commonly symptoms may be present with one partner but not another. Or historically symptoms may not be present before marriage but may appear after marriage. The reverse is just as frequent. In some instances an unresolved Oedipal problem plays a dynamic role. In others, the symptoms seem to result from early life messages that the individual was not to assume an adult sexual role or that the sexual act in some fashion was ugly or dirty. When evaluating these patients, especially patients in whom functional dyspareunia and inhibited orgasm are suspected, a careful medical work-up including history and laboratory tests is indicated, since a number of medical conditions may first be manifest with one of these problems as the primary symptom. Penile erection studies are increasingly being utilized in this regard. Full erections take place during REM sleep. If such are reported or demonstrated, erectile difficulties are most likely psychogenic in origin.

Adjustment Disorder (Transient Situational Reactions)

The diagnosis of adjustment disorder should be used frequently, especially in primary care settings. These patients present with mental, emotional, or behavioral symptoms in response to a given life event, but the criteria of the diagnostic categories outlined above are not met. However, there is evidence of a maladaptive reaction to an identifiable social stressor within 3 months of the onset of the stressor. The maladaptive nature of the reaction is indicated by impairment in social or occupational function or by symptoms that seem in excess of a normal or an expected response to such a stressor. With this diagnosis it is assumed that the symptoms would remit should the stressor cease or a new level of adaptation achieved should the stressor persist.

Depending on the predominant manifestation, the diagnosis of adjustment disorder is modified by one of the following self-explanatory phrases: with anxious mood, with depressed mood, with mixed emotional features, with disturbance of conduct, with mixed disturbance of emotions and conduct, with work or academic inhibition, with withdrawal, and finally with atypical features. These disorders are to be distinguished from normal fear, anger, or grief responses to the stresses of injury, frustration of real need, or loss, respectively.

Most patients with adjustment disorders can be helped with supportive or educational psychotherapy or counseling. In general, pharmacotherapy is not indicated nor is referral for intensive psychotherapy. If a new level of adaptation does not occur or if symptoms persist or become worse, then the diagnosis of adjustment disorder no longer applies; the diagnosis should be changed and treatment strategies developed accordingly.

Psychological Factors Affecting Physical Condition (Psychophysiological Disorders)

Psychologically meaningful environmental stimuli may be temporally related to the initiation or exacerbation of physical conditions, conditions that either have a demonstrable organic pathology or a known pathophysiologic process. An example of the latter would be tension headaches and of the former, ulcerative colitis. A great number of patients fall into this category. The pathophysiology of such illness is increasingly well known and will not be reviewed in detail here. Psychologically significant events or trains of events often linked to situations or events reminiscent of childhood or adolescence are interpreted in the cortex. Then, with involvement of the limbic system, the hypothalamic/pituitary/adrenal axis and the hypothalamic/autonomic nervous system axis trigger pathophysiologic responses or accentuate existing pathologies. Many patients have difficulty in understanding how psychological or social factors can contribute to their illness. A trusting relationship with their physician is of prime importance as is skill in communicating this understanding. Even then patients frequently do not recognize their conflict areas or area of stress. In fact in many instances it is difficult for the clinician to determine these as well. A careful psychosocial history relative to the onset of the illness or the exacerbations or remissions in the illness may be clues in this regard, as may the patient's utilization of "body language," that is, such figures of speech as "pain in the neck," "he makes me sick to my stomach," "it just breaks my heart," and so forth. Therapeutic intervention often requires the cooperation of a number of medical specialties. In addition to traditional medical management, the use of psychotropic medication, behavioral modifying techniques, and psychotherapy may be utilized as well. The following represents a brief outline of the organ systems to which disorders of this category may apply.

SKIN DISORDERS

Psychological factors are prominent in patients with dermatitis factitia, trichotillomania, pruritus, and neurodermatitis and may be significant with alopecia, urticaria, rosacea, psoriasis, herpes, and hyperhidrosis, as well as others.

MUSCULOSKELETAL DISORDERS

Musculoskeletal tension headache is one of the most common symptoms of mankind. Similarly, pain involving skeletal musculature elsewhere whether in the chest or in the back or in the extremities can result from similar underlying psychophysiological mechanisms. Immunologic abnormalities seem significant in rheumatoid arthritis, but it should be remembered that stress reactions acting through the hypothalamus can affect immune mechanisms. The common observation that some patients with rheumatoid arthritis have exacerbations of symptoms under emotional stress should not be ignored.

RESPIRATORY DISORDERS

The hyperventilation syndrome is the most common syndrome in this category. Frequently it is a manifestation of underlying anxiety. However, depressed patients may hyperventilate, and hyperventilation may be a learned response without there necessarily being an underlying psychodynamic conflict of major significance. Psychological factors also seem to play a role in some patients with bronchial asthma and some patients with vasomotor rhinitis.

CARDIOVASCULAR DISORDERS

Some patients with an underlying anxiety syndrome or acute sensitivity to body sensations may become aware of their cardiac function and become alarmed at what is essentially normal tachycardia. Emotional factors may play a role in certain cardiac arrhythmias. The precise relationship between anxiety syndromes and the mitral valve prolapse syndrome requires further study. Certain categories of patients with hypertension, when studied psychiatrically, present evidence for a psychological component in their etiology. Difficulty in handling hostile feelings, difficulty in being assertive, and the presence of obsessive–compulsive traits are not uncommon. Recently, the so-called "Type A personality" has been reported as being particularly prone to angina or coronary artery disease. This personality is characterized by an excessive competitive drive, a chronic sense of time urgency, a tendency to overcommit to a series of responsibilities, achievement orientation, and an immersion in self-imposed deadlines. Emotional factors play a role in vasodepressor syncope. There is evidence that emotional factors may precipitate sudden death in certain patients.

GASTROINTESTINAL DISORDERS

In addition to anorexia nervosa and bulimia, already described, here would be included cardiospasm, nervous vomiting, diarrhea, and constipation. Psychogenic factors play a role in ulcerative colitis in certain patients. In patients with peptic ulcer, most psychiatric investigations have reported a basic conflict between passivity and aggressiveness. Reaction formation is a common defense mechanism. Clinical investigations have estimated that about 80% of gastric hyperactivity and hyperacidity is related to life situations.

GENITOURINARY DISORDERS

In addition to the various sexual dysfunctions already reviewed, psychological factors can play a role in a wide variety of disturbances of genital and urinary functions. In certain individuals life conflict influences menstrual disorders, abortion, leukorrhea, urinary frequency, urgency, retention, and prostatitis. Perhaps most dramatic is the amenorrhea of false pregnancy (pseudocyesis), in which there are other signs of pregnancy including breast changes, weight gain, and abdominal distention. This syndrome is almost entirely psychogenic in origin.

ENDOCRINE DISORDERS

Obesity has been defined as an increase in adipose tissue of 15% or more above the norm for a given height and age. Psychological responses to obesity are nearly universal, and in a majority of patients, psychological factors play a role in etiology. Group therapy seems particularly helpful in the treatment of obesity. Therapy limited to reducing diets and drugs frequently fails or if successful tends, in the overwhelming number of instances, to be followed by weight gain. The course of diabetes mellitus, hyperthyroidism, and myxedema is affected by psychological factors, and some investigators attribute a role in disease onset to such factors.

In contrast to the somatoform and dissociative disorders where the symptom is frequently symbolic of the conflict, this is not the case in this group of disorders. In general, the effort to identify a specific constellation of psychological conflicts and relate them to specific psychophysiological disorders has not been successful. If there is a personality type prone to psychosomatic disease, it would be the compulsive personality. However, all individuals seem more vulnerable to stress in one organ system than another. Genetic predisposition and early developmental factors probably play a more significant role in organ selection than personality type or the category of conflict. With these patients in particular, the conceptual principle of individual response specificity is essential for diagnosis and management. What life situations and life events represent a psychological stress to a specific patient or which long-term psychological conflicts in fact are significant to a psychophysiologic process must be determined on an individual basis. The process of evaluation outlined earlier is helpful in this regard.

Personality Disorders

Each of us has certain characteristic attitudes and reaction patterns in our relationship to the world, to others, and to ourselves that make us a unique individual. For each of us the development of this character structure has a history. It begins in our early years and is elaborated over time. While genetic influences play a role in temperament, there is little evidence that various personality patterns have prominent genetic determinants per se. Much more prominent etiologically are all those events and situations of life to which a person responds over time with learned, acquired response patterns. Early mother/child interactions, familial example, discipline and teaching from significant others, peer relationships, unique personal experiences, cultural shaping, all contribute to our personalities. When these ways of behaving become exaggerated, when behavior to some degree becomes stereotyped regardless of the external reality, the individual then may be said to suffer from a character or personality disorder.

Usually the individual experiences little sense of distress with his personality. More often others find them disturbing, or the individual is distressed by the consequences of his character structure, often without awareness of how his character determined the very consequence he or she finds dis-easing. Each personality pattern disorder to some degree predicts that person's response to stress. A wise physician includes in his thinking the personality diagnosis of his patient. The management of appendicitis in a paranoid character is quite different than the management of appendicitis in a hysterical character. A paranoid character in delirium tends to behave differently from an hysterical character. The adjustment reactions of each to an identical stressful life event will be different. Therapeutic intervention, therefore, in each instance is different.

In reviewing the following personality disorders the reader would do well to ask a series of questions. If this personality disorder decompensated, would there be a tendency for the emergence of a particular mental disorder? If there was superimposed a delirium or a dementia, what would be the manifestations? If this kind of individual would develop an anxiety disorder, what kind of stress, what kind of conflict would be most likely, and how would this affect management and treatment? How would this category of personality tend to respond to pregnancy, bronchoscopy, herniorrhaphy, diabetes mellitus, an intensive care unit, renal dialysis, paraplegia, loss of a job, malignancy in a young son, infidelity, divorce, death of spouse, my characteristic way of opening an interview, my particular style of asking questions and giving suggestions? The list is endless.

Any nosology of personality disorders would be somewhat arbitrary. Many individuals show features of more than one category. Even within categories the principle of individual response specificity still holds. Nonetheless, even when the personality pattern of a given patient does not warrant the label of a disorder, a physician limits his or her therapeutic potential if he or she fails habitually to diagnose the personality traits of his or her patients.

The following group of disorders tends to show greater psychopathology than those that follow, utilize more primitive defense mechanisms, and with decompensation under stress move toward more serious categories of mental illness.

SCHIZOTYPAL PERSONALITY DISORDER

While not meeting the criteria for schizophrenia, this personality type, as the name implies, has certain features of that illness. There tends to be magical thinking, ideas of reference, recurrent illusions, depersonalization not associated with manifest anxiety, and paranoid ideation. There is usually evidence for social isolation and undue social anxiety or hypersensitivity to real or imagined criticism. Their speech is often odd, vague, circumstantial, metaphorical, but without loosening of association or incoherence. There is inadequate rapport in face-to-face interaction with others. These individuals seem to have introjected a semicrazy world. In addition, schizophrenia is commonly present in the extended family.

PARANOID PERSONALITY DISORDER

Individuals of this type show a propensity for using projection as a defense mechanism. They demonstrate pervasive, unwarranted suspiciousness, and mistrust of people. Hence, they are hypervigilant, expect trickery, are guarded or secretive, question the loyalty of others, tend to avoid accepting blame even when blame is warranted, look for hidden motives in the behavior of others, and often show unusual jealousy. In addition, they are often hypersensitive, tending to take offense quickly. They show restricted affectivity, appearing to be cold or unemotional, often taking pride in being, in their view, objective or rational. They often lack a sense of humor, and frequently there is an absence of soft, tender, sentimental feelings. In short, these individuals have been taught to distrust the world.

SCHIZOID PERSONALITY DISORDER

This type of personality is characterized by emotional coldness or aloofness, or absence of tender feelings toward others, and by relative indifference to praise or criticism or to the feelings of others. They tend to have very few if any close friends but may be very attached to animals. They may have outstanding academic records, having spent hours alone in studying. As adolescents they tend to be seen as shy, withdrawn, alone. They give the appearance of being quiet loners. In contrast to the schizotypal personality disorders, there are, however, no major eccentricities in speech, behavior, or thought. In short, these individuals have been taught to expect hurt from the world but defend themselves by becoming indifferent to it.

ANTISOCIAL PERSONALITY DISORDER

Several of the following features are found in the history of these patients with onset before age 15: truancy, expulsion or suspension from school, behavioral delinquency, running away from home, persistent lying, casual sexual intercourse, repeated drunkenness or substance abuse, thefts or vandalism, poor school performance, chronic violation of rules at home, or initiation of fights. After age 18, there are manifestations of the disorder as follows: an inability to sustain consistent work behavior, an inability to function in a consistent way as a responsible parent, failure to accept social norms with respect to lawful behavior, an inability to maintain enduring attachments to a sexual partner, irritability and aggressiveness as indicated by repeated physical fights or assaults, which may include spouse or child beating, failure to honor financial obligations with repeated defaulting on debts, failure to provide child support, failure to plan ahead, impulsively traveling from place to place without a clear goal in mind, disregard for the truth as indicated by lying, using aliases, "conning" others, and recklessness. Current diagnostic criteria require that such a behavioral pattern be present for at least 5 years without any intervening period in which the syndrome is absent. These individuals constitute a major social problem, consuming a considerable percent of the manpower and fiscal resources of law enforcement, social service, and health agencies. To date, this disorder stands alone in this category in there being convincing data suggesting a major genetic factor in etiology. Early psychological factors also play a role. Particularly striking is the finding of a parental disciplinary pattern that is demanding, inflexible, and punitive one moment and permissive and nonpunitive the next. In short, these individuals behave as if they have failed to incorporate any set of value systems; hence, they are often described as without conscience.

The following group of disorders tend to show less psychopathology than those above but more than those that follow.

BORDERLINE PERSONALITY DISORDER

These individuals show many of the following characteristics. First, there tends to be impulsivity in areas that are potentially self-damaging, for example, spending, sex, gambling, shoplifting, overeating, or physically self-damaging acts such as recurring accidents, self-mutilation, or suicide attempts. Drug or alcohol abuse is common. Second, there tends to be a pattern of unstable or intense personal relationships. Third, there is often inappropriate intense anger or a lack of control in the expression of anger. Identity disturbances are commonly manifest by uncertainty over such issues as choice of friends, values, loyalties, or career. There is considerable difficulty, in short, with self-image. Next, there is frequently affective instability with marked shifts from normal mood to depression or irritability, usually lasting several hours but rarely for more than a few days with then a return to normal mood. They tend to be intolerant of being alone and experience chronic feelings of emptiness or boredom. For periods of time they seem to block out incoming stimuli but on other occasions seem exquisitely sensitive to it. Certain of these individuals under stress develop "micropsychotic" episodes. During such episodes the diagnosis of schizophreniform reaction may be appropriate. Many physicians find these patients particularly difficult to understand or treat. They seem neither psychotic nor neurotic, simultaneously both, but also normal from moment to moment. Although there is no convincing evidence to date for a genetic determinant for this disorder, the possibility of CNS dysfunction secondary to maturational lag or early developmental trauma is frequently raised by clinical investigators.

NARCISSISTIC PERSONALITY DISORDER

Narcissists seem to possess a grandiose sense of self-importance or uniqueness and often are preoccupied with fantasies of unlimited success, power, brilliance, or beauty. There may be a quality of exhibitionism, that is, requiring attention. They may show cool indifference or marked feelings of rage, shame, or humiliation in response to criticism by others. Interpersonally, they tend to operate from the posture of entitlement, that is, the expectation of special favors from others without assuming reciprocity. There tends to be, therefore, interpersonal exploitiveness. They lack empathy and tend to relate to others alternating between the extremes of overidealization and devaluation. Having never received or having received without the expectation of reciprocity, psychologically they seem like little babies who simply expect the world to revolve about them; they would be quick to take umbrage with this description.

DEPENDENT PERSONALITY DISORDER

These individuals lack self-confidence and see themselves as helpless or stupid. They tend to subordinate their own needs to those of persons on whom they depend. Their passivity allows others to assume responsibility for major areas of their life because of their inability to function independently. Because they seem so obedient and compliant, they are sometimes viewed by physicians as being "good" patients. Nonetheless, there is a tendency, in order to maintain their dependency, for them to stay "sick" in one fashion or another. They can feel literally devastated with the loss of those upon whom they depend—parent, spouse, employer, son, or daughter. They have been taught that they cannot or should not function in the world as independent beings.

This last group of disorders with decompensation tend to move toward less serious categories of mental illness than do those that precede it. It should be understood that this is a general statement and not applicable in all instances. Further, the hierarchy is ordered with the assumption that "serious" refers to the more psychotic end of the spectrum of mental illness and "less serious" to the more neurotic. There would be those clinicians who would argue, quite appropriately, that this does not necessarily indicate less psychopathology.

PASSIVE–AGGRESSIVE PERSONALITY DISORDER

These individuals express their hostility in an indirect fashion, hence, they resist demands for performance in occupational or social settings through procrastination, dawdling, stubbornness, intentional inefficiency, or forgetfulness. A long-standing history of educational, social, or occupational ineffectiveness and inefficiency is common. These behaviors persist even under circumstances in which more self-assertive behavior would be possible and effective. These individuals tend to evoke frustration, impatience, anger, and eventually rejection from others including, of course, physicians.

COMPULSIVE PERSONALITY DISORDER

These individuals tend to be preoccupied with details, rules, order, organization, schedules, and lists. They often give themselves or are given the appellation of *perfectionist*. The perfectionist is one that attends to details and fails to grasp the larger picture. The compulsive frequently is unduly conventional or formal, has restricted ability to express warm and tender emotions, is unaware of feelings of anger even though the anger may be communicated to others nonverbally, or, if aware of anger, places premium on control of expression, and may be devoted almost excessively to work or studies to the exclusion of pleasure or interpersonal relationships. They tend to insist that others submit to their particular ways of doing things and seemingly are unaware of the feelings elicited in others by this behavior. Nonetheless, quite often they are indecisive, that is, decision making is postponed or avoided or protracted from inordinate fear of making a mistake. In response they adopt rules, principles, and belief systems that they automatically impose on themselves or on others in an arbitrary, unthinking fashion even when the situation does not particularly warrant that approach or response. They lack flexibility. Intellectualization, rationalization, compartmentalization, and reaction formation are typical defense mechanisms. In short, these individuals psychologically seem fixated on that stage of life where great emphasis is placed on "doing things right" or risk punishment, shame, withdrawal of love, or rejection.

AVOIDANT PERSONALITY DISORDER

This pattern of personality is characterized by hypersensitivity to rejection, an unwillingness to enter into relationships unless given strong guarantees of uncritical acceptance, social withdrawal, a desire for affection, and usually extremely low self-esteem. Outwardly they may behave in a manner similar to the schizoid, but these individuals are not indifferent to the world—they are afraid of the world's shame and ridicule.

HISTRIONIC PERSONALITY DISORDER (HYSTERICAL PERSONALITY)

These persons demonstrate behavior that is overly dramatic, reactive, and intensely expressed. This may be manifest by some of the following characteristics: self-dramatization with exaggerated expression of emotions, drawing of attention to self, a craving for activity and excitement, overreaction to minor events, including irrational angry outbursts or tantrums. In addition, there are disturbances in interpersonal relationships. Often they are perceived by others as shallow and lacking in genuineness even if superficially charming, or as egocentric, self-indulgent, vain and demanding, or sometimes dependent and helpless, seeking constant reassurance. They demonstrate considerable denial and repression and at an unconscious level often sexualize their relationships with others, yet find sexual experience incomplete or unrewarding or unsatisfying. These individuals psychologically seem stuck, fixated in the role of staying little boys or little girls.

One characteristic of normal, nonneurotic individuals is a personality structure that is not stuck or fixated into a particular pattern; hence, they demonstrate flexibility and adaptability. These individuals, sometimes called **genital characters,** may show features of any or all of the above personality disorders. But, none of the above patterns predominate or endure when such behavior becomes maladaptive to a given situation. There are those who would insist that no one is normal, that everybody is neurotic or has some kind of neurotic personality disorder. However, this is simply not true. From studies from a variety of sources one can estimate that about 20% to 30% of the adult population are genital characters. The concept of integration of certain features within a personality is useful when working with patients who are genital characters. It is useful to think in such terms as a genital character with integrated compulsive features or a genital character with integrated histrionic features, and so forth.

Conditions Not Attributable to a Mental Disorder

All individuals over a lifetime regardless of diagnosis are confronted with particular problems of one kind or another and frequently turn to their physicians for assistance. When the problem is not due to a mental disorder, when it is not a feature of one of the diagnostic categories described above, this problem should be recognized without attaching a diagnosis of mental disorder. Common examples of such problems which may be a focus of attention or treatment are borderline intellectual functioning, adult antisocial behavior (*e.g.*, manifest in some professional thieves, dealers of illegal substances), academic problems, occupational problems, uncomplicated bereavement (especially common in the practice of medicine), noncompliance with medical treatment, phase-of-life problem, marital problems, parent–child problems, and other interpersonal problems.

PREVENTION

From within the health professions and from without, the growing emphasis on prevention derives from multiple factors: the realization that in some domains of medicine there seems to be almost no limit to the possible growth of treatment programs, the dramatically rising costs of medical care, and a genuine interest in the prevention of disability and suffering. We will consider here the prevention of smoking, obesity, alcohol abuse, and the prevention of behavioral and emotional disorders in children. There is considerable evidence to suggest that successful techniques for prevention in these areas would have considerable impact on the incidence of a whole variety of diseases.

Abstinence can be achieved among heroin addicts, alcohol abusers, and smokers. For those who successfully maintain their abstinence, decreased incidence of certain illnesses has been documented. However, the relapse rates for these three addictions follow essentially a similar curve. After achieving abstinence, at 3 months only 40% remain abstainers and after 12 months the figure falls to approximately 20%. A similar pattern holds for obesity. Programs for prevention too often are judged only in terms of immediate rates.

For example, initial reports on the utilization of behavior therapy compared to conventional programs for weight reduction were impressive with behavior therapy programs outperforming the other approaches by impressive margins. However, more recently, with long-range studies, the overly optimistic expectations in this field have turned to disillusionment and pessimism at least for some. Obesity after all is a lifestyle disorder. To effect the maintenance of weight reduction requires a lifestyle change. Some programs devoted to prevention have failed to confront the complexity of the problem and the repeatedly demonstrated difficulty in effecting major and enduring change in human behavior.

Another example is smoking. When smoking behavior is analyzed, it would appear that the main purpose in smoking technique is to get nicotine into the blood and particularly into the brain as quickly as possible. The usual attempts at primary prevention tend to be educational programs. There is evidence that there has been a decrease of smoking of tobacco in the United States. This has been attributed to a large-scale national education effort. However, the incidence of tobacco smoking has increased among adolescents in recent years in spite of this educational effort, especially among females. Also, if one considers the increasing incidence of marijuana smoking in segments of population, it is highly questionable whether there has in fact been an overall decreased incidence of smoking per se. The proportion of persons 18 to 25 years old who have used marijuana has increased from 4% to 68% since 1962.

The primary prevention of alcohol abuse poses similar problems. Alcohol education programs have been developed in schools. From studies of these programs students do make significant gains in their knowledge of alcohol, but changes in attitude and behavior do not necessarily follow. Actually, broader sociologic techniques may be more effective. For example, it is fairly clear from a variety of studies that those states that have lowered the legal drinking age have seen an increase in traffic accidents and fatalities and an increase in the number of young drinkers in treatment for alcoholism. Some studies suggest that the number of alcohol distribution outlets can be correlated to rates of consumption and of alcoholism.

Other techniques for prevention have been developed to involve the population at risk more directly. An example is an instrument that asks the individual to characterize their lifestyle. Then utilizing that data they determine the likelihood of their succumbing to various diseases, given that lifestyle. Whether this approach effects change remains to be researched. The effect of a book on self health care distributed to 460 families in a prepaid health plan was recently reported. At 6- and 12-month study periods, there was *no* significant effect on the number of physician visits made, even though it was determined that half of the families read most of the book and a third used it specifically for a particular medical problem. All in all in these areas it is clear that prevention on a large scale is a complex problem. Some have concluded that there has been more rhetoric regarding prevention than programs which have been demonstrated to work. Others point to studies showing some success and argue that this is too pessimistic a view.

Various studies suggest that children born into a wanted and nurturant environment tend to receive good parenting and tend to develop fewer behavioral and emotional problems in childhood. By inference this group may show a lower incidence of mental illness as adults. But to actually effect an increase in the likelihood of children being born into such settings is difficult. In fact the number of unwanted pregnancies, especially among teenagers, has increased as has the number of teenagers keeping their babies. Sex education and abortion issues tend to generate very strong opinions. Current trends in the United States do *not* suggest a decrease in the number of unwanted children born into our population. Programs more narrowly focused, however, show promise.

Some observers have suggested rather caustically that society will know when the medical profession takes prevention seriously when we see effective stress reduction programs in medical schools and in health science centers for the health professionals and the staff who work in such centers.

TREATMENT

The Physical Therapies

The most common of the physical therapies is electroconvulsive therapy (ECT) or EST. Although many theories have been postulated, the mode of action of this treatment is not certain. Empirically, there is no question that treatment will produce remission in a high percentage of patients with severe depression. Major depression is almost a universally accepted indication for EST, especially when the depression has not responded to pharmacotherapy. On some occasions, patients with manic episodes also are treated with this modality. Patients with schizophrenia or with severe psychoneurosis are also sometimes treated in this manner, but indications here are controversial.

Historically, treatment was instituted by applying an alternating current through electrodes placed bitemporally, but considerable variations of technique have been introduced, including electrode placement at other sites, changes in the way the current is administered or in the properties of the current and utilization of unidirectional currents and unilateral treatments. The advantages of the various methods are still primarily a matter of opinion; however, seizures, confusion, and memory loss are not necessarily required for therapeutic success. Treatments are typically given 3 times a week up to 8 to 14 in a series. The most common complication is an induced organic brain disorder

with blurring of memory. This clears spontaneously. With modern techniques, the procedure has become exceedingly safe. There is certainly much less risk to the patient than the risk of suicide with unrelenting depression. Fractures and dislocations, especially compression fractures of the spine, have been considerably reduced with the use of muscle relaxants or subconvulsive therapy. Personnel must be prepared to deal with an occasional respiratory arrest or cardiac arrest. EEG changes occur almost universally with slowing in all leads, becoming maximal after 10 to 12 treatments and disappearing in most cases within a few weeks. There would seem to be very few if any absolute contraindications, but special consideration should be given to patients who are pregnant, have bone and joint disease, an aortic aneurysm, coronary artery disease or a brain tumor, or increased intracranial pressure. Other techniques for inducing convulsions are now primarily of historical interest.

With the widespread use of tranquilizing medications, psychosurgery is also now mainly of historical interest. Its most frequent application is in cases of intractable pain. Light therapy is indicated for a seasonal affective disorder, a type of major depressive episode.

Pharmacotherapy

While the treatment of the mentally ill by means of drugs is not new, there has certainly been a renewed interest, even excitement, regarding drug therapy in the last several decades. The era of psychopharmacology came into being with the synthesis of chlorpromazine by Laborit in 1951. Psychopharmacotherapy aims at achieving better control of psychological symptoms. They do not cure patients in the usual sense of the word. When prescribing medication, it must be prescribed on an individual basis with thorough knowledge of the patient's condition, a knowledge of the patient's reaction to the drug in question, and with a clear view of the therapeutic goal in mind. There are many drugs used in the practice of psychological medicine. What follows is a brief and cursory review.

ANTIPSYCHOTIC AGENTS (MAJOR TRANQUILIZERS, NEUROLEPTICS, ATARACTICS)

Like the barbiturates, these agents have a quieting or calming effect, but unlike the older hypnotic agents, this occurs without producing marked drowsiness. Subcortical sites of action are more prominent than cortical effects. In general these drugs cause accumulation of the O-methylated metabolites of dopamine and noradrenalin within the brain, suggesting that they block these brain receptor sites. Highest concentrations of these receptors are in the hypothalamus, the basal ganglia, the thalamus, the hippocampus, and in the septum. In addition to an antipsychotic effect, these drugs have an antiemetic effect, can result in extrapyramidal symptoms such as pseudo-Parkinsonism, akathisia (motor restlessness), dyskinesia, and torsion spasms. Some of these effects may be controlled by synthetic anticholinergic agents (e.g., methanesulfonate, Cogentin; trihexyphenidyl, Artane). Of particular concern is tardive dyskinesia, which has a chronic course and usually appears after prolonged administration of such agents with the symptoms often exaggerated when the drug is withdrawn. The dyskinesia is characterized by Parkinson-type activity of a choreiform character especially involving the tongue and the mouth. Other adverse side effects include gynecomastia, heat intolerance (especially chlorpromazine), pigmentation of the exposed areas of the skin, retinal pigmentation (especially thioridizine), jaundice of the cholestatic type on occasion, and less commonly dermatitis and various blood dyscrasias. A neuroleptic malignant syndrome with cardinal features of elevated temperature and muscle rigidity can be a life-threatening complication. These drugs enhance the effects of central depressants such as barbiturates. This class of drugs is most useful with schizophrenic disorders. They also are utilized to help control the agitated or the hyperactive states of mania and the organic brain disorders. In some patients in particular, they have a marked lessening effect on the intensity of delusions and hallucinations. The accompanying table provides examples of the various categories of antipsychotic agents with the generic name followed by the trade name and in parentheses the daily dose range.

ANTIANXIETY AGENTS (ANXIOLYTICS, MINOR TRANQUILIZERS)

Antianxiety agents are used primarily to control the tension and anxiety seen in patients with anxiety disorders and in patients with depression accompanied by agitation. They have essentially replaced the barbiturates and sedatives in this regard. They have become the most commonly prescribed group of medications in the United States in all categories, psychiatric or otherwise, and are subject to considerable abuse. They are frequently used in suicide attempts and can become addicting. It is increasingly evident that considerable caution should be utilized in prescribing these medications for more than short periods of time but, given that caveat and with careful monitoring, they can be quite helpful. Perhaps the most serious side effect is that long-term use tends to support the patients' tendency to avoid facing their psychological problems and effecting more appropriate solutions. The drugs produce mild sedation without major impairment of psychomotor performance. Physiologic relaxation is another effect. Drowsiness is perhaps the most common side-effect. Patients should be warned about any activity involving skilled motor coordination, for example, driving a car. These drugs have synergistic effects with alcohol and other sedatives, and patients should be forewarned. Other effects include dizziness, headache, dry mouth, and on occasion paradoxical hyperactive, or rage reactions. Less common are hematological, allergic, renal, and hepatic reactions. Table 7-1 gives common examples of these agents.

SEDATIVES AND HYPNOTICS

These drugs are utilized less and less in the practice of psychological medicine but are still employed for nighttime insomnia and severe daytime anxiety. The antianxiety agents or even certain of the phenothiazines are probably better drugs of choice for severe daytime anxiety. After 2 to 3 days, the nighttime sedative effect begins to abate. In sleep laboratories, sedatives can be shown almost universally to have a disrupting effect on the sleep cycle. Earlier reports suggested there might be an exception to the latter statement, namely, flurazepam (Dalmane), but more recent studies raise questions regarding its disruption of the sleep cycle as well. As an adjunct to certain phases of psychotherapy, short-acting barbiturates are used to induce a state of light narcosis (narcotherapy). It appears that all sedative–hypnotic preparations are potentially addicting.

CENTRAL NERVOUS SYSTEM STIMULANTS

There are perhaps only two indications for utilization of this class of drugs in the modern practice of psychological medicine. One is in the management of hyperkinetic children where methylphenidate (Ritalin) and pemoline (Cylert) are widely used. Methylphenidate and other amphetamines are also useful in the treatment of narcolepsy.

TABLE 7-1. Psychopharmacologic Agents

CLASS	GENERIC NAME	BRAND NAME	DAILY DOSAGE
Antipsychotic Agents			
Phenothiazines			
Aliphatic	Chlorpromazine	Thorazine	50–1,000 mg
Piperidine	Thioridazine	Mellaril	50–800 mg
Piperazine	Fluphenazine	Prolixin	1–20 mg
Thioxenthines	Thiothixene	Navane	5–60 mg
Butyrophenone	Haloperidol	Haldol	1–100 mg
Dibenzoxazepine	Doxapin	Loxitane	20–250 mg
Antianxiety Agents			
Benzodiazepines	Alprazolam	Xanax	0.5–6 mg
	Chlordiazepoxide	Librium	15–100 mg
	Diazepam	Valium	4–40 mg
	Oxazepam	Serax	30–120 mg
Azaspirodecanedione	Buspirone	Buspar	15–30 mg
Antihistamines			
	Hydroxyzine	Atarax	50–400 mg
Carbonates			
	Meprobamate	Equanil	200–1,200 mg
Antimanic Agents			
	Lithium carbonate	Eskalith	1,200–1,800 mg
Antidepressants			
Unicyclic	Bupropian	Wellbutrin	100–300 mg
Tricyclics	Imipramine	Tofranil	75–300 mg
	Nortriptyline	Aventyl	75–150 mg
	Desimipramine	Norpramine	75–200 mg
	Amitriptyline	Elavil	75–300 mg
	Doxepine	Sinequan	75–300 mg
Tetracyclic	Maprotiline	Ludiomil	150–225 mg
Monomine oxidase inhibitors			
	Phenelzine sulfate	Nardil	60–90 mg
	Tranylcypromine	Parnate	10–30 mg
Phenylpropylamine	Floxetine	Prozac	20–80 mg

ANTIMANIC AGENTS

Lithium carbonate is considered to be the only specific antimanic drug for use in bipolar depression. Since it requires 7 to 10 days to achieve a threshold level in body tissues, acute episodes are usually managed initially with antipsychotic agents (*e.g.,* Haldol) until the lithium can begin to take effect. Long-term maintenance on lithium of patients with manic attacks is reported to prevent the recurrence of such attacks in 50% to 80% of patients. There is controversy as to whether lithium is effective in preventing recurring episodes of depression. Utilization of lithium requires the monitoring of blood levels. A therapeutic serum level of 0.5 to 1.5 mEq/liter is usually in the therapeutic range. Since lithium competes with the sodium ion, it is not surprising that lithium is contraindicated in patients with renal, hepatic, or heart disease. With long-term administration, asymptomatic thyroid en-largement can occur. The range between a therapeutic level and toxicity is relatively narrow. Most common effects are polyuria, polydipsia, and a fine hand tremor. These tend to be transient in most patients. As more toxic levels are reached, there is progressively the appearance of nausea and diarrhea, malaise, vomiting, muscle weakness, ataxia, abdominal pain, slurred speech, nystagmus, vesiculations, choreoathetoid movements, convulsions, circulatory failure, stupor, coma, and death. Extreme toxic effects have been reported at levels above 2.5 mEq/liter.

ANTIDEPRESSANTS

As a group, antidepressants elevate mood, enhance mental alertness, improve sleep and appetite patterns, increase physical activity, reduce morbid preoccupations, and lower the risk of suicide in patients with depression. Tricyclics act by inhibiting the reuptake of norepinephrine and serotonin by the neuronal terminals. Monoamine oxidase inhibitors block intracellular metabolism of biogenic amines resulting in an increased amine concentration at the terminals. Imipramine, nortriptyline, and desipramine seem to have more effect on norepinephrine systems, whereas amitriptyline and doxepin have a greater impact on serotonin. Patients who may not respond to one class of tricyclics may respond to another. All these compounds require one to three weeks before there is symptomatic response.

Tricyclics can aggravate the symptoms of schizophrenia and may convert depression into mania. Side effects include dry mouth, constipation, hyperhidrosis, and blurred vision. Weight gain has also been reported; less frequently, tachycardia, anorexia, increased ocular tension, urinary retention, and orthostatic hypertension. Monomine oxidase inhibitors are less effective than tricyclics and are usually utilized only after failure with tricyclics or ECT. Careful monitoring is needed because adverse reactions can be serious. These drugs should not be administered to patients taking other sympathomimetic compounds, often present in cold remedies, decongestants, and so forth. Foods with high tyramine content should be avoided since hypertensive crisis may be precipitated. Subarachnoid hemorrhage has been reported. Other adverse reactions include orthostatic hypotension, dizziness, headache, cardiac arrhythmias, fatigue, dryness of mouth, blurred vision, and constipation.

Classes of antidepressants other than tricyclics have been introduced. Whether they have special advantage or fewer side effects is controversial.

At the present time, there is probably a tendency to *overprescribe* all these classes of pharmacotherapeutic agents, especially the antianxiety drugs and the antidepressants. Normal fear responses and normal grief reactions do *not* require medication. Oft times these medications make such individuals feel even worse. A second trend, however, is seen as well. Once a given psychoactive agent is indicated, there is a tendency to *underdose* the patient. Doses should be gradually increased and given for a sufficient length of time so that the patient truly has been given an adequate trial before the drug is discontinued.

Psychotherapy

Interviews are conducted for many purposes—research, education, selling merchandise, and moral persuasion, among others. Even when the interaction is intended to be therapeutic, such may not be the case. A good doctor/patient relationship sets the stage, but whether an interview or a series of interviews has a therapeutic outcome depends on many other factors. Outcome depends on the motivations of both parties, the capacities of both participants, the nature of the communication process, the experiences facilitated by the encounter, the resulting inner permission given by the patient to himself or herself to experiment with new patterns of action, the practice opportunities within the context of the interview to effect change, and the balance between resistance and assistance for change in the patient's environs.

PSYCHOTHERAPY EFFECTS CHANGE

Psychotherapy, if effective, facilitates change, a giving up or a modification of maladaptive responses and the acquisition of more adaptive behaviors. Without change at some level—biochemical, intrapsychic, behavioral, interpersonal—the patient stays sick. He or she holds to a response pattern and maintains a character structure vulnerable to illness. Although therapists may utilize different theoretical frameworks for understanding human behavior, may belong to different schools of therapeutic intervention, and have different styles in their work, they are similar in their effort to facilitate change.

The process of psychotherapy can be described. As is the case with acquiring any new skill, whether walking or talking for a child or farming or performing a surgical operation for an adult, the first step is increased *awareness*. Without awareness for the possibility of change, without awareness of possible options, without awareness of some of the determinants in these options, choices remain elusive. The effective therapist facilitates increased awareness often in the face of resistance and unconscious if not conscious opposition from the patient. The evaluation process described earlier in this chapter not only sharpens diagnostic accuracy and enhances interviewing efficiency, but encourages increased awareness as well.

From this awareness evolves *understanding.* It is not enough for the child to be aware of the possibility of walking. To walk there must also be understanding of that process, whether acquired by imitation or formal study. As therapy proceeds, awareness fosters more complete understanding of the maladaptive process in question. Ultimately, more significant than the physician's understanding is the patient's understanding.

From this understanding, a range of possible alternatives comes into view, and after due consideration, *decision.* To continue our analogy, awareness of the possibility of walking, understanding the process of walking, does not make a walker. Insight in and of itself is not enough. To walk requires the decision to walk. To effect change requires a decision as to the what, the how, and the when of change.

Acquiring and integrating a new behavior requires *practice.* The effective therapist encourages and supports such practice, again often in the face of resistance. Any new behavior is unskilled, awkward, and does not feel natural. The new behavior also opposes, so to speak, the dynamics in the neurotic solution to the conflict. Beyond this, change when manifested may be resisted by the patient's surround. For example, a male patient with a dependent personality recovering from depression may experience resistance from his wife and children as he moves behaviorally toward independence.

Finally, with sufficient practice, the circle is complete. The new behavior now integrated feels natural. The new behavior allows a new level of awareness. Having learned to walk, no longer having to pay attention to the walking per se, the child becomes aware of a whole new world. Many patients avoid change because, to oversimplify, they wait for the feeling to change first. They say, for example, "When I no longer feel so terrified, then I'll be able to get on the elevator." Change in feeling comes after practice, not before. Others avoid change because they obsess, waiting for the "right" decision, the "perfect" solution, the "answer" which has no consequences other than the relief of symptoms.

The emphasis may be different between therapies. Traditional psychoanalysis emphasizes awareness and understanding and tends to assume that the patient will work through the decision/practice part of the change cycle. With appropriately selected patients, this can occur. Certain behavior therapies tend to ignore awareness and understanding, focus on a particular decision often prescribed, and detail a schedule for practice. Again, with appropriate selection, there can be good outcome. Most psychoanalysts and behavior therapists would object to this somewhat stereotyped description and appropriately so. Neither completely ignores the principles of the other. The principle of individual response specificity would suggest that some patients are more likely to benefit from one method than the other and vice versa. Studies of therapeutic

efficacy are beginning to demonstrate the validity of this statement.

CHARACTERISTICS OF EFFECTIVE PHYSICIANS

The following represents a summary of the characteristics of effective physicians based upon outcome studies; that is, given a group of physicians whose patients have an effective outcome by some measure, what are their characteristics compared to those physicians whose patients by the same measure do not have a comparable outcome. Interestingly, the results of these studies suggest comparable characteristics, whether the study relates to pediatricians and the rates of recurring otitis media in their patients, family physicians and maintenance of weight reduction by their patients, surgeons and morbidity rates following gallbladder surgery, psychiatrists and rate of rehospitalization of schizophrenic patients, therapists and measured improvement in their depressed patients with cognitive psychotherapy, and so forth.

It is interesting to notice what is not significantly different between the two groups of physicians in a given study. There do not seem to be significant differences in any cognitive measurement (*e.g.,* I.Q., grades in medical school, or performance on national testing examinations). Apparently the system that selects individuals into medicine and the system that educates them accomplishes the cognitive mission. Physicians learn what they need to know. At least in these studies there appears to be no significant differences between the two groups in this domain. However, there are differences in other dimensions.

First, the effective physician is appropriately nurturant, that is, appropriately supportive. Some physicians tend to be "too nurturant," taking a stance that might be characterized in the following message to their patient: "I care about you. You simply should trust me and place yourself in my hands. Don't worry. I know what is in your best interest." Others tend to be "insufficiently nurturant." Their message may be characterized in this manner: "I know what to do. I intend to do it. You follow my instructions. If you don't get better, it's essentially your fault." Patronizing communication is characteristic of the first example, whereas blaming communication is characteristic of the second. Neither is appropriately nurturant in most instances.

From the data, even more powerful in the statistical sense than the above, is the second characteristic. An effective physician is extraordinarily skilled in providing a cognitive model so that the patient understands the disease process. This is not surprising when considered. The patient who understands hypertension is more likely to follow the antihypertensive regimen than one that does not, especially through periods when there may be no symptoms and in fact even side effects from the medication. With psychotherapy, despite what adamant adherents to given schools of psychotherapy may proclaim, a given theoretical model cannot be shown from data to be consistently more powerful than another. A therapist who uses transactional analysis does not necessarily have better outcome than one who uses the model of Freudian psychoanalysis or another who employs a model from learning theory. The nihilist may jump to the conclusion that it is not necessary to have a model at all. But this is not the case either. Apparently what these good therapists have in common is some model of understanding, a model they understand very well and are able to employ, and especially a model they can communicate to their patients with consistency and from interview to interview.

Finally, what seems to emerge from the evidence is that the effective physician is very skilled in involving the patient in the problem solving. This is in striking contrast to the sick role as defined by Western culture, which tends to exempt patients from being responsible for their illnesses and that simply expects them to comply with the recommendations of the health expert. It is also in striking contrast to the all too frequently observed process of the physician making his or her diagnosis after evaluation and simply prescribing a therapeutic regimen. Involving certain patients in the problem-solving process requires considerable skill.

Recent studies suggest that effective physicians are emotionally healthy themselves compared with their counterparts.

TYPES OF PSYCHOTHERAPY

Before reviewing the various types of psychotherapy, it should be noted that in the last decade studies of therapeutic outcome are demonstrating the significant effect of appropriately conducted psychotherapy. The studies involve control groups, counterbalanced design, reliable measurements, and careful statistical analysis; the usual requirements in scientific medicine. Of course, clinical experience has for years suggested such an effect. This kind of research is just beginning. Much remains to be done. The results of such studies seem to show a greater effect than therapeutic nihilists

might have anticipated but less effect than therapeutic enthusiasts would have predicted.

Hypnotherapy. Historically, hypnosis was one of the earliest psychotherapies. It was utilized initially to effect suggestion during the hypnotic state or to accomplish psychological catharsis and abreaction. The technique also can facilitate dynamic understanding of the pathological process. In the modern era, it is probably used most successfully for control of pain and for early intervention into conversion or dissociative disorders. The technique tends to foster dependent attitudes in certain patients. For others it savors of magic. To others it seems to threaten their need for control. Of course, all effective therapies have potential adverse side effects.

Relaxation Therapy and Biofeedback. The teaching of relaxation techniques also has a long history. A more sophisticated version utilizes biofeedback techniques, although the effect of biofeedback is probably not related simply to skeletal muscle relaxation in all instances. There are reports of therapeutic effect in many kinds of patients, but most consistently in patients with generalized anxiety accompanied by generalized muscular tension and in patients with specific psychophysiologic syndromes, in particular, tension headache, and certain varieties of hypertension.

Individual Psychotherapies. *Psychoanalysis* or psychoanalytic-oriented therapy makes considerable use of the technique of *free association,* which encourages patients to put into words whatever comes to their minds without censuring. At first, this is difficult for most patients to do; however, over time, this technique carries the possibility of fostering more complete understanding of the pathologic process.

Related to psychoanalysis is a variety of *dynamic psychotherapies.* Here also, there is considerable emphasis on increasing awareness and developing understanding. As is the case with psychoanalysis, transference may be fostered and utilized through interpretation to bring greater understanding to the pathological process. Transference refers to the unconscious tendency of the patient to respond to the therapist as if he or she were someone else, a significant other in the patient's present or the patient's past. The concept of fixation is also characteristic of many of these therapies, namely, that maladaptive behavior patterns are old patterns that persist from specific points in time of psychological development and revolve around certain issues. Returning to those situations and events in the patient's past history, reexamining them, reinterpreting them, and identifying their role in the present is a process effecting change.

Supportive psychotherapy emphasizes the development of a more effective support system for the patient in his family setting or work setting. It also seeks to discover the more healthy behaviors in the patient and encourages their elaboration. Uncovering the past, making the unconscious conscious, is not emphasized, even avoided. There is, of course, a supportive element to all effective therapies.

Educational psychotherapy is a term given to that intervention that focuses primarily on educational techniques. There is also an element of education in all therapies.

Behavior therapy using the principles of learning theory also has many variations but focuses specifically in some fashion on a program of practice of behaviors to help the patient extinguish old inadequate responses and/or learn new, more adaptive ones. Some forms of behavior therapy may be particularly helpful to patients who have phobias or in patients who clearly need to alter specific destructive habit patterns (*e.g.*, overeating, smoking, etc.).

Group Psychotherapy.   The group psychotherapies are as varied as the individual therapies. They share in common patients working together in the context of a group. Certain therapists employ a psychoanalytic theoretical background with an emphasis on developing an understanding of each member of the group or an understanding of the group process as a whole. Others may be more active and experiential, for example, those who utilize psychodrama. Conjoint marital therapy, that is, working with both husband and wife, might be viewed as the smallest group possible. Family therapy focuses on therapy with the whole family. Particular indications for these techniques may be in those situations where pathologic interactions occurring between the dyad or between members of the family perpetuate pathologic processes. Group psychotherapy has an advantage in that it provides the patient with a particular opportunity to practice such new behaviors as more openly sharing feelings, responding to angry confrontations, and so forth, in a safe and supportive setting and with individuals who are not part of the patient's family or work group.

Self-help Groups.   These groups can be extraordinarily helpful in some situations in fostering therapeutic outcome. Perhaps the best known is Alcoholics Anonymous. It is effective in helping a

significant percentage of alcoholics maintain abstinence. Other groups have been modeled after Alcoholics Anonymous, including such groups as Narcotics Anonymous and Weight Watchers. There are self-help groups made up of individuals who have recovered from severe mental illness, groups who share in common a particular kind of chronic disease or have undergone similar surgery (*e.g.*, colostomy, mastectomy), or share in common the death of a child or the loss of a marital partner. Finally, given the primary intent of this chapter, indeed the intent of this book, it might be useful in closing to say that self-help groups have been formed by individuals who share in common the anticipated taking of national certifying or competency examinations.

QUESTIONS IN PSYCHIATRY

Multiple-Choice Questions

Choose the *best* answer in the following multiple-choice questions. This does *not* mean, necessarily, that there are only one right answer and four wrong answers.

1. Identify the most accurate statement:
   (a) Rates of admissions and discharges of patients to and from state mental hospitals are decreasing.
   (b) About one in three or four persons during a lifetime will be hospitalized in a psychiatric hospital for mental illness.
   (c) The most common diagnosis for patients with mental illness seen in ambulatory care medical settings is alcoholism.
   (d) Twenty-five percent to thirty percent of all visits to ambulatory care medical care settings in the United States are related directly to mental illness.
   (e) The number of patients resident in county and state mental hospitals over the past decade has increased.
2. A surgical resident making early morning rounds of patients scheduled for elective surgery during that day makes one of the following opening statements to each patient as he enters. Which statement most clearly suggests the concept of stimulus–response specificity?
   (a) "Good morning. How was your night?"
   (b) "I know you are a little anxious about the surgery. Would you like to talk about it?"

(c) "Well, how are you feeling this morning?"

(d) "Anything you would like to ask me this morning?"

(e) "Well, we're all set for your surgery. Are you?"

3. During the first moments of an initial visit to a family physician, a man about 24 licks his lips and with tremulous voice states, "Well, Doctor, it's good to meet you. I suppose you are interested in why I'm here?" The physician nods and the patient continues, "Well, there is no problem really. I'm just here for a regular checkup." Choose the best response.

(a) "You are obviously anxious. What's bothering you?"

(b) "Is there anything in particular you would like me to check?"

(c) "Any particular reason you decided to have a checkup right now?"

(d) "I am wondering if you are feeling a little uneasy."

(e) "So there is nothing in particular and you're just here for a regular checkup. Right?"

4. An experienced pediatrician has completed his initial evaluation of a 9-year-old boy brought to his office by his mother. He has interviewed the mother. Given the evidence from history and physical, he strongly suspects an attention-deficit disorder with hyperactivity. Which of the following is most likely to be helpful to the physician for diagnosis and management of this patient?

(a) Consultation with the patient's teacher

(b) Referral to a clinical psychologist for psychologic tests

(c) Referral to a neurologist for a detailed neurologic examination

(d) Electroencephalographic examination

(e) A blood chemistry battery (especially to rule out hyperthyroidism)

5. While reviewing an electroencephalographic tracing from an adult patient with a long history of epilepsy, a physician notes considerable delta activity. Which is most likely? The patient:

(a) Has diffuse brain damage

(b) Is entering a toxic delirium

(c) Fell asleep during the tracing

(d) May have a space-occupying lesion

(e) Has the petit mal variety of epilepsy

6. Which of the following accounts for the fewest number of cases of mental retardation in the United States?

(a) Perinatal infections and early childhood encephalitides

(b) Prematurity and birth trauma

(c) Primary mental retardation

(d) Down's syndrome

(e) Phenylketonuria, Gaucher's disease, cretinism, Hurler's syndrome, and kernicterus

7. Patients with anorexia nervosa:

(a) More commonly are adolescent boys than adolescent girls

(b) Rarely die from this disorder

(c) Frequently report feeling fat when objectively emaciated

(d) Complain bitterly of nausea

(e) Commonly report symptoms of hypersomnalence and lethargy

8. Of the following childhood disorders, psychogenesis is clearly most prominent in:

(a) The hyperkinetic reaction

(b) A conduct disorder, aggressive socialized type

(c) Tourette's disorder

(d) Infantile autism

(e) The avoidant disorder (withdrawal reaction)

9. A psychiatric house officer is seeing a 30-year-old man in the emergency room. He has been hospitalized previously for a schizophrenic disorder, paranoid type. On this occasion he presents all of the following symptoms. Which is most suggestive of a delirium (acute brain syndrome)?

(a) Visual hallucinations

(b) Speech bordering on incoherence

(c) Persecutory delusions

(d) Concrete thinking

(e) Clouding of consciousness and disorientation

10. In contrast to the alcohol withdrawal syndrome with delirium, alcohol hallucinosis is characterized by:

(a) Clouding of consciousness

(b) Visual hallucinations

(c) The comparative absence of physiological withdrawal symptoms

(d) A disturbed sleep/wakefulness cycle

(e) Autistic thinking

11. For persons over 65 living outside of hospitals, the most common of the dementias is:

(a) Alzheimer's disease

(b) Multiple infarct dementia
(c) Arteriosclerotic dementia
(d) Normal pressure hydrocephalus
(e) Uremic encephalopathus

12. All of the following substances produce a withdrawal syndrome *except:*
    (a) Barbiturates
    (b) Opioids
    (c) Cocaine
    (d) Caffeine
    (e) Tobacco

13. The intoxication most likely confused with an acute schizophrenic disorder is that produced by:
    (a) Barbiturates
    (b) Cocaine
    (c) Amphetamines
    (d) Alcohol
    (e) Lysergic acid diethylmide

14. The possibility of suicide must be considered in all of the following. In which is it *least* likely?
    (a) Dementia with a depression
    (b) Alcoholism
    (c) Delirium (acute brain syndrome)
    (d) Schizophreniform disorder
    (e) Bipolar disorder, mixed type

15. Identify the most accurate statement regarding schizophrenic disorders.
    (a) An example of a primary symptom (Bleuler) is a persecutory delusion.
    (b) Process schizophrenia has a better diagnosis than reactive schizophrenia.
    (c) Hebephrenia is more common than catatonia.
    (d) Schizophrenia affects about 2% of the population.
    (e) Schizophrenia with a chronic course shows deterioration toward dementia.

16. A genetic component probably plays a role in the genesis of all of the following mental disorders. However, the evidence is *least* compelling in:
    (a) Schizophrenia
    (b) Manic–depressive illness
    (c) Alzheimer's disease
    (d) Huntington's chorea
    (e) Panic disorder

17. Compared to the unipolar disorders, bipolar disorders:
    (a) Are less likely to respond to lithium during the acute phase
    (b) Are less likely to benefit prophylactically from lithium treatment

(c) Have an older age of onset
(d) Are more common in women than in men
(e) May have an acute episode precipitated by imipramine (Tofranil)

18. In primary care ambulatory settings, patients frequently have as their presenting complaint "depression." In such instances the most common diagnosis is:
    (a) Manic–depressive illness (bipolar disorder)
    (b) Major depression with melancholia
    (c) Dysthymic disorder (depressive neurosis)
    (d) Adjustment disorder with depressed mood
    (e) Uncomplicated grief in response to loss

19. Imipramine is most likely indicated in patients with:
    (a) Agoraphobia with panic attacks
    (b) Social phobias
    (c) Generalized anxiety disorders
    (d) Obsessive–compulsive disorders
    (e) Posttraumatic stress disorders

20. A patient with a major depression with psychotic features is hospitalized. He is given a trial of imipramine (Tofranil) but is unresponsive. A decision is made to attempt a different drug. Which of the following would probably be the drug of choice?
    (a) Nortriptyline (Aventyl)
    (b) Desipramine (Norpramin)
    (c) Amitriptyline (Elavil)
    (d) Phenelzine sulfate (Nardil)
    (e) Lithium carbonate (Eskalith)

21. A 32-year-old man reports difficulty maintaining erections during intercourse with his wife. This has developed gradually over the past 3 years since his marriage at 29. He had experienced no such difficulty prior to marriage. He reports noting full morning erections with wakening. He has had a sexual experience on a recent business trip and noted no difficulty with erection on that occasion. He says he is embarrassed in having this difficulty, and he frequently looks embarrassed as he gives his history. He volunteers no other symptoms of significance. Given the above, the most appropriate tentative diagnosis would be:
    (a) Psychosexual dysfunction, inhibited sexual excitement
    (b) Psychosexual dysfunction, inhibited male orgasm
    (c) Latent ego-dystonic homosexuality
    (d) Adjustment disorder with anxious mood

(e) Adjustment disorder with depressed mood

22. In which of the following are psychological factors probably *least* significant etiologically?
    (a) Dermatitis factitia
    (b) Urticaria
    (c) Rosacea
    (d) Hyperhidrosis
    (e) Acne

23. In which of the following are psychological factors *most* significant etiologically?
    (a) Dermatitis factitia
    (b) Urticaria
    (c) Rosacea
    (d) Hyperhidrosis
    (e) Pemphigus

24. Which of the following personality disorders is probably *most* prone to psychophysiological disorders?
    (a) Compulsive personality disorder
    (b) Dependent personality disorder
    (c) Histrionic personality disorder
    (d) Narcissistic personality disorder
    (e) Passive–aggressive personality disorder

25. Identify the most accurate statement.
    (a) After 1-year follow-up, heroin addicts who have achieved abstinence are more likely to return to use of heroin than tobacco addicts are likely to return to smoking.
    (b) Patients with obesity who successfully lose a significant amount of weight through behavior therapy techniques tend to maintain the weight loss over the next 2 years.
    (c) In the United States, in response to a national education program, there has been a decreased incidence in smoking.
    (d) Alcohol-abuse educational programs have resulted in a decreased intake of alcohol among high-school students.
    (e) Distribution of self-care health books to families in prepaid health plans to date have not shown significant decreases in number of physician office visits.

26. All of the following statements about electro-shock therapy are correct *except:*
    (a) The most commonly accepted indication is major depression.
    (b) Risk of mortality in patients with depression is considerably less than the risk of mortality in such patients who are untreated.

(c) The most common complication is an organic brain disorder.
(d) The muscle relaxants have decreased the incidence of compression fractures of the spine.
(e) The therapy is absolutely contraindicated in patients with aortic aneurysms or coronary artery disease.

27. Based on patient-outcome studies, therapists with good outcome compared to therapists with poorer outcome are more likely to demonstrate:
    (a) Utilization of the psychoanalytic model of therapy compared with the transactional analysis model of therapy
    (b) A higher performance on the Boards of Psychiatry and Neurology
    (c) A tendency to use patronizing communication
    (d) Skill in involving the patient in the problem-solving process
    (e) A tendency to use psychopharmacological agents less frequently

28. Which of the following therapies emphasize increasing awareness and understanding the *least?*
    (a) Behavior therapy
    (b) Psychoanalysis
    (c) Dynamic psychotherapy
    (d) Educational psychotherapy
    (e) Hypnotherapy

29. Transference refers to:
    (a) The unconscious tendency of the patient to respond to a situation in the present as if in some measure it were a situation from the past
    (b) The unconscious tendency of the patient to respond to the physician as if he or she were someone else
    (c) The unconscious tendency of the physician to respond to the patient as if he or she were someone else
    (d) The conscious tendency of the patient to displace feelings felt toward others toward the physician
    (e) The conscious tendency of the physician to displace feelings felt toward others toward the patient

30. Careful evaluation of a man who complained of feeling discouraged about his marriage indicated that the problem in the main seemed to relate to pathological communication patterns between husband and wife. This sug-

gests referral for evaluation for which of the following?

(a) Psychoanalytically oriented psychotherapy for the patient
(b) Group therapy for the couple
(c) Group therapy for the patient
(d) Conjoint marital therapy
(e) Educational psychotherapy for the couple

Questions 31 to 33 and 34 to 36 are sets.

31. A medical resident enters an emergency room to see a patient. The patient, a man about 43, is sitting on the examining table. His shoulders are slumped. His head and eyes are downcast. His eyes are red. He looks up slowly and after a deep sigh says at the end of inspiration, "I am sorry to bother you, Doctor, but I have to talk to someone. I have been so discouraged again and so depressed lately that I've been afraid I might try to kill myself." At this point, there is:
   (a) Verbal and behavioral evidence for anxiety
   (b) Verbal and behavioral evidence for sadness
   (c) Verbal and behavioral evidence for anger
   (d) Only behavioral evidence for anxiety
   (e) Only behavioral evidence for sadness

32. Given the above, choose the most effective immediate response on the part of the physician.
   (a) "Don't worry, you're not bothering me."
   (b) "Have you ever tried to kill yourself before?"
   (c) "What is it exactly you are afraid might happen?"
   (d) "You look and feel depressed. Do you have any idea what has you so discouraged?"
   (e) "Would you like to talk to a psychiatrist?"

33. Given the available evidence, which of the following is the most likely diagnosis?
   (a) Uncomplicated bereavement
   (b) Organic affective syndrome
   (c) Schizoaffective disorder
   (d) Dysthymic disorder (depressive neurosis)
   (e) Major depressive disorder

34. A well-dressed woman in her early 30s consults a pediatrician for the first time. While fidgeting with her hands she states, "I want to talk to you about my 7-year-old daughter. She has me worried. She hasn't done anything like this since she was 2 or 3. Last week she wet the bed on two nights. I have been reading, and frankly I'm afraid of what this might mean." The patient pauses and looks at the pediatrician with wide-open eyes. Noting the behavioral and verbal evidence for emotion, the pediatrician responds, "Yes, I can see that you are
   (a) concerned. What in particular about this has you worried?"
   (b) concerned. I doubt that this is anything very serious."
   (c) concerned. Has your daughter complained of burning when she goes to the bathroom?"
   (d) concerned. This sometimes is a reflection of tension in the home."
   (e) concerned. Symptoms like this can be alarming."

35. After the above, the physician learns that the daughter has had no urinary tract complaints, has been previously healthy, has been doing well in school, enjoy playing with several playmates, has a younger sister age 5 and recently was very excited about the pending arrival of another sister. She seemed disappointed 1 week ago when her mother returned home from the hospital with a baby boy. Given this information, which of the following is the most likely diagnosis?
   (a) Adjustment disorder
   (b) Functional enuresis
   (c) Occult cystitis
   (d) Conduct disorder
   (e) Age-appropriate behavior

36. Assume that the diagnosis above is supported during the initial visit with additional evidence following evaluation of the mother and the daughter. Which of the following would then be most appropriate therapeutically?
   (a) Referral of mother for psychological evaluation and possible individual psychotherapy
   (b) Referral of child for psychological evaluation and possible individual psychotherapy
   (c) Referral of child to urologist for further diagnostic evaluation
   (d) Referral of child for psychological evaluation and behavior therapy
   (e) Educational psychotherapy by pediatrician

For the following matching questions, an answer may be used *once, more than once,* or *not at all.*

(37–41) Match the following common side effects with the appropriate agent.
(a) Polyuria, fine hand tremor
(b) Dry mouth, hyperhidrosis
(c) Dry mouth, akathisia
(d) Drowsiness, especially subject to psychological addiction
(e) Hypertensive crisis with ingestion of foods with high tyramine content

37. Phenelzine sulfate (Nardil)
38. Imipramine (Tofranil)
39. Lithium carbonate (Eskalith)
40. Diazepam (Valium)
41. Chlorpromazine (Thorazine)

(42–46) For each of the following, assume the presence of the given illness and *match* with the psychiatric disorder *most likely* to be missed as a superimposed disease thereby.
(a) Major depression
(b) Schizophrenia, paranoid type
(c) Generalized anxiety disorder (anxiety neurosis)
(d) Conversion disorder (hysterical neurosis, conversion type)
(e) Dissociative disorder (hysterical neurosis, dissociative type)

42. Multiple sclerosis
43. Mitral valve prolapse syndrome
44. Temporal lobe epilepsy
45. Hypothyroidism
46. Phencyclidine abuse

For the following matching questions a given answer should be used *once* and *only once.*

(47–51) Link the following diagnosis with the defense mechanisms characteristic of each.
(a) Displacement
(b) Projection
(c) Reaction formation
(d) Conversion
(e) Introversion

47. Schizophrenic disorder, paranoid type
48. Phobic disorder
49. Obsessive–compulsive disorder
50. Psychogenic pain disorder
51. Major depression with melancholia

(52–56) Match the following:
52. Eugene Bleuler   (a) Father of psychiatry
53. James Braid   (b) Introduced the term *schizophrenia*
54. Sigmund Freud   (c) Coined the term *hypnosis*
55. Johann Weyer   (d) Elaborated the concept of defense mechanisms
56. Erik Erikson   (e) Emphasized cultural influences in human behavior

(57–61) In an ambulatory setting, a physician asks a 25-year-old man, "What brings you to see me?" The patient responds with a series of statements. *Match* each of the following.
(a) Neologism
(b) Logical thinking
(c) Autistic thinking
(d) Concrete thinking
(e) Clang association

57. "A Ford."
58. "A fine, flashy ford, my lord."
59. "You'd understand if your stomach made as much gas as mine did."
60. "I am an outstanding gasogenic member of *Homo sapiens.*"
61. "That sounds crazy, doesn't it?"

(62–66) Consider five patients, each with a different personality disorder. Assume that each decompensates with what for each is the severe stress of a recent death of a parent. Considering the structure of the personality, *match* with the following responses.
(a) Schizophreniform disorder
(b) Major depression with psychotic features
(c) Panic disorder
(d) Psychophysiological disorder, neck/shoulder/arm syndrome
(e) None of the above

62. Borderline personality disorder
63. Dependent personality disorder

64. Compulsive personality disorder
65. Histrionic personality disorder
66. Genital character

(67–71) Assume that each of the following patients as adults have the following diagnoses. Match with the most likely diagnosis of a childhood disorder made when the patient was a child.
  (a) Sleep terrors
  (b) Overanxious disorder
  (c) Stereotyped movement disorder—tics
  (d) Avoidant disorder
  (e) Conduct disorder, aggressive undersocialized type
67. Antisocial personality disorder
68. Phobic disorder—social phobia type
69. Anxiety neurosis (generalized anxiety disorder)
70. Conversion disorder (hysterical neurosis)
71. Genital character

(72–76) During a formal mental status examination, a physician asks a series of patients, "What does the following proverb mean to you? 'The grass is always greener on the other side of the street.' " Consider the responses. Although a single response to a proverb is not conclusive, given the following choices, *match* with the *most likely* diagnosis.
  (a) Schizophrenia, undifferentiated
  (b) Bipolar disorder, manic phase
  (c) Primary degenerative dementia, senile onset
  (d) Dysthymic disorder (depressive neurosis)
  (e) Bipolar disorder, depressed phase
72. "That means when you look across the street, the grass looks greener."
73. "Well, Doc, sometimes that's true. If you know where to look, you can make a mint, and I'm on my way to a fortune. If you put some of your money in with me, I'll make you a millionaire."
74. "I don't know."
75. "Green is not my color."
76. "That's the story of my life. No matter what I've done, on my side of the street, so to speak, it seems like there's been nothin' but

bad luck. Of course, it's all my fault, I realize."

(77–96) Consider the following five patients, all being seen for the first time by a family physician. In each instance, the physician makes the observations noted. The patient is making his opening statement.
Mrs. Alport, age 42. Average weight. Neat but old-fashioned dress. Sitting comfortably with hands in lap. She speaks with a hint of whine in her voice. "Well, Doctor, I hardly know where to begin. I don't think I've had a well day in my life since I was in high school. I guess the worst are these excruciating headaches. Half the time I can't even fix meals, but my husband and children try to take care of me. It's all very upsetting. They do the best they can, but I get annoyed and irritable sometimes because I don't think they realize how much I suffer! But then I have these dizzy spells and bowel trouble. Unless I'm very careful with what I eat I get sick to my stomach and my periods have never been right."
Mr. Brazil, age 19. Dressed in red sport shirt and white slacks. Sitting with right leg crossed over left. He speaks with considerable inflection. "Well, there's *nothing* serious. I don't know why my parents are so *concerned.* I have this little headache." (Patient smiles.) "It's right here most of the time." (He gestures dramatically with his right hand to an area about 5 cm to 6 cm in diameter over his right ear.) "As you can see, I don't like to touch it because it is sensitive and shoots pains. Sometimes, it's kinda numb, though."
Mr. Cooper, age 54. Dressed in a conservative, expensive suit. Sitting with his right hand in a fist resting on arm of chair. Eyebrows are knit. Forehead is in a scowl. He speaks in a quiet and controlled manner. "I'll be brief. For 4½ years, almost on a daily basis, mainly at work—I'm Vice President of First National Bank, in charge of the loan division—beginning at noon, becoming severe in the late afternoon, I develop rather painful bilateral frontal headaches. I'll be frank with you. You are the third physician with whom I have consulted. I have not been satisfied with my experience in seeking relief from this malady to date." (With the last statement, he points his finger toward the physician.)
Mrs. Duncan, age 37. Dressed in skirt and blouse. Hands fidget somewhat. Patient looks at physician with wide-open eyes, "Doctor, I'm frightened. For

the last 2 weeks, I have been waking up early in the morning with a kind of a dull, throbbing headache mainly over my right eye. I've had headaches before but nothing like these, and this morning while reading the newspaper I happened to shut one eye and I noticed that the print was blurred, especially with my left eye closed.''

Mr. Eagleton, age 41. Sitting in a rumpled sport coat. Hair uncombed. Head and eyes downcast, looking toward the floor. He speaks quietly and with little inflection. ''Well, Doctor, I need help, but I don't think anybody can help me. I know I have to do it myself, but I can't seem to pull myself together since I got laid off at work, almost a year ago now. My wife is very understanding. I don't deserve her. She'd be better off without me. I just sit home and hardly don't want to get up. To be honest, I'm just awfully discouraged. I feel awful, just awful. I don't know what's going to become of me.''

(77–81) Match the following. A given answer may be used *once, more than once,* or *not at all*.
(a) Evidence for anxiety
(b) Evidence for anger
(c) Evidence for sadness
(d) Evidence for disgust
(e) Little evidence for any of the above, either objective or subjective

77. Mrs. Alport
78. Mr. Brazil
79. Mr. Cooper
80. Mrs. Duncan
81. Mr. Eagleton

(82–86) Given the following, choose the most likely diagnosis. Here an answer should be used *once and only once*.
(a) Major depression
(b) Meningioma
(c) Conversion disorder
(d) Somatization disorder (Briquet's syndrome)
(e) Musculotension headache

82. Mrs. Alport
83. Mr. Brazil
84. Mr. Cooper
85. Mrs. Duncan
86. Mr. Eagleton

(87–91) Given the following, choose the most likely character structure. Here also an answer should be used *once and only once*.
(a) Narcissistic character
(b) Compulsive character
(c) Histrionic character
(d) Dependent character
(e) Genital character

87. Mrs. Alport
88. Mr. Brazil
89. Mr. Cooper
90. Mrs. Duncan
91. Mr. Eagleton

(92–96) Recall that objective evidence refers to behavioral data and subjective evidence to verbal data. Identify the physician's most appropriate move in the interview given above. Again, an answer should be used *once and only once*.
(a) Noting neither objective nor subjective evidence for a distressing emotion when one would be expected, physician inquires how the patient is feeling about his or her symptom.
(b) Noting congruence of objective and subjective evidence, the physician acknowledges the emotion and formulates a question attempting to identify the category of stress.
(c) Noting subjective evidence for an emotion but without objective evidence, physician inquires whether the patient is feeling that way right now, intending to then confront the patient with the absence of objective evidence.
(d) Noting objective evidence but an absence of subjective evidence, physician inquires how the patient is feeling about the symptom and the situation just expressed.
(e) Noting congruence between objective and subjective evidence and sensing already a consensus regarding the stress, the physician inquires what in *particular* the patient is distressed about.

92. Mrs. Alport
93. Mr. Brazil

94. Mr. Cooper
95. Mrs. Duncan
96. Mr. Eagleton

ANSWERS TO MULTIPLE-CHOICE QUESTIONS

1. d	**9.** e	**17.** e	**25.** e	**33.** e	**49.** c	**65.** c	**81.** c
2. b	**10.** c	**18.** e	**26.** e	**34.** a	**50.** d	**66.** e	**82.** d
3. d	**11.** a	**19.** a	**27.** d	**35.** a	**51.** e	**67.** e	**83.** c
4. a	**12.** c	**20.** c	**28.** a	**36.** e	**52.** b	**68.** d	**84.** e
5. c	**13.** c	**21.** a	**29.** b	**37.** e	**53.** c	**69.** b	**85.** b
6. e	**14.** d	**22.** e	**30.** d	**38.** b	**54.** d	**70.** c	**86.** a
7. c	**15.** d	**23.** a	**31.** b	**39.** a	**55.** a	**71.** a	**87.** a
8. e	**16.** e	**24.** a	**32.** d	**40.** d	**56.** e	**72.** c	**88.** c
				41. c	**57.** d	**73.** b	**89.** b
				42. d	**58.** e	**74.** e	**90.** e
				43. c	**59.** c	**75.** a	**91.** d
				44. e	**60.** a	**76.** d	**92.** c
				45. a	**61.** b	**77.** b	**93.** a
				46. b	**62.** a	**78.** e	**94.** d
				47. b	**63.** b	**79.** b	**95.** e
				48. a	**64.** d	**80.** a	**96.** b

Index

Page numbers followed by *f* indicate figures; numbers followed by *t* indicate tabular material.

Abdomen
  injury to, 53–54
    blunt, 53–54
    surgery involving, 53–55
ABO incompatibility, 322
Abortion, 209–210, 296
  complete, 209
  incomplete, 209
  inevitable, 209
  missed, 209
  spontaneous, 209
Abruption placenta, 212–214
Abscess
  brain, 168
  ischiorectal, 67
  lung, 116–117
  pancreatic, 131*t*
  peritonsillar, 43–44
  retropharyngeal, 44
  subdiaphragmatic, 56
Accidents, 335–336
  prevention of, 361–362
Acidosis
  metabolic, 121
  renal tubular, 134*t*
  respiratory, 121
Acquired immunodeficiency syndrome
    (AIDS), 120, 148*t*, 149–150, 334,
    355–356
  cases, by year of report—United
    States, 355*f*
Acromegaly, 139
Acute general hospital, 368
Acute tubular necrosis (ATN), 119
Addison's disease, 137–138
Adenoma
  bronchial, 52–53
  islet cell (pancreatic), 61
Adenomatous polyps, 129*t*
Adenomyosis, 265–266
Adjustment disorder(s), 384, 395
  with depressed mood, 391
Adjustment reaction, 382, 383
Administration
  of health care financing, 353
  of health services, 352–354

Adolescence, psychiatric disorders first
    evident in, 381–384
Adolescent sterility, 283
Adrenal cortex, tumors of, 68
Adrenal glands
  cancer of, palliation for, 69
  surgery of, 68–69
    indications for, 68–69
Adrenal hyperplasia
  congenital, 325
  non-salt-losing form, 325
  salt-losing form, 325
Adrenal medulla, tumors of, 68
Adult respiratory distress syndrome, 52
Aerobic gram-negative pneumonia, 113–
    114
Affective disorder(s), 389–391
  major, 389–390
  organic, 391
  unipolar, endogenous, 390
AGA infants. *See* Appropriate-for-gesta-
    tional-age infants
Age, gestational, 321
  assessment of, 319*f*
Aging. *See* Older adults
Agoraphobia, 391
AIDS. *See* Acquired immunodeficiency
    syndrome
AIDS-related complex (ARC), 148*t*
AIHA. *See* Autoimmune hemolytic
    anemia
Alcohol
  abuse of, 131*t*, 362–363
  disorders induced by, 385–386
  effects on fetus, 316*t*
Alcohol amnestic disorder, 386
Alcohol hallucinosis, 386
Alcoholic liver disease, 133*t*
Alcohol intoxication, 385
  idiosyncratic, 385
Alcohol withdrawal syndrome, 385
Aldosteronism, primary, 138
Aliphatic, 404*t*
Alkalosis
  metabolic, 121
  respiratory, 121

Alpha-1-antitrypsin deficiency, 133*t*
Alpha error, 351
Alzheimer's disease, 165, 385
Ambulatory care, 369
Amebiasis, 148*t*, 154
Amenorrhea, 281, 286
  primary, 286
  secondary, 284
Amnesia, 394
Amnestic disorder, alcohol, 386
Amnestic syndrome, 385
Amoebae, 168
Amphetamines, 386
Amputations, 27–28
Amyotrophic lateral sclerosis, 165
Analgesia
  for labor and delivery, 208–209
  obstetric, 208
Anatomy
  of female sex organs, 184–190
  neonatal, 317–323
Anemia(s), 101–107
  acute blood loss, 103
  aplastic, 103
  of chronic disorders, 103
  Cooley's, 101
  due to excess loss of red cells, 103–107
  due to increased or ineffective red-cell
    production, 101–103
  of endocrine insufficiency, 103
  hemolytic, 103–107, 134*t*
    congenital, 326–327
  iron deficiency, 101–102, 326
  of liver disease, 103
  megaloblastic, 102–103
  myelodysplastic, 103
  pernicious, 102
  sickle-cell, 105, 326–327
  of uremia, 103
Anesthesia
  for labor and delivery, 208–209
  obstetric, 208
Aneurysm
  of aorta, dissecting, 101
  of aortic arch, 90
  ventricular, 93

Angiitis, hypersensitivity, 156
Angina
　Ludwig's, 44
　Vincent's, 43
Angina pectoris, 90–91
Ankle, fractures and dislocations of, 41
Ankylosing spondylitis, 159–160
Anorchia, 293
Anorexia nervosa, 383
Anovulation, 281
　chronic, 283–284
Antianxiety agents, 403, 404t
Antibodies
　cold, 106
　warm, 106
Anticancer agents, effects on fetus, 316t
Anticoagulants, effects on fetus, 316t
Antidepressants, 404t, 404–405
Antigen drift, 142
Antigenemia, hepatitis B, 120
Antihistamines, 404t
Antihypertensive therapy, randomized
　trials of, reduction in odds of
　stroke and CHD in, 348t
Antimanic agents, 404t, 404
Antimicrobials, effects on fetus, 316t
Antipsychotic agents, 402–403, 404t
Antisocial personality disorder, 398–
　399
Anus, imperforate, 69
Anxiety disorder(s), 382, 391–393
　generalized, 392
Anxiety neurosis, 392
Anxiety states, 392
Anxiety syndrome, organic, 385
Anxiolytics, 403
Aorta
　aneurysm of, dissecting, 101
　coarctation of, 50, 85–86
　　incidence of, in patients diagnosed
　　with congenital heart disease,
　　84t
　thromboembolic disease of, 100
Aortic arch, aneurysm of, 90
Aortic arch syndrome, 100
Aortic regurgitation, 88, 90
Aortic stenosis, 88, 90
　incidence of, in patients diagnosed
　　with congenital heart disease,
　　84t
Aortitis, leutic, 90
Apgar score, 320–321
Apnea(s)
　central, 117
　mixed, 117
　neonatorum, 235–236
　　treatment of, 235–236
　obstructive, 117
Appendicitis, 63–64
　acute, 333
　recurrent or chronic, 64
Appropriate-for-gestational-age (AGA)
　infants, 321
ARC. See AIDS-related complex
Arterial aneurysm, 34
Arteriosclerosis obliterans, 33
Arteriovenous fistula, 34
Arteriovenous malformations (AVMs),
　129t, 162
Arteritis
　giant-cell, 156–157, 165
　temporal, 156–157

Arthritis, 157–161
　classification of, 157–158
　crystal-induced, 160–161
　rheumatoid, 158–159
Artificial insemination, 290
Ascites, 134t
Asherman's syndrome, 284
L-Asparaginase, 131t
Asphyxia
　intrapartum, 317
　livida, 235
　pallida, 235
Aspirin, effects on fetus, 316t
Asthma
　bronchial, 111–112
　extrinsic, 111
　intrinsic, 111
Astrocytomas, 164
　of cerebellum, 328
Ataractics, 402–403
Ataxia telangiectasia, 334
Atelectasis, lobar or lung, 53
Atherosclerosis, 90, 93
ATN. See Acute tubular necrosis
Atresia
　choanal, 331
　esophageal, 69
　intestinal, 69
Atrial fibrillation (AF), 99
Atrial flutter, 99
Atrial septal defect(s), 51, 85
　incidence in patients diagnosed with
　　congenital heart disease, 84t
Atrial tachycardias, 98–99
Atriohisian (tract) pathways, 99
Atrioventricular (A-V) conduction de-
　fects or block, 99
Atrioventricular (A-V) nodal reentrant
　tachycardia, 98–99
Atrioventricular (A-V) node block, 99
Atrioventricular (A-V) pathway, 99
Attention-deficit hyperactivity disorder,
　382
Autism, infantile, 383
Autoantibodies, 106
Autoimmune hemolytic anemia (AIHA),
　106
AVMs. See Arteriovenous malformations
Avoidant disorder, 382
Avoidant personality disorder, 400
Awareness, 405
Azaspirodecanedione, 404t
Azathioprine, 131t

Bacteremia, 147
Bacterial endocarditis, 89
　acute (ulcerative), 89
Bacterial meningitis, 167
Bacterial sexually transmitted diseases,
　151–152
Barbiturates, 386
Barlow's syndrome, 87
Barrett's esophagus, 122
Bartholin's duct cyst, 249
Bartholin's gland, carcinoma of, 251
Basal-cell carcinoma, 251
Bassini repair, 55
Behavior(s)
　age-appropriate, 384
　health, 365–366
　individual physician, 370

Behavior therapy, 408
Benign late syphilis, 153–154
Benzodiazepines, 404t
Bereavement, uncomplicated, 391
Beta-adrenergic blocking drugs, 88
Beta (β) error, 351
Bile ducts, surgery involving, 58–59
Biliary cirrhosis, 134
　primary, 134
Biliary colic, 58
Biliary obstruction, 125t
Biliary sclerosis, primary, 133t
Biofeedback, 407
Biologic plausibility, 349–350
Biologic variability, 351
Bipolar disorder, 390
Birth process, family-centered, 206
Birth trauma, 330t
Bite(s)
　insect, 27
　snake, 27
　wounds, 26–27
Blackouts, 386
Bleeding
　control of, 28–29
　disorders of, 107–108
　uterine
　　anovulatory, 281
　　arrhythmic, 281–282
Body, mind, brain, and, unified, 377
Böhlers angle, 41
Bone age, pediatric, 312
Bony pelvis, 184–185
Brain
　abscess in, 168
　body, mind, and, unified, 377
　tumors in, 164
Brain disorders, organic, 385
Brain stem, gliomas of, 328
Brain syndromes, organic, 384–385
　treatment of, 387
Brain waves
　alpha, 381
　beta, 381
　delta, 381
　theta, 381
Branchiogenic cysts, 44
Braxton Hicks version, 232
Breast
　carcinoma of, 47–49
　examination of, 47
　fibroadenoma of, 47
　sarcoma of, 48
　surgery involving, 47–49
Breech extraction
　partial, 227
　total, 227
Breech presentation, 227–228
　classification of, 227
　complete, 227
　frank, 227
　incomplete, 227
　vaginal delivery with, 227
Briquet's syndrome, 393
Broad ligaments, 186
Bronchial adenoma, 52–53
Bronchial asthma, 111–112
Bronchiectasis, 116
Bronchiolitis, 332
Bronchogenic carcinoma, 53
Bronchopneumonia, 113
Bronchopulmonary dysplasia, 321

Bryant's triangle, 39
Buccal mucosa, carcinoma of, 45
Budd-Chiari syndrome, 133*t*
Buerger's disease, 33
Bulimia nervosa, 382
Burns, 28
    classification of, rule of nines for, 28
    first-degree, 28
    second-degree, 28
    third-degree, 28
Bursitis, acute subdeltoid, 35
Butyrophenone, 404*t*

Caffeine, 386
Calculus(i). *See* Gallstones; Renal stones
Caloric requirements, 313–314
Cancer. *See* Carcinoma
Candidiasis, 242–243
Cannabis intoxication, 386
Capillary hemangiomata, 317
Carbonates, 404*t*
Carbuncle, 26
Carcinoid, 126–127
Carcinoid syndrome, 65
Carcinoma. *See also* Malignancy
    adrenal glands, palliation for, 69
    Bartholin's gland, 251
    basal-cell, 251
    breast, 47–49
    bronchogenic, 53
    of buccal mucosa, 45
    clear-cell, renal, 72
    colon, 65–66, 129, 129*t*
    endometrial, 257–260
    esophageal, 55–56, 123
    gastric, 57, 125
    gingival, 45
    hepatocellular, 134*t*
    of lips, 45
    of lung, 113
    of mouth floor, 45
    ovarian, 273–275
    pancreatic, 60–61, 125*t*, 131*t*, 131–132
    prostate, 73–74
    rectal, 65–66
    renal-cell, 121
    squamous-cell, 250–251
    of testis, 75
    thyroid, 136
    of tongue, 44–45
    of vagina, 251–252
Cardiac arrest, 50
Cardiac disorders, chronic, effects on
        fetus, 316*t*
Cardiac dysrhythmias, 98–100
Cardiac tamponade, 50
Cardinal ligaments, 185
Cardiology, 83–101
    questions in, 170
Cardiomyopathy, 94, 134*t*
    dilated, 94
    hypertrophic, 94
    restrictive, 94
Cardiorespiratory system, neonatal, 318
Cardiovascular disease, hypertensive,
        96–98
    treatment of, 98
Cardiovascular disorders, 396
    in children, 332–333
Cardiovascular syphilis, 90, 154

Cardiovascular system, physiologic
        changes of, in pregnancy, 193–
        194
Carpals, fractures of, 38
Case control studies, 347–348
Causality, epidemiologic criteria for
        inferring, 349*t*, 349–350
Celiac sprue, 125*t*
Cellular immunity, 334–335
Cellulitis, 25
Central nervous system
    infections of, 330*t*
        neonatal, 320
    stimulants, 403
    tumors of, 328
Cerebellum, astrocytomas of, 328
Cerebral palsy, 331
Cerebrovascular disease, 161–164
Cervical intraepithelial neoplasias (CIN),
        252–254
Cervicitis, 148*t*, 252
    mucopurulent, 150–151
Cervix, 186
    dilatation of, secondary arrest of, 203
    disorders of, 252–255
    dysplasia of, 252–254
    malignancy of, 254–255
Cesarean section, 232
CGD. *See* Chronic granulomatous dis-
        ease
Chancroid, 148*t*, 152, 245
Childbirth
    injuries of
        classification of, 275–276
        remote effects of, 275–281
    natural, 206
Childhood
    idiopathic nephrotic syndrome of, 334
    psychiatric disorders first evident in,
        381–384
Children. *See also* Pediatrics
    average daily nutritional requirements
        for, 314*t*
    recommended immunization schedule
        for, 335*t*
Chlamydial sexually transmitted dis-
        eases, 150–151
Chlamydia trachomatis, 148*t*, 244–245
Choanal atresia, 331
Cholangitis, primary sclerosing, 133*t*
Cholecystitis, 58–59
    acute, 58–59
    chronic, 59
Cholelithiasis, 58, 130–131
Cholera, immunization recommendations
        for, during pregnancy, 196*t*
Cholesterol
    low-density lipoprotein, classification
        and treatment decisions based
        on, 363*t*
    serum, 340*f*
        and first coronary event in men 30 to
            59, relationship of, 347*f*
        total, initial classification and recom-
            mended follow-up based on,
            363*t*
Chorion, 192–193
Chorion frondosum, 191
Chorion laeve, 191
Christmas disease, 107
Chromosomal abnormalities, 330*t*, 330–
        331

Chronic granulomatous disease (CGD),
        335
Chronic lymphocytic leukemia (CLL),
        109
Chronic myelocytic leukemia (CML),
        108–109
Chronic obstructive pulmonary disease
        (COPD), 111
Chronic ulcerative colitis (CUC), 128
Chronic wasting disease, 149
CIN. *See* Cervical intraepithelial neopla-
        sias
Circulation
    diseases of, 83–101
        diagnostic considerations, 83
    fetal, 234–235
Circumvallate placenta, 205
Cirrhosis
    biliary, 134
    complications of, 134*t*
    etiologies of, 133*t*
    of liver, 133–134
    postnecrotic, 134
Clavicle, fractures and dislocations of,
        36
Clear-cell carcinoma, renal, 72
Click–murmur syndrome, 87
Climacterium, 296–297
Clinical trials, 348
    power of, 351
    randomized, of antihypertensive ther-
        apy, reduction in odds of stroke
        and CHD in, 348*t*
CLL. *See* Chronic lymphocytic leukemia
Cluster headaches, 164
CML. *See* Chronic myelocytic leukemia
CNS. *See* Central nervous system
Coarctation of the aorta, 50, 85–86
    incidence of, in patients diagnosed
        with congenital heart disease,
        84*t*
Cocaine intoxication, 386
Coccyx, fracture of, 38
Cold antibodies, 106
Cold sores, 148*t*
Colectomy, in ulcerative colitis, indica-
        tions for, 128*t*
Colic, biliary, 58
Colitis
    ischemic, 128–129, 129*t*
    ulcerative, 66–67
        chronic, 128, 129*t*
Collagen vascular disease, 100
Colles' fracture, 37–38
Colon
    cancer of, 65–66, 129, 129*t*
        risk factors for, 129*t*
    diseases of, 127–130
    diverticular, 66
    polyps of, nonfamilial, 64–65
Common duct obstruction, 59
Community medicine, 339–370
    questions in, 370–374
Compulsive personality disorder, 400
Conduct disorders, 382
Conduplicato corpore, 226
Congenital adrenal hyperplasia, 325
Congenital anomalies
    associated with mental retardation,
        330*t*, 331
    gastrointestinal, 333
    pulmonary, 331

Congestive heart failure, 95–96, 332
  diagnosis by chest x ray, diagnostic
    sensitivity and specificity for,
    350f
  etiology of, 95
  mechanisms underlying, 95t
Congruence, 349
Connective tissue disease, mixed, 157
Consistency, 349
Contraceptives
  intrauterine devices, 295
  oral, 294–295
Contract, making, 379
Contraction, pelvic, 226
Conversion disorder, 393
Cooley's anemia, 101
Coombs test
  direct, 105
  indirect, 105
COPD. *See* Chronic obstructive pulmo-
    nary disease
Coronary arteries, stenosis of, 90
Coronary artery disease, 90–93
Coronary event, first, in men 30 to 59,
    relationship of serum cholesterol
    and, 347f
Cor pulmonale, 94–95
Corpus luteum, 188–189
Corticosteroids, effects on fetus, 316t
Costs. *See* Hospital, rise in costs
Crab lice, 148t, 154–155
Craniotabes, 315
Cretinism, 137
Creutzfeldt-Jakob disease, 166
Crohn's disease, 67, 125t, 128
  surgery in, indications for, 129t
Cryptorchidism, 75
Crystal-induced arthritis, 160–161
  causes of, 161
CUC. *See* Chronic ulcerative colitis
Cushing's disease, 138
Cushing's syndrome, 138
Cyanosis, in newborn, 321
Cyclothymic disorder, 390
Cyclothymic personality, 390
Cyst(s)
  Bartholin's duct, 249
  branchiogenic, 44
  dermoid, 272
  lutein, 272
  neoplastic, 272
  ovarian, 272–273
  pancreatic, 60
  thyroglossal, 44
Cystadenomas
  pseudomucinous, 272
  serous, 272
Cystic fibrosis, 117, 125t, 332
Cystosarcoma phyllodes, 49
Cytomegalovirus, effects on fetus, 316t
Cytoreduction, 274

Death certification, 341–346
  standard-format, 342f
Death rate(s)
  age-adjusted, 343f, 344
  crude, 343, 343f
    seasonal change in, per 1,000 U.S.
      population, by month of calen-
      dar years 1985, 1986, and 1987,
      344f

Decision, 406
Degenerating diseases, 165–167
Delirium, 384
Delirium tremens, 385
Delivery. *See also* Labor and delivery
  breech extraction
    partial, 227
    total, 227
  by forceps, 230–231
  vaginal breech, 227
Delusional syndrome, organic, 385
Dementia, 384, 386
  multi-infarct, 385
  presenile, 385
  senile, 385
Demyelinating diseases, 165–167
Dental health, 362
Dependent personality disorder, 399
Depersonalization disorder, 394
Depressed mood, adjustment disorder
    with, 391
Depression
  major, 390
  reactive, 390
Depressive episode, major, 389–390
Depressive equivalent, 390
Depressive neurosis, 390
Dermatomyositis, 166
Dermatomyositis–polymyositis, 157
Dermoid cysts, 272
DES. *See* Diethylstilbestrol
Desferoxamine, 134t
Development
  disorders of
    pervasive, 383
    specific, 384
  milestones in, 312t, 313t
  pediatric, 312–313
  retardation of, 330–331
Diabetes, gestational, 140
Diabetes insipidus, 140
Diabetes mellitus, 120, 125t, 134t, 140–
    141
  chronic, effects on fetus, 316t
  complicating pregnancy, 222–224
  insulin-dependent (IDDM, Type I), 140
  juvenile, 325
  maternal, 316–317
  non-insulin-dependent (NIDDM, Type
    II), 140
  overt, 140
  type I (juvenile-onset), 325
Diabetic ketoacidosis, 141
Diagnosis-related groups (DRGs), 367
*Diagnostic and Statistical Manual of
    Mental Disorders of the Ameri-
    can Psychiatric Association*
    (DSM-III R), 376
Diagnostic tests
  evaluating, 350
  predictive value of, 350
Diaphragmatic hernia, 55, 56
Diarrhea, 127
Diazepam
  and epilepsy, 163t, 164
Dibenzoxazepine, 404t
Diethylstilbestrol (DES), exposure *in
    utero*, 291–292
DiGeorge's syndrome, 334
Digestive tract. *See also* Gastrointestinal
    system
  pediatric surgery involving, 69–70

Diphtheria, 143–144
Disaccharidase deficiency, 126
Diseases
  of children, 323–335
  of circulation, 83–101
  of esophagus, stomach, and intestines,
    121–130
  of hematopoietic system, 101–110
  infectious, 141–148
  of kidneys, 118–121
  of lungs, 110–118
  metabolic and endocrine, 135–141
  of nervous system, 161–169
  rheumatic, connective tissue, vascu-
    litides, and related disorders,
    155–161
  sexually transmitted, 148–155
  of spleen, pancreas, gallbladder, and
    liver, 130–135
Dislocations, of extremities, 35–42
Disseminated intravascular coagulation,
    28–29
Dissociative disorders, 394
Distal closed space infection, 34
Diverticulosis coli, 127–128, 129t
Doctor/patient interaction, 378, 379
  process of, 378–379
Dose response, 349
Down's syndrome, 330t, 330–331
Dressler's syndrome, 93
DRGs. *See* Diagnosis-related groups
Drug(s). *See also specific drug*
  hepatotoxicity, 135
  maternal use of, effects on fetus, 316t
  misuse of, 362–363
DSM-III R. *See Diagnostic and Statisti-
    cal Manual of Mental Disorders
    of the American Psychiatric
    Association*
Duchenne's dystrophy, 166
Duct papilloma, 47–48
Dumping syndrome, 58
Duodenum
  surgery involving, 56–58
  ulcer of, 57–58
Dysarthria, 134t
Dyslexia, 384
Dysmenorrhea, primary, 266–267
Dyspareunia, functional, 394
Dysphagia, 122–123
Dysplasia
  bronchopulmonary, 321
  cervical, 252–254
Dysrhythmias, 98–100
Dysthymic disorders, 390
Dystocia, 224
Dystrophy
  Duchenne's, 166
  muscular, 166
  myotonic, 166
  vulvar, 247–248

Ear, surgery involving, 43
Eating disorders, 382–383
Ebstein anomaly (of tricuspid valve), 86–
    87
Eclampsia, 212
Economic aspects, of health care, 367–
    370
Ectopic gestation, 269–270

Education Council for Foreign Medical Graduates (ECFMG)
certification, 9
English test, 10
Eisenmenger complex, 86
Ejaculation
premature, 394
reasonable control of, 394
Elbow, dislocations of, 37
Elderly. *See* Older adults
Electroencephalographic examination, 381
Electrolyte abnormalities, 121
Emboli, pulmonary, 112
Empyema, 53
Encephalitis, 168–169
Encephalopathy, portosystemic, 134*t*
Encopresis, functional, 383
Endocarditis, infective (bacterial), 89–90
Endocrine diseases, 135–141
Endocrine disorders, 324, 397
in children, 324–326
Endocrine insufficiency, anemia of, 103
Endocrinology, 135–141
questions in, 171
Endocrinopathies, 125*t*
gynecologic, 281–286
Endogenous disorder, 390
Endometrial carcinoma, 257–260
Endometriosis, 263–265
pharmacologic control of, 265
English language examinations, 10
Entamoeba histolytica, 148*t*
Enteritis
radiation, 125*t*
regional, 67
Enuresis, functional, 383
Environmental factors, effects on fetus, 316*t*
Enzyme defects, 322*t*
Epidemiology, 346–352
factors for inferring causality, 349*t*, 349–350
methods of research, 347–349
reasoning in, 349–352
Epididymitis, acute, 74
Epidural hematomas, 162
Epidural hemorrhage, 162
Epiglottitis, acute, 331–332
Epilepsy, 163–164
international classification of seizures, 163*t*
myoclonic, 329
of infancy, 329–330
treatment guidelines for, 163*t*
Episiotomy, 205–206
Epstein-Barr viral infections, 143
Errors
type I or alpha, 351
type II or beta (β), 351
Erysipelas, 144
Erythroblastosis, 236–238
Erythroblastosis fetalis, 322
Erythrocytosis, 107
Esophagus, 55–56
atresia of, 69
Barrett's, 122
cancer of, 55–56, 123
diseases of, 121–123
diverticulum of, 56
motility disorders of, 123
Estrogens, 131*t*

Ethnicity, 364–365
Etiology, multiple, 377
Evaluation, 377–381
beyond history, mental status, and physical examination, 381
concepts of, 377–378
involvement of family, friends, and health professionals in, 381
process of, 378–379
purpose of, 378
structure of, 379–380
Evaluative tests, of infertility, 287–289
Examination(s)
breast, 47
electroencephalographic, 381
medical qualifying, 1–22
of mental status, 380
physical, 380
of psychological status, 380
Exchange transfusions, in infant, 322
Exercise, 363–364
Expectation, chief, 379
Extremities
fractures and dislocations of, 35–42
general surgical conditions of, 32–35

Face presentation, 228
Facial nerve paralysis, 43
Facilities, 368
Failure to thrive, 324
Fallopian tube(s), 187
disorders of, 271
infertility due to, plastic procedures for, 290
malignancy of, 271
patency of, test of, 287–288
False negative, 350
False positive, 350
Family, involvement in evaluation, 381
Family cancer syndrome, 129*t*
Family-centered birth process, 206
Family planning, 293–296, 356
Farmer's lung, 117
Fasciculoventricular pathways, 99
Fascitis, necrotizing, 26
Federal health services, in United States, 352–354
Federation Licensing Examination (FLEX), 7–9
Feeding, infant, 314
Felon, 34
Female(s)
infertility in, surgical approaches to, 290
lower generative tract of, disorders of, 241–248
non-salt-losing adrenal hyperplasia in, 325
orgasm in, inhibited, 394
pseudohermaphroditism in, 292
sex organs of, anatomy and physiology of, 184–190
Feminization, testicular, 292–293
Femur
fractures of, 39–40
intertrochanteric, 39
neck, fracture of, 39
shaft, fracture of, 40
Fetal heart rate
late deceleration pattern, 201
long-term variability in, 199

mature parameters, 201*t*
monitoring, 199–201
Fetus
circulation in, 234–235
death of, 182
effects of environmental factors on, 316*t*
effects of pregnancy on, 316–317
growth of, disproportionate, 216–217
maturity, laboratory tests of, 198–199
preventive services for, 358*t*
Fibroadenoma, of breast, 47
Fibrocystic disease, 47
Fibrosarcoma, 42
Fibrosis, cystic, 117
Financing, administration of, 353
Fine motor development, milestones in, 313*t*
Fingers, infections of, treatment of, 35
Fissure-in-ano, 68
Fistula(s)
rectovaginal, 281
tracheoesophageal, 331
Fistula-in-ano, 67
Fitz-Hugh–Curtis syndrome, 152, 261
FLEX. *See* Federation Licensing Examination
Flexor tendon sheaths, tenosynovitis of, 34–35
Fluoridation, 362
FMGEMS. *See* Foreign Medical Graduate Examination in the Medical Sciences
Folic acid deficiency, 102–103
Follicular fluid, 188
Forceps delivery, 230–231
Forearm, fractures and dislocations of, 37–38
Foreign Medical Graduate Examination in the Medical Sciences (FMGEMS), 9–10
Fossa ovale, patent, 85
Fracture(s)
bimalleolar, 41
comminuted, 35
delayed union or nonunion of, 41–42
of extremities, 35–42
greenstick, 36
open, 35
simple, 35
trimalleolar, 41
Free association, 407
Friends, involvement in evaluation, 381
Frostbite, 27
Fungal infection(s), 147, 167
Furosemide, 131*t*

Galactosemia, 325–326
Gallbladder, surgery involving, 58–59
Gallstones, 131*t*
Gardnerella vaginalis, 243
Gardner's syndrome, 64
Gas gangrene, 26
Gastric cancer, 57, 125
Gastric ulcer, 56–57
Gastritis, 125
Gastroenteritis, acute, 333
Gastroenterology, 121–130
questions in, 171
Gastroesophageal reflux (GER), 122

Gastrointestinal system
  disorders of, 396
    in children, 333
  infections of, 333
  lower, hemorrhage of, 129–130
  neonatal, 318–320
  physiologic changes of, during pregnancy, 194
  surgery involving, 55–70
  upper, hemorrhage of, 124–125
Gender identity disorders, 394
General hospital, acute, 368
Generative tract, lower, female, disorders of, 241–248
Genetic screening, 357
Genital characters, 400
Genital herpes, 148t
Genitalia
  enlargement of, 74
  surgery involving, 74–75
Genital warts, 148t
Genitourinary system
  disorders of, 396–397
  surgery involving, 70–75
GER. *See* Gastroesophageal reflux
Gestation
  ectopic, 269–270
  multiple, 218–220
  pathology of, 267–270
  very early, 190–193
Gestational age, 321
  assessment of, 319f
Gestational diabetes, 140
Giant-cell arteritis, 156–157, 165
Gigantism, 139
Gilbert's syndrome, 132
Gingival carcinoma, 45
Gliomas, of brain stem, 328
Glomerular disease(s), 119–120
  chronic progressive, 119
Glomerular syndromes, 119
Glomerulonephritis
  acute, 119, 334
  rapidly progressive, 119
Glomerulopathies, 120
Glucose-6-phosphate dehydrogenase (G6PD) deficiency, 105
Glucose tolerance
  abnormalities of
    potential, 140
    previous, 140
  impaired, 140
Goiter, simple colloid, 135
Gonococcal infections, 151
Gonorrhea, 148t, 262–263
Gout, 160–161
G6PD deficiency. *See* Glucose-6-phosphate dehydrogenase deficiency
Graafian follicles, 188
Graded response, 349
Granuloma, eosinophilic, 329
Granuloma inguinale, 245–246
Granulomatosis, Wegener's, 156
Great vessels, 50
Greenstick fractures, 36
Gross motor development, milestones in, 312t
Group psychotherapy, 408
Groups, self-help, 408
Growth
  definition of, 311
  pediatric, 311–312

retardation of, 324
  classification of, 324
Growth charts, 312
Growth curves, intrauterine, for length, head circumference, and weight, 320f
Guillain-Barré syndrome, 169
Gunshot wounds, abdominal, 54
Gynecology, 241–297
  endocrinopathies, 281–286
  questions in, 297–310
  therapy, remote effects of, 275–281

Haemophilus ducreyi, 148t
Hallucinogens, 386
Hallucinosis
  alcohol, 386
  organic, 385
Halsted herniorrhaphy, 55
Hand(s)
  fractures and dislocations of, 38
  general surgical conditions of, 34–35
  infections of, treatment of, 35
  mouth wounds of, 35
Hand-Schüller-Christian syndrome, 329
Hashimoto's thyroiditis, 135–136
Headache(s), 164–165
  cluster, 164
Head circumference
  intrauterine growth curves for, 320f
  pediatric, 312
Head injury, 330t
Health behavior, 365–366
Health care
  ambulatory, 369
  economic aspects of, 367–370
  facilities, 368
  formal and informal organization of, 369–370
  organizations, state and local, 353
  personnel, 369–370
  professional control, 369
  professionals, involvement in evaluation, 381
  voluntary agencies, 353–354
Health Care Financing Administration, 353
Health service(s)
  administration of, 352–354
  federal, in United States, 352–354
  high-priority areas of problem and treatment, 354–366
  public, United States, 353
  study of
    economic approach to, 366
    geographic approach to, 366
    organization approach to, 366
    social–cultural approach to, 366
    social–psychologic approach to, 366
    sociodemographic approach to, 366
Health statistics, 340–346
Heart, 50, 83. *See also under* Cardiac
  lesions of
    congenital, 51–52, 324
    valvular, acquired, 51
  luetic, 90
Heart disease
  complicating pregnancy, 221–222
  congenital, 84–89, 322, 332
    classification of, 84

incidence of defects in patients diagnosed with, 84t
    reduction in odds of, in randomized trials of antihypertensive trials, 348t
  cyanotic, 322
  diagnostic considerations, 83
Hebephrenia, 388
Height, pediatric, 311–312
Hemangiomata, capillary, 317
Hematologic system
  disorders of, in childhood, 326–328
  physiologic changes of, during pregnancy, 194
Hematology, 101–110
  questions in, 170
Hematoma(s)
  epidural, 162
  puerperal, 207
  subdural, 162
Hematopoietic system
  diseases of, 101–110
    malignancies, 108–110
  neonatal, 318
Hematuria, 70
  asymptomatic, 119
Hemochromatosis, 133t, 141
  clinical characteristics of, 134t
  diagnosis of, 134t
  treatment of, 134t
Hemoglobin, neonatal, 318
Hemoglobinopathies, 104, 322t
Hemolysis, isoimmune, 322, 322t
Hemolytic anemia(s), 103–107, 134t
  acquired (or extrinsic), 103
  autoimmune, 106
  classification of, 103–107
  congenital, 326–327
  hereditary (or intrinsic), 103
  immune, 105–106
  laboratory features of, 104
Hemolytic disease, 236–238
Hemolytic icterus, congenital, 62
Hemolytic jaundice, 132
  in newborn, 322
    causes of, 322t
Hemophilia, 327–328
Hemophilia A, 107
Hemophilia B, 107
Hemophilus pneumonia, 114
Hemorrhage
  epidural, 162
  intracranial, 162
  intraparenchymal, 162
  lower gastrointestinal, 129–130
  postpartal, 230
  subarachnoid, 162
  subdural, 162
  upper gastrointestinal, 124–125
  variceal, 134t
Hemorrhoids, 67–68
  external, 67
  internal, 67
Hemothorax, 49
Henoch-Schönlein purpura, 327
Hepatic jaundice, 132–133
Hepatitis
  chronic active, 133t, 134t
  fulminant, 134t
  viral, 149
    acute, 133

Hepatitis A, 133, 148*t*
  immunization recommendations for, during pregnancy, 196*t*
Hepatitis A virus, 148*t*
Hepatitis B, 133, 148*t*
  immunization recommendations for, during pregnancy, 196*t*
Hepatitis B antigenemia, 120
Hepatitis B virus, 148*t*
Hepatitis C, 133
Hepatocellular carcinoma, 134*t*
Hepatolentricular degeneration, 134
Hepatorenal syndrome, 134*t*
Hereditary spherocytosis (HS), 104
Hermaphrodites, 293
Hermaphroditism, male, 293
Hernia, 54–55
  acquired, 54
  congenital, 54
  diaphragmatic, 55, 56
  epigastric, 55
  femoral, 54
  incarcerated, 54
  incarceration of, 55
  inguinal, 54
    direct, 54
    indirect, 54
  obturator, 55
  reducible, 54
  scrotal, 74
  strangulated, 54
  strangulation of, 55
  umbilical, 54–55
Herniorrhaphy
  Bassini repair, 55
  Ferguson, 55
  Halsted, 55
  McVay repair, 55
Herpes simplex virus (HSV), 245
  infection, 148–149
  types I and II, 148*t*
Hidradenoma, 249
High-priority areas, of problem and treatment, 354–366
Hip, dislocations of, 39–40
  congenital, 40
Hirsutism, 285
Histiocytoma, malignant fibrous, 42
Histiocytosis, 329
Histiocytosis X, 329
Histrionic personality disorder, 400
HIV. *See* Human immunodeficiency virus
Hodgkin's disease (HD), 44, 110
Homostructural grafts, 31
Homovital grafts, 31
Hormonal therapy, for infertility, 289–290
Hospital
  acute general, 368
  rise in costs, reasons for, 367
HPV. *See* Human papillomavirus
HSV. *See* Herpes simplex virus
Human immunodeficiency virus (HIV), 148*t*
  infection, 149–150
Human papillomavirus (HPV), 243–244
  infection, 150
Humerus
  fractures and dislocations of, 36–37
    of anatomic neck, 36
    of greater tuberosity, 36

of lower end, 37
of shaft, 37
of surgical neck, 36
upper epiphysis, separation of, 36
Humoral immunity, 334
Hydrocele, 74
Hydrocephalus, 330*t*
Hydrocephaly, 331
Hydronephrosis, 71
Hydrops fetalis, 237
Hydroxylysine, 24
Hydroxyproline, 24
Hyperaldosteronism, 68–69
Hyperalimentation, intravenous, 30–31
Hyperbilirubinemia, 238
Hypercalcemia, 121, 131*t*
Hypercontractility, 224
Hyperemesis gravidarum, 210
Hyperkalemia, 121
Hyperlipoproteinemia, 93
  type I, 93
  type II, 94
  type III, 94
  type IV, 94
  type V, 94
Hypermenorrhea, 281, 296
Hypernephroma, 72, 121
Hyperparathyroidism, primary, 139
Hyperpigmentation, 134*t*
Hypersensitivity angiitis, 156
Hypersplenism, 62
Hypertension, 96–98, 354–355
  accelerated or malignant, 97
  chronic, 212
  essential, 96
  portal, 62–63
  secondary, 96
  treatment of, 98
    randomized trials of, reduction in odds of stroke and CHD in, 348*t*
Hypertensive cardiovascular disease, 96–98
  treatment of, 98
Hypertensive states, of pregnancy, 210–212
Hyperthyroidism, 136–137
  effects on fetus, 316*t*
Hypertriglyceridemia, 131*t*
Hypertrophic cardiomyopathy (HCM), 88
Hyperuricemia
  primary, 160
  secondary, 160
Hypervitaminosis A, 315
Hypervitaminosis D, 315
Hypnotherapy, 407
Hypnotics, 403
Hypocalcemia, 131*t*
Hypochondriacal neurosis, 393–394
Hypochondriasis, 393–394
Hypocontractility, 224
Hypoglycemia, 141
Hypogonadism
  hypergonadotropic, 284
  hypogonadotropic, 284
Hypokalemia, 121
Hypomenorrhea, 281
Hyponatremia, 121
Hypoparathyroidism, 139
  effects on fetus, 316*t*
Hypophosphatemia, 121
Hypopituitarism, 138–139
Hypotheses, testing, 351

Hypothyroidism, 137
  congenital, 324–325
  effects on fetus, 316*t*
Hypoxia, 330*t*
  perinatal, 330*t*
Hypsarrhythmia, 330
Hysterical neurosis
  conversion type, 393
  dissociative type, 394
Hysterical personality, 400

Icterus gravis, 237
IDDM. *See* Diabetes mellitus, insulin-dependent
Idiopathic hypertrophic subaortic stenosis (IHSS), 88
Idiopathic nephrotic syndrome of childhood, 334
Idiopathic thrombocytopenic purpura, 62, 108
Ileal disease, 125*t*
Ileus, 131*t*
Imaging studies, 381
Immune hemolytic anemias, 105–106
  autoimmune, 106
  drug-induced, 106
Immune system, diseases of, in children, 334–335
Immunity
  cellular, 334–335
  humoral, 334
Immunization(s), 359–360
  during pregnancy, current recommendations for, 196*t*
  recommended schedule for, 335*t*
Immunologic system, neonatal, 318
Inborn errors of metabolism, 324, 330*t*
Incidence rate, 342
Individual patient care, 339
Individual psychotherapy, 407
Individual response specificity, 377
Infancy
  myoclonic epilepsy of, 329–330
  psychiatric disorders first evident in, 381–384
Infant(s). *See also* Newborn
  appropriate-for-gestational-age (AGA), 321
  average daily nutritional requirements for, 314*t*
  effects of labor and delivery on, 317
  exchange transfusions in, 322
  feeding of, 314
  full-term, 321
  health of, 356–357
  large-for-gestational-age (LGA), 321
  low-birth-weight, 321
  mortality, top ten causes, by race, United States, 1983, 357*t*
  mortality rates, 344
    by race, specified years, 356*t*
  normal, preventive services for, 359*t*
  postterm, 321
  premature, 182, 238–241
  preterm, 321
  recommended immunization schedule for, 335*t*
  small-for-gestational-age, 321
Infantile autism, 383

Infarction
    ischemic, 161–162
    myocardial, 91–93
Infection(s)
    acquired, in neonates, 323
    of central nervous system, 330t
    in compromised hosts, 147–148
    congenital, 330t
        in neonates, 323
    distal closed space, 34
    of fingers and hand, treatment of, 35
    fungal, 147, 167
    gastrointestinal, 333
    gonococcal, 151
    intrapartal, 225–226
    kidney, 71–72
    listerial, 145
    mycobacterial, 167
    nosocomial, 146–147
    of palmar spaces, 35
    pelvic, 260–263
    postnatal, 330t
    puerperal, 232–234
    pulmonary, 116–117, 331–332
    surgical wound, 146
    urinary tract, 146
    viral, 147. See also Viral infection(s)
    of wounds, 25–26
Infectious diseases, 141–148
    effects on fetus, 316t
    questions in, 171
    surveillance and control of, 357–359
Infectious disorders, of nervous system,
        167–169
Infective (bacterial) endocarditis, 89–90
Infertility, 286–290
    evaluative tests and procedures for,
        287–289
    female, surgical approaches to, 290
    male, procedures for, 290
    treatment of, 289
        hormonal, 289–290
    tubal, plastic procedures for, 290
Inflammatory bowel disease, 128, 129t
    extraintestinal manifestations of,
        128t
Inflammatory myopathies, 166
Influenza, 142–143
    immunization recommendations for,
        during pregnancy, 196t
    type A, 142
    type B, 142
Infranodal block, 99
Injury. See also Trauma
    abdominal, 53–54
    of childbirth, remote effects of, 275–
        281
    control of, 361–362
    head, 330t
    urinary tract, 279–281
Insect bites, 27
Insect sexually transmitted diseases,
        154–155
Insemination, artificial, 290
Internal medicine, 83–178
    questions in, 170–178
Interstitial disease
    lung, 112–113
    renal, 120
Intervention
    developing strategy for, 379
    implementation of, 379

Interview
    priorities for, 378
    process of, 379
Intestines. See also Colon; Small intes-
        tine
    atresia of, 69
    ischemia of, 125t
    lymphoma of, primary, 125t
    obstruction of, 63
    polyposis of, 64–65
    surgery involving, 63–68
Intoxication, 385
    alcohol, 385
        idiosyncratic, 385
    cannabis, 386
    cocaine, 386
    lead, 330t
    opioid, 386
Intracranial hemorrhage, 162
Intraparenchymal hemorrhage, 162
Intrapartal infection, 225–226
Intrapartum asphyxia, 317
Intrauterine contraceptive devices, 295
Intrauterine growth curves, for length,
        head circumference, and weight,
        320f
Intrauterine status, laboratory tests of,
        198–199
Intravenous hyperalimentation, 30–31
Intussusception, 70, 333
in vitro fertilization, 290
Iron deficiency anemia(s), 101–102, 326
Irritable bowel syndrome, 127
Ischemia
    intestinal, 125t
    silent, 91
Ischemic colitis, 128–129, 129t
Ischiorectal abscess, 67
Islet cell adenoma, pancreatic, 61
Isoantibodies, 106
Isoimmune hemolysis, 322t, 322

Jaundice, 132–133
    cholestatic (obstructive), 132
    hemolytic, 132
        in newborn, 322
            causes of, 322t
    hepatic, 132–133
    neonatal, 322
    obstructive, 131t
Joint replacement, 41–42
Juvenile diabetes mellitus, 325

Kallmann's syndrome, 286
Kaposi's sarcoma, 42
Kayser-Fleischer rings, 134t
Kernicterus, 237
    in neonate, 322
Ketoacidosis, diabetic, 141
Kidney(s). See also under Renal
    clear-cell carcinoma of, 72
    diseases of, 118–121
        in children, 333–334
        interstitial, 120
        primary, 119
        secondary, 119
        vascular, 120
    disorders of, chronic, effects on fetus,
        316t

    embryoma of, 72–73
    functions of
        excretory, 118
        regulatory, 118
    infections of, 71–72
    polycystic, 120
    rupture of, 73
    surgery involving, 70–73
    tumors of, 72–73
        benign, 72
Knee, fractures and dislocations of, 40
Koilocytosis, 244

Labor
    active phase, 202
    dysfunctional, 224–225
        primary, 203
    latent phase, 202
        prolonged, 202–203
    pathology of, 224–234
    physiology and conduct of, 201–202
    precipitate, 225
    preterm or premature, 215–216, 317
    second stages, prolonged, 203
Labor and delivery
    analgesia and anesthesia for, 208–209
    breech presentation in, 227–228
    cardinal movements, 203
    effects on infant, 317
    face presentation in, 228
    mechanism of, 203–204
    normal, 202–208
    spontaneous, 227
    stages of, 202–203
Laboratory tests, 381
    during pregnancy, 198–201
Language development, milestones in,
        313t
Laparoscopy, diagnostic, 288–289
Large-for-gestational-age (LGA) infants,
        321
Larynx, surgery involving, 45
Lead
    effects on fetus, 316t
    intoxication, 330t
Leg(s), general surgical conditions of,
        32–34
Legionella pneumonia, 114–115
Leiomyomata, 255–257
Length, intrauterine growth curves for,
        320f
Leprosy, 145
    lepromatous, 145
    tuberculoid, 145
Leptospirosis, 168
Lesions. See also Tumor(s)
    cardiac
        congenital, 51–52, 324
        valvular, acquired, 51
    vulvar
        involving abnormal pigmentation,
            247–248
        malignant, 251
        melanotic, 248
        of syphilis, 246–247
        ulcerative, benign, 245–247
Letterer-Siwe syndrome, 329
Leukemia(s), 328
    acute, 109
    granulocytic, acute, 328
    lymphatic, acute, 328

lymphocytic, chronic, 109
myelocytic, chronic, 108–109
Leukorrhea, 241–245
LGA infants. *See* Large-for-gestational-age infants
LGV. *See* Lymphogranuloma venereum
Lice, pubic, 148*t*, 154–155
Lichen sclerosus et atrophicus, 247
Lichen simplex chronicus, 247
Life expectancy, 345–346
   at birth, by year of birth and by race—United States, 1970–1989, 345*f*
Life table, abridged, United States, 1981, 345*t*
Lipoprotein plasma abnormalities, 93–94
Liposarcoma, 42
Lips, cancer of, 45
Listerial infections, 145
Liver. *See also under* Hepatic
   cirrhosis of, 133–134
   surgery involving, 62–63
Liver disease
   alcoholic, 133*t*
   anemia of, 103
Lobar atelectasis, 53
Local health organizations, 353
Lorazepam
   and epilepsy, 163*t*, 164
Lou Gehrig's disease, 165
Low-birth-weight infants, 321
Low-density lipoprotein cholesterol, classification and treatment decisions based on, 363*t*
Lower extremities
   fractures and dislocations of, 39–41
   general surgical conditions of, 32–34
Lower gastrointestinal hemorrhage, 129–130
   acute, common causes of, 129*t*
Lower generative tract, female, disorders of, 241–248
Ludwig's angina, 44
Luetic aortitis, 90
Luetic heart, 90
Lung(s). *See also under* Pulmonary
   abscess in, 116–117
   atelectasis of, 53
   carcinoma of, 113
   farmer's, 117
   surgery involving, 52–53
   tumors of, 52–53
Lung disease(s), 110–118
   interstitial, 112–113
Lutein cysts, 272
Lyme disease, 145, 168
Lymphadenitis, 25
Lymphangiectasia, 125*t*
Lymphangitis, 25
Lymph node enlargements, in neck, 44
Lymphogranuloma venereum (LGV), 148*t*, 151, 246
Lymphoma
   malignant, 44
   non-Hodgkin's, 110

McCune-Albright syndrome, 282
McVay repair, 55
Malabsorption, 125–126
   causes of, 125*t*
Male(s)
   hermaphroditism in, 293

infertility in, procedures for, 290
non-salt-losing adrenal hyperplasia in, 325
orgasm in, inhibited, 394
Malignancy. *See also* Carcinoma; *specific tumor*
   cervical, 254–255
   in children, 328–329
   of hematopoietic system, 108–110
   of small intestine, 65
   tubal, 271
   vulvar, 251
      invasive, 250–251
Malnutrition, 324
   effects on fetus, 316*t*
Manic–depressive illness, 390
Manic episode, 389
Mastitis, cystic, chronic, 47
Maternal death, 181
   indirect obstetric cause, 181
Maternal diabetes mellitus, 316–317
Maternal mortality, in United States, 1950–1988, 180*f*
Maternal mortality rate, 344–345
Maternal use of drugs, effects on fetus, 316*t*
Mean, regression to, 351–352
Measles, 142
   immunization recommendation for, during pregnancy, 196*t*
Measurement, precision of, effect of repeated observations on, 352*f*
Meconium, 319
Meconium ileus, 69
Medical qualifying examinations, 1–22
   English language, 10
   essay, 3
   examples of questions, 12–22
      objective multiple-choice type, 12–17
         association and relatedness items, 13–14
         case histories, 16–17
         cause and effect, 15–16
         completion type, 12–13
         quantitative values and comparisons, 14–15
         structure and functions, 16
      review, 17–22
         basic sciences, 17–20
         clinical sciences, 20–22
   five points to remember, 11–12
   Foreign Medical Graduate Examination in the Medical Sciences (FMGEMS), 9–10
   innovations in formulating test questions, 11
   Medical Science Examination, 10
   multiple-choice, 3–4
      scoring of, 4
   types of, 3–4
   United States Medical Licensing Examination (USMLE), 10–11
Medical Science Examination, 10
Medical statistics, 350–351
Medulloblastomas, 328
Megacolon
   aganglionic, congenital, 333
   congenital, 70
Meiotic division, 190
Melancholia, 390
Melanotic lesions, of vulva, 248

Membrana granulosa, 188
Menarche, 282
Ménière's syndrome, 43
Meningitis, 167–168, 330
   aseptic, 167
   bacterial, 167
   cryptococcal, 167–168
   tuberculous, 116, 167
Meningomyeloceles, 331
Menopause, 296–297
Menorrhagia, 281
Menstrual cycle, 189–190
Menstruation
   disorders of, 281–282
      classification of, 281–282
      regulation and dysfunction of, 282–286
Mental disorder(s)
   conditions not attributable to, 400–401
   induced by alcohol, 385–386
   induced by CNS-active agents, 386
   organic, 384–387
      treatment of, 387
   secondary, 386–387
Mental retardation, 330–331, 381–382
   major causes of, 330*t*
   perinatal factors, 382
   postnatal factors, 382
   prenatal factors, 382
   primary, 381
   secondary, 381
Mental status examination, 380
   outline, 380
6-Mercaptopurine, 131*t*
Mercury, effects on fetus, 316*t*
Meta-analysis, 348–349
Metabolic acidosis, 121
Metabolic alkalosis, 121
Metabolism
   diseases of, 135–141
   disorders of, 324
      in children, 324–326
   inborn errors of, 324, 330*t*
Metacarpals, fractures of, 38
Methyldopa, 131*t*
Metrorrhagia, 281–282, 296
Microencephaly,. 330*t*, 331
Micropsychotic episodes, 399
Midgut, malrotation of, 70
Migraine, 164
Miliary tuberculosis, acute, 115–116
Mind, brain, and body, unified, 377
Mitral insufficiency, 87
Mitral regurgitation, 87
Mitral valve
   prolapse of, 87
   stenosis of, 87–88
Mixed connective tissue disease, 157
Molluscum contagiosum, 248–249
Mongolian spots, 317
Monoamine oxidase inhibitors, 404*t*
Mood, depressed, adjustment disorder with, 391
Mood syndrome, organic, 385
Morbidity
   puerperal, 232–234
   reporting, 346
Mortality, maternal and perinatal, in United States, 1950–1988, 180*f*
Mortality rate(s)
   infant, 344
   maternal, 344–345

Mother. *See also under* Maternal
 postpartal care of, 206–208
Mouth
 floor, carcinoma of, 45
 trench, 43
Mouth wounds, of hand, 35
Movement disorders, stereotyped, 383
MS. *See* Multiple sclerosis
Mucopurulent cervicitis, 150–151
Mucosa, buccal, carcinoma of, 45
Mucoviscidosis, 117
Multi-infarct dementia, 385
Multiple personality, 394
Multiple sclerosis (MS), 165
Mumps, immunization recommendations
 for, during pregnancy, 196*t*
Muscle diseases, 166
Muscular dystrophy, 166
Musculoskeletal disorders, 396
Myasthenia gravis, 166
Mycobacterial infections, 167
Mycoplasma pneumonia, 114
Myocardial infarction, 91–93
 acute, treatment of, 92–93
 complications of, 93
Myocardial revascularization, 52
Myoclonus, 163
Myopathies
 inflammatory, 166
 noninflammatory, 166
Myotonic dystrophy, 166
Myxedema, 137

Narcissistic personality disorder, 399
Narcotics, maternal use of, effects on
 fetus, 316*t*
National Board of Medical Examiners
 (NBME), 4–7
NBME. *See* National Board of Medical
 Examiners
Neck, 44
 lymph node enlargements in, 44
Necrosis, tubular, acute, 119
Necrotizing fasciitis, 26
Neisseria gonorrhoeae, 148*t*
Nelaton's line, 39
Neonatal death, 182
Neonatal jaundice, 322
Neonatal sepsis, 322
Neoplasias
 cervical intraepithelial, 252–254
 cysts, 272
 vulvar intraepithelial, 248
Nephrology, 118–121
 questions in, 170
Nephropathy, obstructive, 120–121
Nephrotic syndrome, 119–120
Nervous system
 diseases of, 161–169
 infectious disorders of, 167–169
Neuralgia, trigeminal, 164–165
Neuroblastoma, 328–329
Neurodermatitis, 247
Neuroleptics, 402–403
Neurologic diseases, degenerative, 330*t*
Neurologic disorders, 324
 in childhood, 329–331
Neurology, 161–169
 questions in, 171
Neuropathy, peripheral, 166–167

Neurosis
 anxiety, 392
 depressive, 390
 hypochondriacal, 393–394
 hysterical
 conversion type, 393
 dissociative type, 394
 obsessive–compulsive, 392
 phobic, 391
Neurosyphilis, 154, 169
Newborn, 234–241. *See also under*
 Infant(s); Neonatal
 anatomy and physiology of, 317–323
 cardiovascular changes in, 318
 care of, 235, 316
 classification of, 320–321
 diseases of, 321–323
 hemolytic jaundice in, 322
 causes of, 322*t*
 normal, 317–321
 postdate, 217–218
 respiratory changes in, 318
NHL. *See* Non-Hodgkin's lymphoma
NIDDM. *See* Diabetes mellitus, non-
 insulin-dependent
Nines, rule of, 28
Non-beta-cell tumors, of pancreas, 61
Non-Hodgkin's lymphoma (NHL), 110
Nose, surgery involving, 45–46
Nosocomial infections, 146–147
Nosology, 381–401
Nucleus pulposus, herniated, 38–39
Nutrition, 30–31, 313–316, 363
 average daily requirements, for infants
 and children, 314*t*

Obesity, 363
Observational studies, 347
Observations, repeated, effect on preci-
 sion of measurement, 352*f*
Observed experience, 377
Obsessive–compulsive disorder, 392
Obsessive–compulsive neurosis, 392
Obstetrics, 179–241
 analgesia, 208
 anesthesia, 208
 questions in, 297–310
Occiput
 anterior rotation of, 203
 external rotation of, 203
 restitution of, 203
Occiput posterior (OP) position, 226–227
Occupational health, 360–361
ODDS ratio, 347
Older adults, 364
Olecranon fossa, fractures through, 37
Oligomenorrhea, 281
Opioid intoxication, 386
Opioid withdrawal, 386
Oral cavity, surgery involving, 44–45
Oral contraceptives, 294–295
 mini-pill, 294–295
 postcoital or morning-after pills, 295
Orchitis, acute, 74
Orgasm
 female, inhibited, 394
 male, inhibited, 394
Os calcis, fractures and dislocations of,
 41
Osteoarthritis, 159
 differential diagnosis of, 159*t*

Osteoporosis, 139–140, 297
Ostium primum defect, 85
Otitis media, 331
Ovary, 187–189
 carcinoma of, 273–275
 cysts in, 272–273
 torsion of, 273
 disorders of, 271–275
Overanxious disorder, 382
Oviducts, conditions of, 271
Ovulation, test for, 288
Ovum, 188
 fertilization of, 190–191
 implantation of, 191–192

Paget's disease
 of breast, 47–48
 vulvar, 248
Pain disorder, psychogenic, 393
Pain syndrome, chronic benign, 393
Palmar spaces, infections of, 35
Pancreas
 abscess in, 131*t*
 cancer of, 60–61, 125*t*, 131*t*, 131–132
 cysts in, 60
 islet cell adenoma of, 61
 pseudocyst in, 131*t*
 surgery involving, 60–61
 ulcerogenic tumors of, 61
Pancreatitis, 131–132
 acute, 60, 131
 complications of, 131*t*
 etiologies of, 131*t*
 acute edematous or interstitial type, 60
 acute hemorrhagic or necrotizing, 60
 chronic, 60, 125*t*, 131
 drug-induced, 131*t*
 hemorrhagic, 131*t*
Panic disorder, 392
Paranoid disorder, 389
Paranoid personality disorder, 398
Paraovarium, conditions of, 271
Paraphilias, 394
Paraphimosis, 75
Parasitic sexually transmitted diseases,
 154
Parathyroids, surgery involving, 46–47
Parkinsonism, 165–166
Paronychia, 34
Paroxysmal supraventricular tachycardia
 (PSVT), 98
Passive–aggressive personality disorder,
 399–400
Patella, fractures and dislocations of, 40
Patent ductus arteriosus, 50, 85
 incidence in patients diagnosed with
 congenital heart disease, 84*t*
Patient(s)
 chief expectation of, 379
 establishing consensus with, regarding
 stress, 379
 identifying primary emotions and
 obtaining congruence with, 378–
 379
 individual care for, 339
 interaction with, 378
PBC. *See* Primary biliary cirrhosis
Pediatrics, 311–336. *See also* Children;
 Infant(s)
 diseases, 321–323, 323–335

growth and development, 311–313
nutrition, 313–316
preventive, 335–336
questions in, 336–338
surgery involving digestive tract, 69–70
Pelvic congestion syndrome, 266
Pelvic dystocia, 226
Pelvic inflammatory disease (PID), 148t, 152
Pelvis
bony, 184–185
contraction of, 226
floor of, 185–186
fractures and dislocations of, 39
infections of, 260–263
general, 260–262
true, lower or small, 184
Penicillamine, 134t
Pentamidine, 131t
Peptic ulcer disease (PUD), 124
Perfectionists, 400
Pericardial disease, 100
Pericardial effusion, 100
Pericarditis, 89–90
acute benign, 100
uremic, 100
Perihepatitis, 148t
Perinatal mortality, in United States, 1950–1988, 180f
Perinephric abscess, 71–72
Perineum, lacerated, care of, 206
Peripheral arterial disease, 33–34
Peripheral embolization, 34
Peripheral neuropathy, 166–167
Peritonsillar abscess, 43–44
Pernicious anemia (PA), 102
Personality
cyclothymic, 390
hysterical, 400
multiple, 394
Personality disorder(s), 397–398
antisocial, 398–399
avoidant, 400
borderline, 399
compulsive, 400
dependent, 399
histrionic, 400
narcissistic, 399
paranoid, 398
passive–aggressive, 399–400
schizoid, 398
schizotypal, 398
Personality syndrome, organic, 385
Personnel, 369–370
Peutz-Jegher's syndrome, 64
Phalanges, fractures of, 38
Pharmacotherapy, 402–405
Phencyclidine, 386
Phenobarbital
and epilepsy, 163t
Phenothiazines, 404t
Phenylketonuria, 325
Phenylpropylamine, 404t
Phenytoin
effects on fetus, 316t
and epilepsy, 163t
Pheochromocytoma, 138
Phimosis, 75
Phlebitis, 32–33
Phlebothrombosis, 33
Phlebotomy, 134t

Phobia, 391
simple, 391
social, 391
Phobic disorders, 391
Phobic neurosis, 391
Phototherapy, in neonate, 322
Phthirus pubis, 148t, 154–155
Physical condition, psychological factors affecting, 384, 395–397
Physical examination, 380
Physical fitness, 363–364
Physical therapies, psychiatric, 402
Physician(s)
effective, characteristics of, 406–407
individual behavior of, 370
and patient
establishing consensus regarding stress, 379
identifying primary emotions and obtaining congruence, 378–379
interaction between, 378
Physiology
of female sex organs, 184–190
of labor, 201–202
neonatal, 317–323
Pica, 382
Pick's disease, 385
PID. See Pelvic inflammatory disease
Pigmentation, abnormal, lesions of vulva involving, 247–248
Piperazine, 404t
Piperidine, 404t
Placenta, 192–193
abruption of, 212–214
circumvallate, 205
delivery of, 204–205
Placenta previa, 214–215
active treatment of, 214–215
diagnosis of, 214
expectant management of, 215
Plague, immunization recommendations for, during pregnancy, 196t
Plasma cell disorders, 109–110
Plasma lipoprotein abnormalities, 93–94
Plastic procedures, for tubal infertility, 290
Platelet disorders, 108
Pleural effusions, 112
PMS. See Premenstrual syndrome
Pneumonia(s), 113–115, 146–147
aerobic gram-negative, 113–114
hemophilus, 114
legionella, 114–115
lobar, 113
mycoplasma, 114
staphylococcal, 114
streptococcal, 113
Pneumothorax, 49
spontaneous, 117
Poisonings, 335–336
Poliomyelitis, immunization recommendations for, during pregnancy, 196t
Polyarteritis nodosa, 156–157
Polycythemia vera, 107
Polymenorrhea, 281, 296
Polymyalgia rheumatica, 157
Polymyositis, 166
Polyposis
familial, 64
of intestinal tract, 64–65
Polyposis coli, familial, 129t

Polyps
adenomatous, 129t
of colon, nonfamilial, 64–65
Population, world, estimates of, in billions, 341f
Population perspective, 340
Portal hypertension, 62–63
Portosystemic encephalopathy, 134t
Postcoital test, 287
Postdates, 217–218
Posterior occipital position, 226–227
Postmenopausal syndrome, 296–297
Postmyocardial infarction syndrome, 93
Postpartal care, of mother, 206–208
Postterm infants, 321
Posttraumatic stress disorder, 392–393
Pott's fracture, 41
Practice, 406
Preeclampsia
mild, 210
severe, 210
Pre-excitation syndrome, 99
Pregnancy, 356–357
calculation of term, 197
complications of, 209–224
coincidental, 220–224
diagnosis of, 197–198
ectopic, 269–270
effects on fetus, 316–317
hypertensive states of, 210–212
immunizations during, current recommendations for, 196t
laboratory tests during, 198–201
multiple gestation, 218–220
physiologic changes of, 193–194
presentation in, diagnosis of, 197–198
preventive services for woman during, 358t
prolonged, 217–218
toxemia of, 316
Premature beats, 98
Premature infants, 182
Premature labor, 317
Prematurity, 238–241
retinopathy of, 321
Premenstrual syndrome (PMS), 266
Prenatal care, 194–201
preventive services for, 358t
Presenile dementia, 385
Preterm infants, 321
Prevalence ratio, 342
Prevention
of accidents, 361–362
psychiatric, 401–402
Preventive services
for normal infant, 359t
for pregnant woman and fetus, 358t
Primary biliary cirrhosis (PBC), 134
Proctitis, 148t
Professional control, 369
Progesterone, 189
Prolactin-producing tumors, 139
Prolonged rupture of membranes (PROM), 317
PROM. See Prolonged rupture of membranes
Prostate
carcinoma of, 73–74
hypertrophy of, benign, 73
treatment of, 73
surgery involving, 73–74
Proteinuria, asymptomatic, 119

Proteoglycans, 24
Protozoa, 147–148
Pseudocyst, pancreatic, 131*t*
Pseudohermaphroditism, female, 292
Pseudomucinous cystadenomas, 272
Psychiatric disorders
    first evident in infancy, childhood, or
        adolescence, 381–384
    issues in, 384
    with physical manifestations, 383
Psychiatry, 375–408
    evaluation in, 377–381
    history of, 376–377
    nosology, 381–401
    prevention in, 401–402
    questions in, 407–416
    treatment in, 402–408
        physical therapies, 402
Psychoanalysis, 407
Psychodynamics
    primary gain, 393
    secondary gain, 393
Psychological factors, affecting physical
        condition, 384
Psychological status examination, 380
Psychological tests, 381
Psychologization, 376
Psychopharmacologic agents, 404*t*
Psychophysiological disorders, 395–397
Psychosexual disorders, 394–395
Psychotherapy, 405–408
    change effects, 405–406
    dynamic, 407–408
    educational, 408
    group, 408
    individual, 407
    supportive, 408
    types of, 407–408
Psychotic disorders, 389
Pubarche, 282
Pubic (crab) lice, 148*t*, 154–155
Public health, 339–370
    questions in, 370–374
    United States service, 353
Pubourethral ligament, 185
PUD. *See* Peptic ulcer disease
Puerperal hematoma, 207
Puerperal infection, 232–234
    prophylaxis for, 233
    treatment of, 233
Puerperal morbidity, 232
Puerperium, pathology of, 224–234
Pulmonary disorders, in children, 331–
        332
Pulmonary emboli, 112
Pulmonary embolism, 52
Pulmonary function tests, 111
Pulmonary infections, 116–117, 331–332
Pulmonary stenosis, 86
Pulmonary tuberculosis, chronic, 115
    treatment of, 115
Pulmonic stenosis, incidence of, in pa-
        tients diagnosed with congenital
        heart disease, 84*t*
Pulmonology, 110–118
    questions in, 170
Pulseless disease, 100
Pyloric stenosis, 69–70, 333
Pyruvate kinase (PK) deficiency, 105

Q fever, 146
Qualifying examinations, 1–22

Quinine, effects on fetus, 316*t*
Quinsy, 43–44

Rabies, 26–27
    immunization recommendations for,
        during pregnancy, 196*t*
Radiation, 361
    effects on fetus, 316*t*
Radiation enteritis, 125*t*
Radius
    head, fracture of, 37
    shaft, fractures of, 37
Randomized trials, of antihypertensive
        therapy, reduction in odds of
        stroke and CHD in, 348*t*
Rapidly progressive glomerulonephritis
        (RPGN), 119
Raynaud's syndrome, 33–34
Reaction(s)
    adjustment, 382, 383
    situational, transient, 395
Reactive depression, 390
Rectovaginal fistulas, 281
Rectum
    carcinoma of, 65–66
    prolapse of, 68
Red-cell fragmentation syndrome, 106–
        107
Red-cell membrane defects, 322*t*
Red cells
    loss of, excess, anemias due to, 103–
        107
    production of, increased or ineffective,
        anemias due to, 101–103
Regression to the mean, 351–352
Reiter's syndrome, 160
Relaxation therapy, 407
Renal-cell carcinoma, 121
Renal defects, congenital, 333–334
Renal failure, 118–119
    acute, 119
    chronic, 118–119
Renal stones, 70–71, 121
Renal system, neonatal, 318
Renal tubular acidosis, 134*t*
Research, epidemiologic, methods of,
        347–349
Respiratory acidosis, 121
Respiratory alkalosis, 121
Respiratory disorders, 396
Respiratory distress, in newborn, 321–
        322
Respiratory distress syndrome, 321–322
Respiratory disturbances, during sleep,
        117–118
Respiratory failure, 110–111
Respiratory system, physiologic changes
        of, in pregnancy, 193
Retinopathy of prematurity, 321
Retropharyngeal abscess, 44
Rhabdomyosarcoma, 42
Rheumatic fever, 144–145, 332–333
Rheumatoid arthritis, 158–159
    differential diagnosis of, 159*t*
    treatment of, 158–159
Rheumatology, 155–161
    questions in, 171
Rh incompatibility, 322
Rickettsial diseases, 146
Round ligaments, 186
RPGN. *See* Rapidly progressive glomeru-
        lonephritis

Rubella, 142
    effects on fetus, 316*t*
    immunization recommendations for,
        during pregnancy, 196*t*
Rule of nines, 28

Salivary glands, surgery involving, 43
Sarcoidosis, 117
Sarcoma, 257
    of breast, 48
    Kaposi's, 42
    soft-tissue, 42
    synovial, 42
Sarcoptes scabi, 148*t*, 155
Scabies, 148*t*, 155
Scarlet fever, 144
SC disease. *See* Sickle-cell hemoglobin C
        disease
Schizoaffective disorder, 389
Schizoid personality disorder, 398
Schizophrenia
    process, 389
    reactive, 389
Schizophrenic disorders, 387–389
    catatonic type, 388
    disorganized type, 388
    paranoid type, 388
    residual type, 388–389
    undifferentiated type, 388
Schizophreniform disorder, 389
Schizotypal personality disorder, 398
Schwannoma, malignant, 42
SCID. *See* Severe combined immunodefi-
        ciency disease
Scleroderma, 125*t*, 156
Sclerosing cholangitis, primary, 133*t*
Sclerosis
    biliary, primary, 133*t*
    systemic, progressive, 156
Sclerotherapy, 125
Scrotal hernia, 74
Scrotum
    enlargement of, 74
    surgery involving, 74–75
Scurvy, 315
Sedatives, 403
    effects on fetus, 316*t*
Seizure disorders, 329–330
Seizures
    absence, 163
    epileptic, international classification of,
        163*t*
    febrile, 329
    generalized, 163
    partial
        complex, 163
        simple, 163
    tonic–clonic, 163
Self-help groups, 408
Semen, evaluation of, 287
Senile dementia, 385
Sensitivity, 350
    diagnostic, for diagnosing congestive
        heart failure by chest x ray, 350*f*
Separation anxiety disorder, 382
Sepsis, neonatal, 322
Serous cystadenomas, 272
Serum cholesterol, 340*f*
    and first coronary event in men 30 to
        59, relationship of, 347*f*
Severe combined immunodeficiency
        disease (SCID), 334

Sex hormone, effects on fetus, 316*t*
Sex organs, female, anatomy and physiology of, 184–190
Sexual desire, inhibited, 394
Sexual development, abnormal, 290–293
Sexual differentiation, 191
Sexual excitement or arousal, inhibited, 394
Sexually transmitted diseases (STDs), 148–155, 360
  bacterial, 151–152
  chlamydial, 150–151
  etiologic agents and associated disease states, 148*t*
  insect, 154–155
  parasitic, 154
  treponemal, 152–154
  viral, 148–150
SGA infants. *See* Small-for-gestational-age infants
Shock, 29–30
  cardiogenic, 29
  hypovolemic, 29
  neurogenic, 29–30
  septic, 30
Shoulder
  dislocation of, 36–37
  general surgical conditions of, 35
Shoulder–hand syndrome, 93
Sickle-cell anemia, 105, 326–327
Sickle-cell hemoglobin C disease (SC disease), 105
Sickle-cell β-thalassemia (S β thal), 105
Sickle-cell trait, 104
Sick sinus syndrome, 98
Silent ischemia, 91
Silo-filler's disease, 117
Sinoatrial block, 98
Sinusitis, 45–46
Sinus pauses, 98
Sinus venosus defect, 85
Situational reactions, transient, 395
Sjögren's syndrome, 157
Skeletal disorders, congenital, 324
Skin, neonatal, 317–318
Skin disorders, 396
SLE. *See* Systemic lupus erythematosus
Sleep, respiratory disturbances during, 117–118
Sleep terrors, 383
Sleepwalking, 383
Slim disease, 149
Small-for-gestational-age (SGA) infants, 321
Small intestine
  diseases of, 125–127
  tumors of, 126
    malignant, 65
Smoking, 362
Snake bites, 27
Social development, milestones in, 313*t*
Social phobia, 391
Soft-tissue sarcomas, 42
Somatization, 376
Somatization disorder, 393
Somatoform disorders, 393–394
Specificity, 349, 350
  diagnostic, for diagnosing congestive heart failure by chest x ray, 350*f*
  individual response, versus stimulus–response, 377–378
Spherocytosis, hereditary, 104

Spleen
  rupture of, 61–62
  surgery involving, 61–62
Splenectomy, 130
  indications for, 61–62
Splenomegaly, 130
Spondylitis, ankylosing, 159–160
Spondyloarthropathies, seronegative, 159–160
Sprain, 41
Sprue
  celiac, 125*t*
  tropical, 125*t*
Squamous-cell carcinoma, 250–251
Stab wounds, abdominal, 54
Staphylococcal pneumonia, 114
State health organizations, 353
Statistics, 340–346, 350–351
STDs. *See* Sexually transmitted diseases
Stenosis
  aortic, 88, 90
    incidence of, in patients diagnosed with congenital heart disease, 84*t*
  idiopathic hypertrophic subaortic, 88
  mitral, 87–88
  pulmonary, 86
  pulmonic, incidence of, in patients diagnosed with congenital heart disease, 84*t*
  pyloric, 69–70, 333
Stereotyped movement disorders, 383
Sterility, adolescent, 283
Sterilization, 295–296
S β thal. *See* Sickle-cell β-thalassemia
Stimulants, central nervous system, 403
Stimulus–response specific assumption, 377
Stomach. *See also under* Gastric
  diseases of, 123–125
  surgery involving, 56–58
Stork bites, 317
Strength/independence, 349
Streptococcal pneumonia, 113
Streptococcal tonsillopharyngitis, acute, 144
Streptomycin, effects on fetus, 316*t*
Stress, establishing consensus regarding, 379
Stress disorder, posttraumatic, 392–393
Stress ulcer, 58
Stroke, reduction in odds of, in randomized trials of antihypertensive trials, 348*t*
Stuttering, 383
Subarachnoid hemorrhage, 162
Subdiaphragmatic abscess, 56
Subdural hematomas, 162
Subdural hemorrhage, 162
Subjective experience, 377
Substance abuse, 387
Sulfonamides, 131*t*
  effects on fetus, 316*t*
Supratentorial tumors, 328
Surgery, 23–82
  breast, 47–49
  in Crohn's disease, indications for, 129*t*
  ear, 43
  gastrointestinal tract and abdomen, 53–70
  genitourinary system, 70–75
  larynx, 45

  lung, 52–53
  nose, 45–46
  oral cavity, 44–45
  parathyroids, 46–47
  pediatric, involving digestive tract, 69–70
  questions in, 75–82
  response to, 23–24
  salivary glands, 43
  thorax, 49–52
  throat, 43–44
  thyroid, 46
Surgical wound infection, 146
Swyer syndrome, 293
Synovial sarcoma, 42
Syphilis, 74–75, 148*t*, 152, 168
  benign late, 153–154
  cardiovascular, 90, 154
  effects on fetus, 316*t*
  late, benign, 153
  latent, 153
  meningovascular, 169
  primary, 152–153
  secondary, 153
  tertiary, 153–154
  vulvar lesion of, 246–247
Systemic lupus erythematosus (SLE), 120, 155–156
Systolic Hypertension in the Elderly Program, cumulative fatal plus nonfatal stroke rate per 100 participants in, 355*f*

Tachycardia(s)
  atrial, 98–99
  A-V nodal reentrant, 98–99
  paroxysmal supraventricular, 98
  ventricular, 99–100
Takayasu syndrome, 100
Temporal arteritis, 156–157
Temporality, 349
Tenosynovitis, of flexor tendon sheaths, 34–35
Teratomas, benign, 272
Testicular feminization, 292–293
Testis
  carcinoma of, 75
  torsion of, 74
Test of English as a Foreign Language (TOEFL), 10
Tetanus, 25–26
  prophylaxis, in wound management, guide to, 26*t*
Tetanus–diphtheria, immunization recommendations for, during pregnancy, 196*t*
Tetracyclic antidepressants, 404*t*
Tetracycline, 131*t*
  effects on fetus, 316*t*
Tetralogy of Fallot, 50–51, 86, 332
  incidence of, in patients diagnosed with congenital heart disease, 84*t*
Thalassemia, 327
β-Thalassemia
  homozygous, 101
  sickle-cell, 105
Thalassemic syndromes, 101
Theca, 188
Thelarche, 282
Thiazide diuretics, 131*t*
Thioxenthines, 404*t*

Thorax
  basic physiologic mechanisms of, alterations in, 49–50
  surgery involving, 49–52
  trauma to, 49–50
Thrive, failure to, 324
Throat, surgery involving, 43–44
Thromboangitis obliterans, 33
Thrombocytopenia, 108
  idiopathic, 327
Thromboembolic disease of aorta, 100
Thrombolytic therapy, 92
Thrombophlebitis, 32–33
Thyroglossal cysts, 44
Thyroid
  cancer of, 136
  function tests, 135
  radioactive, effects on fetus, 316t
  surgery involving, 46
Thyroid disorders, effects on fetus, 316t
Thyroiditis, 46, 135–136
  Hashimoto's, 135–136
  subacute, 135
Thyroid nodules, 136
Tibia, fractures and dislocations of, 41
Tic douloureux, 164–165
Tics, 383
  chronic, 383
  transient, 383
Tobacco, 386
  use of, effects on fetus, 316t
TOEFL. See Test of English as a Foreign Language
Tongue, carcinoma of, 44–45
Tonic–clonic seizures, 163
Tonsillopharyngitis, streptococcal, acute, 144
Torsades des Points, 100
Torsion, of ovarian cysts, 273
Total cholesterol, initial classification and recommended follow-up based on, 363t
Tourette's disorder, 383
Toxic agents, 330t, 361
Toxic shock syndrome, 245
Toxoplasmosis, effects on fetus, 316t
Tracheoesophageal fistula, 331
Tranquilizers
  major, 402–403
  minor, 403
Transfusions, exchange, in infant, 322
Transplantation, 31–32
  homostructural, 31
  homovital, 31
Transposition of the great arteries, 51
Trauma, 131t, 330t
  birth, 330t
  to thorax, 49–50
Treatment. See also specific therapy
  high-priority areas of, 354–366
Tremor, 134t
Trench mouth, 43
Treponemal sexually transmitted diseases, 152–154
Treponema pallidum, 148t
Trichomonas vaginalis, 148t
Trichomoniasis, 148t, 154, 242
Tricuspid insufficiency, 88–89
Tricuspid valve, Ebstein anomaly of, 86–87
Tricyclics, 404t
Trigeminal neuralgia, 164–165

Trisomy, 330t
Trisomy 21, 330–331
Trophoblast, tumors of, 267–269
Tropical sprue, 125t
True negative, 350
True positive, 350
Tuberculosis, 53, 72, 100, 115–116
  miliary, acute, 115–116
  pathogenesis of, 115
  pulmonary, chronic, 115
  vulvar, 247
Tubular necrosis, acute, 119
Tumor(s)
  adrenal cortex, 68
  adrenal medulla, 68
  brain, 164
  of central nervous system, 328
  kidney, 72–73
  prolactin-producing, 139
  small intestine, malignant, 65
  supratentorial, 328
  trophoblast, 267–269
  vulvar
    benign, 248–250
    solid, benign, 249–250
  Wilms', 329
Typhoid, immunization recommendations for, during pregnancy, 196t
Typhoid fever, 145–146

UGI hemorrhage. See Upper gastrointestinal hemorrhage
Ulcer(s), 32
  duodenal, 57–58
  gastric, 56–57
  peptic ulcer disease, 124
  stress, 58
Ulcerative colitis, 66–67
  chronic, 128, 129t
  colectomy in, indications for, 128t
Ulcerative lesions, of vulva, benign, 245–247
Ulcerogenic tumors, pancreatic, 61
Ulna, shaft, fractures of, 37
Umbilical cord, prolapse of, 229
Understanding, 405
Unicyclic antidepressants, 404t
Unified mind, brain, and body, 377
Unipolar disorder, 390
United States
  abridged life table, 1981, 345t
  AIDS cases, by year of report, 355f
  crude death rate, seasonal change in, per 1,000 people, by month of calendar years 1985, 1986, and 1987, 344f
  federal health services, 352–354
  infant mortality in, top ten causes, by race, 1983, 357t
  life expectancy at birth, by year of birth and by race, 1970–1989, 345f
  maternal and perinatal mortality in, 1950–1988, 180f
  Public Health Service, 353
United States Medical Licensing Examination (USMLE), 10–11
Upper extremities
  fractures and dislocations of, 36–39
  general surgical conditions of, 34–35

Upper gastrointestinal (UGI) hemorrhage, 124–125
Uremia, anemia of, 103
Uremic syndrome, 118
Urethra, stricture of, 74
Urethral syndrome, 150–151
Urethritis, 148t
Urinary system, physiologic changes of, during pregnancy, 194
Urinary tract infection, 146
Urinary tract injuries, 279–281
USMLE. See United States Medical Licensing Examination
Uterine bleeding
  anovulatory, 281
  arrhythmic, 281–282
Uterine constriction rings, 225
Uterine corpus, 186–187
  disorders of, 255–260
Uterosacral ligaments, 185
Uterus, 186–187
  blood supply of, 187
  lymphatics of, 187
  rupture of, 229–230
    causes, 229
    symptoms of, 229–230

Vaccines, 336
Vagina, 186
  cancer of, 251–252
Vaginal breech delivery, 227
Vaginismus, functional, 395
Variceal hemorrhage, 134t
Varicella, immunization recommendations for, during pregnancy, 196t
Varicocele, 74
Varicose veins, 32
Vascular disease(s), 100–101
  renal, 120
Vasculitides, 156–157
Velamentous cord insertion, 205
Venous thrombosis, 32–33
Ventricular aneurysm, 93
Ventricular septal defect, 85, 332
  incidence of, in patients diagnosed with congenital heart disease, 84t
Ventricular septal defects, 51
Ventricular tachycardia (VT), 99–100
Version, 231–232
  Braxton Hicks, 232
  external, 231
  internal, 231–232
Vertebral column, fractures and dislocations of, 38–39
VIN. See Vulvar intraepithelial neoplasia
Vincent's angina, 43
Viral hepatitis, 149
  acute, 133
Viral infection(s), 147
  Epstein-Barr virus, 143
  herpes simplex virus, 148–149
  human immunodeficiency virus, 149–150
  human papilloma virus, 150
  slow, 169
Viral sexually transmitted diseases, 148–150
Vitamin(s), imbalances, 315